Cytopathology

Cytopathology

Grace T McKee

BA, MB, BS
Head of the Department of Cytopathology
Royal Surrey County Hospital
Guildford, Surrey

Foreword by Torsten Lowhagen

Mosby-Wolfe

London Baltimore Barcelona Bogotá Boston Buenos Aires Caracas Carlsbad, CA Chicago Madrid Mexico City Milan New York Philadelphia St Louis Seoul Singapore Sydney Taipei Tokyo Toronto Wiesbaden

*To Phillip, my husband, companion
and best friend*

Published in 1997 by Mosby-Wolfe, an imprint of Times Mirror International Publishers Limited

Printed by Grafos, Arte sobre papel, Barcelona, Spain

ISBN 0 7234 2449 7

For full details of all Times Mirror International Publishers Limited titles, please write to Times Mirror International Publishers Limited, Lynton House, 7–12 Tavistock Square, London WC1H 9LB, England.

A CIP catalogue record for this book is available from the British Library.

Library of Congress Cataloging-in-Publication Data applied for.

Project Manager: Tuan Hô

Designer: Peter Wilder

Layout Artist: Gisli Thor

Cover Design: Ian Spick

Illustration: Lee Smith

Production: Gudrun Hughes

Index: Kathy Croom

Publisher: Fiona Foley

FOREWORD

Clinical cytopathology, as practised today, is a fairly new discipline; this is particularly true in the field of aspiration cytology. During the last decade, we have seen an unprecedented explosion of new knowledge in this context, followed by a wide demand for a clinical diagnostic service. To meet the demand and justify the confidence of our clinicians we, practising cytopathologists, all have a permanent need to broaden our horizons by continued education and ongoing discussion. It is a matter of fact that we all look at morphology differently, yet pool our ideas to arrive at a correct diagnosis.

Experience has demonstrated that a cytopathology service needs to be of excellent quality, otherwise confidence in the method is eroded, which is a retrograde step. The recent emphasis, centred around the complex world of cell biology and immunology, has somewhat, unfortunately, deviated interest from fundamental cell morphology and thus cytopathology.

Grace McKee has now given us a beautiful, high-quality atlas, covering all accessible organs and sites. The reader is presented with an array of cytomorphological features—some, well-known, but repeated for emphasis and yet others that update our knowledge. Rare are cytopathologists who combine a vast experience of cytology in its many facets with the talent, ambition and drive to produce a book of this kind. *Cytopathology* has been written with an emphasis on cytomorphological features, and demonstrates how much information can be obtained from a simple smear or aspirate without recourse to expensive ancillary tests.

This is a substantial textbook which is pleasing to read and, at the same time, would be useful as a bench book. It will make an excellent addition to the library of practising cytopathologists and trainees. I have the greatest respect and praise for this gigantic single-handed undertaking, and I am certain it will find wide acceptance and use by the cytopathology fraternity.

Torsten Lowhagen, MDhc, FIAC
Consultant Cytopathologist
Karolinska Hospital
Stockholm

PREFACE

For many years cytopathology has been the poor relation of histopathology, tucked away in a dark corner and left severely alone by pathologists—except under duress. Times are changing. No longer does cytology mean just tedious screening of cervical smears by technical staff, with abnormalities being checked by reluctant histopathologists. The speciality has made great strides forward, both in the field of gynaecological problems and, even more importantly, in the diagnosis of non-gynaecological lesions. Most laboratories have noticed an ever-increasing workload in the field of fine needle aspirates. This is attributable in part to the Breast Screening Programme with access to stereotactic aspirates, and partly to the courage and expertise of interventional radiologists who insert needles into areas of the body that would intimidate the less bold.

Many excellent histopathologists quake with fear and trembling when faced, for example, with a fine needle aspirate of breast, when the surgeon may rely on the cytological diagnosis to help him decide on management. There are many such pathologists who, even now, request a tru-cut biopsy as well as a fine needle aspirate to help them out of this dilemma. Much of the problem lies in the fact that histopathological diagnoses depend on pattern and the low-power lens, while cytopathology relies more on the detailed study of individual cells, often at high power, including oil-immersion. The only way of relating these two disciplines is by looking at both types of samples together, and developing expertise by looking at as much cytological material as possible. There is a problem in some laboratories where the range of non-gynaecological cytology is limited; the way forward here is to have a ready reference—a comprehensive atlas of cytopathology with clear colour illustrations showing every possible variation of normal and abnormal cells stained by both the Papanicolaou and May–Grünwald techniques.

This textbook provides the reader with examples of all cytological material encountered in a busy laboratory. It is for quick reference, to be used at the bench, both for making a diagnosis and training medical and technical junior staff. The photomicrographs include Papanicoloau and May–Grünwald–Giemsa-stained preparations, so that pathologists using only one of these will relate to the stain they prefer and will become familiar with the other. The emphasis throughout this book is on morphological appearances, rather than on special techniques, since rapid diagnosis is part of the attraction of this discipline. Cytopathology can be a very exciting subject—looking at the detailed structure of the relatively small numbers of cells on a smear and arriving at the correct diagnosis preoperatively is quite a challenge. It is hoped that this book with its exhaustive, high-quality colour illustrations will transmit some of this excitement to the reader and convert more reluctant histopathologists to the up-and-coming field of cytopathology!

Grace T. McKee

ACKNOWLEDGEMENTS

My grateful thanks go to Tuan Hô, Senior Project Manager, responsible for the production of and development work on this book, Gudrun Hughes, Production Controller, Peter Wilder, Design Manager, Lynda Payne, Illustrations Manager and Ian Spick, Cover Designer. Fiona Foley deserves a special mention for inviting me to embark on writing this book. My thanks also go to the others at Mosby–Wolfe who had fleeting but, no doubt, important contact with one or more of the publishing aspects.

I am indebted to my colleagues who supplied me with interesting cases and, even more, to the staff in my department who spent considerable time and effort ferreting out lost slides. My mentors, Professor John Tighe and Dr Chandra Grubb, who guided my first faltering footsteps into the world of cytology, deserve special mention, which also goes to Dr Torsten Lowhagen, not only for his encouragement, but for writing the foreword to this book.

Last, but definitely not least, I thank my husband, Phillip McKee, for his advice (sometimes extreme!) and encouragement, and my children, Stephen, Kathryn and Sharon, who saw very little of me during this undertaking.

CONTENTS

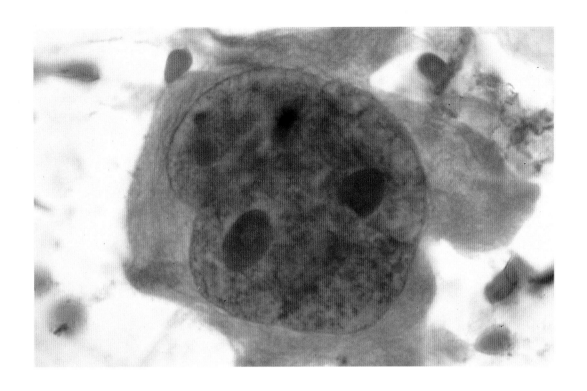

CELL STRUCTURE

1

CELL STRUCTURE

It is important to become familiar with the structure of a normal cell before attempting to make a cytological diagnosis of abnormality. Every organ in the body is composed of cells which, while performing different functions, have a common structure. It is also worth remembering that cells from various parts of the body resemble each other, so it is vital to know from where an aspirate has been taken to ensure one does not diagnose an adenocarcinoma of the breast when the material has been taken from the pancreas.

BASIC CELL

The basic cell is composed of a nucleus and cytoplasm confined by a plasma membrane (**Fig. 1.1**). The sizes of the nucleus and the cell vary from tissue to tissue, but nevertheless maintain a certain nucleo-cytoplasmic ratio (**Fig. 1.2**) The **nucleus**, which contains DNA (deoxyribonucleic acid), is usually located centrally and is limited by a double-layered nuclear membrane, in which gaps, known as nuclear pores, occur at intervals. These are not visible by light microscopy, but are seen clearly on electron microscopy. The nuclear membrane is detectable on light microscopy only because the chromatin attached to it stains with haematoxylin. The nucleus itself is composed of two types of chromatin – inactive heterochromatin, which stains with haematoxylin, and active euchro-

matin, which is represented by the clear pale areas (**Fig. 1.3**). This is why dyskaryotic or malignant cells may occasionally have pale rather than hyperchromatic nuclei (**Fig. 1.4**), although traditional teaching usually emphasizes the hyperchromatic nuclei only.

The **nucleolus** is an area within the nucleus where ribonucleic acid (RNA) is synthesized, and therefore is more prominent in cells which are active or reactive (**Fig. 1.5**). The presence of a small nucleolus (or nucleoli) does not mean that the cell is malignant. However, nucleoli which are abnormally enlarged or irregular in shape and multiple are an indicator of malignancy (**Fig. 1.6**).

The **cell membrane** or **plasma membrane** defines the outer boundary of the cell, separating cells from one another and from the environment. Under the light microscope it appears to be smooth, but on scanning electron microscopy the cell membrane can be very variable, with ruffles in macrophages, microvilli in mesothelial cells, and ridges in squamous cells. In cytological preparations the cell membrane may be sharp and well-defined, as in squamous cells (**Fig. 1.7**), or ill-defined, as in histiocytes (**Fig. 1.8**). It may display microvilli in the form of a frilly or lacy border in the case of mesothelial cells for example (**Fig. 1.9**). The cell membrane is impermeable to some substances and permeable to certain electrolytes and nutrients. It also has the ability to incorporate foreign material, such as bacteria or breakdown products of other cells, into the cell by a process of invaginating and then surrounding the material, known as **endocytosis (Fig. 1.10)**.

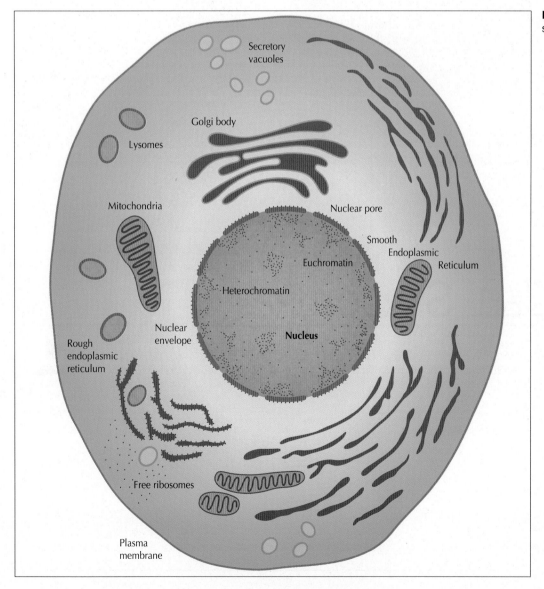

Fig. 1.1 Cell structure. Diagram to show the basic structure of a human cell.

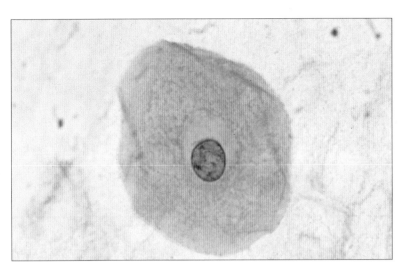

Fig. 1.2 Normal cell – Pap x100. This view of an intermediate squamous cell from the ectocervix demonstrates the comparatively small central nucleus with abundant cytoplasm seen in normal cells. Note the vesicular nucleus.

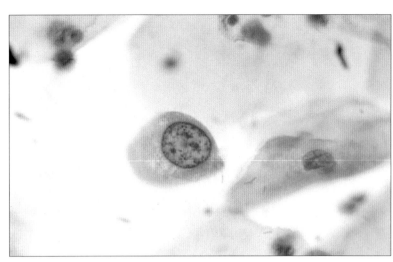

Fig. 1.3 Chromatin pattern – Pap x100. This dyskaryotic squamous cell illustrates clearly the rim of chromatin outlining the nuclear membrane, the dark purple clumps of inactive heterochromatin, and the pale active euchromatin, also known as parachromatinic areas.

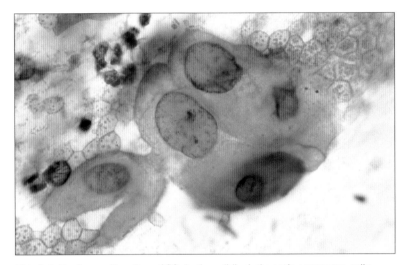

Fig. 1.4 Euchromatin – Pap x100. In the mildly dyskaryotic squamous cells seen in this photomicrograph, the nuclear chromatin consists of pale euchromatin with a few minute specks of heterochromatin, indicating that most of the chromatin is of the active type. The cells are nevertheless dyskaryotic, in spite of the usual emphasis that is put on hyperchromasia as a feature of dyskaryosis.

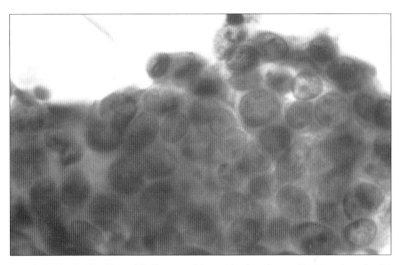

Fig. 1.5 Nucleoli – Pap x40. Illustrated is a cohesive sheet of benign ductal cells aspirated from a fibroadenoma. The nuclei are vesicular and most contain a small, clearly visible nucleolus, indicating a reactive rather than a neoplastic process.

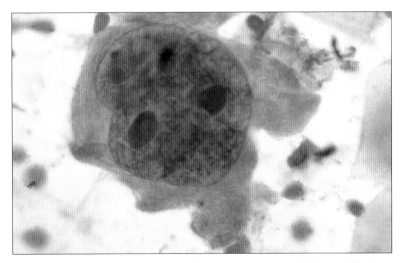

Fig. 1.6 Abnormal nucleoli – Pap x100. In contrast to that in **Figure 1.5**, this adenocarcinoma cell contains two large, red, abnormally shaped nucleoli with smaller indistinct nucleoli, confirming that this is a malignant cell. Other features of malignancy are also seen, such as an increased nuclear–cytoplasmic ratio and abnormally clumped chromatin.

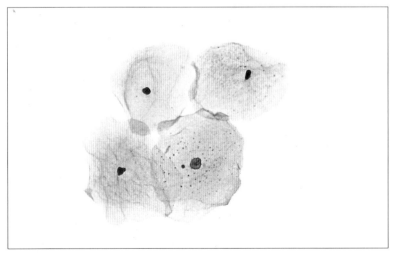

Fig. 1.7 Cell membrane – Pap x40. The superficial and intermediate squamous cells illustrated are from the ectocervix. They have clearly defined, sharp cytoplasmic borders, noticeable even where the cells overlap, this being one of the advantages of the Papanicolaou stain.

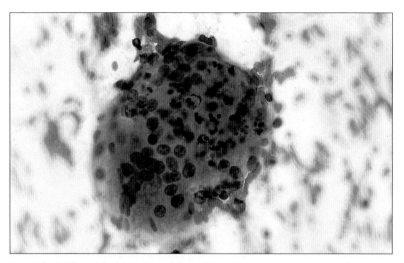

Fig. 1.8 Cell membrane – Pap x40. In this multinucleated histiocyte the plasma membrane is ill-defined and fuzzy, as opposed to the crisp boundaries of squamous cells. Also note the numerous nuclei and the phagocytosed neutrophils within the cytoplasm of this scavenger cell.

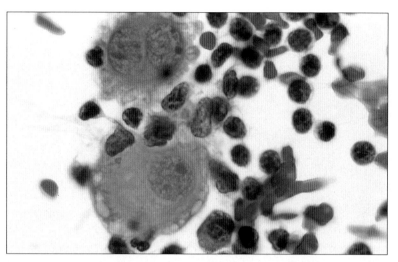

Fig. 1.9 Cell membrane – Pap x100. The two mesothelial cells illustrated show the characteristic lacy or frilly border of this type of cell. These borders represent microvilli (which are only visible on electron microscopy). One of the mesothelial cells is binucleate and both have visible nucleoli. The lymphocytes in the background have imperceptible cytoplasm.

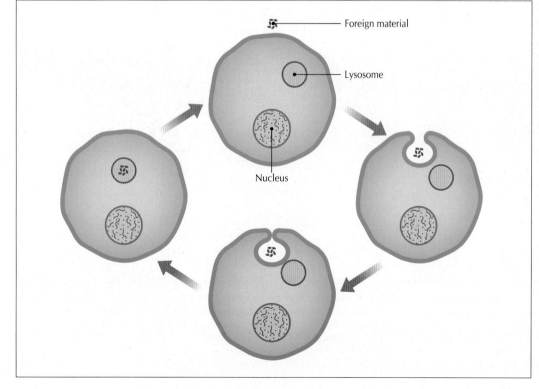

Fig. 1.10 Endocytosis – This diagram illustrates the process of phagocytosis of minute foreign particles (endocytosis), whereby the particle is engulfed by the cell and enclosed in a vacuole which then fuses with a lysosome. The enzymes in the lysosome then digest the particle and any unused material is expelled by a reverse process, known as exocytosis.

The **organelles** within the cytoplasm, such as the endoplasmic reticulum, the mitochondria, and Golgi body, are not visible in cytological preparations, except in certain circumstances. For example, **mitochondria**, which are essential for cell respiration, are abundant in hepatocytes and apocrine cells (**Fig. 1.11**), and also in oncocytic tumours (**Fig. 1.12**). The **Golgi body**, which is responsible for packaging protein products, is represented well in plasma cells on light microscopy in the form of a 'hof' or clear space (**Fig. 1.13**). Secretory products are seen clearly, such as mucin in endocervical cells (**Fig. 1.14**) or in tumour cells, which can be stained with PAS or Alcian blue for confirmation (**Fig. 1.15**). Glycogen is demonstrated well in intermediate squamous cells from the cervix (**Fig. 1.16**). Pigment is detected easily in cytological material, whether melanin in a malignant melanoma (**Fig. 1.17**), haemosiderin in macrophages [after haemorrhage into a cyst, for example (**Fig. 1.18**)], or degenerative pigments, such as lipofuschin in urothelial cells (**Fig. 1.19**). Other intracellular material, such as keratin, is seen not only in cells which produce it, such as well-differentiated squamous carcinoma cells (**Fig. 1.20**), but also in the macrophages closely associated with a metastasis from a keratinizing carcinoma (**Fig. 1.21**).

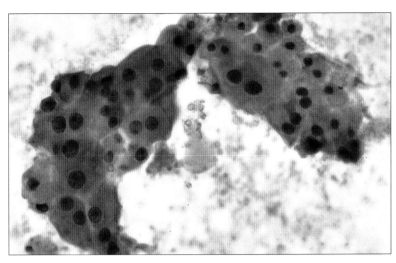

Fig. 1.11 Mitochondria – Pap x40. The apocrine cells illustrated are from a breast cyst. They contain numerous mitochondria which are represented by the abundant pinkish orange granular cytoplasm.

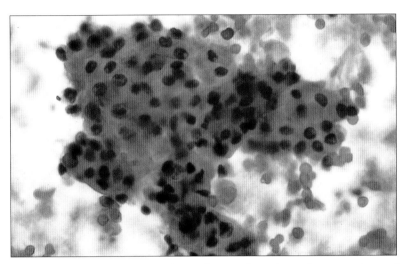

Fig. 1.12 Oncocytoma – Pap x40. This fine needle aspirate of an oncocytoma of the kidney is seen to be composed of cells with abundant orange granular cytoplasm. They , like apocrine cells, contain numerous mitochondria.

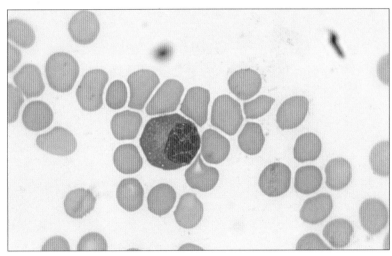

Fig. 1.13 Golgi body – MGG x100. This photomicrograph shows a plasma cell with an eccentric nucleus, 'clock-face' chromatin, and a clear area between the nucleus and cytoplasm, known as the 'hof'. This represents the Golgi body, which is responsible for protein packaging. Plasma cells are involved in producing antibodies which are proteins.

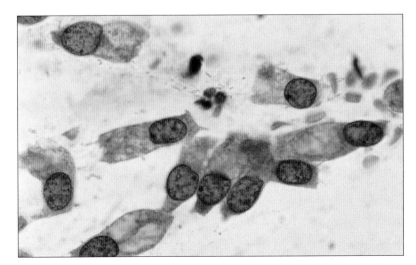

Fig. 1.14 Mucin-containing endocervical cells – Pap x100. The endocervical cells illustrated in this field are tall columnar cells with basal nuclei. Mucin can be seen distending the cytoplasm of a few of the cells. Mucin is not seen clearly with the Papanicolaou stain.

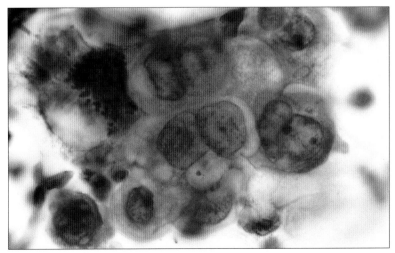

Fig. 1.15 Mucin in tumour cells – Pap x100. This cluster of large adenocarcinoma cells demonstrates mucin within the vacuoles in the cells, seen as pale pink, almost granular, material. Note also the abnormal, irregular nuclear margins and pale chromatin of the neoplastic cells, as well as the mitotic figure.

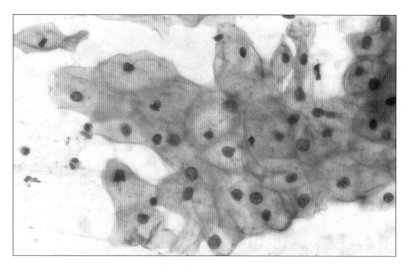

Fig. 1.16 Glycogen – Pap x40. The intermediate squamous cells illustrated in this field are from a cervical smear taken during the secretory phase of the menstrual cycle. They contain glycogen, seen as bright yellow material within the cytoplasm.

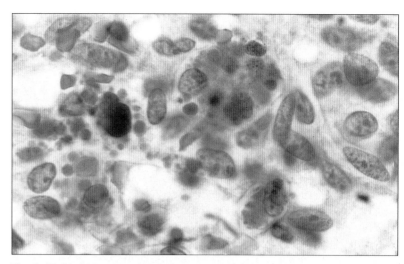

Fig. 1.17 Melanin – Pap x100. This is a fine needle aspirate of a metastatic melanoma in an inguinal node. It contains spindle-shaped melanoma cells without characteristic intranuclear inclusions and huge red nucleoli, but melanin is present in the form of large yellowish brown granules within both neoplastic cells and macrophages.

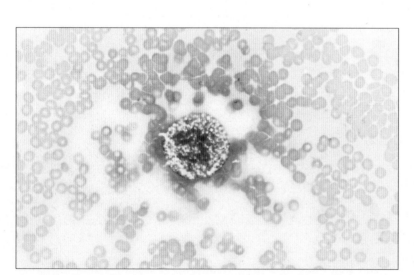

Fig. 1.18 Siderophages – MGG x100. Haemosiderin-laden macrophages are seen commonly where there has been haemorrhage into a lesion, such as a breast or thyroid cyst, or in nipple discharges from a duct papilloma. The macrophages have abundant vacuolated cytoplasm containing blue–black granular haemosiderin.

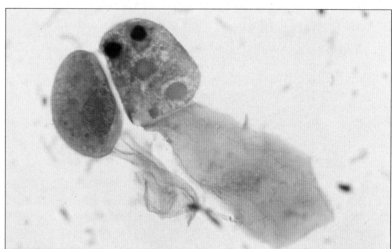

Fig. 1.19 Degenerative pigment – Pap x100. Urothelial cells commonly undergo degeneration, resulting in bright red cytoplasmic globules of lipofuschin breakdown products. In this field, the degenerate urothelial cell contains pigment, while the viable cell does not.

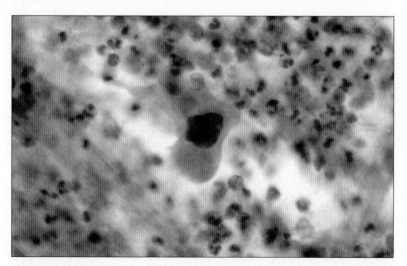

Fig. 1.20 Keratin – Pap x100. The squamous carcinoma cell seen in the centre of the field is from an aspirate of a cavitating squamous carcinoma of the lung, hence the neutrophils in the background. Keratin is produced by mature squamous cells in the skin, but not normally by those in the cervix; it is also produced by well-differentiated squamous carcinoma cells. It is bright orange and refractile with the Papanicolaou stain.

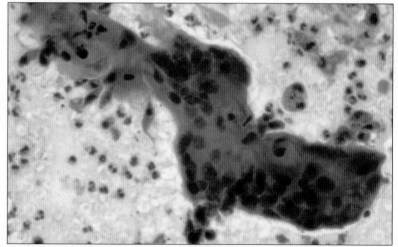

Fig. 1.21 Keratin – Pap x100. This lymph node aspirate from the same case as in **Figure 1.20** shows a huge multinucleated histiocyte containing several ingested keratinized squamous carcinoma cells, as well as some free keratin. The keratin stains a bright orange compared with the pinkish blue cytoplasm of the histiocyte.

A cell function that is commonly associated with polymorphonuclear leucocytes and macrophages is **phagocytosis**, which corresponds to endocytosis, but refers to the ingestion of large particles. This process is seen in other cells, too, at a light microscope level. For example, in endometrial adenocarcinoma, tumour cells are seen stuffed full of polymorphs (**Fig. 1.22**), dyskaryotic squamous cells not infrequently contain other ingested cells (**Fig. 1.23**), and even apparently normal squamous cells can be seen to have phagocytosed bacteria (**Fig. 1.24**).

The **cytoskeleton** is the cellular framework by which cells maintain their shape and, in some cases, movement. It is seen only on electron microscopy, but cilia (**Fig. 1.25**), sperm tails (**Fig. 1.26**), and the flagella of organisms, such as trichomonas vaginalis (**Fig. 1.27**), are all intimately related to the cytoskeleton and visible on light microscopy.

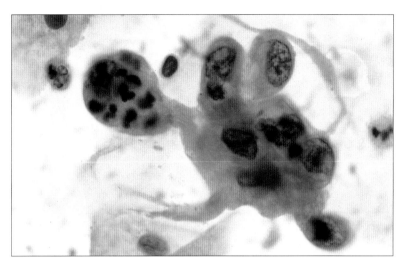

Fig. 1.22 Phagocytosis – Pap x100. This clump of adenocarcinoma cells, derived from an endometrial adenocarcinoma, contains a cell which has phagocytosed several neutrophils. This is a common occurrence with endometrial neoplasms.

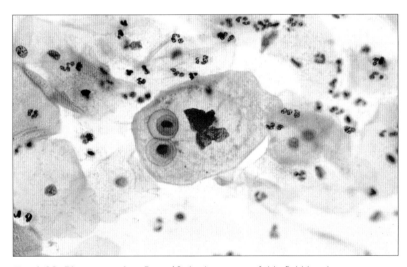

Fig. 1.23 Phagocytosis – Pap x40. In the centre of this field is a large binucleate mildly dyskaryotic cell with two phagocytosed cells within vacuoles in its cytoplasm. Phagocytosis is not uncommon with squamous cell dyskaryosis and carcinoma.

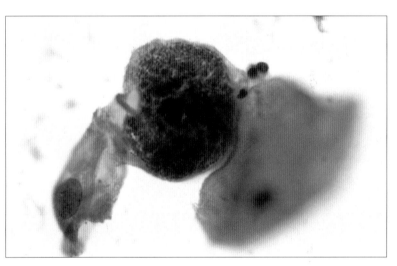

Fig. 1.24 Phagocytosis – Pap x100. This field shows a rare occurrence – a benign squamous cell with ingested bacteria seen in an otherwise normal cervical smear. Note the absence of neutrophils.

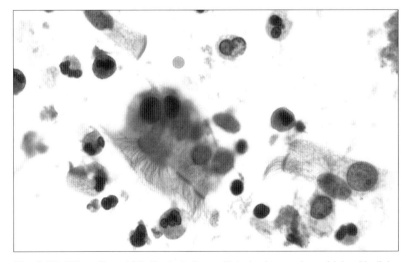

Fig. 1.25 Cilia – Pap x100. Illustrated are ciliated columnar bronchial epithelial cells from a bronchial wash specimen. The cilia, which stain bright pink, are attached to the luminal surface of the cells and are controlled by the cytoskeleton. Cilia are very delicate and are often lost during processing. They are also seen in endocervical and tubal epithelial cells.

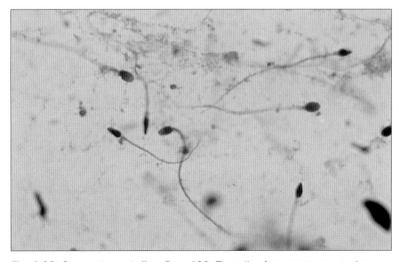

Fig. 1.26 Spermatozoa tails – Pap x100. The tails of spermatozoa are also regulated by their cytoskeletons. The sperm seen in cervical smears have often lost their tails and only the heads are noticeable.

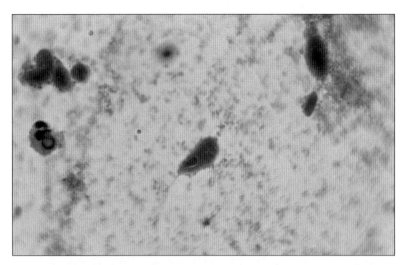

Fig. 1.27 Trichomonas vaginalis flagellum – Pap x100. In the centre of the field is a trichomonas vaginalis organism containing a red nucleus and a barely perceptible flagellum, which enables it to be motile.

Cell junctions are vitally important for the integrity of tissues. These are not visible in cytological preparations, but the principle that benign cells usually stay attached in sheets **(Fig. 1.28)** while malignant cells lose their cohesive qualities **(Fig. 1.29)** is an important one. It must be remembered, however, that in many specimens, such as urine **(Fig. 1.30)**, cells are exfoliated and therefore seen singly, unless brushed off by instrumentation **(Fig. 1.31)**.

Mitotic figures are clearly seen in cytological samples **(Fig. 1.32)**. They usually denote cellular activity, unless the mitoses are abnormal. The various stages of mitosis – prophase **(Fig. 1.33)**, metaphase **(Fig. 1.34)**, anaphase **(Fig. 1.35)**, and telophase **(Fig. 1.36)** – can be identified. Tripolar or abnormal mitoses, however, are an indicator of malignancy **(Fig. 1.37)**.

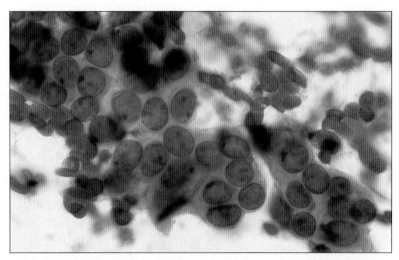

Fig. 1.28 Cell junctions – Pap x100. The sheet of benign ductal cells seen in this photomicrograph does not display the intercellular junctions which hold the cells together. There are more clearly demonstrated in histological sechons of squamous epithelium for example. When cells become malignant they lose their cohesive tendency and tend to dissociate.

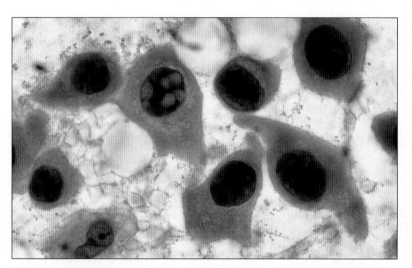

Fig. 1.29 Carcinoma cells – Pap x100. The malignant cells seen here, in an aspirate from a breast carcinoma, show loss of cohesion with the cells lying separately. Other features of malignancy are also present, such as irregular nuclei and hyperchromasia.

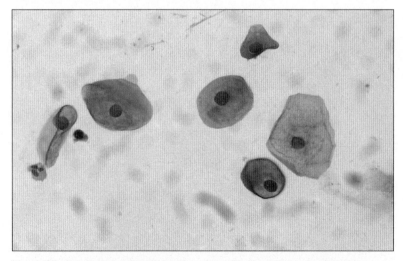

Fig. 1.30 Exfoliated urothelial cells – Pap x40. Urothelial cells which have exfoliated into urine are seen as single cells, but this is not an indication of malignancy.

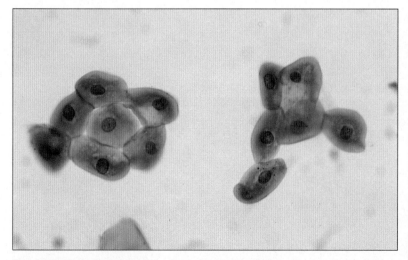

Fig. 1.31 Catheterized urine – Pap x40. The urothelial cells seen in this field are in sheets as they have been removed by instrumentation rather than shed by exfoliation.

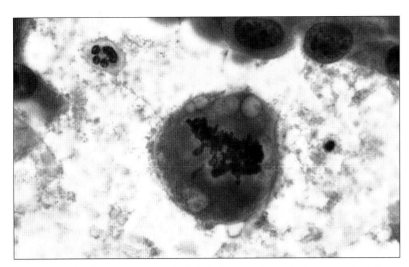

Fig. 1.32 Mitotic figure – Pap x100. This fine needle aspirate of a metastatic adenocarcinoma in liver shows a large malignant cell in mitosis.

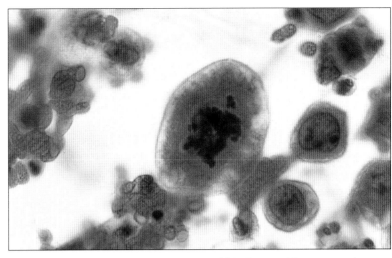

Fig. 1.33 Mitotic figure, prophase – Pap x100. Illustrated is a metastatic adenocarcinoma cell in a pleural effusion demonstrating prophase, when the chromosomes have become visible and the nuclear membrane is no longer seen. The apparent frilly border around the cell does not represent true microvilli, as in a mesothelial cell, because the cell membrane is smooth and the clear areas are within the cytoplasm.

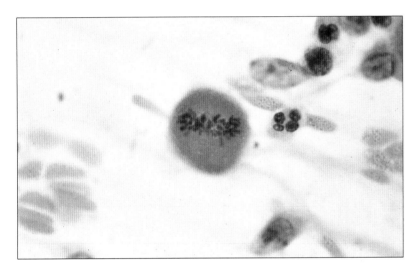

Fig. 1.34 Mitotic figure, metaphase – Pap x100. In this phase of mitosis the chromosomes are arranged along the equator of the cell, as illustrated in this benign mesothelial cell from a reactive pleural effusion.

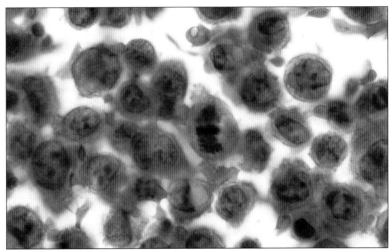

Fig. 1.35 Mitotic figure, anaphase – Pap x100. This photomicrograph demonstrates the two groups of identical duplicated chromosomes moving apart to opposite ends of the cell. The cells illustrated are from a high-grade lymphoma which metastasized to the pleural cavity.

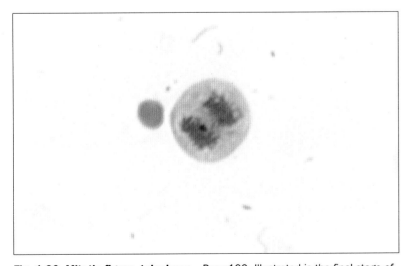

Fig. 1.36 Mitotic figure, telophase – Pap x100. Illustrated is the final stage of mitosis, where the two sets of identical chromosomes have completely separated, before their nuclear membranes have re-formed. The cell seen here is a normal mesothelial cell in ascitic fluid.

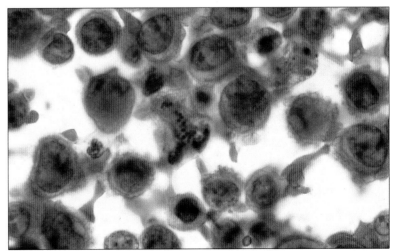

Fig. 1.37 Tripolar mitosis – Pap x100. In the centre of the field is a cell showing a tripolar mitotic figure, a sign of malignancy. This aspirate is from the same case of high-grade lymphoma as in **Figure. 1.35**.

CELL TYPES

Cells from various tissues show different characteristics:
- Squamous and urothelial cells tend to be large and flat, often polygonal in shape, with translucent to dense cytoplasm, depending on their maturation (**Figs 1.38, 1.39**).
- Glandular epithelial cells are either tall and columnar with the nucleus at the base of the cell, as in endocervical cells (**Fig. 1.40**), or cuboidal, as in thyroid epithelium (**Fig. 1.41**).
- Hepatocytes are large cells with striking nuclei, either single or binucleate, a sharp nuclear margin, and a prominent nucleolus. Their cytoplasm tends to be granular and may contain pigment (**Fig. 1.42**). They are often seen in sheets and groups in aspirates.
- Pancreatic acinar cells tend to be smaller than hepatocytes and are seen arranged in small acinar groups. The cells are wedge-shaped and appear to have granular cytoplasm (**Fig. 1.43**).
- Endocrine cells are small with round nuclei and delicate granular cytoplasm (**Fig. 1.44**).

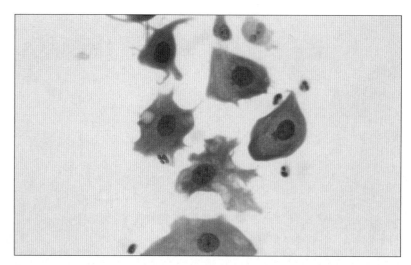

Fig. 1.38 Squamous metaplasia – Pap x40. The metaplastic squamous cells illustrated here vary from immature small ones, with a high nuclear–cytoplasmic ratio, to those which are more mature, containing more abundant cytoplasm. The tails of cytoplasm seen in some of the cells represent the desmosomes or intercellular junctions which hold the cells together in the epithelium. Note the dense cytoplasm of metaplastic cells, which is unlike the translucent delicate cytoplasm of the larger, more mature squamous cells (see **Figure 1.7**).

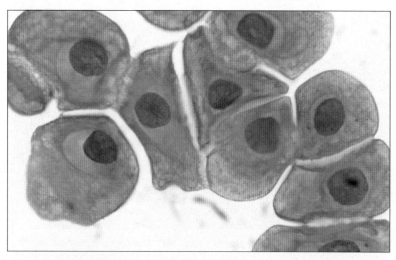

Fig. 1.39 Urothelial cells – Pap x100. The urothelial cells seen in this field are flat with clearly defined outlines and translucent cytoplasm, containing glycogen. These cells are slightly more mature than deep-layer urothelial cells, which tend to be smaller with denser cytoplasm.

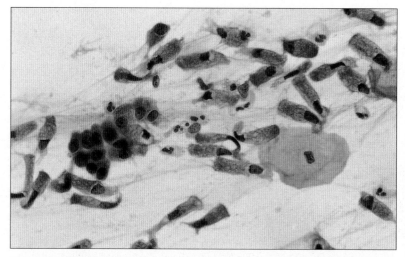

Fig. 1.40 Endocervical cells – Pap x40. These glandular cells from the endocervix are tall and columnar in type, with basal nuclei. The cells are small in comparison with the intermediate cell in the field, but the nuclei are approximately the same size.

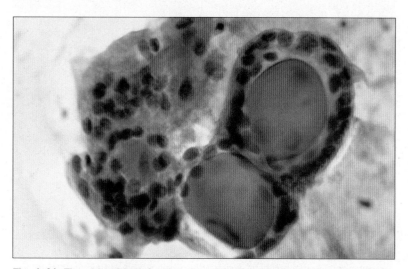

Fig. 1.41 Thyroid epithelial cells – Pap x100. The glandular cells seen here from an aspirate of a colloid nodule of thyroid are cuboidal in shape, with nuclei that are in the centre of the cell.

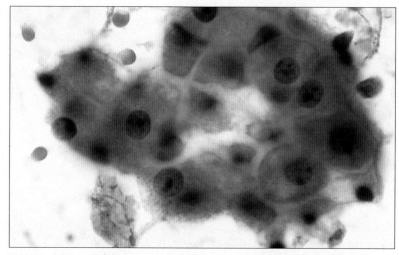

Fig. 1.42 Hepatocytes – Pap x100. These benign hepatocytes, noted in a liver aspirate, have round, central, clearly defined nuclei with prominent nucleoli and abundant granular cytoplasm. The cytoplasmic borders are well-demarcated. Hepatocytes may contain intracytoplasmic pigment; in this field the bile pigment is extracellular.

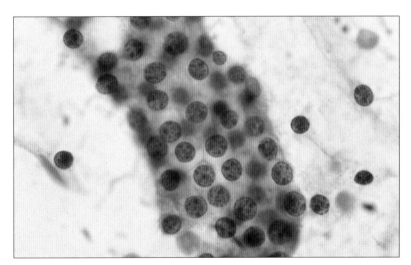

Fig. 1.43 Pancreatic acinar cells – Pap x100. Acinar cells from the normal pancreas are often wedge-shaped and arranged in small acinar groups or clusters. They also have granular cytoplasm. Benign islet cells of pancreas are rarely seen in aspirates.

- Striated muscle is seen in aspirates as thick strips of deeply staining tissue with dark nuclei at the periphery. Faint striations are visible on lowering the condenser **(Fig. 1.45)**.
- Mesenchymal cells are usually spindle-shaped with irregular nuclei, which are usually also spindle-shaped **(Fig. 1.46)**.
- Lymphoid cells are small with deeply staining nuclei and a thin rim of cytoplasm **(Fig. 1.47)**.
- Cells of the monocyte–macrophage type contain delicate cytoplasm and have ill-defined cell boundaries. Their nuclei are often reniform, with sharp outlines and a clearly visible nucleolus **(Fig. 1.48)**.
- Fat cells are very large with clear cytoplasm and peripheral nuclei t.b. **(Fig. 1.49)**.

Cells from various tissues retain their specific characteristics in benign neoplastic conditions, but tend to lose them as they become less differentiated – for example, poorly differentiated squamous cell carcinomas do not keratinize **(Fig. 1.50)** and poorly differentiated adenocarcinomas may not produce mucin **(Fig. 1.51)**. Special stains may be necessary in poorly differentiated tumours, but even these may not provide the answer, in which case immunocytochemistry would be of use.

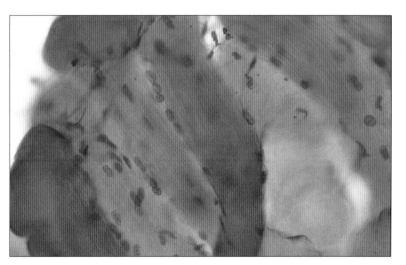

Fig. 1.44 Chief cell adenoma, parathyroid – Pap x100. Endocrine cells tend to be small with very pale, almost imperceptible, cytoplasm. Cell borders are difficult to determine, and the nuclei are small and round, with vesicular chromatin and visible nucleoli.

Fig. 1.45 Striated muscle cells – Pap x100. Striated muscle cells are seen in thick bands, staining orange with the Papanicolaou stain. The cross striations are usually visible with careful focusing and the nuclei are small and situated at the periphery of the muscle fibres.

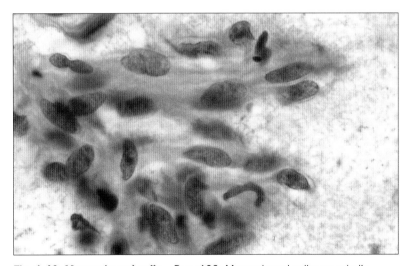

Fig. 1.46 Mesenchymal cells – Pap x100. Mesenchymal cells are spindle-shaped with delicate cytoplasm and ovoid-to-spindle nuclei. The nuclei are vesicular, but may show some irregularities of the margin. This field illustrates an aspirate from benign mesenchymal neoplasm of the breast.

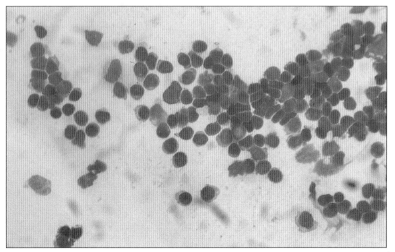

Fig. 1.47 Lymphocytes – MGG x40. Lymphocytes are small with a narrow, often difficult to visualize, rim of cytoplasm. Shown here are benign lymphocytes in a normal lymph node.

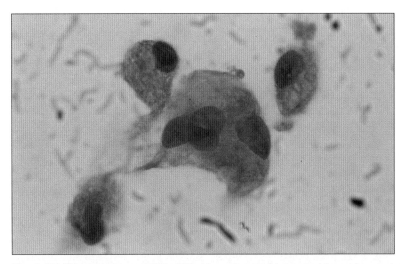

Fig. 1.48 Macrophages – MGG x100. Macrophages (histiocytes) have abundant foamy, delicate cytoplasm with hazy cell borders. The nuclei may be bean-shaped or round, the cells may be multinucleated, and can exhibit a variety of phagocytosed materials, such as pigment or dead cells. This field of macrophages is from a nipple discharge specimen in duct ectasia.

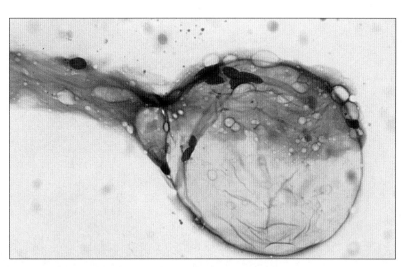

Fig. 1.49 Fat cells – MGG x100. Mature fat cells are large and often in clusters that resemble soap suds, as the cells are clear and have sharp, fine cytoplasmic margins. The nucleus is at the periphery of the cell.

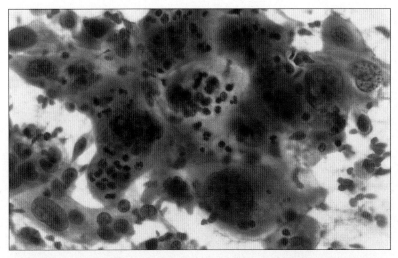

Fig. 1.50 Poorly differentiated squamous carcinoma – Pap x100. This field of a fine needle aspirate of a lung neoplasm illustrates pleomorphic cells with abnormal nuclei and fairly dense cytoplasm, exhibiting phagocytosis of neutrophils. Although this latter feature is commonly seen in adenocarcinomas, it is noted rarely in squamous cell carcinomas. No keratinization is seen here, but in other fields there were occasional keratinized single squamous carcinoma cells.

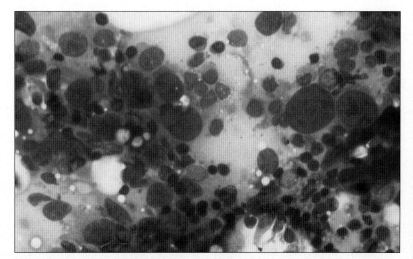

Fig. 1.51 Poorly differentiated adenocarcinoma – MGG x100. This fine needle aspirate of a poorly differentiated adenocarcinoma metastasis in a lymph node shows large pleomorphic malignant cells in a background of lymphocytes. No vacuolation or extracellular mucin is evident. The primary tumour was a high-grade carcinoma of breast.

SUGGESTED READING

Kelly DE, Wood RL, Enders AC. *Bailey's Textbook of Microscopic Anatomy*, 18th ed. Baltimore: Williams & Wilkins; 1985:17–63.

Stevens A, Lowe J. *Histology*. London: Mosby; 1993: 7–25.

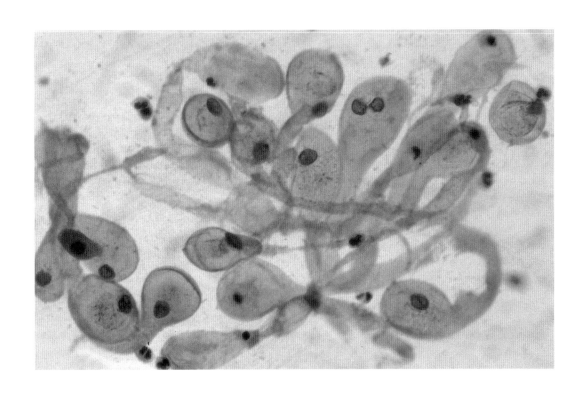

CONSTITUENTS OF
NORMAL CERVICAL SMEARS

2

A working knowledge of the anatomy and histology of the female genital tract is essential in order to properly identify the various cells and material seen in normal cervical smears.

ANATOMY OF THE FEMALE GENITAL TRACT

The female genital tract consists of a uterus with a cervix and two fallopian tubes, each ending in close proximity to an ovary (**Fig. 2.1**). The **ovary** is a small oval organ composed mostly of whorls of connective tissue stroma, which support the oocytes or germ cells, and covered by a layer of cuboidal epithelial cells. The **fallopian tubes** are lined by glandular epithelium which is partly ciliated. Tubal cells are rarely seen in cervical smears. The uterine cavity is lined by endometrium composed of stroma and cuboidal endometrial cells. The **endometrium**, under hormonal influences, undergoes cyclical changes during the various phases of the menstrual cycle. Endometrial cells are not normally seen in a cervical smear, except during menstruation and for 10 days after the last menstrual period (LMP).

The **cervix uteri** is lined by two different types of epithelium – glandular in the **endocervical canal** and squamous in the **ectocervix**, this being continuous with the squamous epithelial lining of the vagina. The **squamo-columnar junction (Fig. 2.2)** varies in its location, depending on the age of the woman. It is at the external os and therefore easily sampled in young and pregnant women but recedes higher up the endocervical canal in older, postmenopausal women. The ectocervix is composed of **stratified squamous epithelium (Fig. 2.3)**. The deepest layer is the basal, regenerative layer of small, darkly staining cells, which are arranged perpendicular to the basement membrane. Above this are the parabasal cell layers, the intermediate cell layers, including navicular cells, and,

at the surface, the superficial cell layer. The cells are seen to enlarge and contain more cytoplasm as they mature towards the surface. No keratinization is seen on the surface in a normal cervix. Beneath the epithelium and separated from it by the basement membrane is the stroma of the cervix, composed of connective tissue containing small blood vessels and lymphatics. The thickness of the squamous epithelium depends upon the age of the patient, being quite atrophic and thin in postmenopausal women.

CELLS SEEN IN SMEARS

A cervical smear which is taken properly should include components of the squamo-columnar junction as well as cells from the ectocervix. It will contain squamous epithelial cells, a few neutrophil polymorphs, histiocytes, endocervical or squamous metaplastic cells, and mucin (**Fig. 2.4**).

Superficial squamous cells are large polygonal cells with abundant cytoplasm which are derived from the superficial layer of the epithelium (**Fig. 2.5**). Each contains a small dark pyknotic central nucleus and translucent cytoplasm, which is usually acidophilic (**Fig. 2.6**), but may be cyanophilic (**Fig. 2.7**). The more mature cells may take up a pinkish orange to pale brown hue (**Fig. 2.8**) and some cells contain keratohyaline granules (**Fig. 2.9**). Superficial cells appear flat on light microscopy, showing no evidence of the ridges that are identifiable under the electron microscope.

Intermediate squamous cells are approximately the same size as superficial cells (**Fig. 2.10**) and are also polygonal, but contain slightly larger, vesicular nuclei which are approximately the size of a neutrophil polymorph (**Fig. 2.11**). The less mature intermediate cells (**Fig. 2.12**) are slightly smaller than those that are more mature. The cytoplasm usually appears cyanophilic (**Fig. 2.13**), but

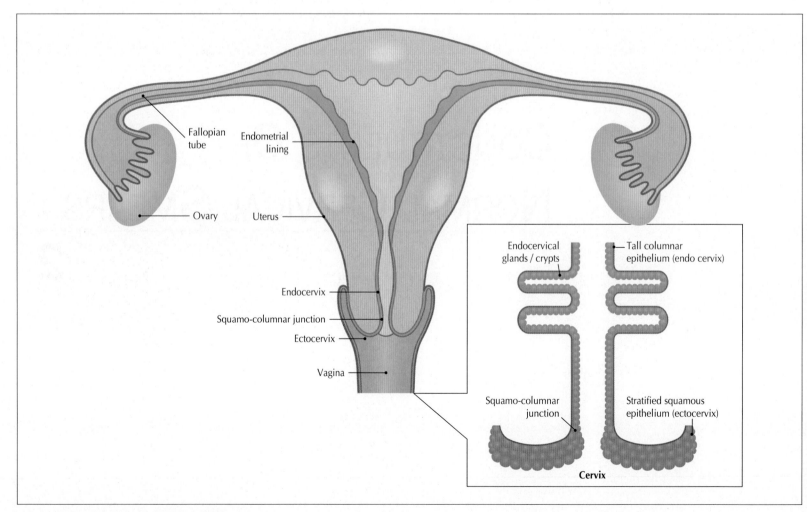

Fig. 2.1 Diagram of the female genital tract.

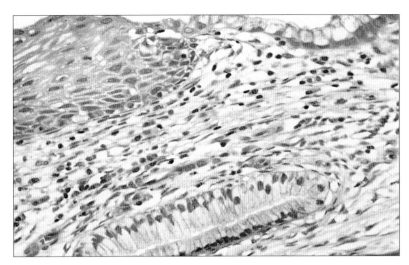

Fig. 2.2 Squamo-columnar junction – H&E x10. The tall columnar endocervical epithelium on the right of the photomicrograph changes abruptly to stratified squamous epithelium of ectocervix.

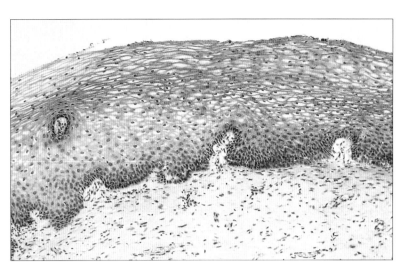

Fig. 2.3 Stratified squamous epithelium – H&E x4. This section illustrates the various layers of stratified squamous epithelium comprising the ectocervix. The layer of small dark cells just above the basement membrane consists of basal cells which mature and enlarge as they reach the surface.

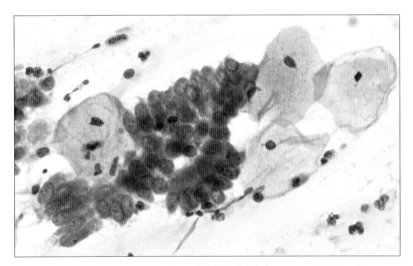

Fig. 2.4 An adequate smear – Pap x40. This field shows superficial and intermediate squamous cells together with a few rows of tall columnar endocervical cells, demonstrating that the squamo-columnar junction has been sampled.

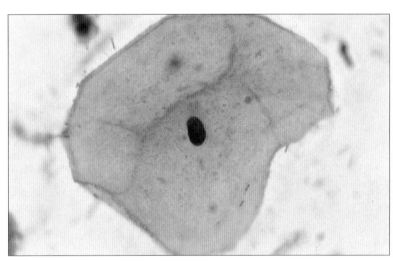

Fig. 2.5 Superficial squamous cell – Pap x100. The superficial cell illustrated here is polygonal with a small pyknotic nucleus and abundant acidophilic cytoplasm. Oestrogen is required for the maturation of immature squamous cells from the deeper layers of the epithelium.

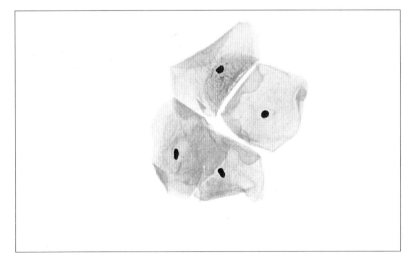

Fig. 2.6 Superficial squamous cells – Pap x40. These superficial squamous cells show characteristic delicate translucent acidophilic cytoplasm and pyknotic nuclei.

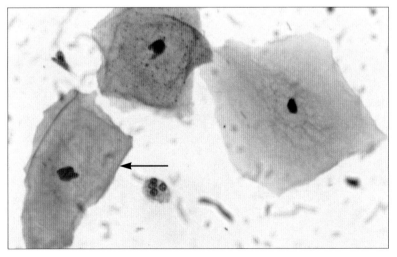

Fig. 2.7 Superficial squamous cells – Pap x40. One of the superficial cells in this group of three shows cyanophilic staining (arrowed). It is distinguished from an intermediate cell by its pyknotic nucleus.

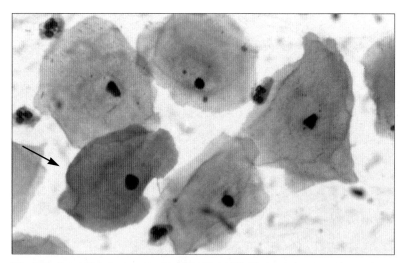

Fig. 2.8 Superficial squamous cells – Pap x40. The variation in cytoplasmic staining is well-illustrated here, with one acidophilic cell (arrowed) and the rest showing the pale beige–brown shade of more mature cells.

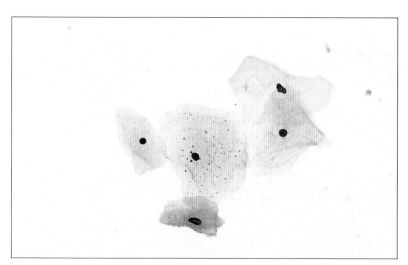

Fig. 2.9 Superficial squamous cells – Pap x40. These superficial cells contain fine keratohyaline granules within their cytoplasm.

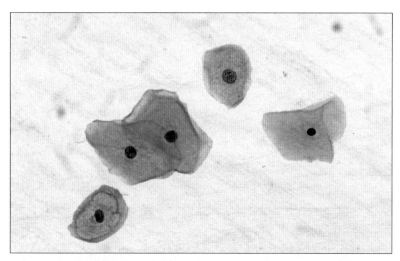

Fig. 2.10 Intermediate squamous cells – Pap x40. This field illustrates the similarity in size between the cyanophilic intermediate cells and the acidophilic superficial cells.

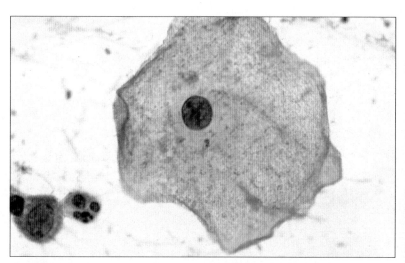

Fig. 2.11 Intermediate squamous cell – Pap x100. This high-power view of an intermediate cell displays a nucleus which is approximately the size of the neutrophil next to it. A small histiocyte is also present.

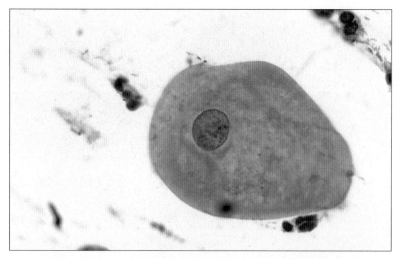

Fig. 2.12 Intermediate squamous cell – Pap x100. The intermediate cell pictured here is slightly smaller than the more mature cell in **Figure 2.11**, with slightly denser cytoplasm, but the nuclei are about the same size.

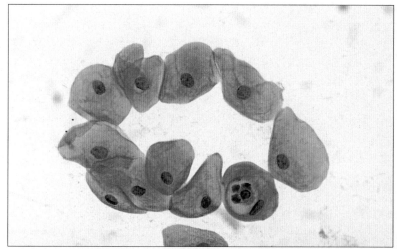

Fig. 2.13 Intermediate squamous cells – Pap x40. The intermediate cells in this field are cyanophilic with slightly varying shapes. One of the cells is displaying phagocytosis.

may occasionally be eosinophilic **(Fig. 2.14)**. The nucleus often contains a visible Barr body **(Fig. 2.15)** and the cytoplasm may contain keratohyaline granules **(Fig. 2.16)**. During the second or secretory part of the menstrual cycle (post ovulation), the squamous epithelium of the ectocervix shows predominantly intermediate cells containing glycogen, referred to as a basket-weave pattern **(Fig. 2.17)**. A smear taken at this time shows intermediate cells arranged in a similar basket-weave fashion **(Fig. 2.18)** and often containing yellow intracytoplasmic glycogen **(Fig. 2.19)**.

Navicular cells are less mature and therefore, are smaller than intermediate cells **(Fig. 2.20)**. They are most commonly seen in smears taken during pregnancy **(Fig. 2.21)**, but not exclusively so. Navicular cells are typically boat-shaped with eccentric nuclei and thick cytoplasmic edges **(Fig. 2.22)**. They, too, may contain glycogen **(Fig. 2.23)**.

Parabasal cells are seen predominantly in cervical smears taken from post-menopausal women. The epithelium does not mature due to a lack of oestrogen and progesterone and is often quite thin **(Fig. 2.24)**. Parabasal cells are

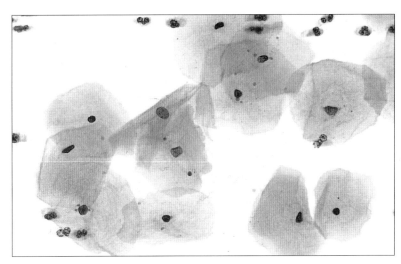

Fig. 2.14 Intermediate squamous cells – Pap x40. This photomicrograph illustrates acidophilic superficial cells as well as acidophilic and cyanophilic intermediate cells. The vesicular nuclei are the only distinguishing feature intermediate of acidophilic cells.

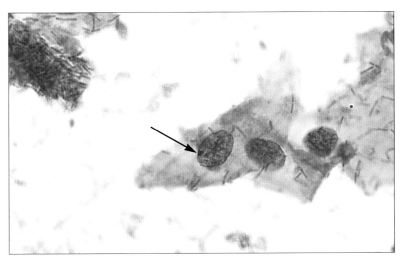

Fig. 2.15 Intermediate squamous cell – Pap x100. The intermediate cell in the centre of this field contains a Barr body at the edge of the nucleus (arrowed).

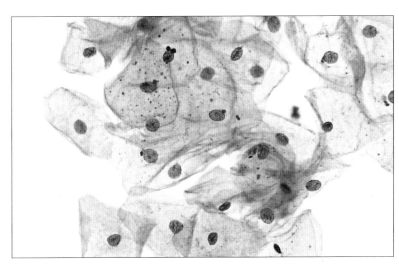

Fig. 2.16 Intermediate squamous cells – Pap x40. Some of the cells in this illustration contain keratohyaline granules similar to those in superficial cells.

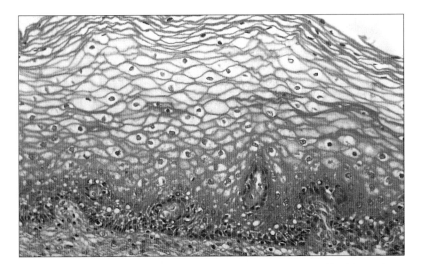

Fig. 2.17 Ectocervix showing basket-weave pattern – H&E x10. This section of ectocervix shows cells with a basket-weave appearance due to the glycogen within the cells in the upper layers.

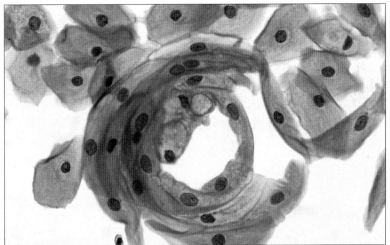

Fig. 2.18 Intermediate cells – Pap x40. The intermediate cells seen in this field show a basket-weave pattern similar to that demonstrated in the biopsy specimen in **Figure 2.17**.

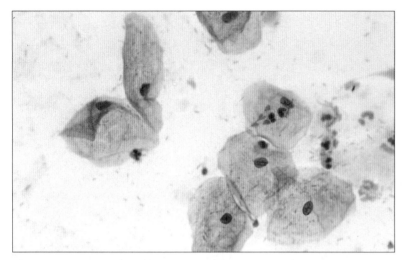

Fig. 2.19 Intermediate cells – Pap x40. Glycogen is frequently seen in intermediate cells, which eventually undergo cytolysis due to the action of lactobacilli.

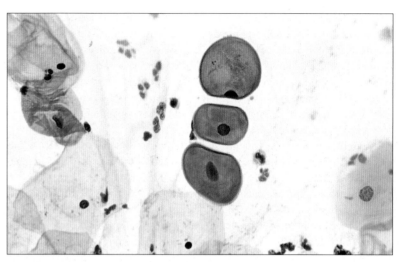

Fig. 2.20 Navicular cells – Pap x40. The navicular cells in the centre of this field are smaller than the neighbouring acidophilic superficial and cyanophilic intermediate cells.

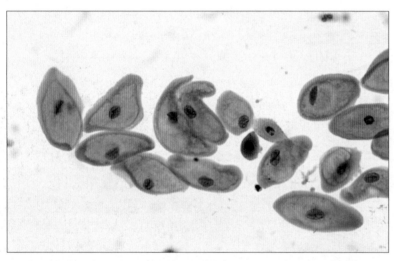

Fig. 2.21 Navicular cells – Pap x40. This field from a smear of a pregnant woman shows navicular cells only; these are characteristically boat-shaped, with a thickened rim of cytoplasm and eccentric nuclei. These cells may be mistaken for koilocytes.

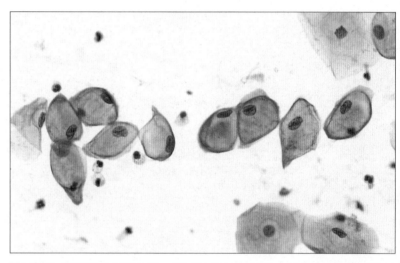

Fig. 2.22 Navicular cells – Pap x40. Illustrated here is a mixture of intermediate cells and navicular cells with eccentric nuclei and thickened margins, seen in a cervical smear taken from a non-pregnant woman.

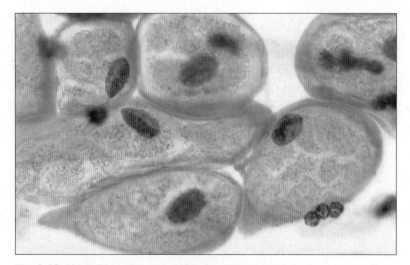

Fig. 2.23 Navicular cells – Pap x100. This high-power view of navicular cells illustrates clearly the glycogen often seen in these cells.

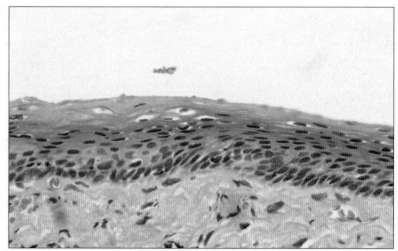

Fig. 2.24 Ectocervix (postmenopausal) – H&E x10. This stratified squamous epithelium is rather thin compared with normal ectocervix from a premenopausal woman (see **Figure 2.3**). This is due to a lack of oestrogen and progesterone.

smaller than navicular cells, but have relatively larger nuclei. They are rounded with a central nucleus and acidophilic or cyanophilic cytoplasm (**Fig. 2.25**). Parabasal cells in smears taken from postmenopausal women are often poorly preserved and show degenerative changes (**Fig. 2.26**). These cells are also seen in young women on the combined oral contraceptive pill, and in postnatal smears, but tend to be better preserved in these cases (**Fig. 2.27**).

Endocervical cells are derived from endocervical epithelium, which is single-layered, lining the surface of the endocervix while being continuous with the crypts or glands of the endocervix (**Figs 2.28, 2.29**). Endocervical cells are tall and columnar in type with basal nuclei (**Fig. 2.30**), and show a variety of appearances in smears. They may be seen in the form of sheets (**Fig. 2.31**), which often exhibit a neat palisaded appearance at one edge (**Fig. 2.32**) and a honeycomb pattern on focusing up and down (**Fig. 2.33**). Not infrequently, ciliated endocervical cells are seen (**Fig. 2.34**), the nuclei showing a vesicular or 'open' pattern. The cells may be distended with mucin (**Fig. 2.35**), the amount of mucin

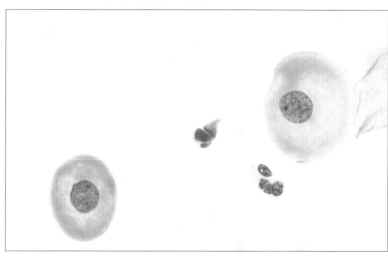

Fig. 2.25 Parabasal cells – Pap x100. The two parabasal cells seen in this field are rounded with central round nuclei. These cells are smaller than navicular cells, being less mature.

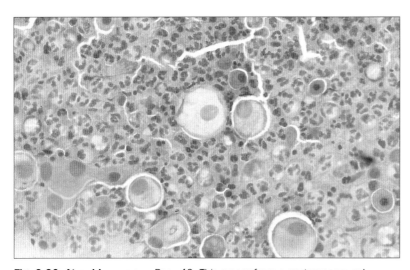

Fig. 2.26 Atrophic smear – Pap x40. This smear from a postmenopausal woman shows the typical poor preservation associated with these cases. The parabasal cells are air-dried with hazy nuclei and degenerative changes, including pyknosis and vacuolation. The neutrophils also show the effect of air-drying.

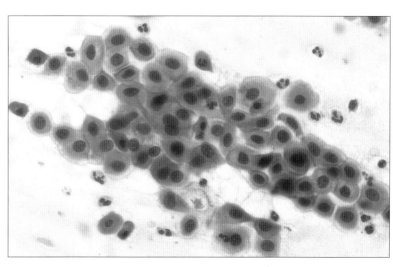

Fig. 2.27 Atrophic smear, combined pill effect – Pap x40. The parabasal cells in this photomicrograph are well preserved, unlike those seen in postmenopausal smears.

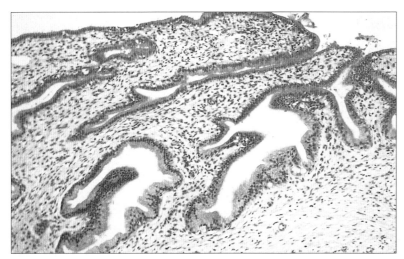

Fig. 2.28 Endocervical epithelium – H&E x4. The epithelium lining the endocervix is tall and columnar in type. Note the crypts and glands of the endocervix lined by similar cells.

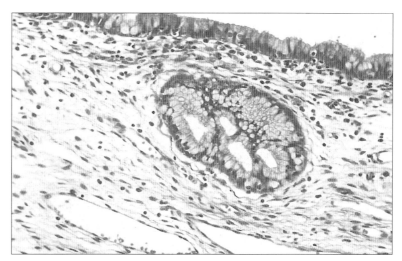

Fig. 2.29 Endocervical epithelium – H&E x10. This section shows in greater detail the tall columnar cells that constitute this epithelial lining. Similar cells line the endocervical glands. Capillaries and lymphatics are seen in the stroma, close enough to the glands to show how easily invasive carcinoma can spread to the blood stream and lymphatics.

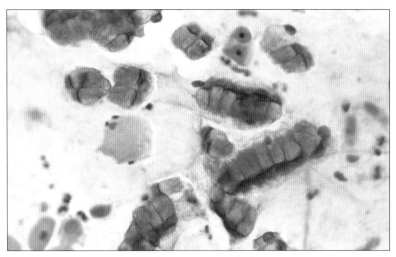

Fig. 2.30 Endocervical cells – Pap x40. The endocervical cells seen in this field are tall columnar cells with basal nuclei showing slight depressions due to the accumulation of mucin within the delicate cytoplasm. Note the picket-fence type of arrangement of the cells.

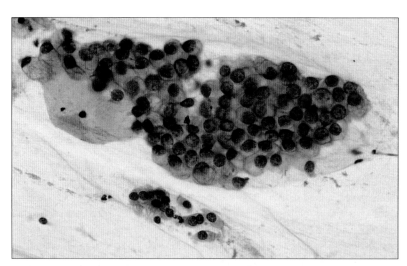

Fig. 2.31 Endocervical cells – Pap x40. This sheet of endocervical cells shows vesicular nuclei and delicate cytoplasm. The cells are much smaller than the adjacent superficial cell. Note also the small ciliated endocervical cells in the background.

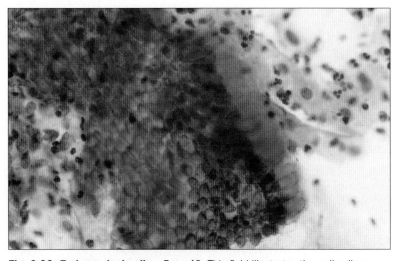

Fig. 2.32 Endocervical cells – Pap x40. This field illustrates the palisading often seen at the edge of a sheet of endocervical cells.

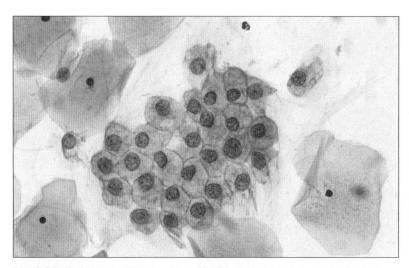

Fig. 2.33 Endocervical cells – Pap x40. The sheet of endocervical cells in the centre of this field exhibits honeycombing, with the outline of the cytoplasmic borders clearly visible. The vesicular nuclei and delicate pale cytoplasm are illustrated clearly.

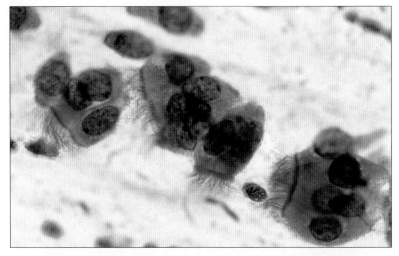

Fig. 2.34 Endocervical cells – Pap x100. The endocervical cells seen here show well-preserved pink cilia.

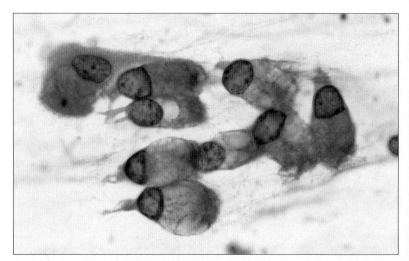

Fig. 2.35 Endocervical cells – Pap x100. In this field the endocervical cells are seen distended with mucin, becoming almost goblet-shaped.

present varying with the phase of the menstrual cycle. They may even be mult-inucleated when reactive (**Fig. 2.36**). If the cervical scrape has been vigorous many sheets of endocervical cells may be seen (**Fig. 2.37**). Mitoses may be seen occasionally in endocervical cells (**Fig. 2.38**).

Endometrial cells are seen during the menstrual phase of the cycle, being derived from endometrium that is being shed. They are often seen as sharply defined clusters of small, hyperchromatic stromal cells surrounded by larger, clearer glandular cells (**Fig. 2.39**). Endometrial cells are approximately the size of a polymorph and have a vesicular nucleus and clear cytoplasm (**Fig. 2.40**). They may be seen as three-dimensional mulberry-like clusters composed of glan-

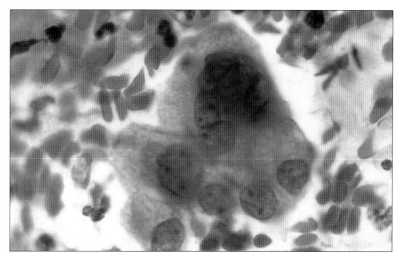

Fig. 2.36 Endocervical cells – Pap x100. The endocervical cells seen here are enlarged and multinucleated, changes attributable to a reactive process. The nuclei are still vesicular and there is no evidence of neoplastic change.

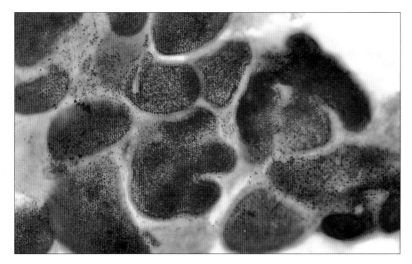

Fig. 2.37 Endocervical cell sheets – Pap x4. Rarely, a vigorous cervical scrape produces microbiopsies composed of sheets of endocervical cells. Even at this low power the peripheral palisading around the clusters is evident.

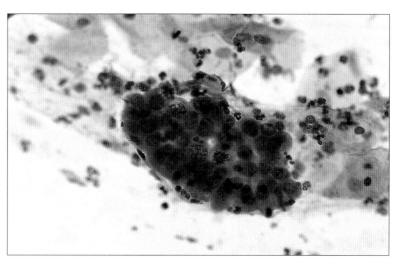

Fig. 2.38 Endocervical cells – Pap x40. Mitotic figures are not uncommon in normal endocervical cells. Three mitoses are seen in the sheet of endocervical cells illustrated here.

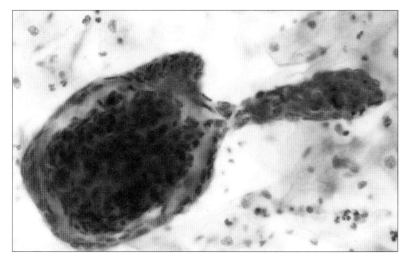

Fig. 2.39 Endometrial cells – Pap x40. The cluster of endometrial cells seen in this field contains small dark stromal cells in the centre and paler glandular cells with abundant cytoplasm around them.

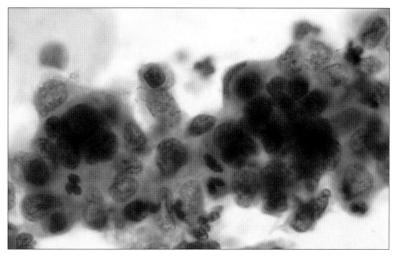

Fig. 2.40 Endometrial cells – Pap x100. This cluster of endometrial cells demonstrates the nuclear size, which is approximately that of a neutrophil polymorph. The nuclei are vesicular, but several show degenerative crinkling of the margins and hyperchromasia.

dular cells alone (**Fig. 2.41**) or accompanied by masses of small histiocytes – the exodus (**Fig. 2.42**). Not infrequently, endometrial cells show degenerative changes, including vacuolation and crinkled nuclei (**Fig. 2.43**).

Neutrophil polymorphs are common components of cervical smears (**Fig. 2.44**). They are often present in small numbers, but may be present in abundance, especially if the smear includes the blobs of mucus seen sometimes at the cervical os. In such cases, the smear is usually unsatisfactory for evaluation as the polymorphs obscure all other cellular detail.

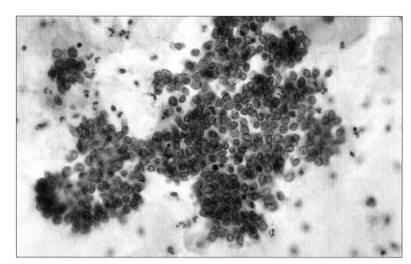

Fig. 2.41 Endometrial cells – Pap x40. In this field the endometrial cells are in well-spread clusters overlying some squamous cells. They are about the size of the neutrophils in the background.

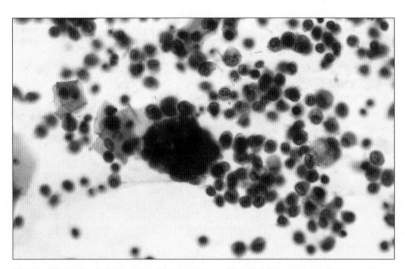

Fig. 2.42 Endometrial cells, the exodus – Pap x40. The exodus is a term used for the large numbers of histiocytes which accompany endometrial cell clusters in menstrual smears. The endometrial cells in this field are small, hyperchromatic, and clustered while the histiocytes have abundant cytoplasm and tend to be single.

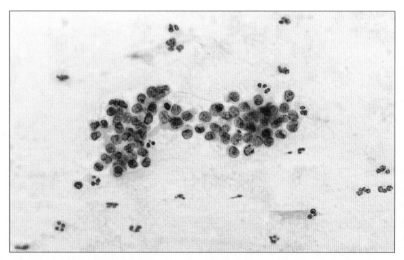

Fig. 2.43 Endometrial cells – Pap x40. Endometrial cells are exfoliated and therefore tend to be degenerate in menstrual smears. Here, the clusters of endometrial cells seen in the centre of the field show vacuolation due to degeneration.

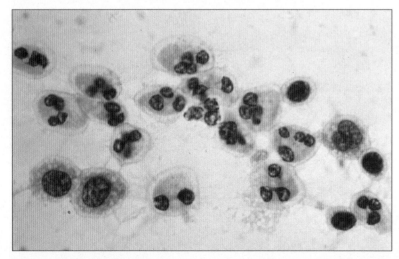

Fig. 2.44 Neutrophils – Pap x100. Neutrophil polymorphs are invariably seen in smears in small numbers. Here they are accompanied by three small histiocytes and some lymphocytes.

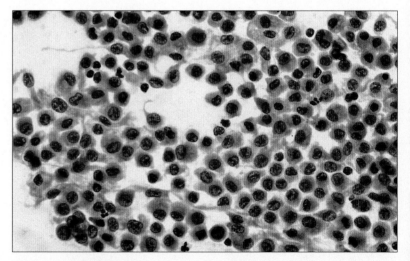

Fig. 2.45 Small histiocytes – Pap x40. The whole field is occupied by small histiocytes with clearly defined nuclear margins, but hazy cytoplasmic borders. At low magnification they may be mistaken for lymphocytes or endometrial cells.

Histiocytes are frequently seen in smears. They may be small histiocytes, the size of endometrial cells **(Fig. 2.45)**, or larger with typical bean-shaped or reniform nuclei **(Fig. 2.46)**. Quite often histiocytes have round or oval nuclei **(Fig. 2.47)**. Their cytoplasm is delicate with ill-defined cell borders and may contain ingested material or dead cells **(Fig. 2.48)**. In smears from postmenopausal women there are usually many large multinucleated histiocytes, sometimes with just a few nuclei **(Fig. 2.49)**, sometimes forming enormous cells with 20 or more nuclei **(Fig. 2.50)**.

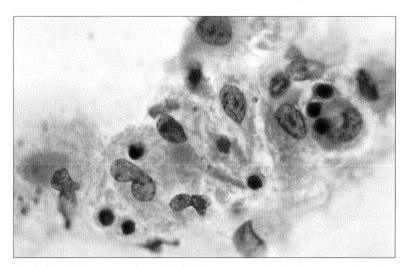

Fig. 2.46 Histiocytes – Pap x100. Histiocytes often display bean-shaped nuclei with clear nuclear margins and delicate ill-defined cytoplasmic borders, as illustrated here.

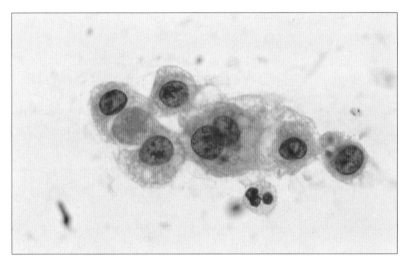

Fig. 2.47 Histiocytes – Pap x100. These histiocytes all have rounded nuclear margins.

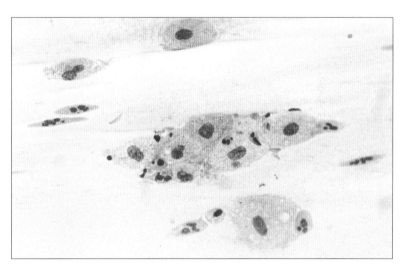

Fig. 2.48 Histiocytes – Pap x40. This field contains histiocytes which have engulfed polymorphs and other cellular debris.

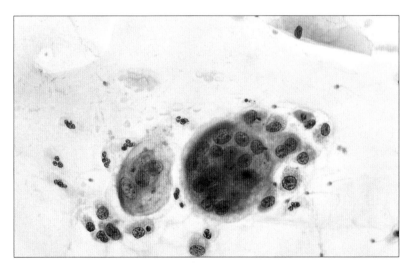

Fig. 2.49 Multinucleated histiocyte – Pap x40. The multinucleated histiocytes pictured here contain several round nuclei and are very closely positioned to small histiocytes, apparently confirming the theory that multinucleated histiocytes are formed by the aggregation of several small histiocytes.

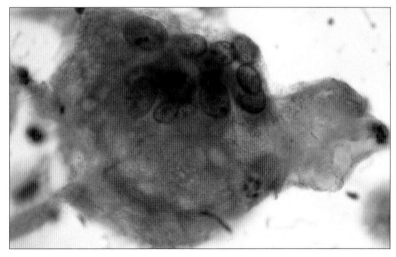

Fig. 2.50 Multinucleated histiocyte – Pap x100. The large multinucleated histiocyte seen here has about 12 nuclei in this plane, but several more come into view on changing the focus.

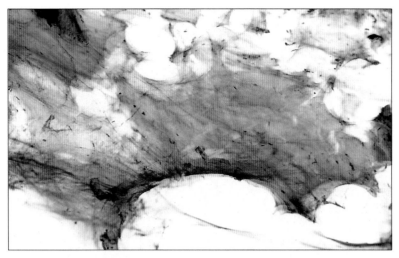

Fig. 2.51 Mucin – Pap x40. Mucin is seen in the form of a pinkish orange wash across the field. If excessive, it can occupy much of the slide, making the sample unsatisfactory for screening. The presence of mucin does not indicate that the squamo-columnar junction has been sampled.

Mucin, which is secreted by endocervical cells, is invariably seen in cervical smears. It usually stains pink with the Papanicolaou stain (**Fig. 2.51**), but may stain blue (**Fig. 2.52**). It often exhibits delicate patterns, such as 'ferning' (**Fig. 2.53**).

Spermatozoa may be noted in smears, although women are usually advised to refrain from sexual activity for 48 hours prior to having a smear taken. They typically have heads and tails (**Fig. 2.54**), although the tails are very fragile and are often lost, the result mimicking candida spores. A problem that could arise in such smears is that seminal vesicle cells may also be present which, with their large apparently abnormal nuclei, could mimic dyskaryosis (**Fig. 2.55**). A distinguishing feature is the presence of lipofuchsin pigment in seminal vesicle cells.

SQUAMOUS METAPLASIA

Squamous metaplasia is a constantly occurring physiological process in the cervix. Under the influence of external stimuli, either chemical or bacterial,

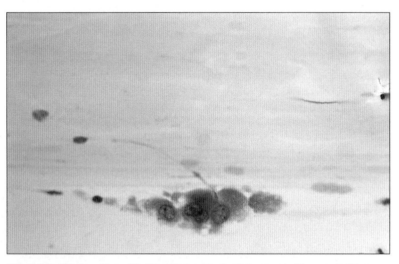

Fig. 2.52 Mucin – Pap x40. Sometimes mucin stains a pale blue, as in this illustration, making it difficult to identify.

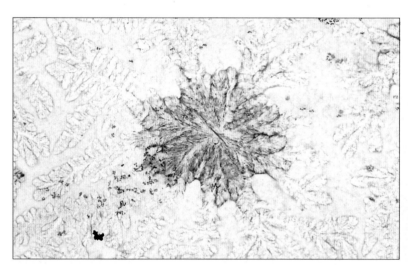

Fig. 2.53 Mucin – Pap x10. Mucin often forms delicate patterns on smears, one of which, 'ferning', is seen in this field.

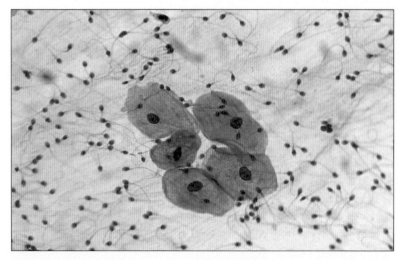

Fig. 2.54 Spermatozoa – Pap x40. Illustrated here are numerous spermatozoa with intact heads and tails, some overlying the intermediate cells in the centre of the field.

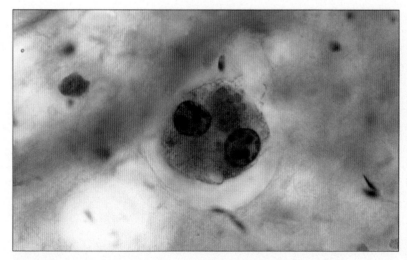

Fig. 2.55 Seminal vesicle cells – Pap x100. The cell pictured here is binucleate with abnormal chromatin and could be mistaken for dyskaryosis, but for the orange cytoplasmic pigment.

the basal reserve cells of the endocervix mature into squamous rather than endocervical cells. Instead of the usual single, columnar cell layer overlying the reserve cell layer (**Fig. 2.56**), a multilayered epithelium is formed with several layers of immature metaplastic squamous cells being topped by columnar endocervical cells in patches (**Fig. 2.57**). Squamous metaplasia can occur within endocervical gland crypts (**Fig. 2.58**). These immature metaplastic cells can appear alarming on a smear, as they are small with an increased nuclear–cytoplasmic ratio and may be mistaken for severe dyskaryosis (**Figs 2.59, 2.60**). As the metaplastic epithelium matures, the cells become larger and more closely resemble native squamous epithelium. In a smear, metaplastic cells have a typical appearance (**Fig. 2.61**). Sometimes they are seen with one, two, or more 'tails' of cytoplasm (**Figs 2.62, 2.63**). The tadpole (**Fig. 2.64**) and spindle-shaped varieties should not be confused with similar cells seen in invasive squamous carcinoma. Metaplastic squamous cells, including those with bizarre shapes, often contain glycogen (**Fig. 2.65**). Squamous metaplastic cells may be seen in close proximity to endocervical cells. They may, on occasion, mimic parabasal cells.

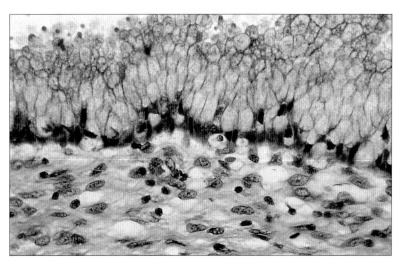

Fig. 2.56 Endocervical epithelium – H&E x25. This section demonstrates the usual single-layered epithelium, composed of tall columnar cells, which forms endocervical epithelium. The basal reserve cell layer is not clearly defined.

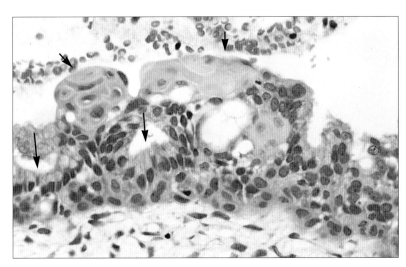

Fig. 2.57 Squamous metaplasia – H&E x10. In this section of endocervix the endocervical cells (long arrows) are interspersed with areas of metaplastic squamous epithelium (short arrows). This process is quite common, so the position of the squamo-columnar junction changes according to the area of the endocervix that has undergone squamous metaplasia.

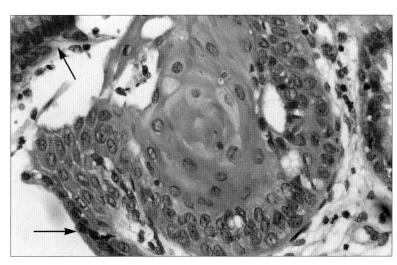

Fig. 2.58 Squamous metaplasia – H&E x40. Illustrated here is an area of squamous metaplastic change in an endocervical gland crypt. Note the normal tall columnar lining epithelium at the surface on the left of the section (arrowed).

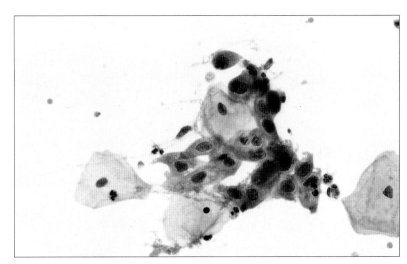

Fig. 2.59 Metaplastic squamous cells – Pap x40. This field shows a group of immature squamous metaplastic cells surrounded by superficial and intermediate cells. The small size and relatively large and hyperchromatic nuclei of the metaplastic cells may be interpreted as dyskaryosis at this magnification.

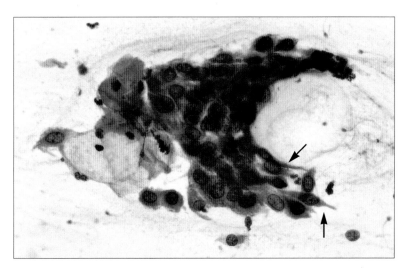

Fig. 2.60 Metaplastic squamous cells – Pap x40. This group of immature metaplastic squamous cells shows a high nuclear–cytoplasmic ratio and hyperchromasia, so may be mistaken for severe dyskaryosis. However, some of the cells in the group show the typical 'tails' of cytoplasm associated with metaplastic cells (arrowed).

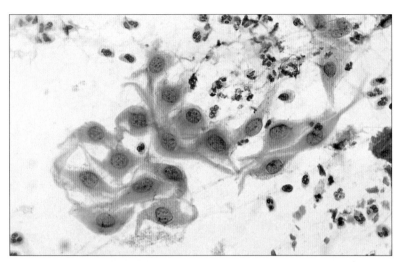

Fig. 2.61 Metaplastic squamous cells – Pap x40. Metaplastic cells in cervical smears have a characteristic shape, with their cytoplasm extending in tails. Most of the cells seen here have only two tails.

RESERVE CELL HYPERPLASIA

Reserve cell hyperplasia is an important process because of its apparent potential for malignant change. Endocervical reserve cells, as discussed above, are small basal cells which can develop along different lines: they normally mature into columnar endocervical cells, but can also produce metaplastic squamous cells and, finally, are thought to be responsible for the development of small cell severe dyskaryosis as well as endocervical adenocarcinoma (**Fig. 2.66**).

In contrast to the single layer of endocervical columnar cells above a patchy layer of reserve cells seen in the normal endocervix, reserve cell hyperplasia forms several layers of small reserve cells beneath the endocevical cells (**Figs 2.67, 2.68**). This is quite different from the appearances of squamous metaplasia (see **Figure 2.57**). On a cervical smear, reserve cell hyperplasia is demonstrated as sheets of small hyperchromatic cells (**Fig. 2.69**), which may be mistaken for endometrial cell clusters. On higher magnification, the cells are seen to have ovoid or elongated nuclei with distinct nuclear grooves and very little cytoplasm (**Figs 2.70, 2.71**). They are not accompanied by blood or histiocytes.

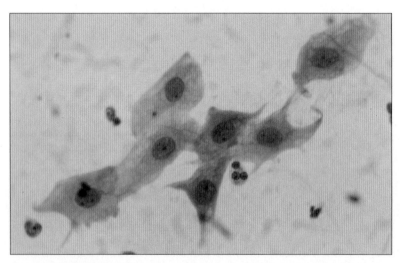

Fig. 2.62 Metaplastic squamous cells – Pap x40. Some of these metaplastic cells have three or four tails, while others resemble parabasal cells.

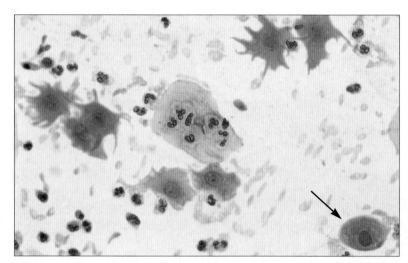

Fig. 2.63 Metaplastic squamous cells – Pap x40. Most of the metaplastic cells in this field have several tails, but the one in the bottom right-hand corner with its smooth outline resembles a parabasal cell (arrowed).

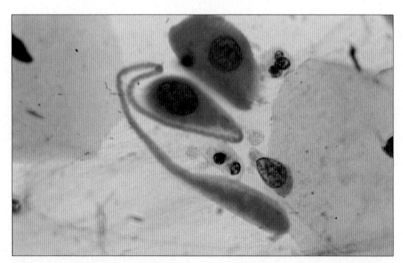

Fig. 2.64 Metaplastic tadpole cell – Pap x40. In this field yet another variation of metaplastic cells is seen, in the form of a tadpole cell. The nucleus, however, is that of a benign metaplastic cell and therefore this should not be interpreted as invasive squamous carcinoma.

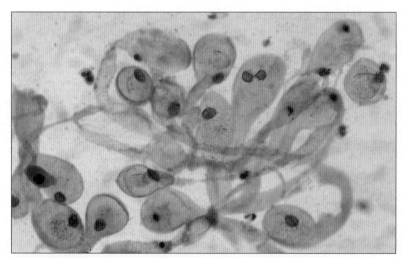

Fig. 2.65 Metaplastic tadpole cells – Pap x40. This photomicrograph illustrates a group of tadpole cells, all metaplastic, most of them containing glycogen. Note the difference in staining reaction, with some cells showing acidophilia, others cyanophilia.

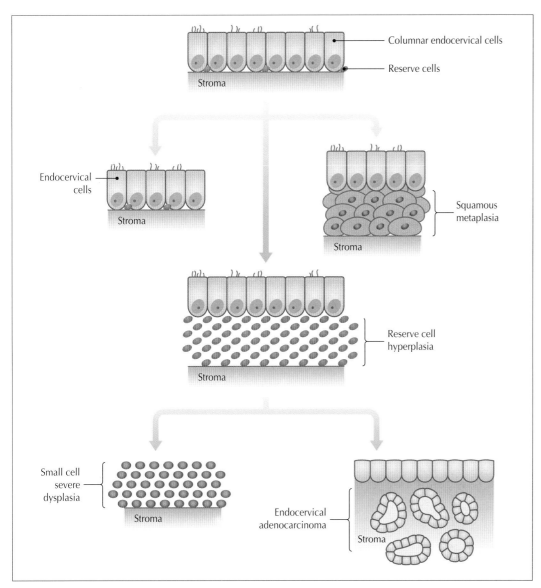

Fig. 2.66 **Reserve cell pathways of differentiation.**

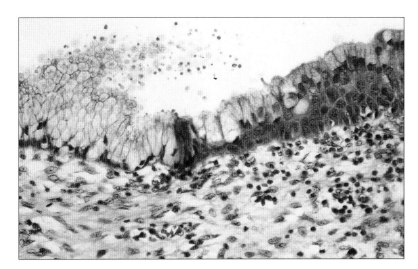

Fig. 2.67 **Reserve cell hyperplasia** – H&E x10. This section of endocervix shows normal endocervix on the left and tall columnar endocervical cells overlying two or three layers of reserve cells on the right. A cervical smear from this area would show mainly endocervical cells.

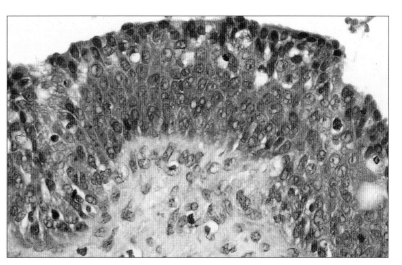

Fig. 2.68 **Reserve cell hyperplasia** – H&E x25. In this section of endocervix there are four to five layers of reserve cells with no superficial columnar cells. A smear from this area would therefore contain reserve cells.

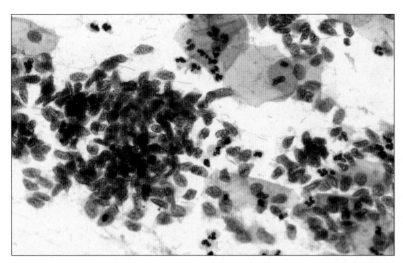

Fig. 2.69 Reserve cells – Pap x40. This field illustrates loose groups of small hyperchromatic reserve cells with no discernible cytoplasm.

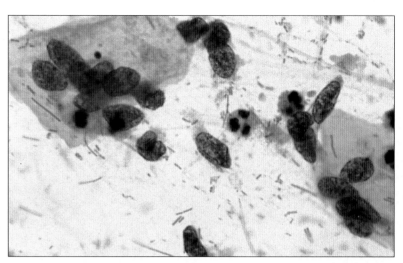

Fig. 2.70 Reserve cells – Pap x100. Reserve cells, as illustrated in this field, have ovoid to spindle-shaped nuclei, granular chromatin, and nuclear grooves. Cytoplasm is not visible. These cells should not be interpreted as endometrial glandular cells.

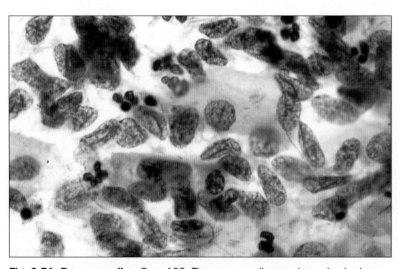

Fig. 2.71 Reserve cells – Pap x100. The reserve cells seen here clearly show nuclear grooves, with nuclei about twice the size of a neutrophil.

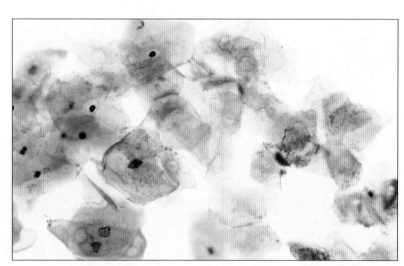

Fig. 2.72 Anucleate squames – Pap x40. In this field there are pale yellowish orange squamous cells without nuclei – anucleate squames – together with superficial and intermediate cells.

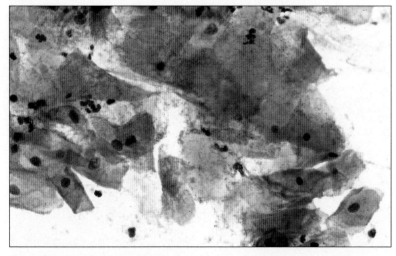

Fig. 2.73 Anucleate squames – Pap x40. Large clumps of anucleate squames warrant follow-up to eliminate underlying dyskaryosis.

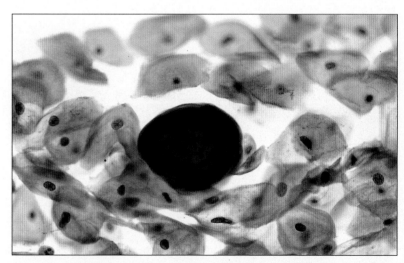

Fig. 2.74 Squamous pearl – Pap x40. Illustrated here in the centre of the field is a squamous pearl composed of a tight cluster of superficial cells with pyknotic nuclei.

OTHER CONSTITUENTS OF SMEARS

Anucleate squames may be seen in normal smears as a few single cells **(Fig. 2.72)**. Their nuclei are lost through normal degenerative processes, as described in Chapter Three. When anucleate squamous cells are keratinized or seen in abundant large clumps **(Fig. 2.73)** there may be other reasons for their presence, such as contamination of the smear by cells from the lower part of the vagina, reaction to a ring pessary, procidentia (prolapse of the uterus), the presence of human papilloma virus infection, or underlying dyskaryosis.

Squamous pearls are small tight whorls of benign squamous cells with pyknotic nuclei **(Figs 2.74, 2.75)**. After careful examination to ensure that they are not composed of dyskaryotic cells, they may be safely ignored.

Psammoma bodies may be seen in normal cervical smears, their significance being unknown **(Figs 2.76, 2.77)**. However, they may also be seen in smears containing metastatic endometrial or ovarian adenocarcinoma cells.

Curschmann's spirals, which are common in sputum and bronchial wash samples, are rarely seen in cervical smears **(Fig. 2.78)**. They may be of varying lenghts and are composed of mucin.

Haematoidin crystals are very occasionally noted. They are bright yellowish orange in colour **(Fig. 2.79)**.

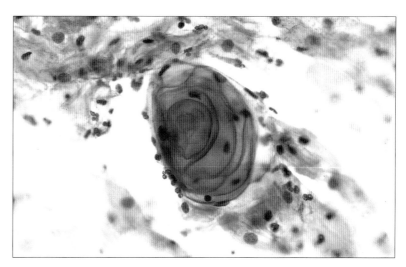

Fig. 2.75 Squamous pearl – Pap x40. This squamous pearl is composed of larger keratinized superficial cells with abundant cytoplasm.

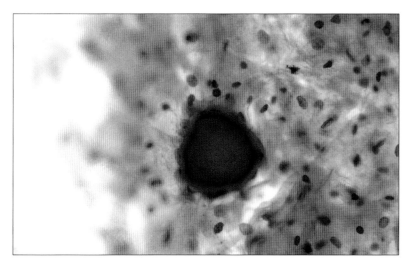

Fig. 2.76 Psammoma body – Pap x40. These calcified structures are not commonly seen in normal cervical smears. If found, a careful search must be made for any evidence of metastatic adenocarcinoma.

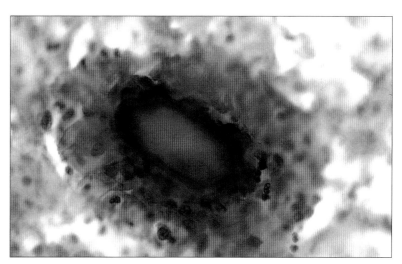

Fig. 2.77 Psammoma body – Pap x40. Psammoma bodies in cervical smears are occasionally walled off by inflammatory cells.

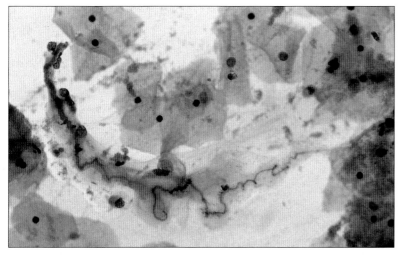

Fig. 2.78 Curschmann's spirals – Pap x40. These spiral structures are identical with those seen in bronchial washings. Their significance is unknown.

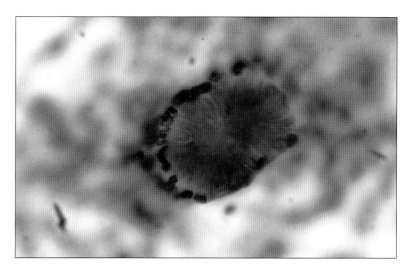

Fig. 2.79 Haematoidin crystals – Pap x40. These crystals are very occasionally noted in cervical smears. In this example the crystals are partially surrounded by neutrophils.

SMEAR PATTERNS

Smear patterns vary with the age of the woman and the phase of the menstrual cycle. The physiological variations in premenopausal and postmenopausal women are discussed below.

Premenopausal Women

Proliferative phase pattern

The smear is composed predominantly of superficial squamous cells, due to the maturation effect of oestrogen, with some intermediate cells (**Fig. 2.80**). Parabasal cells are not usually seen. The background is clean. Endocervical cells should be present if the smear is taken correctly.

Ovulation

At ovulation the smear contains only superficial cells, often with folded edges, again with a clean background. The superficial cells may show

acidophilic or cyanophilic staining (**Figs 2.81, 2.82**).

Secretory phase pattern

In the early part of this phase of the menstrual cycle the effect of progesterone is seen in that the smear is composed of intermediate cells which often contain glycogen (**Fig. 2.83**). In the late secretory phase the smear shows the cytolytic effect of Doderlein bacilli (lactobacilli), with shreds of cytoplasm, few intact cells, and numerous lactobacilli (**Figs 2.84, 2.85**). The bare nuclei in the background should not be mistaken for *Trichomonas vaginalis*. Excessive cytolysis renders the smear inadequate for interpretation and the report should include a request for a repeat smear mid-cycle.

Menstrual smear pattern

This type of smear can be very difficult to interpret because of the large amount of blood and clusters of endometrial cells and histiocytes which are often seen. Endometrial cells may be seen in clusters on their own or accompanied by masses of small histiocytes (**Fig. 2.86**). It is often impossible to dif-

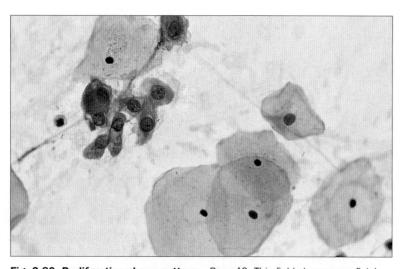

Fig. 2.80 Proliferative phase pattern – Pap x40. This field shows superficial cells with an intermediate cell and some endocervical cells. Oestrogen is responsible for the maturation of squamous epithelium of the cervix.

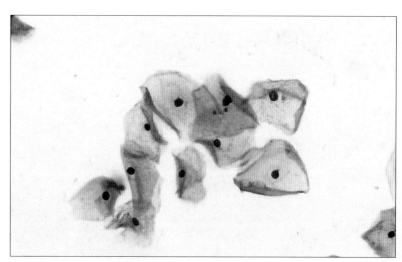

Fig. 2.81 Smear pattern at ovulation – Pap x40. At this time of the menstrual cycle the superficial cells show some folding of their cytoplasmic margins. In this field the cells are all acidophilic.

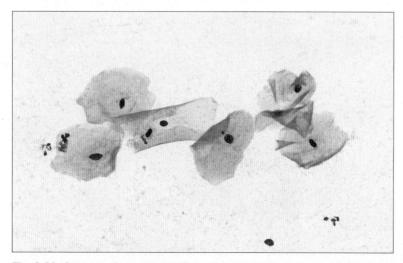

Fig. 2.82 Smear pattern at ovulation – Pap x40. These folded superficial cells, illustrative of smears at ovulation, are cyanophilic.

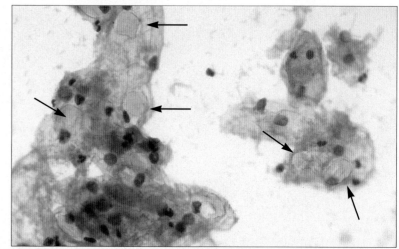

Fig. 2.83 Secretory phase pattern – Pap x40. Many of the intermediate cells in this field contain bright yellow intracytoplasmic glycogen (arrowed).

ferentiate between a single endometrial cell and a histiocyte. Endometrial cells can appear degenerate and vacuolated. The blood in the background may obscure the squamous and endocervical cells and a repeat smear mid-cycle may be necessary.

Intrauterine contraceptive device (IUCD) effect

Smears taken from some women with these devices may contain endometrial cells more than 10 days after the LMP, which is the norm. The endometrial cells may be seen in large clusters, and may appear atypical (**Fig. 2.87**). A common accompaniment is colonies of Actinomyces-like organisms (**Fig. 2.88**), with or without inflammatory changes.

Oral contraceptive pill pattern

Oral contraceptive pill patterns vary with the type of pill. The combined pill (oestrogen and progesterone) produces an atrophic smear pattern even in young girls (**Fig. 2.89**). The progesterone-only pill is associated with a smear showing mainly intermediate cells (**Fig. 2.90**).

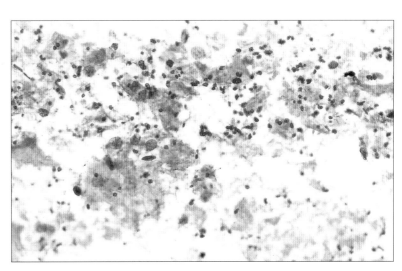

Fig. 2.84 Secretory phase pattern – Pap x40. Illustrated here is cytolysis with shreds of cytoplasm and bare nuclei. The degree of cytolysis renders the smear unsatisfactory for accurate assessment.

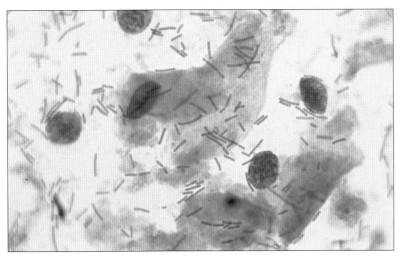

Fig. 2.85 Secretory phase pattern – Pap x100. Lactobacilli are clearly visible at high magnification, together with the bare nuclei and cytoplasmic remnants of cytolysed cells.

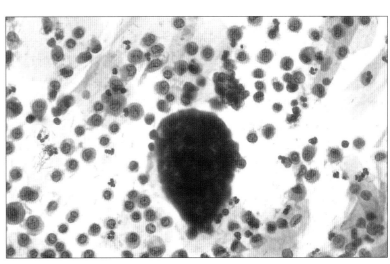

Fig. 2.86 Menstrual phase pattern – Pap x40. This field illustrates the exodus which consists of an endometrial cell cluster accompanied by single histiocytes.

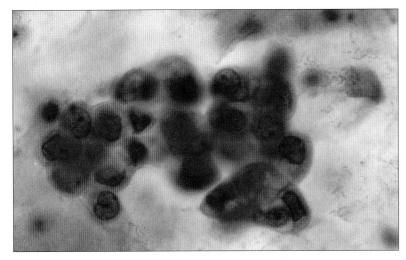

Fig. 2.87 IUCD effect – Pap x100. The endometrial cells in this cluster appear to be abnormal with vacuolation and visible nucleoli. This sort of change is often a result of the IUCD.

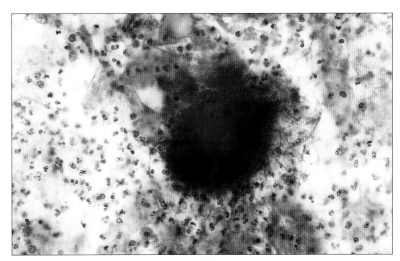

Fig. 2.88 IUCD effect, Actinomyces-like organisms – Pap x40. A clump of Actinomyces-like organisms is seen in the centre of this field, with numerous neutrophils in the background.

Pregnancy pattern

The smear during the early stages shows gradually increasing numbers of intermediate cells. Later in the pregnancy, the smear is usually composed of intermediate cells which contain glycogen and may show cytolysis. Large numbers of navicular cells are often noted (**Fig. 2.91**).

Postnatal smears

Postnatal smears are usually atrophic, composed of parabasal cells (**Fig. 2.92**), often blood-stained, and may contain endometrial cells as well as inflammatory cells (**Fig. 2.93**). They differ from postmenopausal atrophic smears in that they do not show the air drying, multinucleated histiocytes and degenerative features so commonly seen in the latter. Endocervical cells are practically always present. Trophoblastic cells may be noted in postnatal smears; they resemble multinucleated histiocytes.

Perimenopausal smears

Perimenopausal smears show a mixed cellularity pattern with superficial, intermediate, and parabasal cells (**Fig. 2.94**). Later on the smear is composed of intermediate cells only.

Postmenopausal smears

Postmenopausal smears show a variety of appearances. The typical postmenopausal smear is atrophic, air-dried, and composed of parabasal cells showing degenerative changes (**Fig. 2.95**). Occasionally, the smear is well-preserved, containing sheets of parabasal cells with clear cytoplasm resembling endocervical cells, and with bare nuclei in the background (**Figs 2.96, 2.97**). There may be a predominance of small round bare nuclei in clumps and groups; these may be misinterpreted as endometrial cells, but they are actually parabasal cell nuclei (**Fig. 2.98**). 'Blue blobs' are sometimes noted, these being interpreted by some as mucin, by others as degenerate cells (**Fig. 2.99**). Atrophic smears occasionally contain small keratinized cells, which should not be interpreted as squamous carcinoma cells (**Fig. 2.100**).

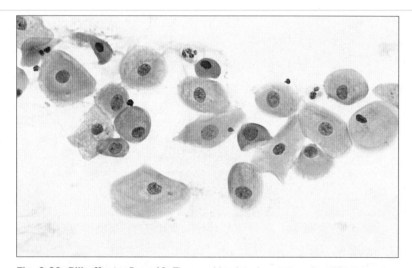

Fig. 2.89 Pill effect – Pap x40. The combined oral contraceptive pill can produce an atrophic smear pattern showing predominantly parabasal cells, as illustrated in this field.

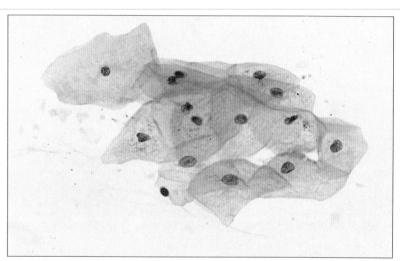

Fig. 2.90 Pill effect – Pap x40. The progesterone-only oral contraceptive pill produces maturation of the epithelium up to the intermediate cell stage, resulting in a smear containing predominantly intermediate cells, as seen here.

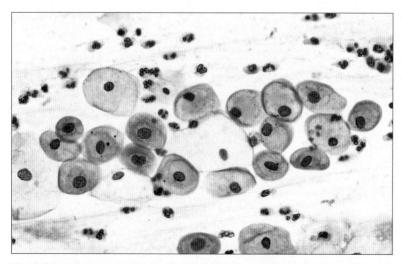

Fig. 2.91 Pregnancy pattern – Pap x40. This photomicrograph illustrates the large numbers of navicular cells often seen in pregnancy.

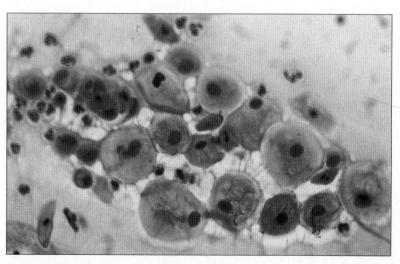

Fig. 2.92 Postnatal smear pattern – Pap x40. This smear is composed mainly of parabasal cells with a few inflammatory cells in the background.

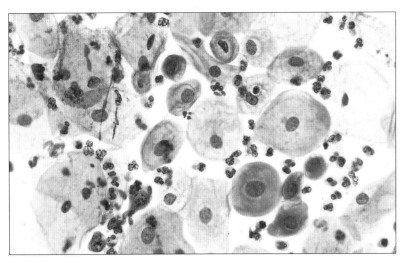

Fig. 2.93 Postnatal smear pattern – Pap x40. This postnatal smear contains intermediate and parabasal cells, the latter being of variable size. Many neutrophil polymorphs are also present.

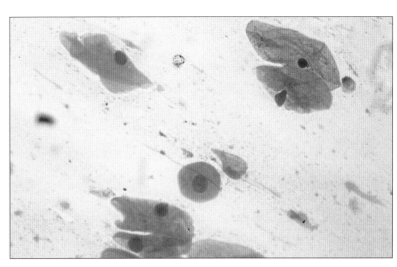

Fig. 2.94 Mixed cellularity smear pattern – Pap x40. Illustrated here is a mixed pattern of superficial, intermediate, and parabasal cells, as seen in the perimenopausal period.

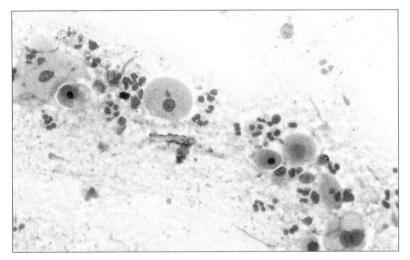

Fig. 2.95 Postmenopausal smear pattern – Pap x40. This smear contains poorly preserved parabasal cells and some inflammatory cells. Note the small, apparently keratinized, cells degenerate squamous cells.

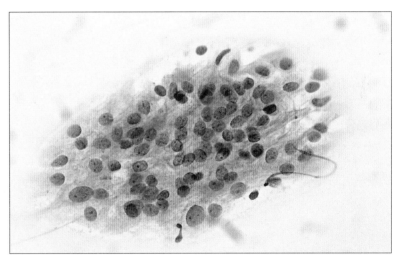

Fig. 2.96 Postmenopausal smear pattern – Pap x40. This field illustrates a common pattern in postmenopausal smears with parabasal cells resembling endocervical cells.

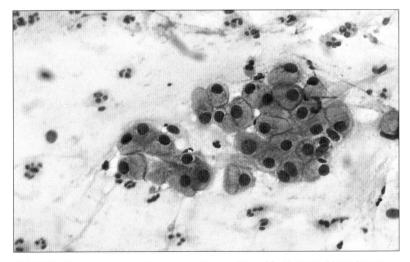

Fig. 2.97 Postmenopausal smear pattern – Pap x40. Illustrated here is yet another postmenopausal smear pattern with parabasal cells mimicking endocervical cells, to the extent that they apparently show honeycombing.

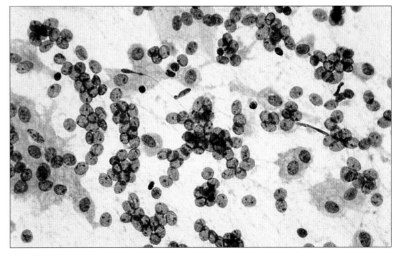

Fig. 2.98 Postmenopausal smear pattern – Pap x40. Atrophic smears may occasionally show this pattern of small bare nuclei. They may be mistaken for endometrial cells, but for the fact that the intact parabasal cells in the background have identical nuclei.

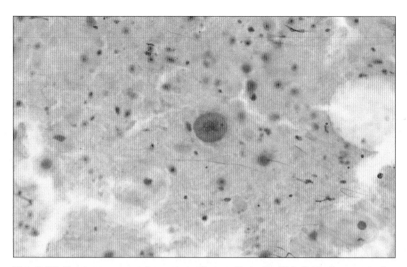

Fig. 2.99 Postmenopausal smear pattern – Pap x40. This field shows granular debris and some degenerate nuclei with a so-called 'blue blob' (staining pink here) in the centre of the field, possibly a degenerate cell.

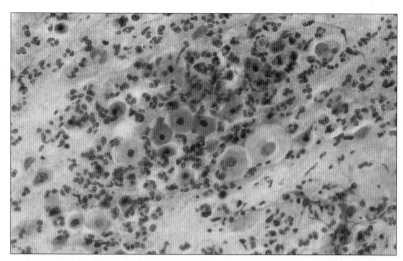

Fig. 2.100 Postmenopausal smear pattern – Pap x40. In the centre of this field of parabasal cells and neutrophils are two small cells with orange-staining cytoplasm and pyknotic nuclei, a fairly common feature in atrophic smears.

SUGGESTED READING

Chang AR. *Obtaining the Ideal Cervical Smear*. Cancer Society of New Zealand (Inc.), Professional Bulletin; 1991: Report No. 2.

Koss LG. *Diagnostic Cytology and its Histopathologic Bases*, 4th ed. Philadelphia: J.B. Lippincott Co.; 1992: 251–281.

Mitchell H, Medley G. The role of an indocervical component in improving the accuracy of cervical cytology. *Cytopathol Ann* 1994; 3: 83–90.

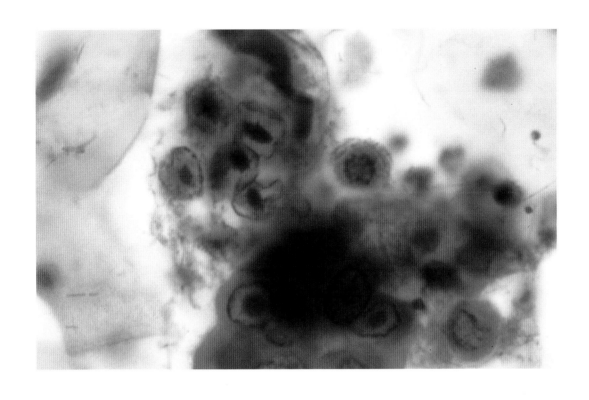

INADEQUATE SMEARS,
INFLAMMATION AND INFECTIONS

3

INADEQUATE OR UNSATISFACTORY SMEARS

Guidelines have been set for defining inadequate or unsatisfactory smears, with most of the emphasis being placed on the absence of material from the squamo-columnar junction. The concern is that smears which do not contain endocervical or squamous metaplastic cells may not have sampled dysplastic areas of the cervix. However, dyskaryotic cells are not infrequently indentified in such smears and therefore they are not necessarily unsatisfactory.

There are several other reasons for placing a smear in this category (**Fig. 3.1**). Poor fixation is usually due to poor preparation before taking the smear, such as not laying out the glass slide and fixative beforehand, delay in applying fixative to the smear, or not leaving fixative on the slide for long enough. The material dries on the side, with the cells becoming enlarged and flattened, producing blurred nuclear details (**Fig. 3.2**). Benign cells can therefore appear to be dyskaryotic and poor fixation can also mimic keratinization. Smears that are thickly spread are difficult to read (**Fig. 3.3**), so smear-takers must be shown how to spread a smear thinly. Technology is now available for the preparation of thin smears, or monolayers. This is an alternative to the usual smear spreading technique commonly practised, but cost is a major implication. Too much blood on the smear can obscure all cellular detail (**Fig. 3.4**); this is commonly the case in smears taken during menstruation. Contact bleeding during smear-taking does not often result in an unsatisfactory smear. Some bleeding is to be expected in the presence of an erosion. Heavy blood-staining is frequently seen in smears from patients with invasive carcinoma of the cervix. In such instances, carcinoma cells can usually be found with a careful search, so such smears should not be categorized as inadequate.

Smears that are prepared too vigorously are often unsatisfactory because of cell disruption or streak artefact (**Fig. 3.5**). This is often seen combined with scanty samples from atrophic cervices. Another reason for poor-quality smears is the presence of lubricant usually due to excessive amounts being applied to the speculum during smear-taking (**Fig. 3.6**). This can be avoided by applying

Cause	Prevention
Poor fixation	Apply fixative to the slide immediately
Smear too thick	Spread material thinly and rapidly on the slide
Too much blood	Avoid taking smears during menstruation
Streak artefact	Smear material gently but rapidly on slide
Excessive cytolysis	Take smear at or before time of ovulation
Excessive lubricant	Use lubricant sparingly, or use warm water for speculum
Too many polymorphs	Swab off mucus plug gently before taking smear

Fig. 3.1 Inadequate smears.

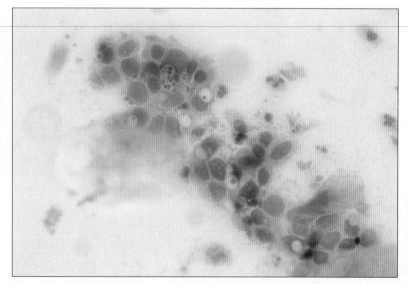

Fig. 3.2 Unsatisfactory smear, poor fixation (air drying) – Pap x40. This field shows a group of epithelial cells with indistinct cytoplasmic margins and homogeneous nuclei with no chromatin detail. The nuclei appear somewhat enlarged due to air drying. This was possibly due to delay in applying fixative to the smear.

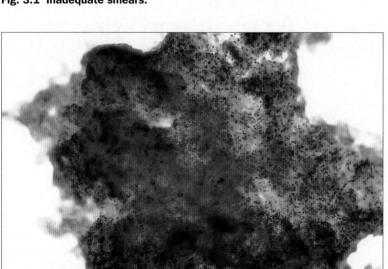

Fig. 3.3 Unsatisfactory smear, thickly spread – Pap x10. Illustrated here is a thick clump of material containing numerous cells which cannot be identified, making this smear unsatisfactory.

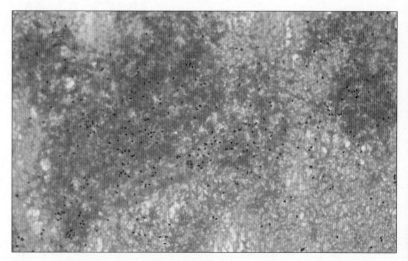

Fig. 3.4 Unsatisfactory smear, heavily blood-stained – Pap x10. Smears taken during menstruation tend to be heavily blood-stained and therefore more likely to be inadequate for interpretation, as illustrated here.

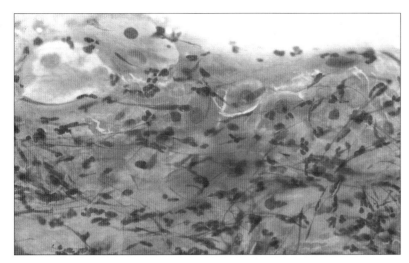

Fig. 3.5 Unsatisfactory smear, streak artefact – Pap x40. This atrophic smear is partially air-dried, but also shows nuclear chromatin pulled out in streaks due to vigorous smearing. This is more likely to occur with a wooden spatula than with the soft flexible plastic variety. Atrophic smears are also more likely to be unsatisfactory than smears from premenopausal women.

just a small amount of lubricant to the outside of the speculum (or by using warm water instead for lubrication), and by performing the smear **before** the bimanual examination. Another cause of extraneous material on the slide is spermicide jelly. Women should be advised to refrain from sexual intercourse for at least 48 hours before a smear test, not only to avoid excessive amounts of spermicide jelly on the smear, but also because seminal vesicle cells can mimic dyskaryosis. Yet another reason for an unsatisfactory smear is the presence of neutrophil polymorphs that obscure all other detail **(Fig. 3.7)**. Neutrophils tend to stick to cervical mucus; therefore, any plugs of mucus that are seen at the cervical os when the speculum is inserted should be gently swabbed off (not scraped off) **before** the spatula is used to take the smear.

As mentioned in Chapter 2, excessive cytolysis with a lack of intact cells makes smear interpretation difficult **(Fig. 3.8)**; this can be prevented by taking the smear mid-cycle. Occasionally, numerous starch or talc granules from glove powder are seen scattered over the smear, obscuring the cells **(Fig. 3.9)**;

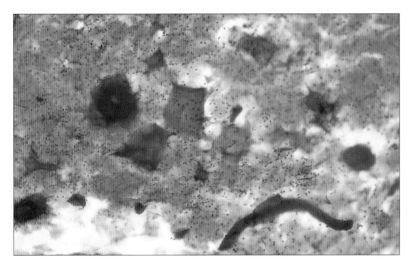

Fig. 3.6 Unsatisfactory smear, excessive lubricant – Pap x10. Illustrated here are large quantities of lubricant, in this case KY jelly applied liberally to the speculum, which obscure much of the cellular detail.

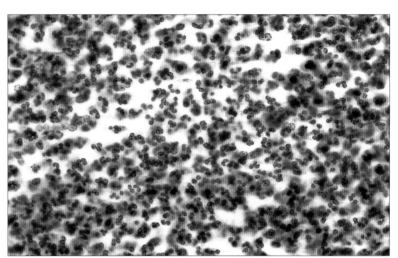

Fig. 3.7 Unsatisfactory smear, excess of neutrophils – Pap x40. This field shows only neutrophil polymorphs and no epithelial cells.

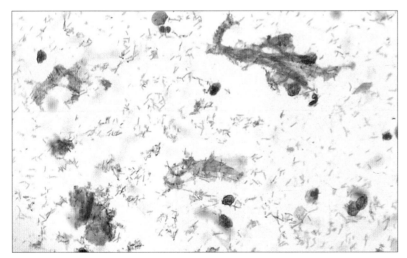

Fig. 3.8 Unsatisfactory smear, excessive cytolysis – Pap x40. The normal physiological process of cytolysis due to lactobacilli has caused disintegration of the squamous cells, so they cannot be assessed.

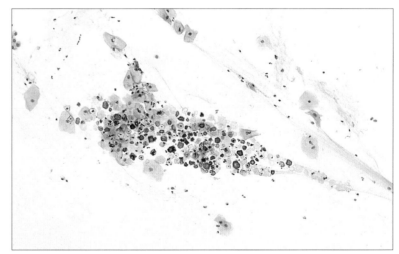

Fig. 3.9 Unsatisfactory smear, contamination by talc – Pap x10. Smear detail can be obscured by deposits of talc from glove powder, as seen here.

these exhibit a Maltese cross birefringence under polarized light **(Fig. 3.10)**. Other problems with smears are related to poor laboratory practice. For example, poor staining is inexcusable in this day of automatic staining machines. 'Cornflake artefact' **(Fig. 3.11)** and stain crystals **(Fig. 3.12)** are problems due to lax laboratory procedures and can be avoided by the meticulous processing of smears. Processing smears next to an open window can lead to an overlay of pollen grains **(Fig. 3.13)**. Other contaminants, either air- or water-borne, can render a smear unsatisfactory **(Figs 3.14, 3.15)**.

While not strictly a cause of unsatisfactory smears, Alternaria should be recognized as this is a not uncommon contaminant **(Fig. 3.16)**.

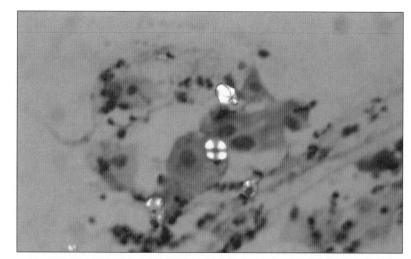

Fig. 3.10 Maltese cross birefringence – Pap x10 (polarized light). Starch granules in talc exhibit Maltese cross birefringence under polarized light.

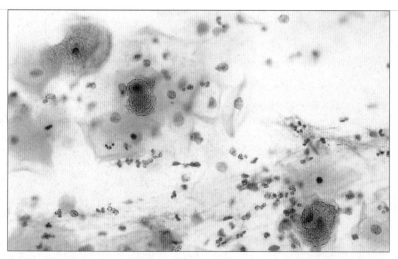

Fig. 3.11 'Cornflake' artefact – Pap x40. This is seen as a dark brown deposit over the cells, rendering them impossible to screen. This is preventable if correct laboratory technique is observed.

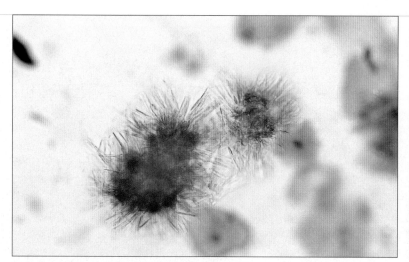

Fig. 3.12 Crystal deposit – Pap x40. These stain crystals are the result of to poor technique; they can obscure cellular detail if present in large amounts.

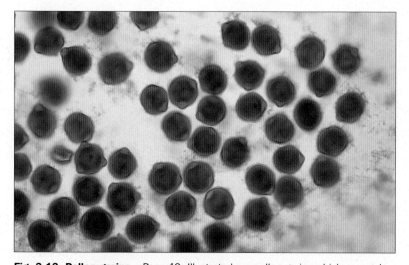

Fig. 3.13 Pollen grains – Pap x40. Illustrated are pollen grains which covered most of the smear, making it unsatisfactory.

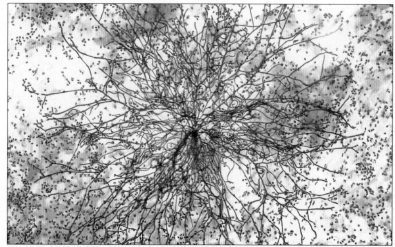

Fig. 3.14 Fungal contaminant – Pap x10. Fungal contaminants, such as the variety pictured here, can obscure all cellular detail.

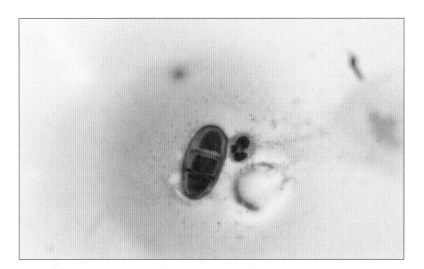

Fig. 3.15 Fungal contaminant – Pap x10. Pictured here is another type of fungal contaminant that rendered the smear inadequate.

DEGENERATIVE CHANGES

Degenerative changes are common and should be recognized. They are most frequently seen in parabasal and squamous metaplastic cells, but are also seen in other epithelial cells. The changes include cellular and nuclear enlargement with variability in the staining pattern, most often demonstrated by amphophilia **(Fig. 3.17)**. There is loss of crispness of the nuclear margin, which may show occasional gaps. Also, the chromatin detail is lost, being replaced by a bland homogeneous appearance **(Fig. 3.18)**, with no sharp demarcation between euchromatin and heterochromatin. The nucleus often shows a crinkled, hyperchromatic appearance **(Fig. 3.19)**, which must be distinguished from dyskaryosis (see **Figure 4.9–4.14**). The end stage of this degenerative process is a small, dark pyknotic nucleus, as in superficial cells **(Fig. 3.20)**. In some cells undergoing degeneration, the nucleus starts to disintegrate,

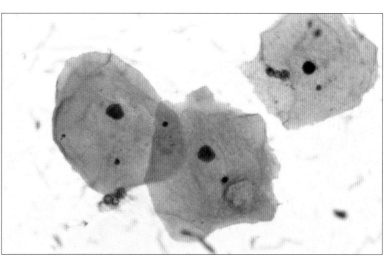

Fig. 3.16 Alternaria – Pap x40. Alternaria are often seen, not only in smears, but also in other cytological preparations.

Fig. 3.17 Amphophilia – Pap x40. Illustrated in this field are three superficial cells of which two show abnormal staining reactions, with a mixture of both acidophilic and cyanophilic staining. This is often seen in degeneration, especially in parabasal cells.

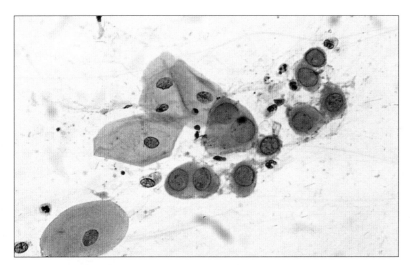

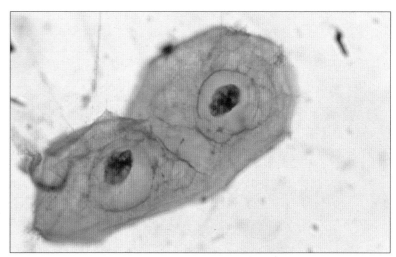

Fig. 3.18 Degenerative changes, homogeneous chromatin – Pap x40. In this photomicrograph the intermediate cells are normal, but the endocervical cells exhibit a bland homogeneous nuclear appearance, with no clear distinction between euchromatin and heterochromatin.

Fig. 3.19 Degenerative changes, irregular nuclear outline – Pap x100. Illustrated here are two intermediate cells showing degenerative and inflammatory changes, including a crinkled hyperchromatic nucleus and perinuclear halo. The sharp irregularity of the nuclear outlines distinguishes this from dyskaryosis.

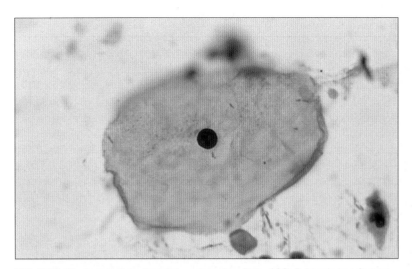

Fig. 3.20 Degenerative changes, pyknosis – Pap x100. Pyknosis is a feature of degeneration, illustrated here by a normal superficial squamous cell.

a process known as karyorrhexis (**Fig. 3.21**). In other cells, the nuleus begins to fade or dissolve away karyolysis (**Fig. 3.22**), with the cell ultimately becoming an anucleate squame. Degenerative cytoplasmic changes include vacuolation, either a few vacuoles (**Fig. 3.23**) or a honeycomb type of vacuolation (**Fig. 3.24**). Degenerative changes are usually irreversible and lead to cell death.

INFLAMMATORY CHANGES

The mere presence of a few neutrophil polymorphs in a smear does not signify

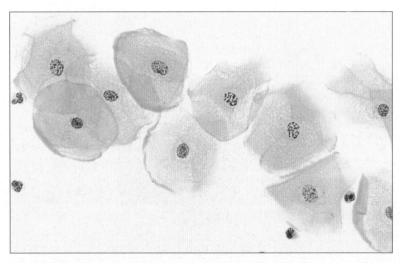

Fig. 3.21 Degenerative changes, karyorrhexis – Pap x40. The intermediate cells seen in this field show loss of the nuclear membrane and breaking up of the nucleus into small fragments, a process known as karyorrhexis.

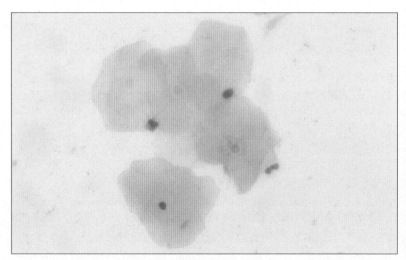

Fig. 3.22 Degenerative changes, karyolysis – Pap x40. In this field the superficial cells show varying degrees of dissolving away of their nuclei, termed karyolysis.

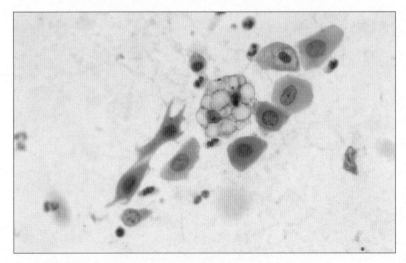

Fig. 3.23 Degenerative changes, vacuolation – Pap x40. This photomicrograph shows metaplastic squamous cells. The two cells in the centre of the field show vacuolar degeneration of their cytoplasm, while an adjacent cell shows a perinuclear halo.

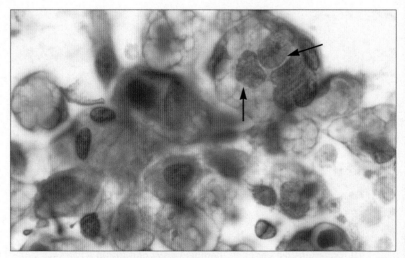

Fig. 3.24 Degenerative changes, vacuolation – Pap x100. Honeycomb vacuolation of the cytoplasm of all the cells is Illustrated in this field. One of the cells is multinucleated and may be dyskaryotic, but the nuclei also show degenerative changes in the form of patchy loss of the nuclear membrane (arrowed).

inflammation. Large numbers of neutrophils are often associated with an inflammatory process, but cellular changes are essential for the diagnosis of inflammation. These changes are reversible. They may be non-specific or associated with a specific organism. Non-specific inflammatory changes include nuclear enlargement (**Fig. 3.25**) and sometimes binucleation (**Fig. 3.26**). Hyperchromasia may be noted with margination of the chromatin in some instances (**Fig. 3.27**). A small perinuclear halo is often present (**Fig. 3.28**), which should not be confused with the large empty perinuclear space of koilocytes (see **Figure 3.56**). The cytoplasm may show vacuolation (**Fig. 3.29**).

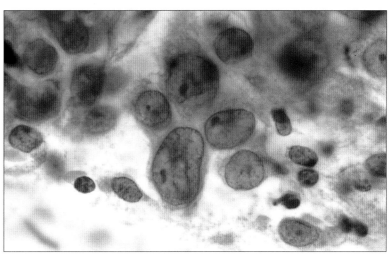

Fig. 3.25 Inflammatory changes, nuclear enlargement – Pap x100. The endocervical cells seen here show marked nuclear enlargement, with accentuation of the nuclear margins and some of the nucleoli. In this case, these inflammatory changes are a result of herpes simplex infection (seen elsewhere in the smear).

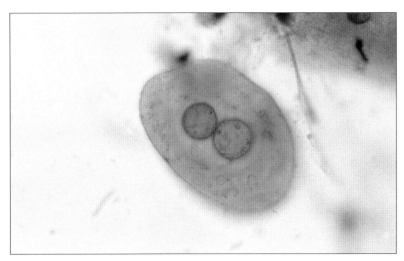

Fig. 3.26 Inflammatory changes, binucleation – Pap x100. This is an intermediate cell showing binucleation with some margination of the chromatin and the faintest hint of a perinuclear halo, all of which are inflammatory changes.

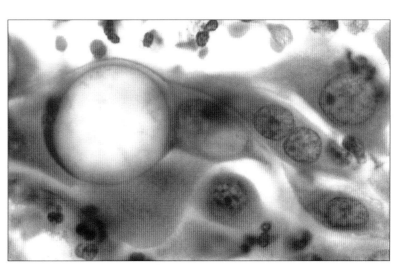

Fig. 3.27 Inflammatory changes – Pap x100. The squamous metaplastic cells illustrated show several features of inflammation – nuclear enlargement, margination of chromatin, and vacuolation. Neutrophils are seen in the background.

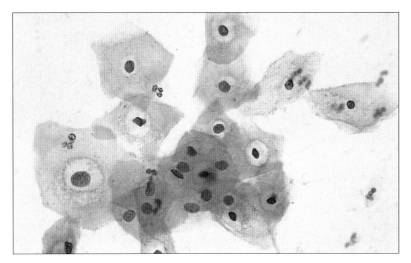

Fig. 3.28 Inflammatory changes, perinuclear haloes – Pap x40. In this field both the superficial and intermediate cells show inflammatory perinuclear haloes. *Trichomonas vaginalis* is a common cause for both the acidophilia and inflammatory changes.

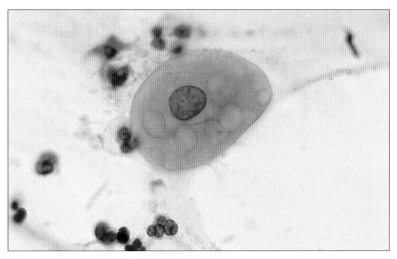

Fig. 3.29 Inflammatory changes, cytoplasmic vacuolation – Pap x100. This squamous metaplastic cell shows degenerative vacuolation of the cytoplasm. The nucleus shows margination of chromatin.

Inflamed endocervical cells show similar changes. They may display multi-nucleation (**Figs 3.30, 3.31**), nuclear enlargement, and margination of chromatin, with prominent nucleoli being a common feature (**Fig. 3.32**). Sheets of endo-cervical cells or metaplastic cells may show infiltration by polymorphs (**Fig. 3.33**), reflecting the histological features of cervicitis. Endocervical polyps are often associated with inflamed endocervical cells (**Fig. 3.34**). Similar inflam-matory changes are noted in squamous metaplastic cells, with vacuolation, enlarged nuclei, and prominent nucleoli. A bacterial background may be present in association with inflammatory cellular changes, but specific bacteria cannot be reliably identified by cytology alone. These cellular changes are often accom-panied by increased numbers of neutrophil polymorphs and histiocytes – occa-sionally, the former are seen surrounding organisms (**Fig. 3.35**).

Many organisms are associated with inflammatory changes in squamous and endocervical cells. A careful search should be made to detect these so that the woman can be treated appropriately. For non-specific inflammatory changes no recommendations can be made for treatment.

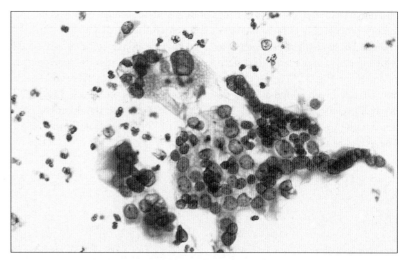

Fig. 3.30 Inflammatory changes, multinucleation – Pap x40. This cervical smear from a woman with cervicitis contains multinucleated and variably sized endocervical cells. The chromatin pattern is still vesicular.

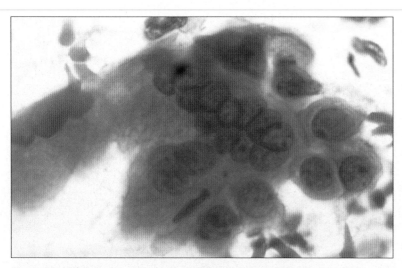

Fig. 3.31 Inflammatory changes, multinucleation – Pap x100. This field shows multinucleation in otherwise normal endocervical cells. Multinucleation may be seen with inflammatory changes, but also in reactive and/or reparatory processes.

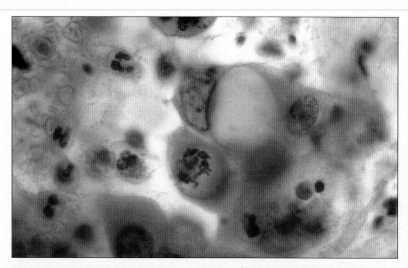

Fig. 3.32 Inflammatory changes, margination of chromatin – Pap x40. The endocervical cells seen in this field show nuclear enlargement, margination of chromatin (especially noticeable in the cell with the large vacuole), prominent nucleoli, and vacuolation. Note the mitotic figure.

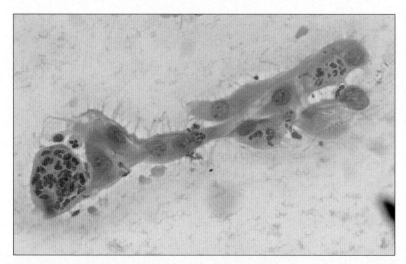

Fig. 3.33 Inflammatory changes, endocervical cells – Pap x40. Pictured here is a group of endocervical cells in a smear taken from a woman with cervicitis. The cells contain neutrophil polymorphs within the cytoplasm, similar to the appearance in histological sections of cervicitis.

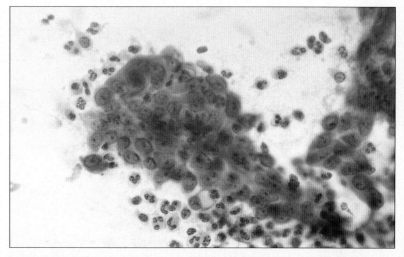

Fig. 3.34 Inflammatory changes, endocervical cells – Pap x40. The endocervical cells seen in this field show noticeable nucleoli and some vacuolation, and are closely associated with acute inflammatory cells. This is characteristic of cells scraped off an endocervical polyp.

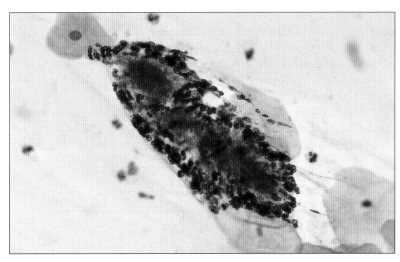

Fig. 3.35 Inflammatory cells – Pap x40. In the centre of the field is a colony of Actinomyces-like organisms surrounded by a barrier of neutrophil polymorphs. The squamous cells in the background do not show any inflammatory changes.

Candida (also known as Monilia), which is responsible for thick white vaginal discharge and itching, is often diagnosed clinically. Candida albicans is a common variety seen in cervical smears. Candida infection is associated with antibiotic usage (as this destroys the normal commensals in the vagina and cervix, thus altering the pH), diabetes, and the use of oral contraceptives. It is seen in smears in the form of pink-staining hyphae (**Fig. 3.36**) and spores (**Fig. 3.37**), which may be missed if the staining is suboptimal. The epithelial cells in the background usually exhibit severe inflammatory changes with perinuclear haloes and margination of the chromatin. *Torulopsis glabrata* is another Candida species which is seen in cervical smears (**Fig. 3.38**).

Trichomonas vaginalis infection is another cause of profuse vaginal discharge with intense itching. Trichomonads are sometimes difficult to identify in smears, since the organisms appear as small ill-defined blobs in the background and may only be recognized under high magnification (**Fig. 3.39**). They are rounded, oval, or pear-shaped with red cytoplasmic granules and a 'Mongoleye' nucleus (**Fig. 3.40**). Oil immersion highlights their delicate flagella

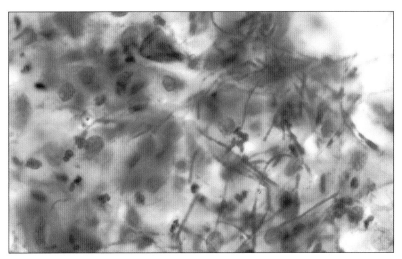

Fig. 3.36 Candida – Pap x40. Illustrated here is Candida in the form of pink septate hyphae overlying intermediate cells.

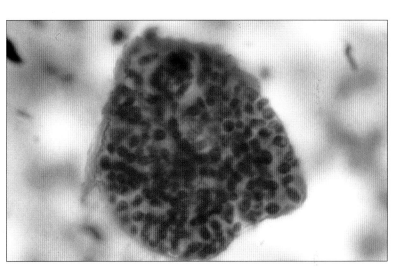

Fig. 3.37 Candida – Pap x100. Candida spores are seen clustered together in the centre of this field. If staining is poor and the spores are not pink they might be mistaken for spermatozoa heads.

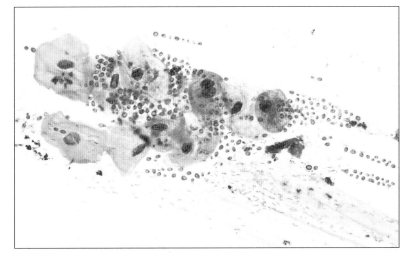

Fig. 3.38 *Torulopsis glabrata* – Pap x40. *Torulopsis glabrata* is a species of Candida that may be noted in cervical smears. Only the spores are seen in this field, scattered among intermediate cells which show inflammatory changes in the form of nuclear enlargement and hyperchromasia.

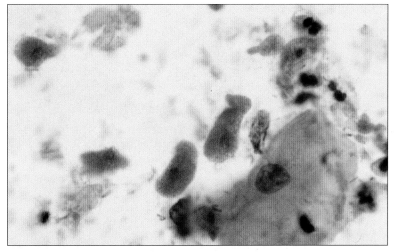

Fig. 3.39 *Trichomonas vaginalis* – Pap x100. At least four large trichomonads are seen in this field, each with a conspicuous nucleus. They stain the same shade of blue–green as intermediate cells and are often difficult to see, especially in a cytolytic smear. Occasionally, air-dried polymorphs can resemble trichomonads, so it is important to identify the nucleus.

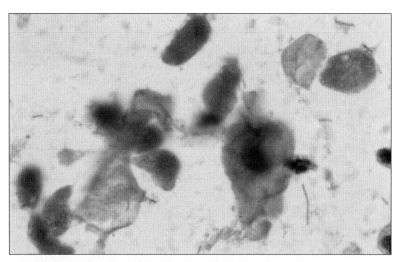

Fig. 3.40 *Trichomonas vaginalis* – Pap x100. In this field the nuclei are not clearly visible, but the red cytoplasmic granules characteristic of trichomonads are well illustrated.

(**Fig. 3.41**). The cells in the smear show inflammatory changes and an acidophilic reaction in the presence of trichomonads, staining pink irrespective of their maturity (**Fig. 3.42**). A harmless commensal which is often associated with Trichomonas, but may be seen on its own, is **Leptothrix**. These are long filamentous organisms which stain dark blue and resemble a child's scribbles on paper (**Fig. 3.43**).

Actinomyces-like organisms are common in smears from women who use intrauterine contraceptive devices (IUCDs). Under low power they appear as dark purplish clumps (**Fig. 3.44**) and under high power are seen to be composed of peripheral filamentous and central, small, dot-like structures (**Fig. 3.45**). These

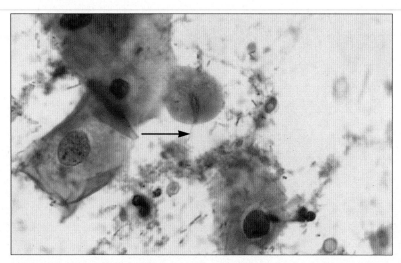

Fig. 3.41 *Trichomonas vaginalis* – Pap x100. Illustrated here is a pear-shaped trichomonad with a well-preserved 'Mongol-eye' nucleus and a faint flagellum attached adjacent to the nucleus (arrowed). The intermediate cells also present exhibit inflammatory perinuclear haloes and hyperchromasia.

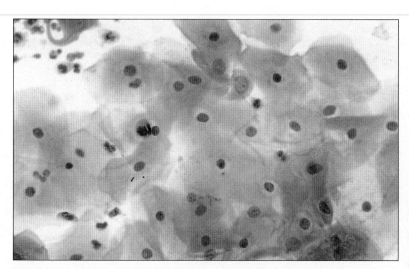

Fig. 3.42 Staining pattern, Trichomonas infection – Pap x40. A common finding in smears with trichomonads is the acidophilic staining reaction of most of the squamous cells, as illustrated here. Note also the perinuclear inflammatory haloes.

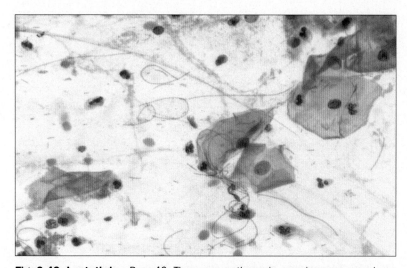

Fig. 3.43 Leptothrix – Pap x40. These non-pathogenic organisms are seen in the form of long delicate threads which usually stain blue. They are not septate and are much thinner than Candida hyphae.

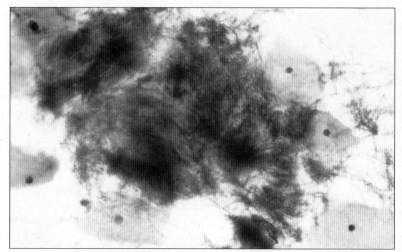

Fig. 3.44 Actinomyces-like organisms – Pap x40. These organisms, which typically have a clumped centre with small bacterial bodies and filaments around the periphery of the colony, are associated with use of IUCDs.

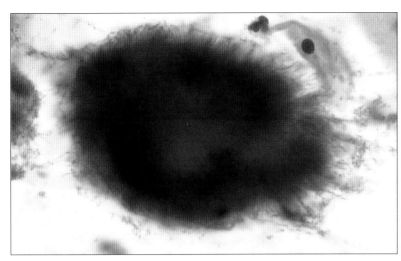

Fig. 3.45 Actinomyces-like organisms – Pap x40. This is another clump of Actinomyces-like organisms, the filamentous shapes at the periphery being demonstrated clearly.

organisms are sometimes, but not always, associated with inflammatory changes.

Chlamydial changes are difficult to diagnose with certainty. Typically, they affect endocervical and squamous metaplastic cells. Cellular changes which are suggestive of Chlamydia infection include cytoplasmic vacuoles (**Fig. 3.46**), which may contain minute bodies (**Fig. 3.47**). Many cases of chlamydial infection are associated with follicular cervicitis (**Fig. 3.48**). The smear in these cases shows an inflammatory picture with streaks and groups of lymphoid cells, including follicle centre cells (**Fig. 3.49**) and tingible body macrophages (**Fig. 3.50**). The mixed population of lymphoid cells should prevent an erroneous diagnosis of lymphoma being made.

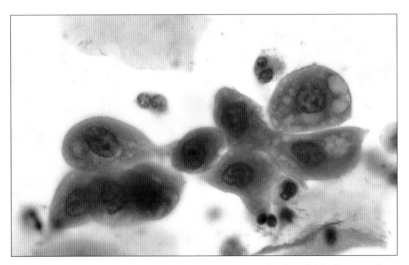

Fig. 3.46 Chlamydia – Pap x100. There are no completely reliable features that can be used to diagnose chlamydial infection on a smear. This field shows a group of squamous metaplastic cells with cytoplasmic vacuoles of varying sizes and nuclei showing prominent margination of chromatin, features that may be due to chlamydial infection.

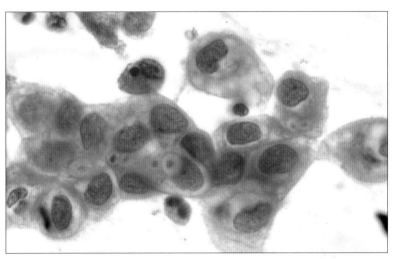

Fig. 3.47 Chlamydia – Pap x100. The metaplastic cells illustrated here display vacuoles, some empty and others containing small bodies which may represent chlamydial infection, but this is not diagnostic.

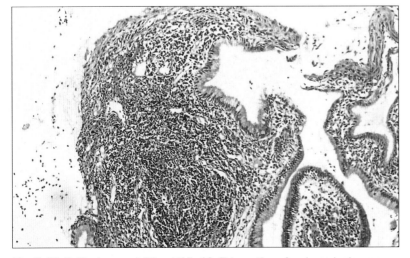

Fig. 3.48 Follicular cervicitis – H&E x10. This section of endocervix shows a heavy infiltrate of lymphoid cells within the stroma, including a well-formed lymphoid follicle, characteristic of follicular cervicitis. This is often associated with chlamydial infection.

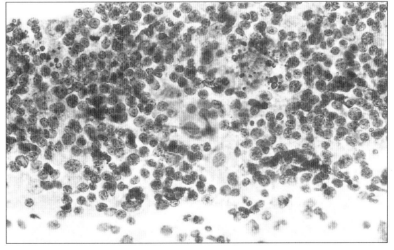

Fig. 3.49 Follicular cervicitis – Pap x40. The abundance of lymphoid cells seen in this field is indicative of follicular cervicitis. Lymphocytes are otherwise seldom seen in cervical smears. The differential diagnosis is lymphoma, but a careful search under higher magnification usually reveals a mixed population of cells, including tingible body macrophages.

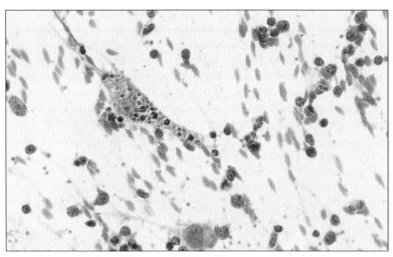

Gardnerella infection (formerly known as *Corynebacterium vaginalis* then as *Haemophilus vaginalis*) is represented in cervical smears by the clue cell – a superficial or intermediate squamous cell, the surface of which is completely covered by small bacteria (**Fig. 3.51**). Similar bacteria may be seen in the background.

Herpes simplex (type II) is responsible for genital herpes, while type I causes cold sores. This virus, which is believed to be an initiator in the development of carcinoma of the cervix (as is cigarette smoking), produces cytopathic changes which are well-recognized. In the early stages of infection only severely inflamed endocervical cells are present (see **Figure 3.25**). Later, the typical multinucleated cells are seen with their moulded nuclei (**Fig. 3.52**). There may be only a few nuclei or several in each cell. These nuclei are characteristically ground-glass in appearance with no chromatinic detail (**Fig. 3.53**). Prominent red intranuclear inclusions are frequently seen (**Fig. 3.54**). A pitfall that should be avoided is to mistake multinucleated endocervical cells for cells infected with herpes simplex virus.

Fig. 3.50 Follicular cervicitis – Pap x40. In the centre of the field is a large tingible body macrophage containing cellular debris, surrounded by lymphoid cells.

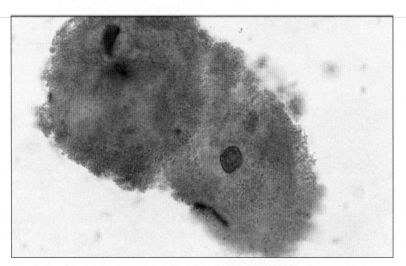

Fig. 3.51 Clue cells – Pap x100. The two intermediate cells seen here are covered by small bacteria and are known as clue cells. They are the diagnostic feature of Gardnerella infection.

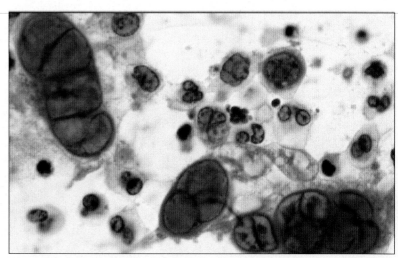

Fig. 3.52 Herpes simplex – Pap x100. Illustrated here are multinucleated cells characteristic of herpes simplex infection. Note the nuclear moulding and the surrounding inflammatory cells.

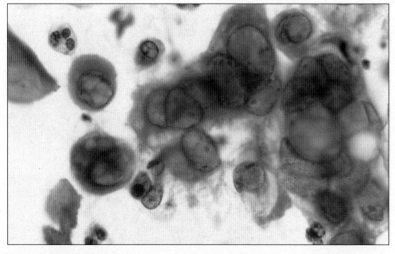

Fig. 3.53 Herpes simplex – Pap x100. This field contains multinucleated herpes-infected cells showing 'ground-glass' chromatin.

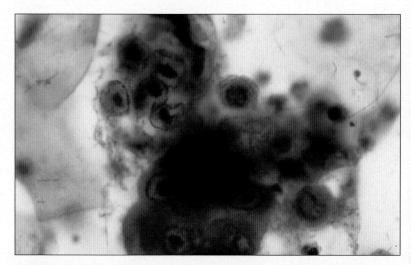

Fig. 3.54 Herpes simplex – Pap x100. Note the spectacular intranuclear red inclusions, which are typical of herpes virus infection.

Human papilloma virus (HPV) or **wart virus** infection is rapidly becoming more commonplace and is seen far more frequently in cervical smears than herpes virus infection. This virus is believed to be a promoter of the development of squamous carcinoma of the cervix, acting on cells previously affected by an initiator, either smoking or herpes virus infection. Wart virus is also implicated in the developement of adenocarcinoma of the cervix. There are over 60 known types of wart virus, the most important genital types being 16 and 18, which are associated with invasive squamous carcinoma. The most characteristic feature of HPV infection in cervical smears is the koilocyte – a squamous cell with three essential features (**Fig. 3.55**):

- An abnormal nucleus.
- A large perinuclear halo or clear space.
- A thickened uneven rim of dense cytoplasm.

The nuclear abnormality may be binucleation (**Fig. 3.56**), pyknosis (**Fig. 3.57**), or multinucleation (although multinucleated koilocytes invariably have dyskaryotic nuclei). The halo represents absence of cytoplasmic organelles. Koilocytes are frequently associated with dyskaryosis (**Fig. 3.58**), which is discussed in Chapter 4. Secondary features associated with HPV infection include parakeratotic cells (**Fig. 3.59**) seen in sheets and clumps and small keratinized cells, which probably represent the dyskeratosis noted in histological sections.

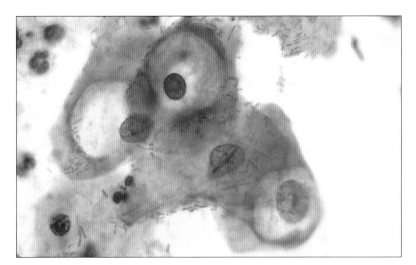

Fig. 3.55 HPV changes – Pap x100. Illustrated here are squamous cells showing the characteristic features of koilocytes – an abnormal nucleus, a substantial perinuclear halo, and a thickened rim of cytoplasm. The staining reaction of the koilocyte may be acidophilic or cyanophilic. The abnormal nucleus may be either pyknotic or dyskaryotic, but is very often binucleate.

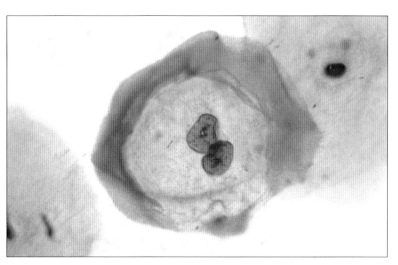

Fig. 3.56 HPV changes – Pap x100. This is a typical koilocyte showing binucleation with slightly enlarged nuclei, a large halo, and a thick rim of cytoplasm.

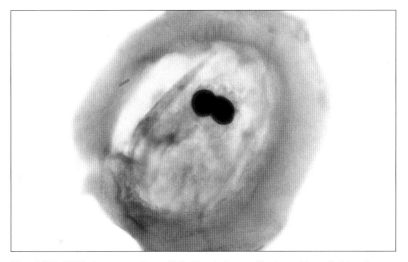

Fig. 3.57 HPV changes – Pap x100. The koilocyte illustrated here is binucleate, but both nuclei are pyknotic. The halo and thick rim of cytoplasm are clearly visible.

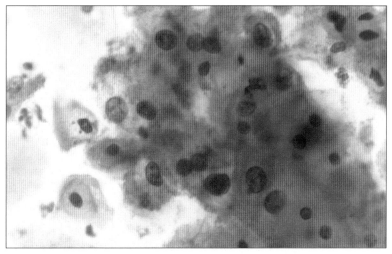

Fig. 3.58 HPV changes with dyskaryosis – Pap x40. This field shows a cluster of mildly dyskaryotic cells with perinuclear haloes suggesting associated wart virus infection.

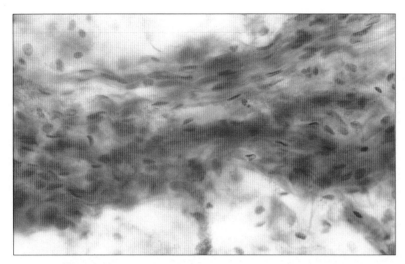

Fig. 3.59 Parakeratosis – Pap x40. This somewhat thickly spread smear displays groups of squamous cells with flattened nuclei, representing the parakeratosis often seen in histological sections of HPV-infected cervix. The presence of this feature alone is insufficient to make a diagnosis of wart virus infection.

Enterobius vermicularis **(pinworm)** ova are occasionally seen in cervical smears, often being transferred from schoolchild to parent because of poor hygiene. They have thick coats and are almost oval with one flat and one convex side (**Fig. 3.60**). They stain yellowish-brown and appear refractile. The numbers of ova seen in smears vary widely.

Schistosome ova in smears are rarely seen, except in those who have travelled to endemic areas. The smear contains numerous large ova, which are larger than those of *Enterobius vermicularis* and stain a distinctive blue–mauve colour (**Fig. 3.61**). Ova with terminal spines characterize *Schistosoma haematobium* (**Fig. 3.62**), which affects the urinary bladder and also the cervix. Large numbers of neutrophils and severely inflamed endocervical cells often accompany these ova.

Lice may very occasionally be seen in cervical smears (**Fig. 3.63**).

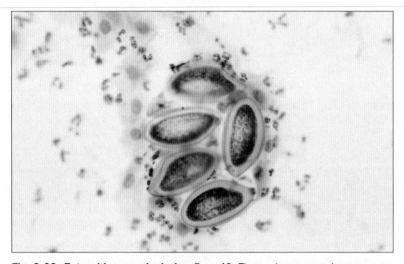

Fig. 3.60 *Enterobius vermicularis* – Pap x40. These pinworm ova have one characteristic flat side, the other being convex. The thick shells which stain yellowish brown are not empty, but contain larvae.

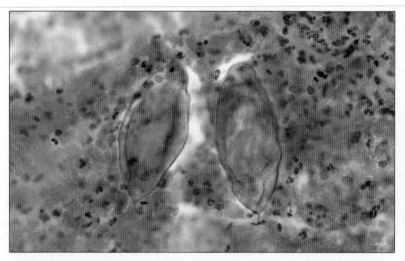

Fig. 3.61 Schistosome ova – Pap x40. Two *Schistosoma haematobium* ova with delicate terminal spines are visible in this field. Note the large size of these blue–mauve-staining ova compared with the *Enterobius vermicularis* ova (**Fig. 3.60**). The smear is blood-stained and showed severe inflammatory changes elsewhere.

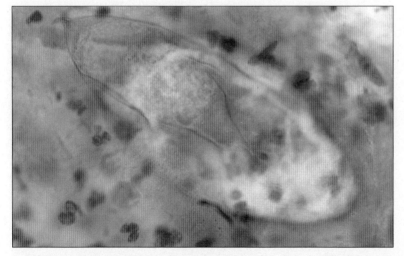

Fig. 3.62 Schistosome ovum – Pap x100. This high magnification field illustrates the small curved terminal spine of this ovum.

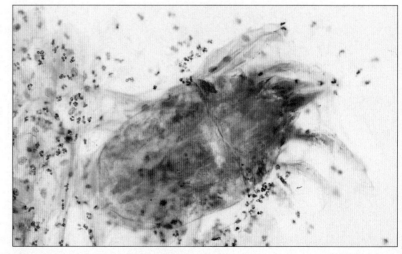

Fig. 3.63 Louse - Pap x10. Lice may occasionally be seen in a cervical smear.

REPAIR

Repair processes follow any sort of trauma to the cervix, including biopsy, curettage, cryotherapy, laser treatment, and even a vigorous cervical smear! The cellular changes are characteristic and should be recognized as such, not mistaken for dyskaryosis or malignancy. The cells that show these changes are endocervical and squamous metaplastic cells. They are often in sheets and contain enlarged nuclei with prominent nucleoli (**Fig. 3.64**). Multinucleation is common (**Fig. 3.65**), but the nuclei retain their vesicular chromatin pattern. Fibroblasts are also seen in smears following surgical procedures. They are elongated, spindle-shaped cells with spindle-shaped nuclei which do not cause a bulge in the cell (**Figs 3.66, 3.67**), unlike the fibre cells of invasive carcinoma (*see* **Fig. 4.41–4.43**).

NEOPLASIA

Neoplasia (new growth) may be benign or malignant, but the term 'neoplastic' is often used loosely to indicate malignant tumours. The cellular features of neoplasms are quite different from those of the degenerative and inflammatory changes described above and obviously are dependent on whether the neoplasm is benign or malignant. Benign neoplasms of the cervix are uncommon. Malignant neoplasms are commonly either squamous or glandular although other types of tumours do occur. It can sometimes be difficult to distinguish between reactive processes and neoplasia; the most important feature to assess is the nucleus. However, bare nuclei cannot be used to make a diagnosis, as it is impossible to recognize the cell type without the cytoplasm. **Figure 3.68** compares the various features seen in the above cellular processes, namely, degeneration, inflammation, repair and neoplasia.

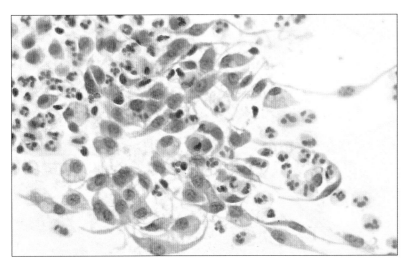

Fig. 3.64 Repair cells – Pap x40. Repair cells, such as these squamous metaplastic cells, show visible nucleoli, even at this low power. They are frequently seen after therapeutic procedures to the cervix, as healing takes place by the process of metaplasia.

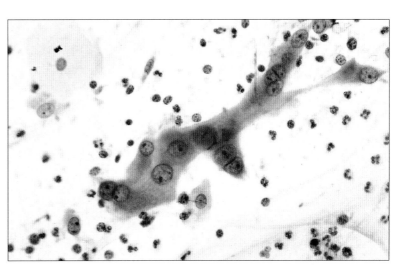

Fig. 3.65 Repair cells – Pap x40. This group of repair cells displays the translucent cytoplasm of metaplastic squamous cells and the vesicular, crisp nuclei of endocervical cells. Note the multinucleation and nucleoli that are associated with active and/or reactive cells.

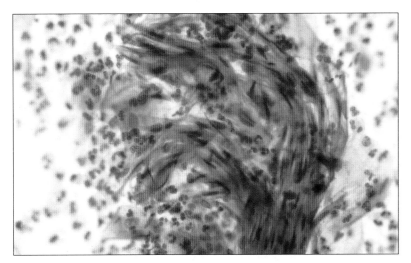

Fig. 3.66 Fibroblasts – Pap x40. Pictured here is a bundle of fibroblasts with thin elongated nuclei that do not cause the cytoplasm of the cell to bulge.

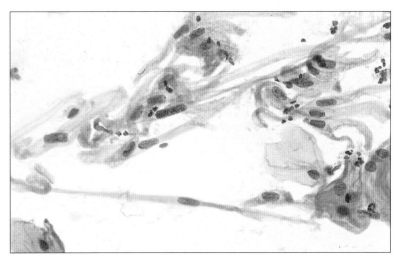

Fig. 3.67 Fibroblasts – Pap x40. Individual fibroblasts are clearly seen in this illustration. They have elongated cigar-shaped nuclei, which are of the same width as the cell.

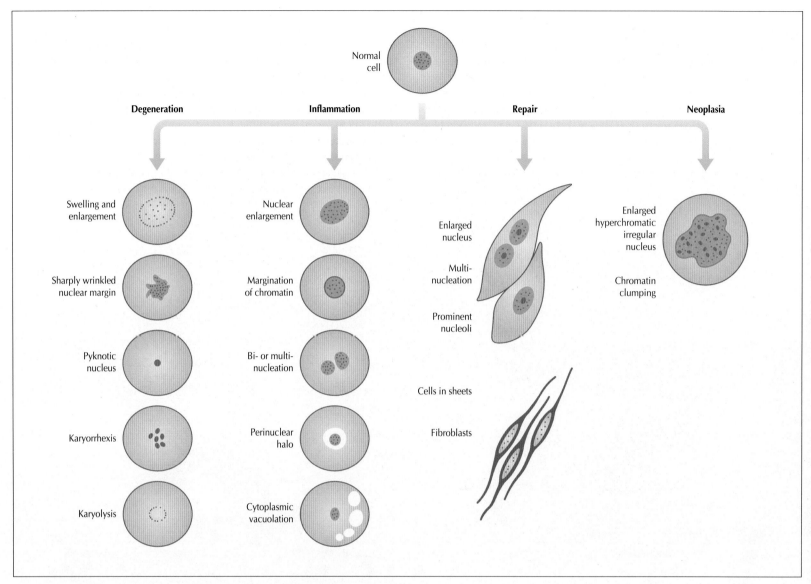

Fig. 3.68 Cellular changes in degeneration, inflammation, repair, and neoplasia.

SUGGESTED READING

Bibbo M, Wied GL. Microbiology and inflammation of the female genital tract. In: *Compendium of Diagnostic Cytology,* 6th ed. Chicago: Tutorials of Cytology; 1988: 54–62.

Bibbo M, Keebler CM, Wied GL. Tissue repair. In:*Compendium of Diagnostic Cytology*, 6th ed. Chicago: Tutorials of Cytology; 1988: 69–70.

Crum CP Nuovo GJ. *Genital Papilloma Viruses and Related Neoplasms.* Raven Press, New York, 1991.

Mitchell H, Medley G. Longtidunal study of women with negative smears according is endocervical statuc. *Lancet* 1991; **367**: 265–267.

The British Society for Clinical Cytology and the NHS Cervical Screening Programme. Achievable Standards, Benchmarks for Reporting, Criteria for Evaluating Cervical Cytopathology. Report of a Working Party. *Cytopathology* 1995; **6 (suppl. 2)**: 7–32.

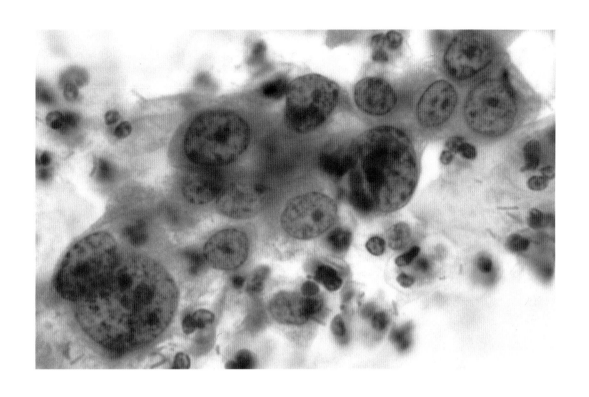

SQUAMOUS ABNORMALITIES
OF THE CERVIX AND VAGINA

4

The rationale behind the UK National Cervical Screening Programme is to reduce the mortality from carcinoma of the cervix by regular screening of all women aged between 20 and 65 years. Smears are recommended at least once every 5 years, but in practice are repeated every 3 years in many districts. In other countries, cervical smears Pap smears) are performed annually. Approximately 4000 new cases of carcinoma of the cervix are diagnosed annually in the UK, but the mortality rate has come down to under 1500 per year from 2000 in 1990.

Squamous carcinoma of the cervix develops from early precursor lesions, although not all precursor lesions progress to invasive cancer. These precancerous changes were, at one time, graded histologically as mild, moderate, and severe dysplasia, then as cervical intraepithelial neoplasia (CIN) grades 1, 2, and 3. Each of these grades is reflected by the type of abnormality seen on the cervical smear – mild, moderate, or severe dyskaryosis, the term being derived from Greek meaning bad nut or nucleus. In 1988 a new system of terminology was introduced in the US and refined in 1991 – the Bethesda System for reporting cervical and/or vaginal cytological diagnosis, whereby squamous abnormalities are classified into low grade and high grade squamous intraepithelial lesions. A comparison of the different classifications is shown in **Figure 4.1**.

Descriptions of the various grades of dyskaryotic cells are well-documented, but there are some cells which do not fit into neat categories – borderline cells in the UK or atypical cells of undetermined significance (ASCUS), as they are known in the US. **Borderline changes** (ASCUS) fall short of those required for a diagnosis of mild dyskaryosis, but are worse than those seen with inflammation. The cells show nuclear enlargement without irregularity of the nuclear margin and the chromatin pattern is vesicular, rather than granular or clumped (**Fig. 4.2**). The cells are often seen in sheets or groups (**Figs 4.3, 4.4**). A common mistake is to label immature squamous metaplastic cells as borderline. The term borderline indicates that there is uncertainty about the potential of these cells and therefore the woman needs follow-up. It should not be used as a dumping category for difficult cases. Most borderline changes disappear on follow-up with subsequent negative smears, but a small percentage of cases develop dyskaryosis. As there are no strictly defined criteria for borderline smears, their numbers vary greatly from laboratory to laboratory and it is not possible to quantify the outcome.

In the UK, human papilloma virus (HPV) changes without dyskaryosis are classified as borderline smears and in the USA as low-grade squamous intraepitheal lesion (**Fig. 4.5**), but the histology of such cases shows just wart virus change.

CYTOLOGY		HISTOLOGY	
BSCC terminology	**Bethesda system**	**Historical**	**CIN**
Borderline changes	ASCUS	–	–
Borderline changes (wart virus changes)	LSIL	Wart virus changes	Wart virus changes
Mild dyskaryosis	LSIL	Mild dysplasia	CIN 1
Moderate dyskaryosis	HSIL	Moderate dysplasia	CIN 2
Severe dyskaryosis	HSIL	Severe dysplasia/carcinoma-in-situ	CIN 3
Severe dyskaryosis/?invasive carcinoma	Squamous carcinoma	Squamous carcinoma	Squamous carcinoma
BSCC = British Society of Clinical Cytology, ASCUS = atypical cells of undetermined significance, CIN = cervical intraepithelial neoplasia,		*LSIL = low grade squamous intraepithelial lesion, HSIL = high grade squamous intraepithelial lesion.*	

Fig. 4.1 Comparison of classifications of cervical abnormalities.

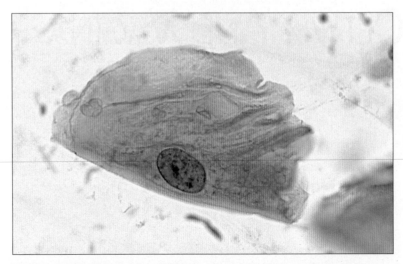

Fig. 4.2 Borderline changes (ASCUS) – Pap x100. The intermediate cell illustrated here displays a nucleus which is slightly enlarged, but still smooth in outline and with vesicular chromatin. The changes fall short of dyskaryosis and are termed borderline. No inflammatory halo is seen.

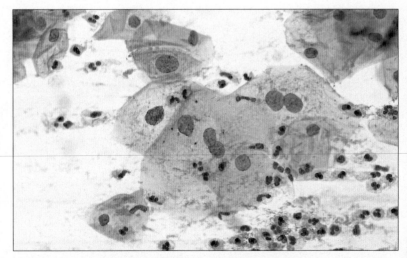

Fig. 4.3 Borderline changes (ASCUS) – Pap x40. In the centre of this field is a group of intermediate cells showing nuclear enlargement and binucleation. There is mild granularity of chromatin, without the coarse clumping seen in dyskaryosis. These changes fall into the borderline category and follow-up smears are needed.

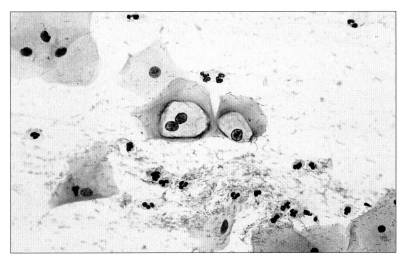

Fig. 4.4 Borderline changes (ASCUS) – Pap x40. Illustrated are intermediate and superficial cells. A few cells contain enlarged nuclei with smooth outlines and vesicular chromatin, not amounting to mild dyskaryosis, yet not showing any evidence of inflammation, and therefore termed borderline changes.

CERVICAL INTRAEPITHELIAL NEOPLASIA 1 (CIN 1)/LOW GRADE SQUAMOUS INTRAEPITHELIAL LESION (LSIL)

The histological lesion (also known as mild dysplasia) shows undifferentiated basal-type cells occupying the lower third of the epithelium, with mitoses confined to this layer, and maturing but abnormal cells occupying the upper two-thirds (**Fig. 4.6**). CIN is often associated with HPV changes. The cytological term dyskaryosis is used when cellular changes are being described, as opposed to the histological term dysplasia, which refers to tissues. Mildly dyskaryotic cells are mature cells of superficial or intermediate type with an enlarged nucleus up to half the size of the cell (**Figs 4.7, 4.8**). Dyskaryotic cells may be multi-inucleated (**Fig. 4.9**). The nuclear outline is irregular (**Fig. 4.10**) and the chromatin is coarsely clumped (**Fig. 4.11**), producing hyperchromasia, although hypochromatic dyskaryotic nuclei do occur, their pale staining being indicative of a predominance of euchromatin (**Fig. 4.12**). The nuclear abnormalities are more clearly visible under oil immersion. Mildly dyskaryotic cells may exhibit phagocytosis (**Fig. 4.13**). They are often associated with HPV infection (**Fig. 4.14**), when they not infrequently show keratinization. Mild dyskaryosis can be seen in metaplastic cells.

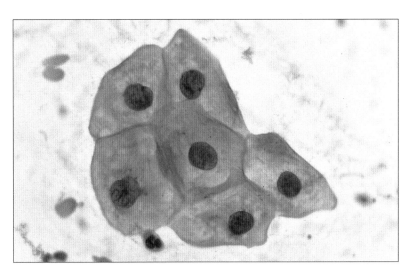

Fig. 4.5 Wart virus (HPV) changes (borderline changes), (LSIL) – Pap x40. There are two koilocytes in the centre of this field, one with a single nucleus and the other binucleate, both with large clear haloes and thickened rims of cytoplasm.

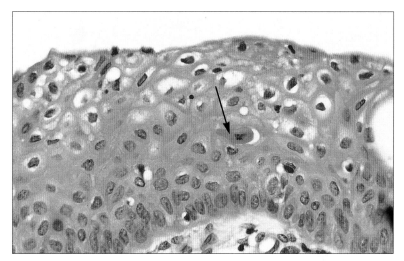

Fig. 4.6 CIN 1, mild dysplasia (LSIL) – H&E x40. This histological section of cervix shows primitive, basal-type cells occupying the lower third of the epithelium with abnormal, maturing cells in the upper two-thirds. Note the dyskeratotic cell within the epithelium (arrowed).

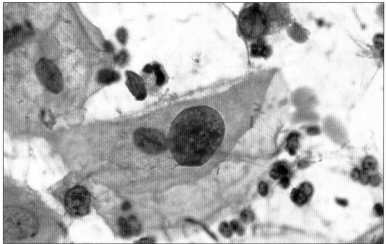

Fig. 4.7 Mild dyskaryosis (LSIL) – Pap x100. The squamous cells in this field show enlarged, hyperchromatic nuclei with some granularity of their chromatin. The cells are the size of intermediate cells and the nuclei are less than half the size of the cell, so they are graded as mildly dyskaryotic.

Fig. 4.8 Mild dyskaryosis (LSIL) – Pap x100. Although mildly dyskaryotic cells typically have irregular nuclear outlines, the cell in the centre of the field has a fairly smooth nuclear margin.

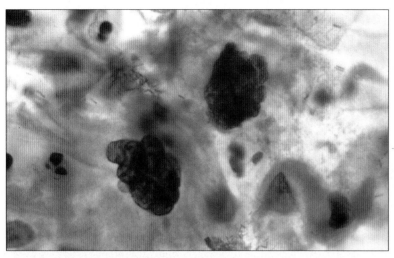

Fig. 4.9 Mild dyskaryosis (LSIL) – Pap x100. This is an example of mildly dyskaryotic cells which are multinucleated with the nuclei occupying about half the size of each cell (although the cytoplasmic margins are ill-defind).

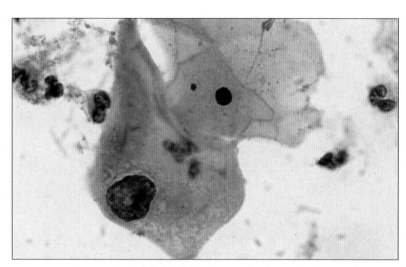

Fig. 4.10 Mild dyskaryosis (LSIL) – Pap x100. The cyanophilic mildly dyskaryotic cell is the same size of the neighbouring superficial cell and has an irregular hyperchromatic nucleus.

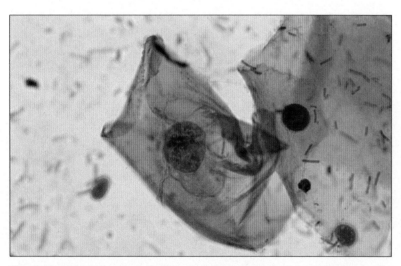

Fig. 4.11 Mild dyskaryosis (LSIL) – Pap x100. Illustrated is a mildly dyskaryotic cell displaying hyperchromasia, with chromatin clumping and a slightly irregular, enlarged nucleus.

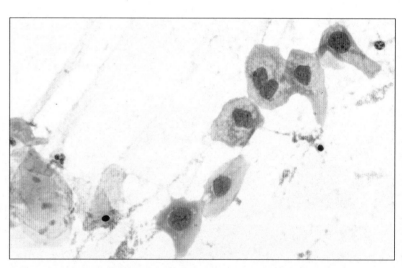

Fig. 4.12 Mild dyskaryosis (LSIL) – Pap x40. Although mild dyskaryosis is usually accompanied by hyperchromasia, the cells in this photomicrograph display pale nuclei, representing active euchromatin.

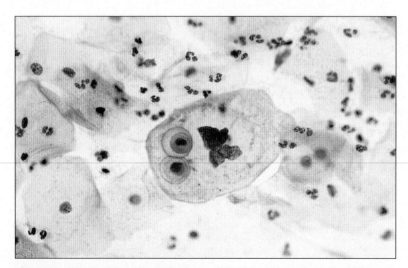

Fig. 4.13 Mild dyskaryosis (LSIL) – Pap x40. This mildly dyskaryotic cell is binucleate and has phagocytosed two dead cells, each of which lies within its own vacuole.

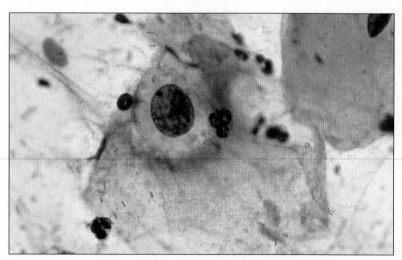

Fig. 4.14 Mild dyskaryosis, HPV changes (LSIL) – Pap x100. Mildly dyskaryotic cells may also show HPV changes, as illustrated here.

CERVICAL INTRAEPITHELIAL NEOPLASIA 2 (CIN 2)/HIGH GRADE SQUAMOUS INTRAEPITHELIAL LESION (HSIL)

On histological examination, a CIN 2 lesion (moderate dysplasia) appears to have the lower two-thirds of its epithelium occupied by undifferentiated basal cells, including mitotic figures (Fig. 4.15). As in mild dysplasia, the whole of the epithelium is abnormal, but the cells in the upper third show some maturation, up to the parabasal cell stage. CIN 2 may also be associated with wart virus (HPV) changes. Moderately dyskaryotic cells show similar features to those of mildly dyskaryotic cells, but of greater severity . The cells are less mature, about the size of parabasal cells (Fig. 4.16).

The nucleus is enlarged up to two-thirds of the size of the cell and is irregular in outline (Fig. 4.17). It is usually hyperchromatic, showing marked clumping and clearing of chromatin, but hypochromic, bland nuclei are also seen (Fig. 4.18). Multinucleation and phagocytosis (Fig. 4.19) may also be noted. It is not uncommon to find koilocytotic change in moderately dyskaryotic cells, indicating HPV infection (Fig. 4.20). Metaplastic cells may show moderate dyskaryosis (Fig. 4.21), which should not be confused with immature squamous metaplasia (see Figure 2.60). In the latter the nuclei may be hyperchromatic, but do not show irregular margins or chromatin clumping. Epithelial pearls composed of dyskaryotic cells may be seen in smears showing mild or moderate dyskaryosis (Fig. 4.22).

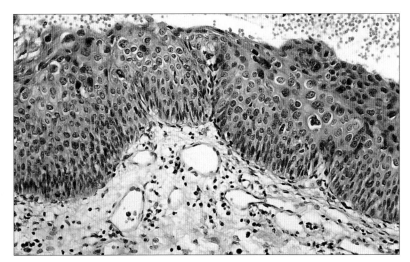

Fig. 4.15 CIN 2, moderate dysplasia – H&E x25. This histological section of cervix shows CIN 2, namely basal undifferentiated cells occupying the lower two-thirds of the epithelium with abnormal but maturing cells involving the upper third.

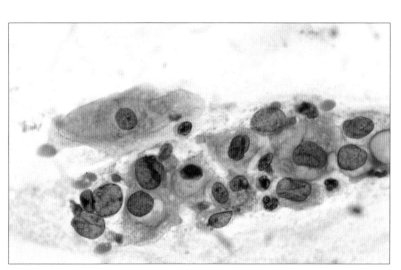

Fig. 4.16 Moderate dyskaryosis (HSIL) – Pap x40. The cells illustrated here show the features of moderate dyskaryosis, namely nuclear enlargement up to two-thirds the size of the cell and irregular hyperchromatic nuclei. The cells are approximately the size of parabasal cells.

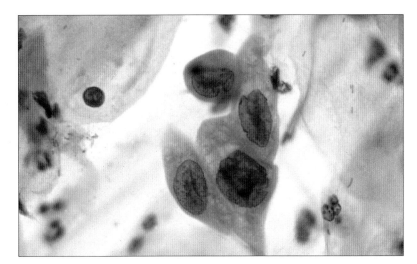

Fig. 4.17 Moderate dyskaryosis (HSIL) – Pap x100. These moderately dyskaryotic cells have markedly irregular hyperchromatic nuclei, with indentations and grooves simulating pecan nuts.

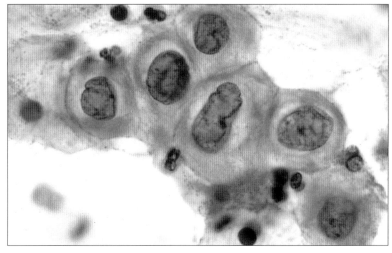

Fig. 4.18 Moderate dyskaryosis (HSIL) – Pap x100. In this field the moderately dyskaryotic cells show pale chromatin (euchromatin) within irregular enlarged nuclei.

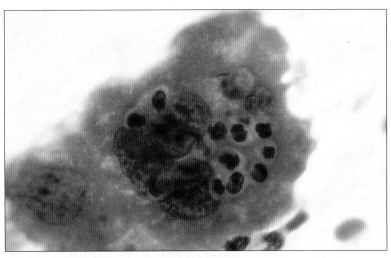

Fig. 4.19 Moderate dyskaryosis (HSIL) – Pap x100. The moderately dyskaryotic cell pictured here has phagocytosed several neutrophil polymorphs. Phagocytosis is observed frequently in dyskaryotic cells.

CERVICAL INTRAEPITHELIAL NEOPLASIA 3 (CIN 3)/HIGH GRADE SQUAMOUS INTRAEPITHELIAL LESION (HSIL)

This category, which is also called carcinoma-in-situ, includes what was formerly known as severe dysplasia. A histological section of such a lesion shows the whole thickness of the epithelium occupied by small undifferentiated basal-type cells, with mitotic figures seen even at the higher levels (Fig. 4.23). There is no maturation of the squamous cells; indeed, if the stroma was missing it would be almost impossible to determine which was the base and which the surface of the lesion. CIN 3 can affect the endocervical glands or crypts while the overlying epithelium appears normal (Fig. 4.24). This is one reason for false negative cytology.

Severely dyskaryotic cells can be loosely subdivided into three types:

- Small-cell type, believed to arise from endocervical reserve cells.
- Large-cell type, arising from the squamo-columnar junction.
- Keratinizing type, thought to arise from the ectocervix.

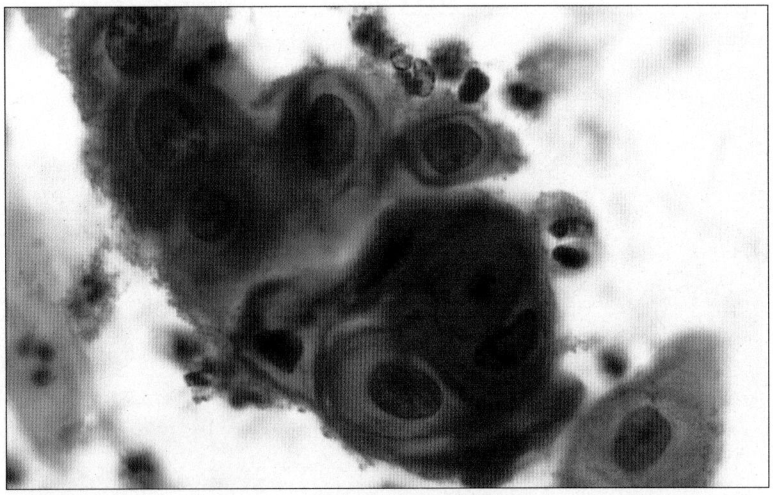

Fig. 4.20 Moderate dyskaryosis, HPV changes (HSIL) – Pap x100. Dyskaryosis is associated frequently with wart virus changes. In this field, all the moderately dyskaryotic cells also show koilocytosis and some are keratinized.

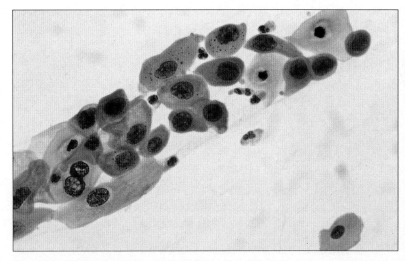

Fig. 4.21 Moderate dyskaryosis (HSIL) – Pap x40. The squamous metaplastic cells illustrated here are all moderately dyskaryotic with enlarged, irregular, hyperchromatic nuclei.

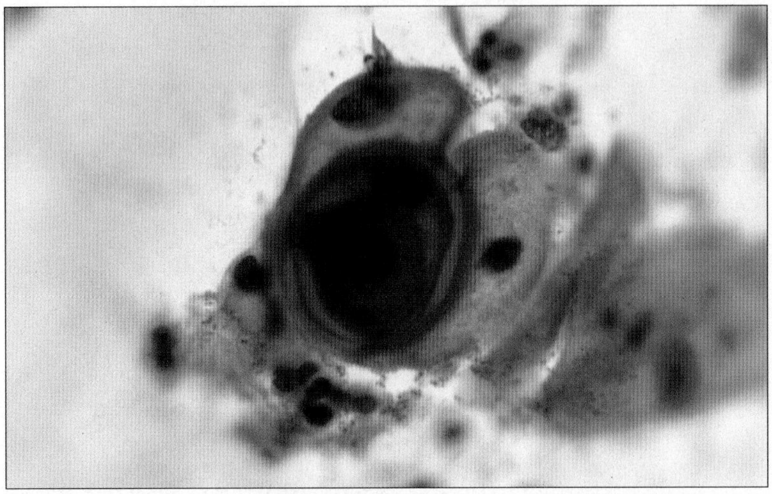

Fig. 4.22 Dyskaryotic pearl – Pap x100. This squamous pearl is composed of dyskaryotic cells rather than the flattened superficial cells of a benign epithelial pearl (see **Figure 2.74** for comparison).

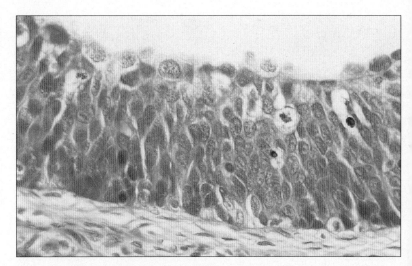

Fig. 4.23 CIN 3, severe dysplasia (HSIL) – H&E x40. This section of cervix shows the epithelium completely occupied by small undifferentiated basal-type cells. No maturation of the surface cells is seen.

The small-cell type of severe dyskaryosis is seen most commonly in the author's laboratory. The cells are smaller than parabasal cells **(Fig. 4.25)** and the nucleus fills most of the cell, leaving only a thin rim of cytoplasm **(Fig. 4.26)**. The nuclear margin is irregular, with coarse chromatin clumping and hyperchromasia **(Fig. 4.27)**, but may be very pale and hypochromic **(Fig. 4.28)**. The nuclear outline may on occasion be quite smooth and the cells may resemble endocervical cells **(Fig. 4.29)**, but careful examination of the rest of the smear usually reveals severely dyskaryotic cells in syncytial groups **(Fig. 4.30)**. When only a few severely dyskaryotic cells are present in a smear they can easily be overlooked or be mistaken for histiocytes **(Fig. 4.31)**. With large-cell severe dyskaryosis the nuclear–cytoplasmic ratio is not as high as in the small-cell type **(Fig. 4.32)**. Keratinized severely dyskaryotic cells are seen in the third type of severe dyskaryosis **(Figs 4.33, 4.34, 4.35)**. Severely dyskaryotic cells may also be associated with wart virus change.

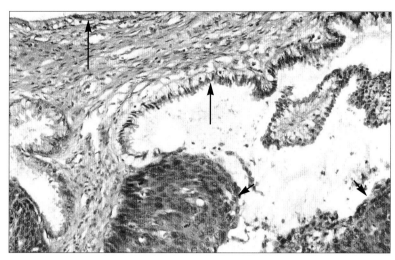

Fig. 4.24 CIN 3 in endocervical glands – H&E x40. In this section the surface epithelium is composed of benign, tall, columnar endocervical cells (long arrows), while in the gland crypts the epithelium is partially replaced by the small severely dyskaryotic cells of CIN 3 (short arrows).

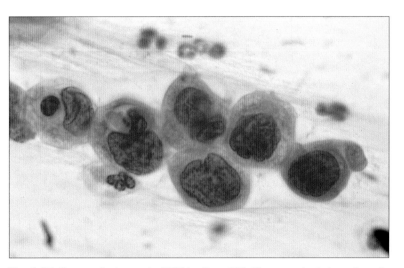

Fig. 4.25 Severe dyskaryosis (HSIL) – Pap x100. The severely dyskaryotic cells illustrated in this photomicrograph are very small, but contain large, very irregular, hyperchromatic nuclei.

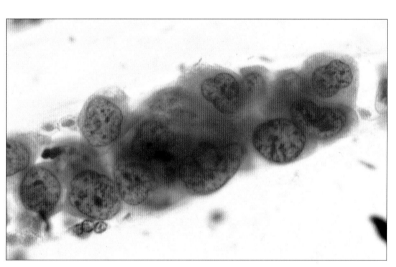

Fig. 4.26 Severe dyskaryosis (HSIL) – Pap x100. These severely dyskaryotic cells contain very little cytoplasm. Note the irregular nuclear outlines and the clumping and clearing of chromatin.

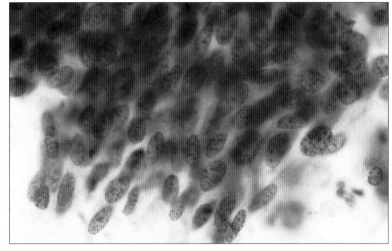

Fig. 4.27 Severe dyskaryosis (HSIL) – Pap x100. Severely dyskaryotic cells can be very small, as illustrated in this cluster, with no visible cytoplasm and prominent chromatin clumping.

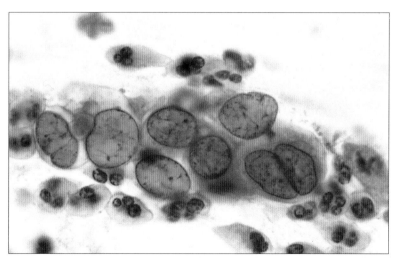

Fig. 4.28 Severe dyskaryosis (HSIL) – Pap x100. In contrast to the example in **Figure 4.27**, these severely dyskaryotic cells exhibit very pale nuclei composed mainly of euchromatin, with a few dots of heterochromatin.

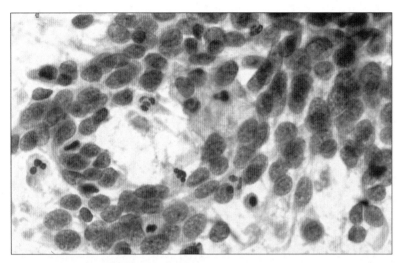

Fig. 4.29 Severe dyskaryosis (HSIL) – Pap x63. These severely dyskaryotic cells may easily be mistaken for endocervical cells on screening. However, the chromatin is abnormal, being stippled, unlike the vesicular chromatin of normal endocervical cells.

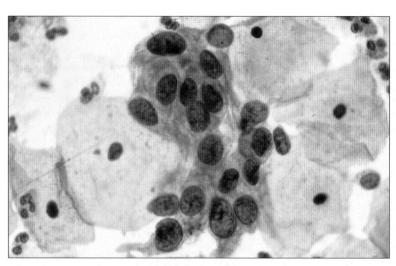

Fig. 4.30 Severe dyskaryosis (HSIL) – Pap x40. This field shows a mixture of superficial and intermediate cells with a syncytial group of small, severely dyskaryotic cells in the centre.

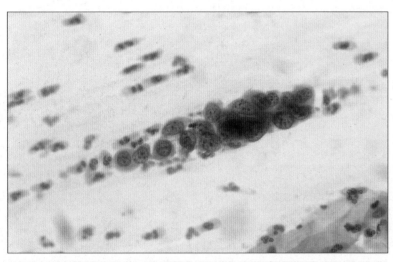

Fig. 4.31 Severe dyskaryosis (HSIL) – Pap x10. This low-power view shows how easy it would be to assume that the small severely dyskaryotic cells in the centre of the field are probably histiocytes. In fact, these are the abnormal cells, illustrated under higher magnification in **Figure 4.26**.

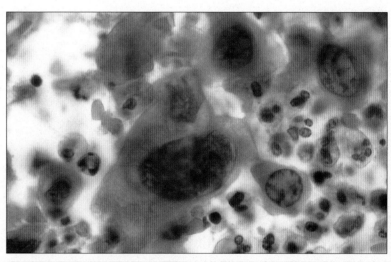

Fig. 4.32 Severe dyskaryosis (HSIL) – Pap x100. In this field there are severely dyskaryotic cells of varying shapes and sizes, including a very large cell with abundant cytoplasm. This is a feature of large cell severe dyskaryosis.

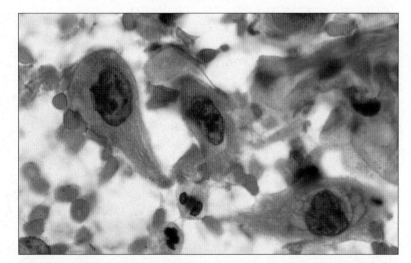

Fig. 4.33 Severe dyskaryosis (HSIL) – Pap x100. The cells in this field are large with abundant cytoplasm and abnormal nuclei. Two of the cells show bright orange keratinied cytoplasm.

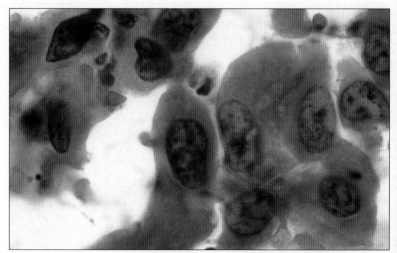

Fig. 4.34 Severe dyskaryosis (HSIL) – Pap x100. Keratinizing severe dyskaryosis is very similar to large-cell dyskaryosis, except that the former shows much keratinization, as illustrated here by the cells with bright orange cytoplasm.

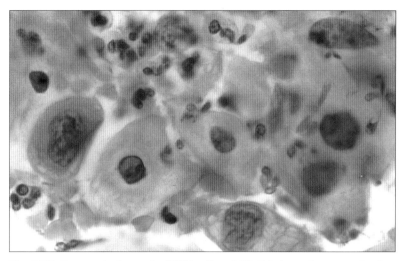

Fig. 4.35 Severe dyskaryosis (HSIL) – Pap x100. This is another example of keratinizing severe dyskaryosis. Note that there may also be cells displaying lesser degrees of dyskaryosis in a severely dyskaryotic smear.

MICROINVASIVE CARCINOMA OF THE CERVIX

A large CIN3 lesion may show only a tiny focus of microinvasion with small buds of tumour breaching the basement membrane and invading the stroma (**Fig. 4.36**). The cells seen on the smear, therefore, will be severely dyskaryotic. However, if severely dyskaryotic cells are seen to contain nucleoli the possibility of microinvasion must be considered (**Figs 4.37, 4.38**). The background is frequently clean, unlike that in invasive squamous carcinoma (see **Figure 4. 46**). An intersting feature noted in histological sections is that the invasive buds or tongues are composed of more differentiated cells with more abundant cytoplasm than those in the dyskaryotic epithelium above.

SEVERE DYSKARYOSIS/?INVASIVE CARCINOMA

Invasion cannot reliably be diagnosed on a cervical smear, although there are usually very strong indications that it is present. On histology, invasion is obvious, with neoplastic cells growing into the stroma and often forming tumour nests or islands. The surface epithelium may show only CIN3, but invasion may be widespread from an invasive focus in the crypts or, occasionally, the area sampled may show normal epithelium overlying invasive carcinoma (**Fig. 4.39**).

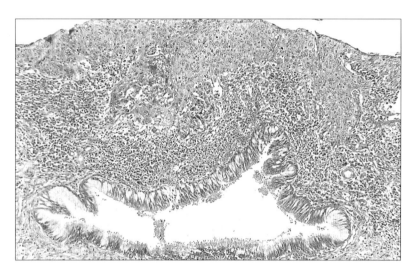

Fig. 4.36 CIN 3 with microinvasion – Pap x25. The section of cervix illustrated here shows CIN 3 with microinvasion. The surface of this lesion would yield only severely dyskaryotic cells when sampled.

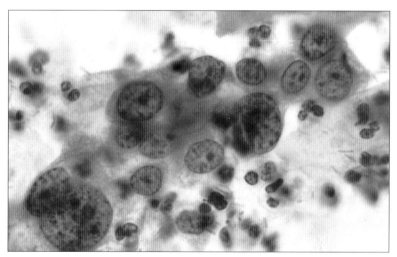

Fig. 4.37 Microinvasion (HSIL) – Pap x100. The severely dyskaryotic cells seen in this field contain prominent red nucleoli, which are a feature of invasion in this context.

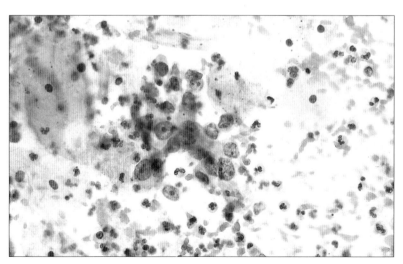

Fig. 4.38 Microinvasion (HSIL) – Pap x40. Illustrated here is a group of small, severely dyskaryotic cells with prominent red nucleoli. The cells are so small that they could easily be missed. The background of neutrophils should arouse suspicion of invasive disease.

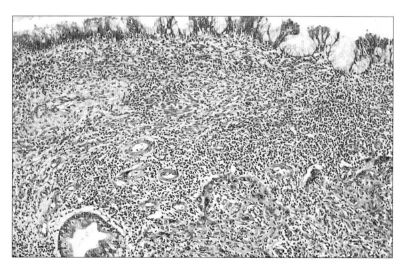

Fig. 4.39 Invasive squamous carcinoma (squamous cell carcinoma) – H&E x25. In this histological section, note the normal endocervical surface epithelium overlying nests of squamous carcinoma deep in the stroma. This is one reason for false negative cytology.

The smear shows severely dyskaryotic cells (**Fig. 4.40**), often with much pleomorphism (**Fig. 4.41**), spindle cells (**Fig. 4.42**), fibre cells (**Fig. 4.43**), tadpole cells, and abnormal mitoses (**Fig. 4.44**). Tumour diathesis (malignant diathesis) is usually present, composed of necrotic cellular material, blood, and polymorphs (**Fig. 4.45**). In fact, the tumour diathesis may be so prominent that the tumour cells are camouflaged and the smear interpreted as showing inflammatory changes (**Fig. 4.46**). The salient features of the various grades of dyskaryosis are shown in **Figure 4.47**.

Rare neoplasms may arise in the cervix, such as **lymphomas**, **sarcomas**, **melanomas**, and **oat cell carcinoma** (**Fig. 4.48**). Cytological features particular to each tumour are usually present and provide clues to the correct diagnosis. In the case of undifferentiated neoplasms, the correct diagnosis may only be searched by performing special stains on biopsy material.

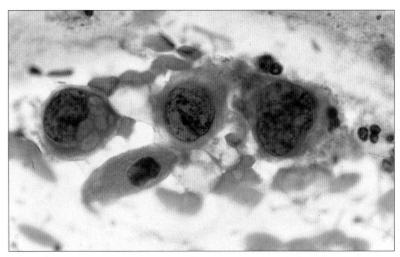

Fig. 4.40 Invasive squamous carcinoma (squamous cell carcinoma) – Pap x100. Note the small severely dyskaryotic cells in this field, displaying markedly abnormal chromatin. These features alone are insufficient to suggest invasion, although these cells are from a smear showing the characteristics of invasion elsewhere.

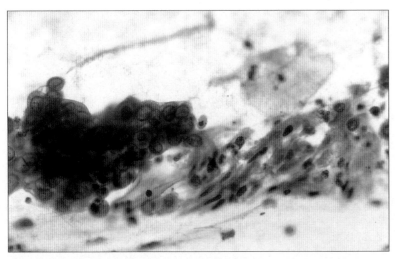

Fig. 4.41 Invasive squamous carcinoma (squamous cell carcinoma) pleomorphism – Pap x40. The severely dyskaryotic cells illustrated here show marked pleomorphism with a cluster of small round cells and fibre cells nearby, characteristic of invasive squamous carcinoma.

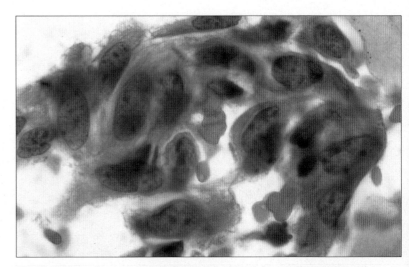

Fig. 4.42 Invasive squamous carcinoma (squamous cell carcinoma) spindle cells – Pap x100. The cells seen in this field are spindle-shaped with prominent nucleoli, multiple in some cells.

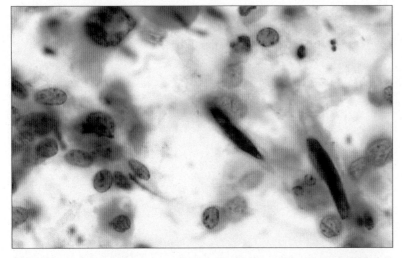

Fig. 4.43 Invasive squamous carcinoma (squamous cell carcinoma) fibre cells – Pap x100. Note the two thin fibre cells with hyperchromatic nuclei, a common feature of invasive squamous cell carcinoma.

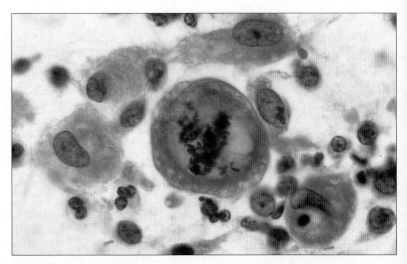

Fig. 4.44 Invasive squamous carcinoma (squamous cell carcinoma) abnormal mitosis – Pap x100. This field, from a smear of a case of invasive carcinoma, shows an abnormal, tripolar mitosis. Histiocytes and neutrophil polymorphs are seen in the background.

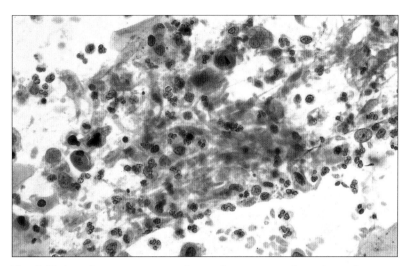

Fig. 4.45 Invasive squamous carcinoma (squamous cell carcinoma) tumour diathesis – Pap x40. This photomicrograph illustrates the characteristic findings in invasive carcinoma – pleomorphic carcinoma cells, degenerate cells with pyknotic nuclei, necrotic cellular debris, erythrocytes, and polymorphs.

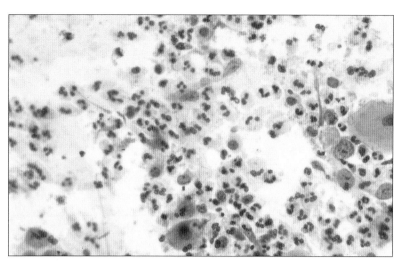

Fig. 4.46 Invasive squamous carcinoma (squamous cell carcinoma) tumour diathesis – Pap x40. In this field the polymorphs and histiocytes predominate and the neoplastic cells with pale nuclei appear insignificant. This type of smear pattern can be interpreted as inflammatory changes and can lead to a false negative smear report.

FEATURE	MILD DYSKARYOSIS	MODERATE DYSKARYOSIS	SEVERE DYSKARYOSIS
Cell size	Superficial or intermediate cell size	Parabasal cell size	Basal cell size
Nuclear size	Less than half cell size	Half to two-thirds cell size	Almost fills cell
Nuclear margin	Irregular	Irregular	Irregular
Chromatin	Hyper/hypochromatic	Hyper/hypochromatic	Hyper/hypochromatic
Chromatin clumping	Fine, granular or coarse	Usually coarse	Coarse, with clear areas
Nucleoli	Absent	Absent	Absent
Cytoplasm	Fairly dense	Fairly dense	Dense or delicate
Cell arrangement	Single or small sheets	Single or small groups	Single or syncytial groups
Pleomorphism	Minimal	Moderate	May be marked
Wart virus	May be present	May be present	May be present
Glandular neoplasia	May be present	May be present	May be present
Follow up	Repeat smear	Repeat early or refer to gynaecologist	Immediate referral to gynaecologist

Fig. 4.47 Cytological features of the various grades of dyskaryosis.

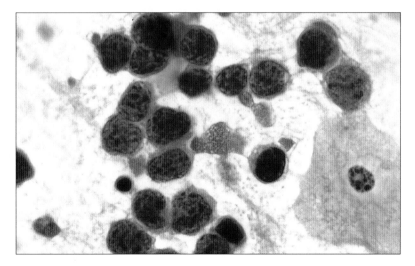

Fig. 4.48 Undifferentiated small-cell neoplasm – Pap x100. The group of hyperchromatic small cells seen here show very little cytoplasm, granular chromatin, and no nucleoli. The differential diagnosis must include small-cell anaplastic carcinoma (oat cell type) and lymphoma. In this case biopsy and subsequent immunocytochemical stains confirmed that this was a small-cell anaplastic carcinoma.

VAGINAL VAULT SMEARS

Vaginal vault smears are performed on women who have had a hysterectomy for CIN 3 or invasive carcinoma. Patients with invasive carcinoma may have radiotherapy rather than surgery and are usually followed up annually by the oncologist. Recently published guidelines (see Suggested Reading) state that vault smears are unnecessary after a hysterectomy for benign disease or mild grades of dysplasia. However, in our experience a small percentage (approximately 5% over the 3-year period studied) of patients who have had a hysterectomy, irrespective of the reason, benign or malignant, develop vaginal intraepithelial neoplasia (VAIN).

Vaginal vault smears often show cytolysis or an atrophic pattern. However, routine follow-up smears may show cytopathic changes suggestive of HPV either with or without dyskaryosis (**Fig. 4.49**), borderline nuclear changes, or mild, moderate, or severe dyskaryosis amounting to **VAIN 1 (Fig. 4.50)**, **VAIN 2 (Fig. 4.51)**, or **VAIN 3 (Fig. 4.52)**. The cytological features of dyskaryosis are exactly the same as those in dyskaryosis of the cervix (see above). Many of these women have no history of previous cervical dysplasia or carcinoma and have had a hysterectomy for fibroids or dysfunctional uterine bleeding. Some of our cases had a hysterectomy following adenocarcinoma of the ovary or endometrium, with no cervical abnormality on histological examination of the cervix. There is, as yet, no explanation for the occurrence of dysplasia in the vaginal vault in these women. A few cases in our study had previously had CIN 3 which had been treated by hysterectomy and the vaginal disease could therefore be postulated as field change.

Cervical smears are the only reliable method of diagnosing VAIN as there are no changes in the vaginal wall detectable by the naked eye. Confirmation by biopsy is therefore not always possible. Treatment is extremely difficult, consisting of laser ablation of any visible lesions, or 5-fluoruracil.

Primary squamous carcinoma of the vagina is rare. The vagina is not uncommonly the site of metastatic tumour deposits from transitional cell carcinoma of the bladder, and adenocarcinoma of the ovary and the breast. The features are similar to those of the primary tumour.

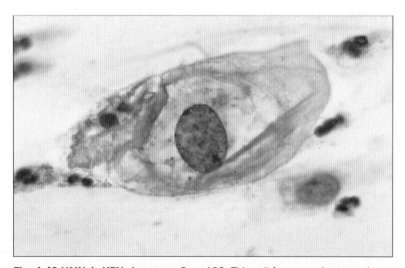

Fig. 4.49 VAIN 1, HPV changes – Pap x100. This cell from a vault smear shows a mildly dyskaryotic nucleus and perinuclear halo with a thick rim of cytoplasm, suggestive of VAIN 1 with wart virus changes.

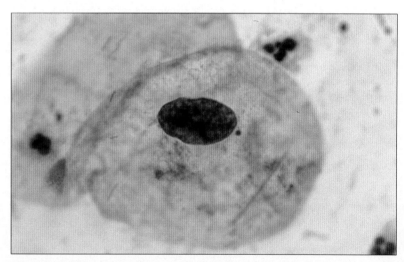

Fig. 4.50 VAIN 1 – Pap x100. Illustrated here is a mildly dyskaryotic cell showing hyperchromasia and an irregular nuclear margin.

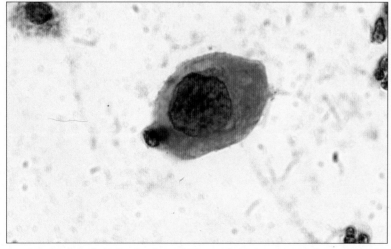

Fig. 4.51 VAIN 2 – Pap x100. This moderately dyskaryotic cell was seen in a vault smear taken from a woman who had a hysterectomy for fibroids 3 years previously, and had no cervical pathology.

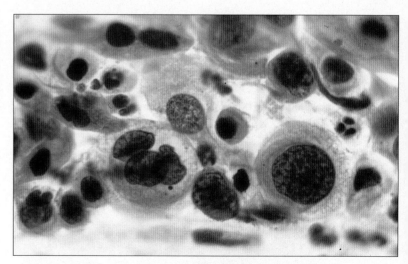

Fig. 4.52 VAIN 3 – Pap x100. This photomicrograph shows many pleomorphic, severely dyskaryotic cells suggestive of VAIN 3.

SUGGESTED READING

Anderson MC, Brown CL, Buckley CH, *et al*. Current views on cervical intraepithelial neoplasia. *J Clin Pathol* 1991; **44**: 969–978.

Bethesda Workshop. The Bethesda system for reporting cervical/vaginal diagnoses. *Acta Cytol* 1993; **37**: 115–124.

Buckley CH, Butler EB, Fox H. Cervical intraepithelial neoplasia, *J Clin Pathol*, 1982; **35**: 1–13.

Duncan ID. Guidelines for clinical practice and programme management. Oxford: National Co-ordinating network for the NHS Cervical Screening Programme; 1992.

Evans DMD, Hudson EA, Brown CL, *et al*. Terminology in gynaecological cytopathology: Report of the Working Party of the British Society for Clinical Cytology. *J Clin Pathol*, 1986; **39**: 933–944.

Hudson E. The borderline cervical smear-Editorial. *Cytopathol* 1995; **6**: 135–139.

National Cancer Institute Workshop. The 1988 Bethesda System for reporting cervical/vaginal cytological diagnoses. *J Am Med Assoc* 1989; **262**: 931–934.

O'Sullivan JP, Ismail SM, Barnes WSF, et al. Interobserver variation in the diagnosis and grading of dyskahryosis in cervical smears: Specialist cytopathologists compared with non-specialists. *J Clin Pathol* 1994; **47**: 515–518

Richart RM. Cervical intraepithelial neoplasia: A review. *Path Ann* 1973; **8**: 301.

Robb JA. The 'ASCUS' Swamp – Editorial. *Diagn Cytopathol* 1994; **11**: 319–320.

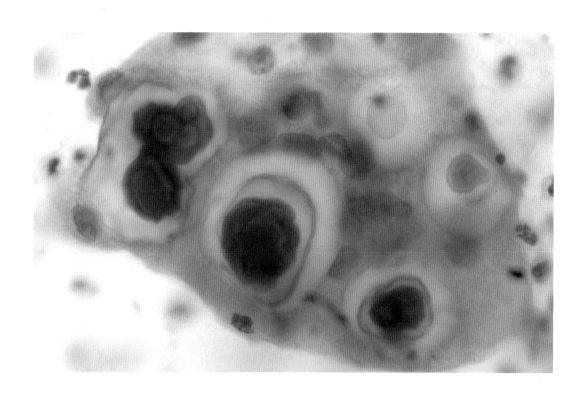

Glandular Abnormalities Of The Cervix And Endometrium, Iatrogenic Changes

5

GLANDULAR ABNORMALITIES OF THE CERVIX

Approximately 10% of all cervical carcinomas are adenocarcinomas, but a relatively high percentage of abnormal smears are diagnosed as '?glandular abnormality' and referred for colposcopy and biopsy. Some of these are glandular atypias on histology, while others are related to endocervical polyps, or endometrial or tubal metaplasia, and yet others show no pathology. It is important to be aware of changes in the cervix that may be misdiagnosed as neoplastic. In the UK the standardized cervical cytology report form has only one diagnostic category for glandular abnormalities – '?glandular neoplasia'. This includes *in situ* and invasive endocervical adenocarcinoma and endometrial adenocarcinoma, and also metastatic adenocarcinoma. It also includes smears that inappropriately contain endometrial cells in postmenopausal women. The Bethesda system subdivides glandular cell abnormalities into three categories:

- Endometrial cells, cytologically benign, in a postmenopausal woman.
- Atypical glandular cells of undetermined significance (AGUS).
- Adenocarcinoma, including endocervical, endometrial, extrauterine, and NOS (not otherwise specified).

The squamo–columnar junction and endocervix can usually be sampled adequately using a spatula with a long tip, such as the Aylesbury spatula or, preferably, the Cervex brush. If there is any suspicion that there is an endocervical lesion, the endocervix is sampled separately using an endocervical brush sampler. Care must be taken when transferring the material to the slide, because too much pressure results in streak artefacts and air drying is often noted (leading to an erroneous impression of enlarged, abnormal endocervical cells). Routine use of the endocervical brush rather than either of the above samplers for cervical smears is to be discouraged as insufficient numbers of squamous cells will be obtained.

Cervicitis

Inflamed endocervical cells are seen commonly in cervicitis. They are somewhat enlarged cells in sheets, with smooth round nuclei, sometimes multinucleated, a prominent nuclear margin, and conspicuous nucleoli (**Fig. 5.1**). The chromatin pattern remains vesicular, as in normal endocervical cells, but may be finely granular . Occasionally, sheets of endocervical cells infiltrated by neutrophils may be noted, reflecting the histology which shows only non-specific cervicitis with acute inflammatory cells within the epithelium and stroma.

Endocervical polyp

These polyps frequently protrude through the cervical os and are scraped when the smear is performed. Sheets of inflamed endocervical cells are seen in the smear (**Fig. 5.2**) often with similar features to those noted in cervicitis (see **Figure 5.1**). The biopsy shows similar changes, the polyp being covered by glandular cells with an acute or chronic inflammatory cell infiltrate.

Endocervical glandular dysplasia or atypia (atypical glandular cells of undetermined significance – AGUS)

Smears from these lesions contain endocervical cells which show enlarged nuclei, sometimes slightly irregular in outline, but without prominent nucleoli (**Fig. 5.3**). The chromatin pattern is finely granular, rather than the usual vesicular type (**Fig. 5.4**). These changes are so subtle that the diagnosis of endocervical glandular dysplasia on cytology is unreliable, although the histological features are more robust (**Fig. 5.5**). Tubal and endometrial metaplasia occur not infrequently and are represented in the smear by clusters of hyperchromatic glandular cells which can look atypical. The presence of cilia aids correct indentification of these cells which, otherwise, resemble cells derived from endocervical dysplasia (see **Figures 5.4, 5.5**).

Endocervical adenocarcinoma-in-situ (AIS)

Wart virus is believed to be implicated in the development of this disease. Endocervical glandular neoplasia may not be represented on cervical smears if the lesion is high up in the endocervical canal and therefore out of reach. The histological features of this condition include crowding of endocervical glands which are composed of abnormal elongated hyperchromatic cells with nuclei situated in the centre of the cell rather than at the base (**Fig. 5.6**) and pseudo-stratification. The cytological features of AIS are similar and clearly defined, making this diagnosis relatively straightforward (**Fig. 5.7**). A striking feature

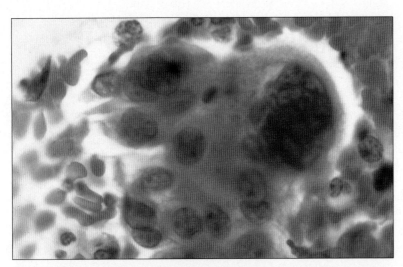

Fig. 5.1 Inflamed endocervical cells – Pap x100. This field shows endocervical cells which are multinucleated, contain visible nucleoli, and show slight irregularity of the nuclear margins.

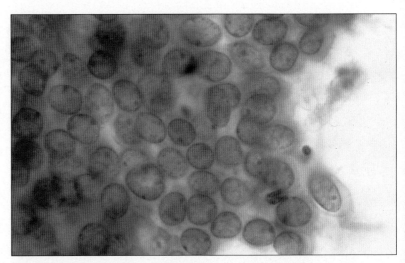

Fig. 5.2 Inflamed endocervical cells – Pap x100. The cluster of endocervical cells seen here shows slightly enlarged nuclei and an abundance of pale active chromatin – euchromatin. The nuclear margins are sharply defined and nucleoli are not prominent. Note the cells are clustered, rather than in the usual flat sheets.

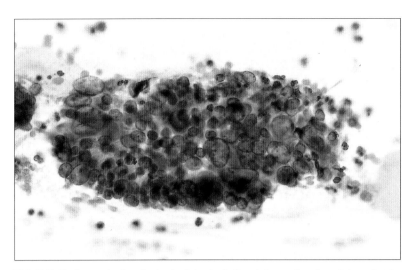

Fig. 5.3 Endocervical cell atypia (atypical glandular cells of undetermined significance) – Pap x40. Many of the cells in this endocervical group show marked nuclear enlargement with an abnormal chromatin pattern. Prominent nucleoli are not a feature.

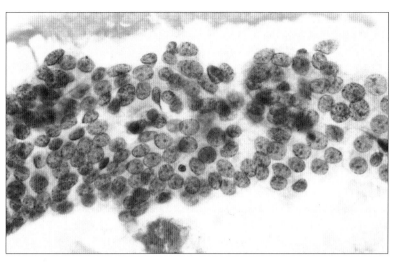

Fig. 5.4 Endocervical cell atypia (atypical glandular cells of undetermined significance) – Pap x40. Illustrated is a loosely cohesive cluster of endocervical cells which show some overlapping, rather than the usual flat sheet arrangement. No honeycombing is evident. The nuclei are round and contain abnormal speckled chromatin with small red nucleoli.

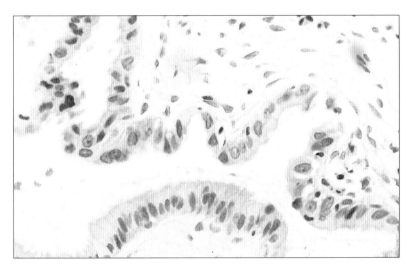

Fig. 5.5 Endocervical dysplasia – H&E x40. This histological section of endocervix shows a gland crypt lined below by normal tall columnar epithelium and above by abnormal endocervical cells with enlarged nuclei (nearer the luminal surface of the cells), displaying red nucleoli and hyperchromasia.

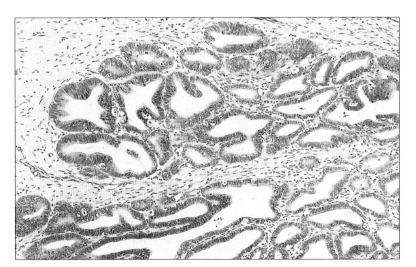

Fig. 5.6 Adenocarcinoma-in-situ (AIS) – H&E x10. In this section there are a number of endocervical glands which are crowded together and lined by abnormal epithelial cells.

FEATURES	NORMAL ENDOCER-VICAL CELLS	ADENOCARCINOMA-IN-SITU
Endocervical groups	Scanty to moderate	Abundant
Cell arrangement	Flat sheets	Clusters
Edges of cell groups	Palisading	Feathering/fraying
Cell strips	Single row (picket fence)	Multilayered pseudostratified strips of cells
Gland openings	Absent	Present
Rosettes	Uncommon	Common
Nuclei	Round or ovoid	Elongated
Nuclear pleomorphism	Absent	Present
Chromatin pattern	Vesicular	Granular or speckled
Nucleoli	Occasionally seen	May be seen
Cilia	Occasionally seen	Never seen
Mitotic figures	Occasionally seen	Frequent

Fig. 5.7 Features of adenocarcinoma-in-situ.

is the cellularity of the smear, with numerous sheets and clusters of endocervical cells (**Fig. 5.8**). Under higher magnification, the sheets show feathering or fraying of their edges (**Figs 5.9, 5.10**), unlike the neatly palisaded edges of normal endocervical sheets (see **Figure 2.32**). The nuclei show overlapping (**Fig. 5.11**), rather than the normal flat honeycombing (see **Figure 2.33**), and the chromatin pattern of the cells is granular or hyperchromatic (**Fig. 5.12**), in contrast to the normal vesicular pattern (see **Figure 2.31**). The nuclei are often elongated and, together with the pseudostratification (**Fig. 5.13**), which is usually regarded as a histological feature, are well-demonstrated in cytological material (**Fig. 5.14**). The endocervical sheets display gland openings (**Fig. 5.15**). Another typical feature is the presence of endocervical cells in rosettes (**Figs 5.16, 5.17**). Caution must be exercised here as endocervical brush smears can occasionally contain small rosettes of poorly preserved cells. Nucleoli are not a particular feature of AIS.

AIS may be seen in association with mild, moderate, or even severe dyskaryosis (**Fig. 5.18**), so smears should be carefully screened for dual pathology. It may also be noted in conjunction with HPV changes (**Fig. 5.19**).

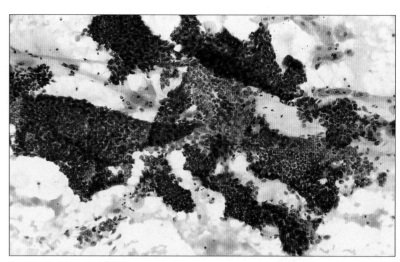

Fig. 5.8 AIS, cellularity – Pap x10. A feature frequently seen in AIS is an over-representation of endocervical cell sheets in the smear, as illustrated here. Such an abundance of large sheets is unusual for a normal cervical smear.

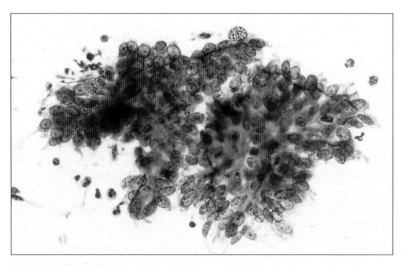

Fig. 5.9 AIS, feathering – Pap x40. The two clusters of endocervical cells seen here exhibit fraying or feathering of their edges. The cells show some elongation of their nuclei and speckled chromatin.

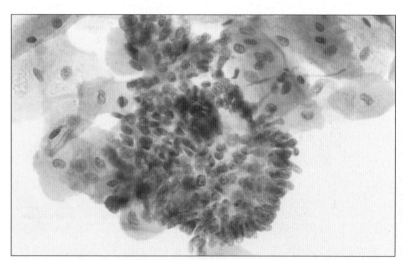

Fig. 5.10 AIS, feathering – Pap x40. This is another example of feathering of the edges of endocervical clusters in AIS. The nuclei are not hyperchromatic and may be judged to be normal under low power.

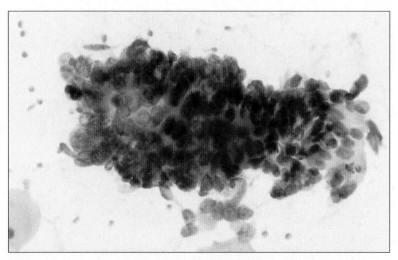

Fig. 5.11 AIS, nuclear crowding – Pap x40. In this field there is a cluster of hyperchromatic endocervical cells which show overlapping of nuclei, as opposed to the flat sheets associated with normal endocervical cells.

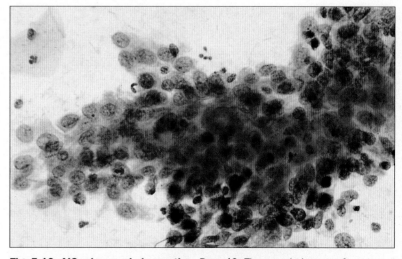

Fig. 5.12 AIS, abnormal chromatin – Pap x40. The crowded group of endocervical cells illustrated displays granular, hyperchromatic nuclei. The edges of the group show slight fraying, rather than the palisading often seen with benign endocervical cells.

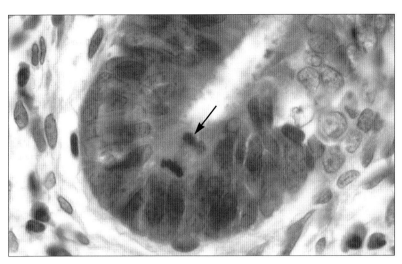

Fig. 5.13 AIS, pseudostratification – H&E x40. This section, showing part of a gland involved by AIS, contains abnormal, elongated, hyperchromatic nuclei in cells arranged in a pseudostratified fashion. Note the mitotic figure (arrowed).

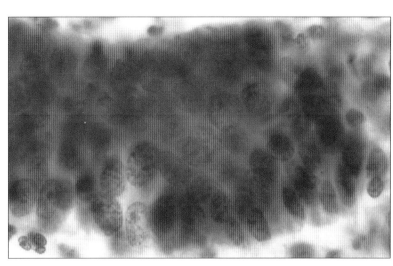

Fig. 5.14 AIS, pseudostratification – Pap x100. This cervical smear shows a fragment composed of elongated abnormal endocervical cells arranged in a pseudostratified fashion, corresponding to the histological arrangement seen in **Figure 5.13**.

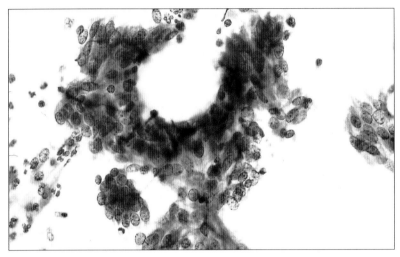

Fig. 5.15 AIS, gland opening – Pap x40. Demonstrated here is a cluster of abnormal endocervical cells showing hyperchromasia, elongated nuclei, speckled chromatin, and a gland opening.

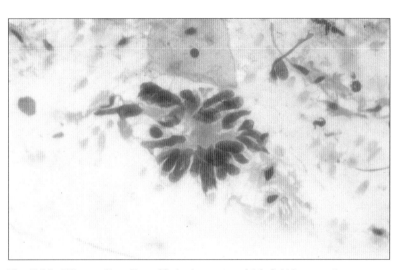

Fig. 5.16 AIS, rosette – Pap x40. In the centre of this field is a rosette composed of elongated hyperchromatic endocervical cells, suggesting a daisy.

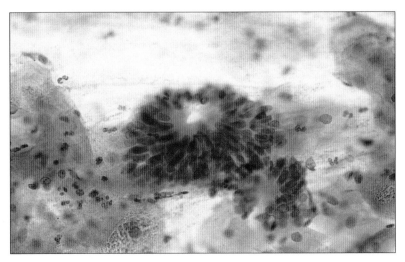

Fig. 5.17 AIS, rosette – Pap x40. This photomicrograph shows two rosettes, the larger one resembling a dahlia with multiple layers of hypochromatic nuclei for petals, and a smaller, incomplete rosette just below it.

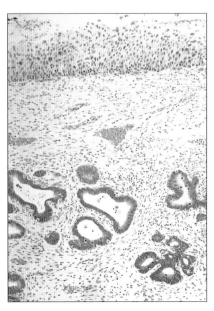

Fig. 5.18 AIS with CIN – H&E x10. This histological section of cervix shows moderately dysplastic surface epithelium (CIN 2) overlying AIS.

Adenocarcinoma of the endocervix

Invasive adenocarcinoma of the endocervix is readily diagnosable on histology (**Fig. 5.20**). The smear shows clusters of adenocarcinoma cells which are enlarged, show vacuolation with abnormal nuclei pushed to the periphery of the cell (**Fig. 5.21**), and contain huge red nucleoli (**Fig. 5.22**) – in other words, typical features of adenocarcinoma from any site in the body. The cytoplasm may contain phagocytosed neutrophils (**Fig. 5.23**). The cells are larger than endometrial adenocarcinoma cells and the woman is usually premenopausal and asymptomatic, among other differences (**Fig. 5.24**).

ABNORMALITIES OF THE ENDOMETRIUM

Adenocarcinoma of the endometrium

This is a neoplasm of older, postmenopausal women who usually present with postmenopausal bleeding. A cervical smear is not the best method for collecting diagnostic material in these cases – a posterior fornix sample has a better pick-up rate. Another sampling method is endometrial aspiration, discussed below. The histological features of this endometrial adenocarcinoma (**Fig. 5.25**) are well-reflected in the cytological appearances. The smears are usually heavily blood-stained and atrophic, making them air-dried and difficult to interpret. Clusters of cells that resemble normal endometrial cells are often seen and might be disregarded if the woman is on hormone-replacement therapy (**Fig. 5.26**). There may be clusters of small adenocarcinoma cells with vacuoles (**Fig. 5.27**) or larger cells with abnormal nuclei containing prominent red nucleoli (**Fig. 5.28**). Single malignant cells may be seen. Neutrophils may be seen within the carcinoma cells (**Fig. 5.29**), resembling the histological appearances (see **Figure 5.25**). Rarely, the smear may show psammoma bodies surrounded by carcinoma cells (**Fig. 5.30**). The first danger signal in a smear is the presence of numerous small histiocytes, not the multinucleated giant histiocytes usually associated with atrophic smears, even when neoplastic cells are not present.

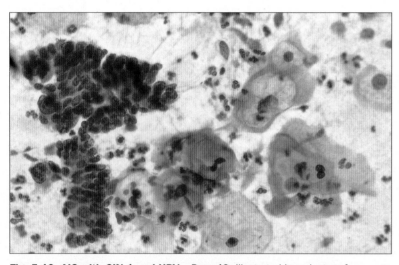

Fig. 5.19 AIS with CIN 1 and HPV – Pap x40. Illustrated is a cluster of abnormal endocervical cells from AIS together with koilocytes, some showing mild dyskaryosis.

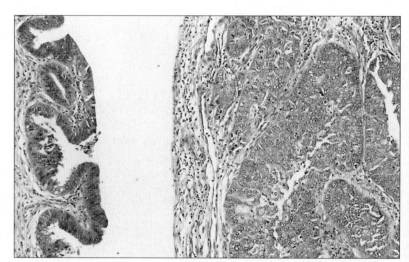

Fig. 5.20 AIS and adenocarcinoma – H&E x10. This section of endocervix shows AIS affecting the surface epithelium on the left, while on the right invasive adenocarcinoma is seen beneath the denuded epithelium.

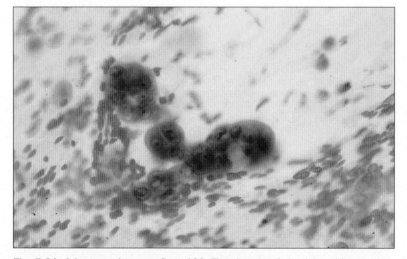

Fig. 5.21 Adenocarcinoma – Pap x100. The clusters of glandular cells seen in this field show nuclei pushed to the periphery and intracytoplasmic vacuoles. Red nucleoli are visible, even at this magnification.

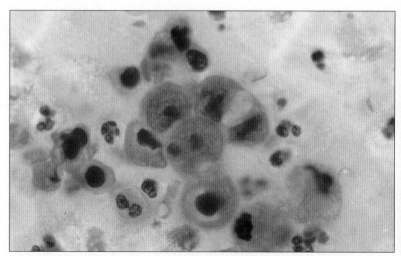

Fig. 5.22 Adenocarcinoma – Pap x100. Note the enormous red central nucleoli in these adenocarcinoma cells.

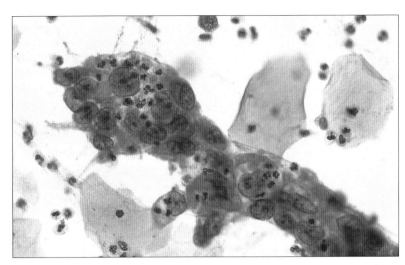

Fig. 5.23 Adenocarcinoma – Pap x100. This cluster of adenocarcinoma cells shows phagocytosis of neutrophils, vacuolation, red nucleoli, and granular chromatin. It is obvious that the smear is from a premenopausal woman by the superficial cells in the background.

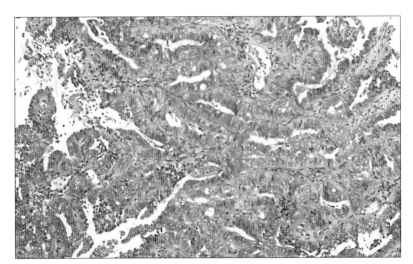

Fig. 5.25 Endometrial adenocarcinoma – H&E x10. This section of an endometrial adenocarcinoma shows closely packed abnormal glands, some of which contain neutrophils.

FEATURES	ENDOCERVICAL	ENDOMETRIAL
Age	Younger, pre-menopausal women	Older, postmenopausal women
Symptoms	Often none	Postmenopausal bleeding
Smear pattern	Mature	Atrophic
Background	Not usually blood-stained	Heavily blood-stained
Endometrial cells	Not usually present	Often present
Cell size	Larger	Smaller
Vacuoles	Present	Present
WBC in vacuoles	Not always present	Usually present
Large nucleoli	Usually present	Usually present
Single tumour cells	Not usually present	Often present
Normal endocervical cells	Not usually present	May be present

Fig. 5.24 Comparison of endocervical and endometrial adenocarcinoma.

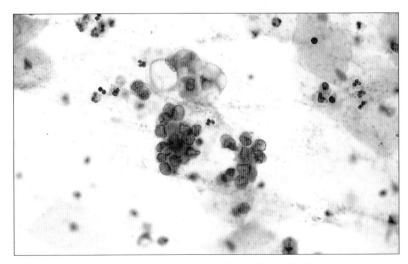

Fig. 5.26 Endometrial adenocarcinoma – Pap x40. In this field are clusters of small endometrial cells, with one cluster showing large vacuoles. No evidence of malignancy is visible in these cells, but other areas of the smear showed adenocarcinoma. The squamous cells seen are mature because this woman was on hormone-replacement therapy.

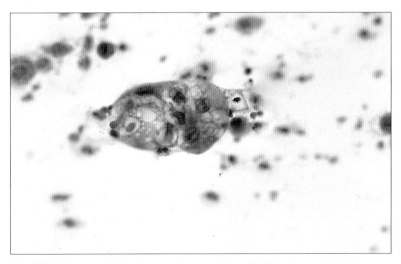

Fig. 5.27 Endometrial adenocarcinoma – Pap x40. This cluster of mildly pleomorphic adenocarcinoma cells shows marked vacuolation and small irregular nuclei.

Adenosquamous carcinoma of the endometrium

This is not common and the cytological sample shows some cells with features of adenocarcinoma and others showing squamous differentiation.

Other endometrial neoplasms cannot be diagnosed reliably on cytology.

Squamous carcinoma of the endometrium

This is an extremely rare entity and is indistinguishable from squamous carcinoma of the cervix on cervical smears.

Pure squamous carcinomas of the endometrium are very rare.

Endometrial aspirate samples

Endometrial aspirate samples are increasingly being used for diagnosis in cases of postmenopausal bleeding when the woman is unfit for a curettage. Cores of tissue are usually produced and sent for histological examination, but when very little material is obtained it is spread on a slide for cytology. In desperate cases, the formol–saline (in which an inadequate core has been despatched to the laboratory) may be spun down and the cells examined. The fixative does not affect the cell preservation. The cytological appearances of aspirated samples are quite different from those of a normal smear. In a cervical or vaginal smear, endometrial cells are usually in small, mullberry-type clusters or in clusters comprising hyperchromatic stromal cells surrounded by larger, paler glandular cells. They are often accompanied by histocytes (see **Figure 2.39–2.42**). Normal endometrium in aspirate smears is seen in the form of rectangular flat sheets, sometimes with a scattering of stromal cells on the surface (**Fig. 5.31**), reminiscent of the 'sesame seeds' appearance of myoepithelial cells in a fibroadenoma (see **Figure 8.94**). Endometrial cells appear uniform with round-to-ovoid nuclei and sharply delineated nuclear margins (**Fig. 5.32**). In simple hyperplasia, the size of the endometrial sheets increases with a corresponding increase in cell size (**Fig. 5.33**), but without any features of neoplasia. In atypical hyperplasia the cells tend to be in clusters rather than in sheets and show nuclear enlargement and mild irregularity in outline (**Fig. 5.34**). The features of adenocarcinoma are the same as those in ordinary smear samples – clusters of enlarged cells with prominent nucleoli, showing vacuolation (**Fig. 5.35**). Histiocytes and multinucleated histiocytes accompany the epithelial cells and single stromal cells may be noted in both benign and malignant aspirates.

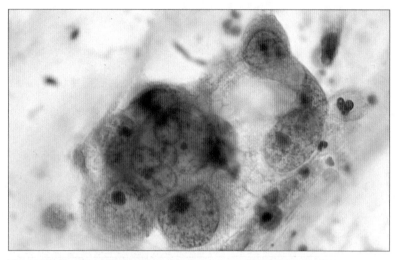

Fig. 5.28 Endometrial adenocarcinoma – Pap x100. Endometrial adenocarcinoma cells are usually small, but in this case are large with huge red nucleoli and some vacuolation.

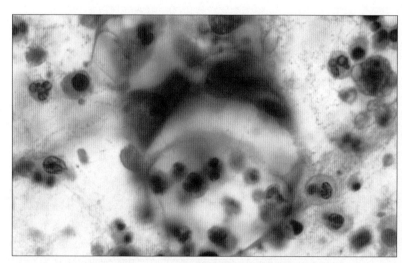

Fig. 5.29 Endometrial adenocarcinoma – Pap x100. This cluster of adenocarcinoma cells shows vacuoles pushing the nuclei to the periphery of the cluster, red nucleoli, and neutrophils within the vacuoles.

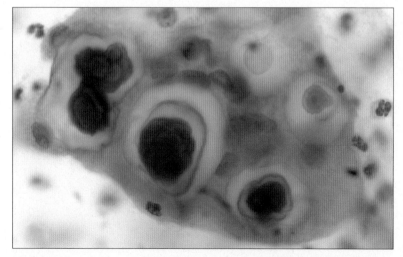

Fig. 5.30 Psammoma bodies – Pap x100. There are laminated psammoma bodies within vacuoles in this cluster of adenocarcinoma cells exfoliated from an endometrial adenocarcinoma. The tumour cells appear hypochromatic in this field.

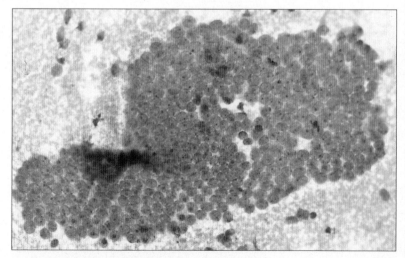

Fig. 5.31 Benign endometrial cells, Pipelle sample – Pap x40. This flat sheet of benign endometrial cells shows round uniform nuclei and a scattering of stromal cells on the surface, like sesame seeds on a bun.

Endometriosis

Endometriosis of the cervix or vaginal vault cannot be distinguished on a routine smear from endometrial cells shed during menstruation. However, if the woman has an endometriotic cyst, aspiration cytology shows the presence of endometrial cell clusters and haemosiderin-filled macrophages **(Fig. 5.36)** in a background of fresh and altered blood.

DES (diethylstilboestrol) exposure

DES was administered to women with threatened miscarriages in the 1960s, resulting in live babies but with the possibility of daughters developing abnormalities in the vagina – vaginal adenosis. Vaginal smears in such patients would include clusters of grandular cells with the usual squamous population. There is an increased incidence of adenocarcinoma of the cervix and vagina in women exposed to DES *in utero*.

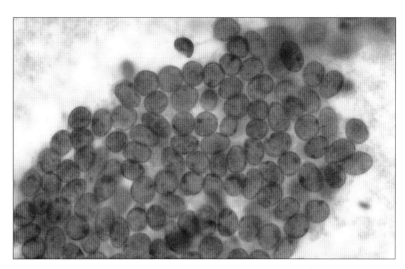

Fig. 5.32 Benign endometrial cells, Pipelle sample – Pap x100. At higher magnification, endometrial cells are seen to have vesicular nuclei with sharply defined nuclear margins.

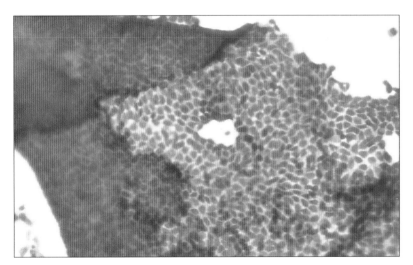

Fig. 5.33 Endometrial cells, simple hyperplasia – Pap x40. This very large folded sheet of benign endometrial cells has been aspirated from hyperplastic endometrium.

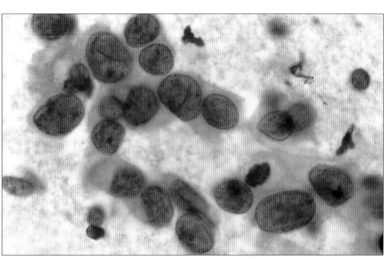

Fig. 5.34 Endometrial cells, atypical hyperplasia – Pap x100. These cells differ from the normal endometrial cells shown in **Figure 5.33** by their larger size and mildly pleomorphic nuclei, some with nuclear grooves.

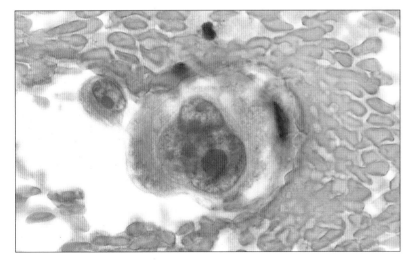

Fig. 5.35 Endometrial adenocarcinoma – Pap x100. This field shows a small cluster of adenocarcinoma cells with huge red nucleoli, abnormal chromatin, and foamy cytoplasm.

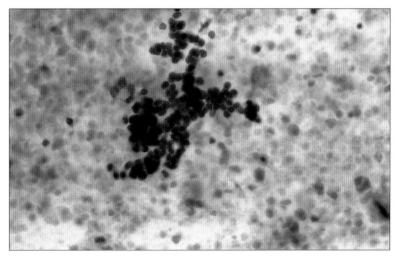

Fig. 5.36 Endometriosis – Pap x40. This aspirate, from an endometriotic cyst of the vagina, shows clusters of small endometrial cells in a background of cellular debris and blood. No siderophages are seen in this field, but they are usually present.

IATROGENIC CHANGES

These are physician-induced effects which are a consequence of diagnostic procedures or treatment, such as curettage, cryocautery, biopsy, laser ablation, chemotherapy and radiotherapy. The cellular changes are detectable on smears and should be recognized, and not mistaken for malignancy.

The first changes to be noted following such procedures are inflammatory, with the characteristic features of nuclear enlargement and margination of chromatin (see Chapter 3), accompanied by masses of neutrophils and large multinucleated histiocytes (Fig. 5.37). Degenerative changes follow, including cytoplasmic vacuolation and amphophilia (Fig. 5.38), and karyorrhexis and karyolysis (Fig. 5.39). Healing takes place by repair, with the smear showing repair cells and fibroblasts, followed by squamous metaplasia which matures into normal squamous epithelium. Smears should not be taken too soon after any diagnostic or curative procedure – 6 months is an acceptable interval.

Radiotherapy produces the most spectacular iatrogenic effects on both benign and malignant cells, the changes being detectable even after 15–20 years. Acute radiation changes include an inflammatory cell infiltrate consisting of neutrophils and histiocytes with accentuation of the features of malignancy. Smears should never be taken at this stage. Chronic radiation changes affect both the nuclei and cytoplasm of cells. The epithelial cells develop bizarre shapes (Fig. 5.40) and exhibit amphophilia (Fig. 5.41). Nuclei appear enlarged, but the chromatin is bland and homogeneous (Fig. 5.42). The nuclei of malignant cells show degenerative changes, including karyorrhexis (Fig. 5.43) and vacuolation. If there is any suspicion that the nuclear changes may represent recurrence, a 5-day course of oestrogen cream should

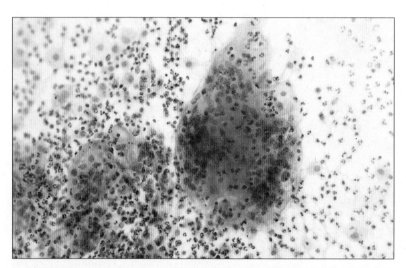

Fig. 5.37 Iatrogenic changes, inflammation – Pap x40. This smear shows the features associated with inflammation following therapeutic procedures to the cervix. Note the large multinucleated histiocyte in the centre of the field, with small histiocytes in the background, accompanied by neutrophil polymorphs.

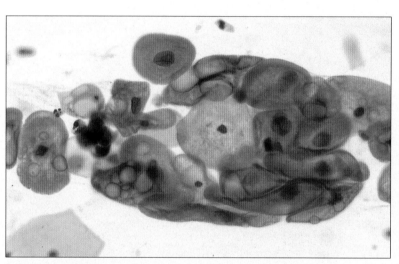

Fig. 5.38 Iatrogenic changes, degeneration – Pap x40. The superficial cell in the centre of this group is surrounded by squamous metaplastic cells showing cytoplasmic vacuolation, amphophilia, and varying degrees of karyolysis.

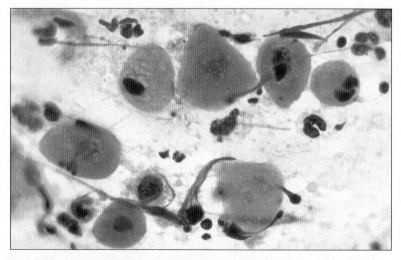

Fig. 5.39 Iatrogenic changes, degeneration – Pap x40. The parabasal cells seen in this field show karyolysis and karyorrhexis, with one cell containing a pyknotic nucleus.

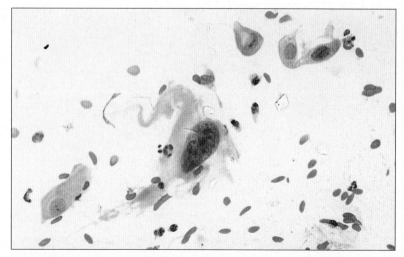

Fig. 5.40 Radiation changes – Pap x40. This smear, from a woman who had radiotherapy for cervical carcinoma 15 years previously, shows an enlarged squamous cell with a bizarre cytoplasmic shape. The nucleus is also enlarged, but its margin is incomplete in places, indicating degeneration rather than dyskaryosis.

be administered before repeating the smear. This matures the epithelium and thus highlights any abnormalities that may be present **(Fig. 5.44)**.

Post-radiation dysplasia is a different entity from recurrent carcinoma of the cervix. It may develop at any time from 6 months to 21 years after treatment of carcinoma of the cervix by radiotherapy. The first warning sign is the change in smear appearance from atrophy to a mature pattern. Dyskaryotic cells of varying severity are noted **(Fig. 5.45)**.

Chemotherapy, such as busulphan treatment, can affect the cells of normal organs, such as the lung, bladder, and cervix. The smear shows a few individual, abnormal enlarged epithelial cells with nuclei that appear dyskaryotic, but the rest of the smear appears perfectly normal. The cell outlines are abnormal **(Fig. 5.46)** and the nuclei often exhibit degenerative changes, such as vacuolation **(Fig. 5.47)**. The changes revert to normal after cessation of treatment.

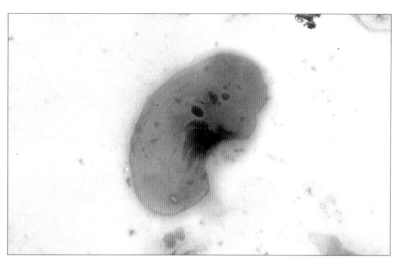

Fig. 5.41 Radiation changes – Pap x40. The cell illustrated here shows amphophilia and degenerative nuclear changes.

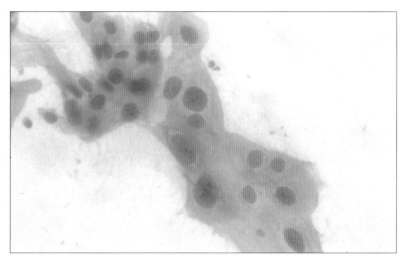

Fig. 5.42 Radiation changes – Pap x40. The nuclei in this group of squamous cells are enlarged, but the chromatin pattern is homogeneous and bland, indicating degenerative changes.

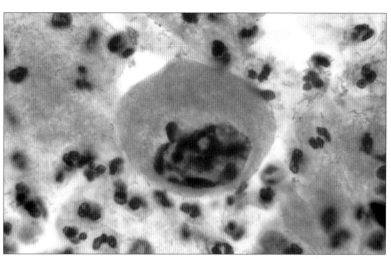

Fig. 5.43 Radiation changes – Pap x100. This dyskaryotic cell shows the effects of radiotherapy – the nuclear margin is incomplete and the chromatin fragments have a structureless, pyknotic appearance.

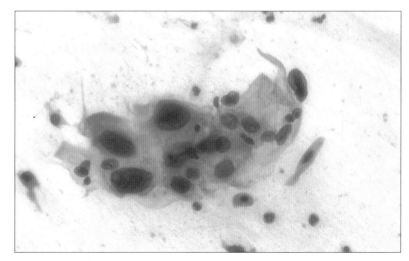

Fig. 5.44 Radiation changes – Pap x40. Occasionally, as in this case, it may be difficult to decide whether the nuclear changes seen (enlargement and irregularity) are due to recurrence of disease. A 5-day course of oestrogen cream applied locally will mature the epithelium and identify clearly any dyskaryotic cells that are present.

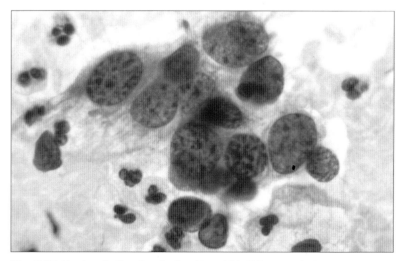

Fig. 5.45 Post-radiation dysplasia – Pap x100. This smear is from a woman who had been treated 15 months previously with radiotherapy for carcinoma of the cervix. The smear shows severely dyskaryotic cells with abnormally clumped chromatin and an intermediate cell, indicating a mature smear pattern, consistent with post-radiation dysplasia.

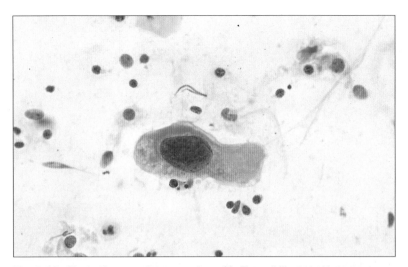

Fig. 5.46 Chemotherapy changes – Pap x40. The cell illustrated here was one of a few seen in a cervical smear that was taken from a woman on busulphan. The cell has an irregular shape and an enlarged, but otherwise bland, nucleus.

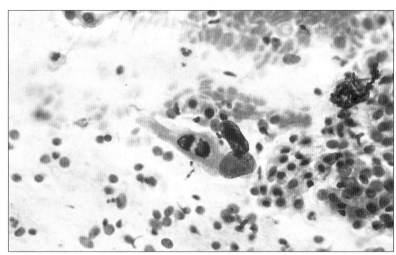

Fig. 5.47 Chemotherapy changes – Pap x40. In the centre of the field are a few enlarged cells with hyperchromatic nuclei, which at first appear dyskaryotic. However, one nucleus has a pale area where the chromatin is homogeneous and the other two nuclei are degenerate.

SUGGESTED READING

Ayer B, Pacey F, Greenberg M. The cytologic diagnosis of adenocarcinoma *in situ* of the cervix uteri and related lesions II. Microinvasive adenocarcinoma. *Acta Cytol* 1988; **32**:318–324.

Ayer B, Pacey F, Greenberg M, Bousfield L. The cytologic diagnosis of adenocarcinoma *in situ* of the cervix uteri and related lesions I. Adenocarcinoma *in situ*. *Acta Cytol* 1987; **31**: 397–411.

Buckley CH, Fox H. Carcinoma of the cervix. In: *Recent Advances in Histopathology, 14*. Edinburgh: Churchill Livingstone; 1989: 63–78.

Cooper K, Herington CS, Lo ES-F, *et al*. Integration of human papillomavirus 16 and 18 in cervical adenocarcinoma. *J Clin Pathol* 1992; **45**: 382–384.

Lee KR, Manna EA, Jones MA. Comparative cytologic features of adenocarcinoma *in situ* of the uterine cervix. *Acta Cytol* 1991; **35**: 117–126.

Pacey F, Ayer B, Greenberg M. The cytologic diagnostic of adenocarcinoma in situ of the cervix uteri and related lesions III. Pitfalls in diagnosis. *Acta Cytol* 1988; **32**: 325–329.

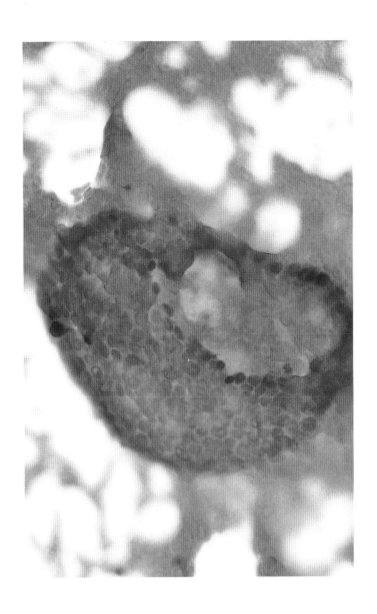

FINE NEEDLE ASPIRATION CYTOLOGY

6

Cytology has made great strides forward in the diagnosis of palpable masses and impalpable lesions. It is no longer the poor relation of histopathology, but rather a refined technique that is broadening horizons, with fine needle aspiration cytology reaching organs that once were only accessible at surgery.

The initial role of cytology was to distinguish between benign and malignant lesions; it was then expanded to elaborate on the type of benign lesion, whether inflammatory or proliferative, and also on the type of malignant lesion. It is now possible to grade certain tumours, such as breast, urothelial, and renal carcinomas, using the results of fine needle aspirates. Fine needle aspiration cytology has made frozen sections and tru-cut biopsies redundant in many centres.

Fine or thin needles have several advantages over core and tru-cut biopsies: they are less painful, sample a wide area, need no anaesthetic, can be reported within half an hour, are more economical and are much less likely to spread tumour cells along the needle track. With practice, excellent sampling is achievable on the part of the aspirator, and confident diagnoses can be made by the cytopathologist.

The practice of cytopathology requires a solid foundation in histopathology and then further training in cytology, including exposure to the multitude of cytological variations seen in every pathological condition. The best way to learn is to examine as much material as possible, because even normal tissues vary enormously. It is not possible to recognize abnormality unless one is familiar with normal appearances; hence, every site discussed in the following chapters starts with a description of normal cells before proceeding to the abnormalities. Looking at marked slides is not as good a method of learning as screening unmarked slides. The diagnostic process of cytopathology is quite different from that of histopathology, as the latter examines patterns (usually under low power)

and the former examines cells, usually under high power (even using oil immersion for difficult cases).

Methods used to procure fine needle aspiration samples vary widely. In many centres, clinicians perform the aspirate and send the sample to the cytopathology laboratory. Increasingly, however, the aspirate is taken by the cytopathologist, who then has the added dimension of the feel of the lesion to help in making a diagnosis. In busy laboratories, the cytopathologist is responsible for all the routine reporting and may not have the time to perform aspirates. He or she should then ensure that there are written protocols for aspiration, preparation and fixation of smears to maintain high standards (**Fig. 6.1**).

Palpable lesions are sampled more easily than are impalpable ones. The latter, in deep-seated organs such as the liver, adrenal, and kidney, are routinely aspirated by radiologists using computerized axial tomography, while lesions in the breast are sampled with the help of stereotaxis or ultrasound. The size of the fine needle used depends on the technique employed for impalpable lesions. With palpable masses, the finer the needle used, the better the sample obtained. A 23-gauge needle is frequently used, but a 25- or 27-gauge needle is often more effective because less bleeding is induced. The mass can be sampled either by the capillary action method, in which the needle is inserted and moved within the lesion with no suction being applied, or by aspirating with a syringe (attached to a syringe holder if preferred). The capillary method is advocated for vascular lesions and thyroid lumps. It is not necessary to use local anaesthetic; in fact, it is preferable not to do so in case it affects the cells being sampled.

Some air should be drawn into the syringe before attaching the needle. The skin is cleansed, and the lesion is then immobilized with the fingers of one hand while the needle is inserted through the skin into the lesion. Once the needle is in place, suction can be applied, moving the needle in several different directions within the lesion without removing it from the skin (**Fig. 6.2**). Suction should cease when blood or fluid is seen in the hub of the syringe, as any cells that enter the syringe are difficult to retrieve. The needle is then withdrawn and a drop of the aspirate expelled gently on to the centre of the already labelled slide. If a cytotechnologist is at hand, the material can be spread in the same way as a blood film. There are other methods, such as using a cover slip to spread the aspirate, which work with practice. The simplest method, which is also the least destructive to the cells, is to use a microbiology loop to rapidly, but gently, spread the material in a circular, controlled fashion in the centre of the slide (**Figs 6.3, 6.4**). The advantages of the loop-spreading method are shown in **Figure 6.5**. It is important that too much material should not be expelled on to

---

Fine needle aspiration method

1. Fill in clinical details on request card.

2. Label frosted ends of two glass slides in pencil with patient's name, date of birth, and WF (wet-fixed) or AD (air-dried).

3. Prepare Coplin jar or other container with alcohol for fixation, and label a universal container.

4. Clean skin over lesion, immobilize lump, and follow procedure 5 or 6 below.

5. **Capillary action:** Insert a needle alone (23-, 25-, or 27-gauge) through the skin into the mass, and move the needle in different directions within lesion. Withdraw the needle, attach a syringe containing 2 ml of air, and prepare smear as in 7 below.

6. **Aspiration:** Insert a needle attached to a syringe containing 2 ml of air and sample the mass as described in 5 using suction. Stop aspirating when fluid is seen in the hub of the syringe and withdraw the needle.

7. Expel one drop of aspirate on to the centre of the glass slide labelled WF, and spread with a microbiology loop gently and rapidly. Immerse **immediately** in alcohol and leave for 15 minutes.

8. Prepare a second smear with another drop of aspirate on the slide labelled AD and wave rapidly to dry.

9. Detach the needle from the syringe, draw 1–2 ml of alcohol into syringe, re-attach the needle, and gently flush alcohol through needle into the labelled universal container.

10. Send wet-fixed and air-dried slides in separate boxes with the universal container and request form to the cytopathology laboratory.

Fig. 6.1 Fine needle aspiration method.

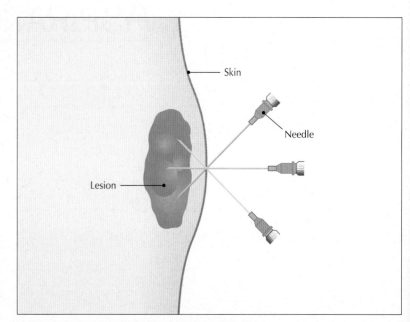

Fig. 6.2 Sampling technique for palpable lesions.

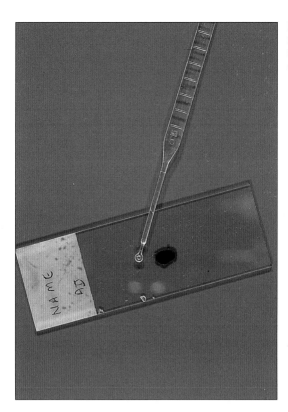

Fig. 6.3 The microbiology loop used for spreading aspirates.

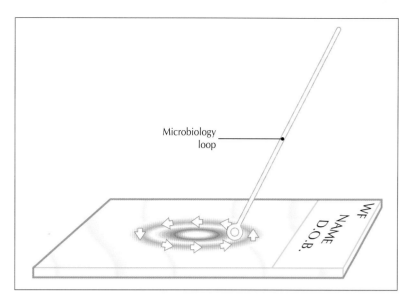

Fig. 6.4 Spreading technique using a microbiology loop.

Smear made with a microbiology loop

Cell clusters

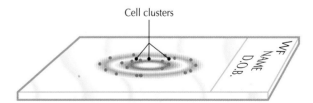

1. Controlled spread of material in the centre of the slide with even scattering of cells

2. Cells not damaged by plastic loop

3. Material not too thinly spread so less likely to air-dry

4. If too much material expelled on first slide, loop can be used to transfer small amounts to clean glass slides and prepare additional smears

Smear made with a glass slide

Cell clusters

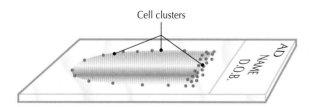

1. Difficult technique with most of the cells at the edges of the smear

2. Cells easily damaged by vigorous smearing

3. Much of the smear is thinly spread, therefore air-dries very quickly

4. Difficult to transfer material with a glass slide

Fig. 6.5 Comparison of spreading techniques.

the slide as it will flow off the edges. **Figure 6.6** demonstrates the appearances of stained smears spread by various techniques.

Once the smear has been spread it is imperative that it is fixed immediately, preferably by immersion into a Coplin or other jar containing alcohol, or by flooding the slide with fixative, or by spray fixation (**Figs 6.7, 6.8**). The slide should be in contact with alcohol for 15 minutes before it is ready to be despatched to the laboratory, either wet, in a leak-proof container, or dry, in a slide box. While the smear is being fixed the second slide should be prepared in the same way, using the material remaining in the needle, and rapidly waved to dry it. A gently blowing hair dryer on a cool setting may be used for this purpose. The needle is then disconnected from the syringe, alcohol (1–2 ml) drawn into the syringe, and the needle reconnected and gently rinsed into a universal container to collect any material that has remained in the needle (**Fig. 6.9**). In some centres this is the only way aspirates are sent to the laboratory, in fluid, as this eliminates the possibility of poorly prepared smears. This technique, however, means that no air-dried slides can be prepared and the pattern of cell clustering seen on normal smears is lost. In our experience, the first two smears prepared contain most of the diagnostic material (unless a lot of blood is aspirated into the syringe) and the subsequent needle washings contain the remaining cells, so that no part of the aspirate is wasted. The air-dried and wet-fixed smears should be transported in separate slide boxes to the laboratory (**Fig. 6.10**).

When the aspirate is performed by the cytopathologist and reported in the clinic, the aspirate can be repeated immediately if it is inadequate. However, if clinicians perform the aspirate and there is no technical help available to perform a DiffQuik stain for cellularity, a useful alternative is to use a simple toluidine blue staining method (**Fig. 6.11**). Clinicians can perform this test to check whether

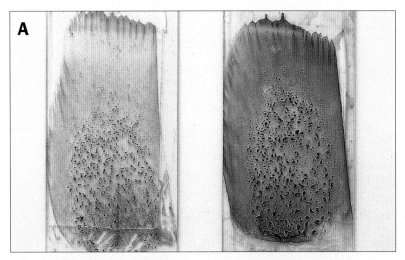

Fig. 6.6 Stained smears prepared by different techniques. Fig. 6.6A demonstrates smears prepared by staff trained in haematology. The dark dots are clusters of cells which are evenly spread. However, most aspirators cannot prepare such good smears and the material tends to flow off the edges of the slide.

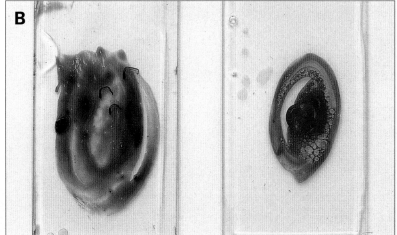

Fig. 6.6B demonstrates the types of smears produced using a microbiology loop. The material is in the centre of the slide, so easily screened when scanty and there is no danger of any artefact due to air-drying.

Fixation methods

1. Immerse prepared slide in alcohol (75%, 90%, or 95%) in a Coplin jar or leak-proof slide container and leave for 15 minutes.

2. Flood slide with alcohol or cervical smear fixative after laying it down on a flat surface and leave for 15 minutes or until dry.

3. Hold spray fixative can 15–30 cm away from slide and spray gently. Leave to dry.

Fig. 6.7 Fixation methods.

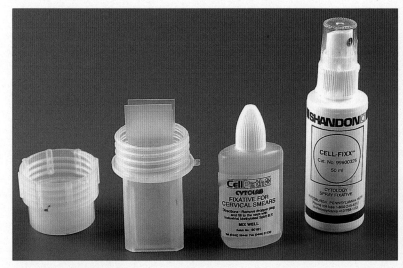

Fig. 6.8 Types of fixatives.

the aspirate is cellular or needs repeating. With toluidine blue cells stain blue, and mucin and stroma stain pink. The great advantage of this method is that the smear can then be replaced in alcohol and sent to the laboratory for a Papanicolaou stain.

In the laboratory, wet-fixed smears are stained using the Papanicolaou method, which has several advantages (Fig. 6.12). The air-dried smears are stained with a modification of the Romanowsky method – the May Grunwald Giemsa stain. If an immediate report is desired, wet-fixed smears are stained using a rapid Papanicolaou method (Fig. 6.13). Another rapid staining method that is used is the DiffQuik stain on wet-fixed material, but we find the rapid Papanicolaou method superior to this. For those who prefer interpreting air-dried smears the DiffQuik stain is useful. The needle washings are prepared using a cytospin, one slide is stained with the Papanicolaou technique, and the others are stored for immunocytochemical stains and research purposes.

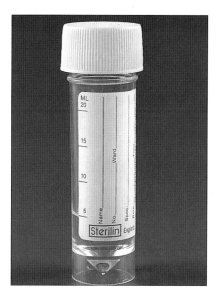

Fig. 6.9 Universal container for needle washings.

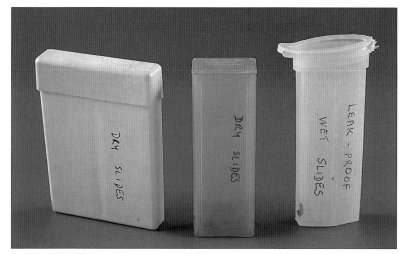

Fig. 6.10 Slide transport boxes.

Toluidine blue rapid staining method

1. Fix smear immediately in alcohol for 30 seconds.

2. Place slide in 1% toluidine blue in 20% alcohol for 10 seconds.

3. Rinse in tap water.

4. Dry back of slide and examine under the microscope for cellularity.

5. Replace slide in alcohol for 10 minutes before staining by the Papanicolaou method.

Fig. 6.11 Toluidine blue rapid staining method. Adapted from the protocol used in the Edinburgh Breast Clinic.

Wet-Fixed	Air-Dried
Stained by the Papanicolaou method	Stained by the May Grunwald Giemsa method
The cells remain three dimensional	The cells flatten out and enlarge
Cells within clusters can be seen on focusing	Cells within clusters are difficult to see clearly
Cytoplasm stains pale blue and is transluscent	Cytoplasm stains blue to pale purple, and is dense
Nucleus stains a bluish purple	Nucleus stains purple
Nuclear margins sharply defined	Nuclear margins not as sharp
Chromatin pattern clearly visible	Chromatin pattern not as well seen
Nucleoli blue or red	Nucleoli seen as pale areas
Apocrine cells have red granular cytoplasm	Apocrine cells have blue granular cytoplasm
Erythrocytes stain red	Erythrocytes stain grey
Altered blood stains deep red	Altered blood stains blue–black
Mucin stains pale pink or blue	Mucin stains bright pink
Keratin stains bright refractile orange	Keratin stains azure blue
Stroma stains pale blue	Stroma stains bright pink
Hyaline material stains pale pink	Hyaline material stains bright pink/purple
Haemosiderin stains greenish yellow	Haemosiderin stains bluish black
Melanin stains greenish black	Melanin stains bluish black
Calcium stains dark red	Calcium stains deep purple
Colloid stains pale pinkish yellow	Colloid stains mauve to deep blue
Bile stains bright yellowish green	Bile stains bluish black

Fig. 6.12 Comparison of Papanicolaou and May Grunwald Giemsa stains.

With the Papanicolaou stain, the wet-fixed cells, which remain three-dimensional, display subtle variations in chromatin pattern, nucleoli are clearly visible, and the cytoplasm is translucent (**Fig. 6.14**). This enables close examination of all the cells at various levels within the clusters. Architectural patterns, such as bowl-shaped arrangements of cells, are clearly seen in wet-fixed smears (**Fig. 6.15**). The May Grunwald Giemsa method stains nuclei purple so that cells are obvious in a scanty aspirate. However, nuclear details, such as chromatin pattern and nucleoli, are not always visible (**Fig. 6.16**).

Reports of fine needle aspirates should not be limited to a brief 'benign' or 'malignant'. It is important to mention the cellularity (whether scanty, moderate or cellular), and the preservation of the specimen (whether well or poorly preserved) and whether it is heavily blood-stained. The types of cells present are then described and the appropriate diagnosis is given. Attention should be drawn to the absence of clinical details, if appropriate, as this has a bearing on the final diagnosis. For example, knowing that the patient is pregnant or lactating aids the interpretation of a difficult breast aspirate. Even benign reports can provide the clinician with important information; for instance, the presence of epithelioid histiocytes in a lymph node aspirate may be the only clue to a granulomatous process.

Inadequate specimens are inevitable unless a few experts only perform all the aspirates. When describing a sample as inadequate the reason must be made clear, i.e., the specimen contains only blood, or is too poorly preserved, or contains too few cells for reliable assessment. Generally, the presence of five to six clusters of well-preserved epithelial cells is essential for an aspirate to be adequate. Obviously, when lipomas or lymph nodes are aspirated, epithelial cells need not be present for the sample to be adequate. If the samples are consistently poorly preserved, it is often helpful for the pathologist to attend and demonstrate good techniques when the next aspirate is performed.

Place fixed smear in the following stains:	
1. 70% alcohol and rinse.	8. Alcohol and rinse.
2. Water and rinse.	9. EA 50 for 1.5 minutes.
3. Haematoxylin for 6 seconds.	10. Alcohol and rinse.
4. Running water for 2–3 minutes.	11. Alcohol and rinse.
5. Alcohol and rinse.	12. Xylene and rinse.
6. Alcohol and rinse.	13. Xylene and rinse.
7. OG 6 for 1 minute.	The staining times can be reduced if necessary

Fig. 6.13 Rapid Papanicolaou method.

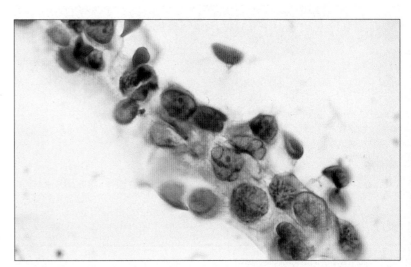

Fig. 6.14 Staining characteristics – Pap x100. The cells seen in this field demonstrate the translucency of cytoplasm and clarity of nuclear detail obtained with this stain.

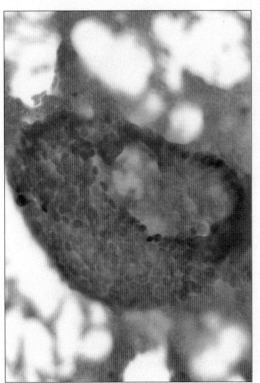

Fig. 6.15 Cell arrangement – Pap x40. These benign ductal cells from a benign proliferative breast lesion are in the form of a bowl with a well-defined opening. Three-dimensional architecture is well preserved with wet fixation.

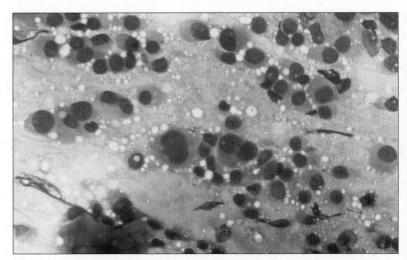

Fig. 6.16 Staining characteristics – MGG x40. These carcinoma cells in a breast aspirate have dark purple nuclei which are easily seen, but the more subtle nuclear characteristics are not well-defined.

BREAST SCREENING CYTOLOGY

Fine needle aspiration cytology is a particularly useful tool in the diagnosis of impalpable mammographic abnormalities as well as the more obvious lesions. There are well-defined national guidelines in the UK for reporting breast cytology specimens. These include the use of reporting categories C1 to C5, where C1 indicates inadequate or unsatisfactory specimens, C2 normal breast aspirates or benign lesions, such as cysts or fibroadenoma, C3 lesions which show cytological atypia, but are probably benign, C4 lesions which are suspicious of malignancy, and C5 an unequivocally malignant diagnosis.

Reporting of breast cases is thus standardized, which is important for the National Breast Screening Programme as women have their mammograms and cytology performed at Regional Assessment Centres and the surgery sometimes performed at their local hospitals. The procedures followed to report breast screening cytology can be used for aspirates from clinically detected breast lesions.

C1 aspirates are repeated if the mammographic or clinical features cause concern. C3 cases have early repeat mammograms and aspiration cytology if the other two modalities are normal, C4 specimens are repeated if the sample contains only a few abnormal cells or poorly preserved but suspicious cells. All C5 cases, and those in the other categories for which the mammographic or clinical impression is of malignancy, are referred to the breast surgeon. A C2 result enables the patient to return to routine three-yearly screening. Surgery is not performed on the basis of a C5 report if the other two modalities are normal.

An important element in the breast screening process is communication between the various disciplines. A weekly meeting between the radiologists, radiographers and cytopathologists is extremely useful for deciding patient management in the case of screen-detected lesions, especially the suspicious ones (C3 and C4). A weekly meeting of the breast team including radiologists, cytopathologists, histopathologists, surgeon, oncologist and breast care nurse is an excellent forum for clinico–pathological correlation and audit. These meetings have the added bonus of providing the cytopathologists with the opportunity to discuss problems with smear preparation and fixation and to recommend solutions.

SUGGESTED READING

Anderson JB, Webb AJ. Fine needle aspiration biopsy and the diagnosis of thyroid cancer. *Br J Surg* 1987; **74:** 292–296.

Christ ML, Haja J. Intranuclear cytoplasmic inclusions (invaginations) in thyroid aspirations. *Acta Cytol* 1979; **23:** 327–331.

Dixon JM, Lamb J, Anderson TJ. Fine needle aspiration of the breast: Importance of the aspirator. *Lancet* 1983; **2 (8349):** 564.

Elston CW, Ellis I0. Pathology and breast screening. Invited review. *Histopathology* 1990; **16:** 109–118.

Frable WJ. Fine needle aspiration biopsy: A review. *Hum Pathol* 1983; **14:** 9–28.

Kline TS. Survey of aspiration biopsy cytology of the breast. Review article. *Diagn Cytopathol* 1991; **7:** 98–105.

NHS. *Breast Screening Programme Guidelines for Cytology Procedures and Reporting in Breast Cancer Screening.* Sheffield: NHS; 1993: NHSBSP publication no. 22.

Zajdela A, Zillhardt P, Vuillemot N. Cytological diagnosis by fine needle sampling without aspiration. *Cancer* 1987; **59:** 1201–1205.

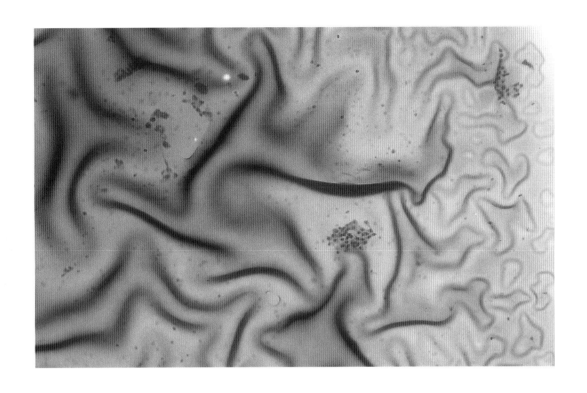

THE THYROID GLAND

7

THE THYROID GLAND

The thyroid gland consists of two lateral lobes connected by an isthmus (**Fig. 7.1**). When enlarged it is easily palpable and therefore accessible to fine needle aspiration techniques. Interpretation of the aspirate is always enhanced by clinical details, such as the age of the patient, symptoms, and description of the lesion (whether it is a solitary nodule or a diffuse enlargement, whether it is tender, whether it is fixed to adjacent structures, and whether the nodule is hot or cold). The results of any autoimmune studies performed are also helpful in interpreting aspirates, as are ultrasound findings. Diagnostic accuracy is extremely high when the samples are examined by experts.

Aspiration of the thyroid should be performed using as fine a needle as possible, for example a 25- or even a 27-gauge needle. Vascular lesions are best sampled using a technique developed in France, that of capillary action without suction. The needle, with no syringe attached, is inserted into the immobilized lesion and moved in several different directions within the mass without withdrawing the needle from the skin. After several passes have been made the needle is then withdrawn, a syringe with a small amount of air in it attached, and the aspirate gently expelled on to the centre of a glass slide. If the lesion is cystic, it is preferable to use a syringe and a slightly larger needle, such as 23-gauge, for aspiration. Suction may be necessary to obtain sufficient material from nodules or thyroid masses which feel solid on palpation. It is essential to stop suction as soon as material is seen at the hub of the needle. Once the aspirated material enters the barrel of the syringe it is impossible to retrieve it.

There are several methods of spreading the material on the slide: by using a second glass slide and preparing a smear in the form of a blood film, by using a cover slip, by using the needle itself, or by using a microbiology loop to allow controlled spread of the material on the slide. The last technique is the simplest one and requires little or no expertise. If much blood is aspirated, great care should be taken not to expel too much material on to the slide. In expert hands (Lowhagen, personal observation) the blood is removed from the slide by carefully using a piece of gauze, leaving only the solid cellular material. This technique can be mastered with practice.

After spreading the aspirate quickly the slide is waved in the air to achieve rapid drying. In some centres a hair dryer is used on a cold setting for this purpose. Any remaining material can be used to make wet-fixed slides and the needle is then gently rinsed with alcohol (1 ml) into a universal container, so that no cells are lost. Air-dried smears stained with May Grunwald Giemsa are best for thyroid aspirates, as is demonstrated later. However, wet-fixed smears also show features that are useful and are always complementary to the air-dried samples. Wet-fixed smears are stained by the Papanicolaou technique, familiar to those involved in reporting cervical smears. The needle washings are spun down and stained with the Papanicolaou stain. The relative merits of each staining method are detailed in **Figure 7.2**.

The normal thyroid gland is composed of numerous colloid-filled follicles of various sizes lined by cuboidal epithelial cells (**Fig. 7.3**). An aspirate from a normal thyroid shows colloid which stains blue or purple on the air-dried smear and pale pink to orange in the wet-fixed sample. The appearance of colloid is variable. It may be seen as discrete, sharply defined blobs (**Figs 7.4, 7.5**), or as ill-defined, wispy material (**Figs 7.6, 7.7**), and sometimes as a layer of pale blue, varnish-like material in the background in air-dried smears. The aspirate also contains small groups of epithelial cells with delicate cytoplasm and round monomorphic nuclei. The bland chromatin pattern is best appreciated on the wet-fixed smear (**Fig. 7.8**), as air-drying tends to obscure the chromatin detail of these small cells (**Fig. 7.9**).

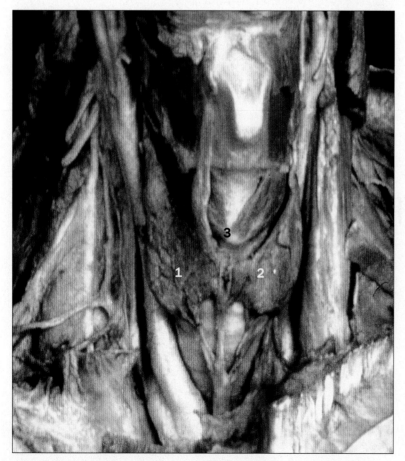

Fig. 7.1 Thyroid gland – This illustration shows the two lobes of the thyroid gland, right (1) and left (2), which are connected by a bridge of thyroid tissue called the isthmus (3). (Reproduced with permission from *A Colour Atlas of Human Anatomy*, 3rd ed. RMH McMinn, RT Hutchings, J Pegington and P Abrahams, Mosby–Wolfe, 1993.)

Features	May Grunwald Giemsa	Papanicolaou
Colloid	Dark blue to purple	Pale pink to orange
Thin colloid	Easily seen	Difficult to identify
Cytoplasm	Blue, translucent	Pale blue, transparent
Nuclei	Purple	Bluish purple
Chromatin	Dense	Details identifiable
Stroma	Bright pink	Pale pink or blue
Haemosiderin	Bluish black	Greenish yellow
Erythrocytes	Grey	Red
Fire flares	Visible	Difficult to identify
Psammoma body	Dark blue	Reddish purple
Nuclear grooves	Not visible	Clearly defined
Amyloid	Purplish blue, birefringent	Pale blue, birefringent
Keratin	Azure blue	Refractile orange
Parathyroid adenoma	Background secretion ill-defined	Clearly visible background secretion

Fig. 7.2 Staining characteristics.

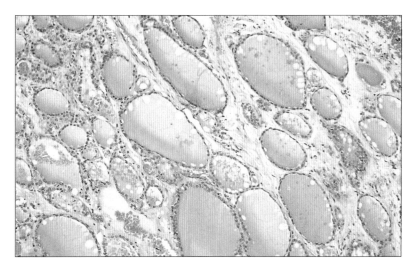

Fig. 7.3 Histology of normal thyroid gland – H&E x10. This section of normal thyroid shows colloid-filled follicles of different sizes, lined by cuboidal epithelial cells. The calcitonin-secreting C cells are not identifiable on H&E-stained sections.

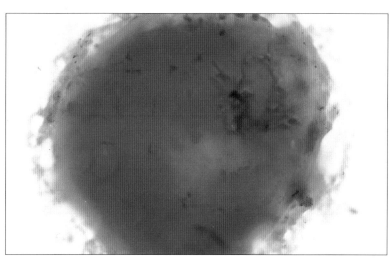

Fig. 7.4 Colloid – MGG x40. On air-dried material treated with May Grunwald Giemsa, the colloid stains a deep blue or purplish blue. In this field the colloid is of the 'thick' variety, which is easily identified. Colloid is not always as well-defined as in this illustration.

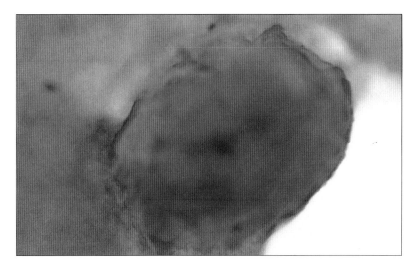

Fig. 7.5 Colloid – Pap x40. In wet-fixed smears, colloid stains a pale, translucent, pinkish shade, as illustrated in this field. Problems arise with heavily blood-stained aspirates, as the bright red erythrocytes obscure the delicate collections of colloid.

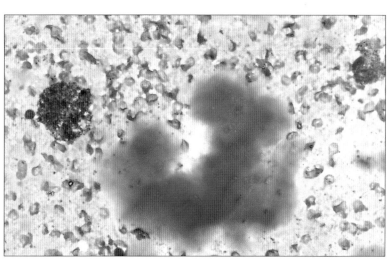

Fig. 7.6 Colloid – MGG x40. The colloid seen here is of the paler, wispy, or fluffy type with poorly defined edges. It is a pale mauve in colour and may be overlooked unless present in substantial amounts.

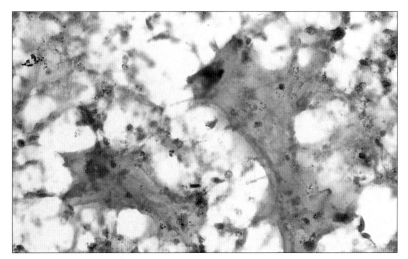

Fig. 7.7 Colloid – Pap x40. This field illustrates delicate, wispy colloid in a wet-fixed, Papanicolaou-stained thyroid aspirate. The pale, pinkish blue colloid may be mistaken for debris in this preparation.

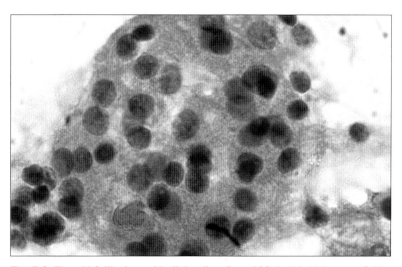

Fig. 7.8 Thyroid follicular epithelial cells – Pap x100. In this high-power field the epithelial cells are seen to have delicate, pinkish blue cytoplasm, round nuclei, a vesicular chromatin pattern, and a small but visible nucleolus. The cytoplasmic margins of individual cells are not well-defined.

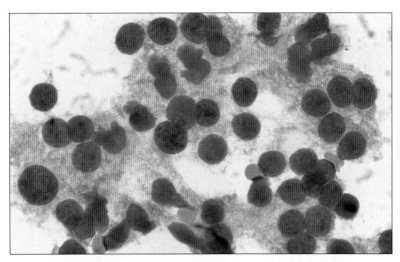

Fig. 7.9 Thyroid follicular epithelial cells – MGG x100. With May Grunwald Giemsa the epithelial cell nuclei stain a deep pinkish purple. They are round with bland, almost structureless chromatin and just visible nucleoli. The cytoplasm is pale blue and ill-defined in this field.

COLLOID GOITRE, MULTINODULAR GOITRE AND COLLOID NODULE

These entities basically show the same cytological features to differing degrees: an abundance of colloid, varying numbers of clusters of follicular epithelial cells, bare nuclei in the background, wisps of stroma, and foamy macrophages. The relative amounts of these constituents depend on whether the lesion is predominantly cellular (e.g., an adenomatous or hyperplastic goitre), whether it is composed mainly of colloid-distended follicles, or whether cystic degenerative changes have occurred. However, problems in interpretation may arise when the aspirate is hypercellular, mimicking a neoplastic process.

A histological section of a colloid nodule shows typical features, with colloid-filled follicles of varying sizes and degenerative changes (**Fig. 7.10**).

The thyroid epithelial cells seen in aspirates are uniform with vesicular nuclei, smooth nuclear margins, and delicate cytoplasm. The sheets may be extremely

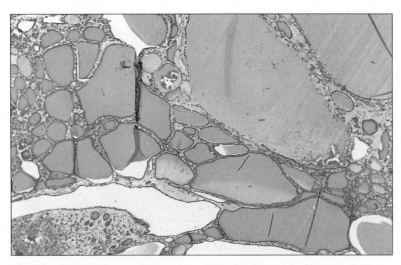

Fig. 7.10 Histology of colloid goitre – H&E x10. This section from a colloid goitre of thyroid shows greatly distended follicles filled with colloid, and other smaller follicles, as well as areas of cystic and degenerative change and small areas of haemorrhage.

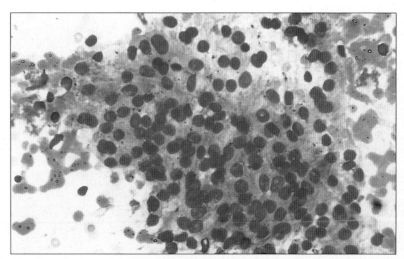

Fig. 7.11 Sheet of benign follicular epithelial cells – MGG x40. Illustrated here is a large sheet or group of benign epithelial cells with delicate cytoplasm. The nuclei appear to be of the same size as the grey erythrocytes in the background.

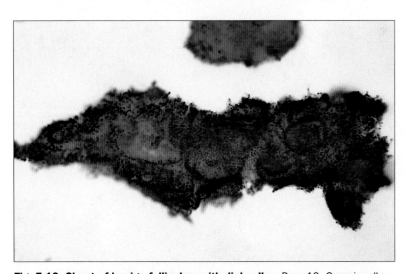

Fig. 7.12 Sheet of benign follicular epithelial cells – Pap x10. Occasionally, quite large cohesive groups of epithelial cells may be seen in aspirates from colloid goitres, as in this field. It is unusual to see no bare nuclei or colloid in the background.

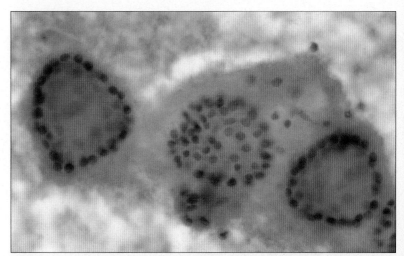

Fig. 7.13 Intact follicles – Pap x40. A good, well-spread aspirate not infrequently contains intact follicles composed of benign follicular epithelial cells. They vary in size and number, and are sometimes situated within large sheets of epithelial cells. It is not possible in this field to discern colloid within the follicles, as there is much blood in the background, obscuring the delicate hue of colloid stained by the Papanicolaou method.

large (**Figs 7.11, 7.12**) or in the form of small groups. Not infrequently, intact acini are aspirated. These are unmistakable as they are sharply defined and spherical, better appreciated on the wet-fixed Papanicolaou-stained smear (**Figs 7.13, 7.14**). These intact follicles should not be mistaken for multinucleated histiocytes. The latter have delicate, ill-defined cytoplasm and are not normally perfectly spherical (see **Figures 7.30 and 7.31**). Intact follicles containing colloid may be seen (**Figs 7.15, 7.16**). Epithelial cells often lose their cytoplasm and are seen as single, bare nuclei in the background (**Figs 7.17, 7.18**). They may be mistaken for lymphocytes and vice versa, but careful examination of the single cells, under oil immersion if necessary, will show that the lymphocytes have a small rim of cytoplasm and a more pronounced chromatin pattern (see **Figures 7.47 and 7.48**). A feature that is sometimes noted is hyalinized stroma attached to the epithelial cells. This is more readily detectable in the air-dried smear, in which the material stains pink, while it is pale blue and can be missed on the

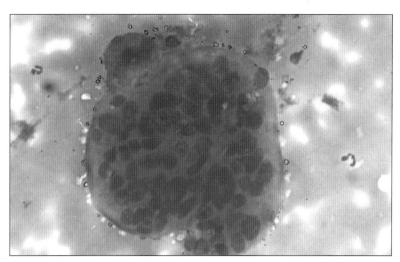

Fig. 7.14 Intact follicle – MGG x40. This illustration shows a well-defined follicle containing numerous benign epithelial cells with indistinguishable cytoplasmic borders. The structure is too sharply demarcated to be a multinucleated giant histiocyte.

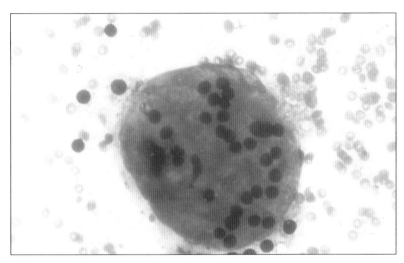

Fig. 7.15 Intact follicle containing colloid – MGG x40. The follicle pictured here shows uniform epithelial cells surrounding colloid. The border of the follicle is sharp and there are a few bare nuclei outside it. As with the case shown in **Figure 7.14**, this should not be confused with a multinucleated giant histiocyte.

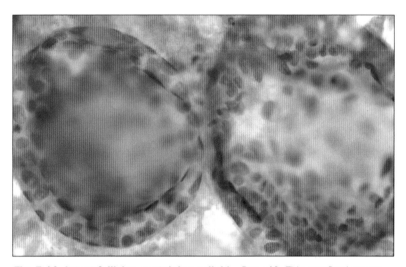

Fig. 7.16 Intact follicles containing colloid – Pap x40. This wet-fixed smear shows two distended follicles containing colloid, surrounded by small uniform epithelial cells. The colloid is pale violet and fairly easily identifiable by its translucent sheen.

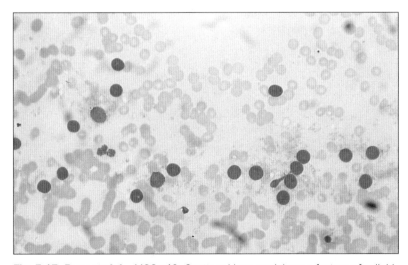

Fig. 7.17 Bare nuclei – MGG x40. Scattered bare nuclei are a feature of colloid goitre. The cytoplasm of the cells is not apparent. The nuclei bear a superficial resemblance to lymphocytes, but the latter can be distinguished by their thin rim of blue cytoplasm in air-dried smears.

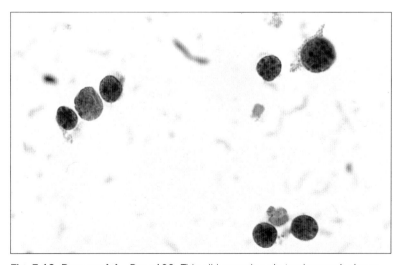

Fig. 7.18 Bare nuclei – Pap x100. This oil immersion photomicrograph shows the details of the bare nuclei seen in aspirates from colloid goitres. The chromatin is well-displayed in the Papanicolaou-stained material. No cytoplasm is apparent, highlighting the difference between these nuclei and lymphocytes.

wet-fixed smear (**Figs 7.19, 7.20**). Askanazy (or Hurthle) cells are occasionally seen in colloid goitre. These cells have abundant cytoplasm, which is well-defined and pale pink on the wet-fixed smear (**Fig. 7.21**) and bluish grey on the air-dried smear (**Fig. 7.22**). Hurthle cells are oncocytic, the cytoplasm being stuffed with mitochondria. Their nuclei are enlarged and may appear atypical, but should not be mistaken for malignancy.

The colloid in these aspirates, while usually abundant, is variable in appearance, from satiny sheets showing folds [best seen in the air-dried smear (**Fig. 7.23**)] to thin sheets exhibiting cracks (**Figs 7.24, 7.25**). Foamy macrophages are almost inevitably present in aspirates from colloid nodules representing degenerative changes. They have pale foamy cytoplasm and nuclei which vary from round to oval to bean-shaped. The nuclei have a sharp margin and a well-defined small nucleolus (**Figs 7.26, 7.27**). In the presence of long-standing haemorrhage the macrophages are seen to contain intracytoplasmic haemosiderin, the granules being a greenish yellow colour in the wet-fixed smear and blue–black in the air-dried smear (**Figs 7.28, 7.29**). Multinucleated giant histiocytes may also be seen. These cells have ill-defined cytoplasmic borders and

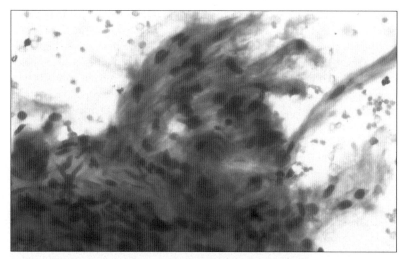

Fig. 7.19 Stromal strands – MGG x40. Stromal fragments stain a bright pinkish purple with May Grunwald Giemsa. Epithelial cells may be seen attached to these stromal strands in colloid goitre.

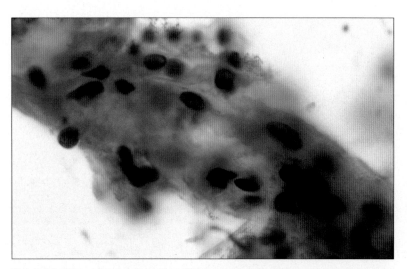

Fig. 7.20 Stromal strands – Pap x100. In wet-fixed preparations, stroma takes on a pink-to-blue tinge with the Papanicolaou stain. It appears more delicate here than in the corresponding air-dried smear shown in **Figure 7.19**. Epithelial cells are seen to be closely associated.

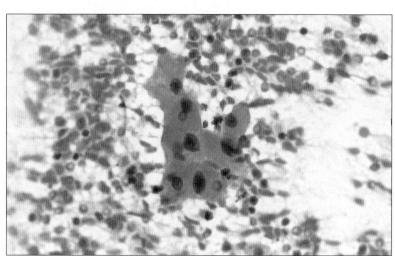

Fig. 7.21 Askanazy (Hurthle cells) – Pap x40. These cells contain numerous mitochondria in their abundant cytoplasm, which stains pink by the Papanicolaou method. The nuclei are somewhat variable in size. The cells may be seen in small groups or may lie singly in aspirates from colloid goitres. They bear a similarity to oncocytic cells in other organs.

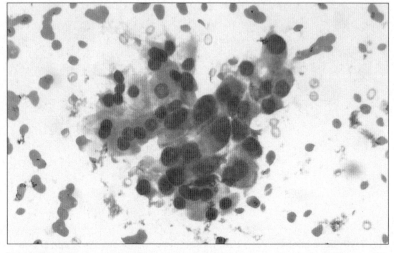

Fig. 7.22 Askanazy (Hurthle cells) – MGG x40. The variability of Askanazy cells is well-illustrated here. The cells have abundant cytoplasm, but the nuclear size is not uniform.

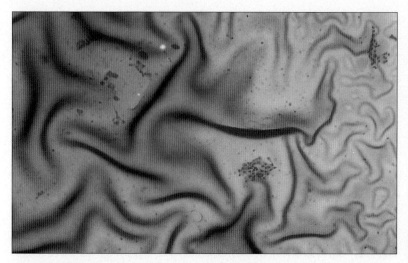

Fig. 7.23 Colloid – MGG x40. Colloid in aspirates from colloid goitres can take many appearances, one of the most attractive resembling a satin sheet draped in folds.

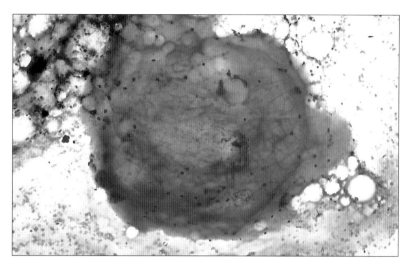

Fig. 7.24 Colloid – MGG x10. This field demonstrates colloid exhibiting 'pavementing', which is just perceptible at this power. Paler fluffy colloid is seen at the periphery.

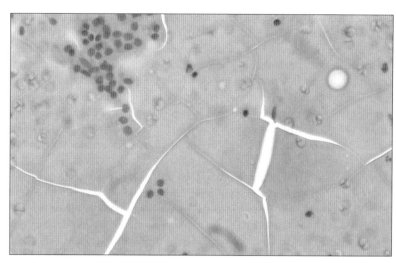

Fig. 7.25 Colloid – Pap x10. The yellowish colloid forming the background of this field would not be noticed except for the obvious cracks seen in its surface. This is one of the disadvantages of the wet-fixed, Papanicolaou-stained smear.

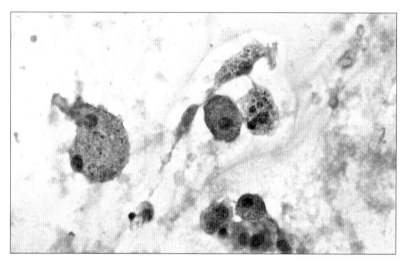

Fig. 7.26 Foamy macrophages – Pap x40. The variation in size of macrophages is well-illustrated here. The cytoplasm is foamy and variable in amount, some containing debris. The cytoplasmic margins are indistinct in areas. The nuclei are small and round in these cells, but are occasionally bean-shaped. Note the debris in the background, which often accompanies cystic degenerative changes in colloid goitres.

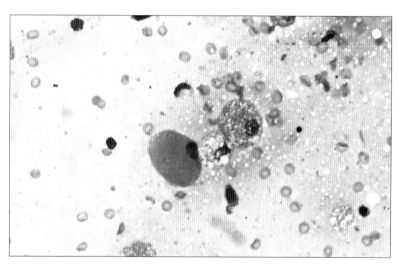

Fig. 7.27 Foamy macrophages – MGG x40. One of the macrophages in this field displays denser cytoplasm than the others, in which the cytoplasm is foamy. A few erythrocytes and bare nuclei are seen in the background.

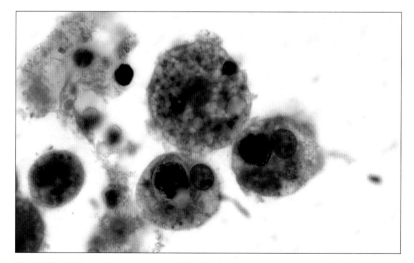

Fig. 7.28 Siderophages – Pap x100. The haemosiderin-laden macrophages shown here have sharply outlined nuclei and foamy cytoplasm containing large granules of greenish yellow haemosiderin. Variation in the size of the macrophages is marked. These cells are an indication of previous haemorrhage.

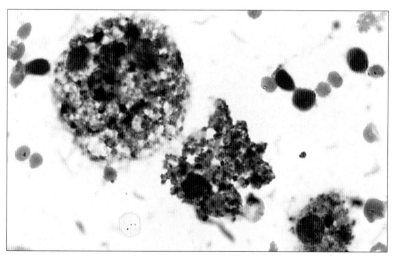

Fig. 7.29 Siderophages – MGG x100. In air-dried smears haemosiderin takes on a bluish black hue with the May Grunwald Giemsa stain. The cells are variable in size and there are some bare nuclei in the background.

scattered nuclei (**Figs 7.30, 7.31**). Even multinucleated histiocytes may be seen to contain haemosiderin (**Figs 7.32, 7.33**).

Cystic degenerative changes are common in multinodular and colloid goitres. The cystic lesions produced may be clinically palpable and can be aspirated, usually producing dark brown or greenish brown fluid. This fluid can be cyto-centrifuged, stained, and shown to contain altered blood, many foamy macrophages, siderophages, and varying amounts of colloid and cholesterol crystals (**Fig. 7.34**). Crystals are best identified by examining a drop of unstained cyst fluid under polarized light. Although they look most spectacular when polarized, these crystals, with their square shapes and missing corners, are readily identified on air-dried smears by examining the edge of the smear where the outlines of the crystals may be seen (**Fig. 7.35**). Indeed, these outlines of cholesterol crystals may also be observed in Papanicolaou-stained wet-fixed smears. The shape of cholesterol crystals in a histological section of thyroid showing degenerative cystic changes, however, is quite different (**Fig. 7.36**). Although oxalate crystals are identifiable in colloid in histological sections (**Fig. 7.37**), they are not readily visualized in cytological preparations.

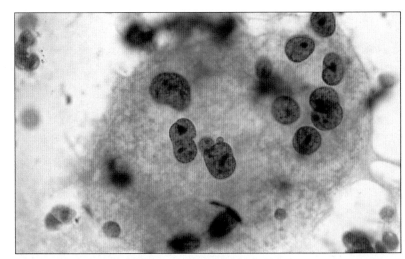

Fig. 7.30 Multinucleated giant histiocyte – Pap x100. This enormous cell shows the characteristic delicate, foamy cytoplasm of histiocytes with scattered nuclei, some round, others bean-shaped, but all exhibiting sharp nuclear margins and conspicuous nucleoli. The cytoplasmic border is indistinct.

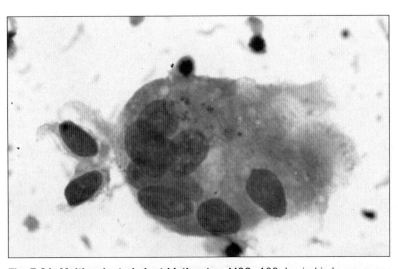

Fig. 7.31 Multinucleated giant histiocyte – MGG x100. In air-dried smears these cells appear to have more substantial cytoplasm, although the cytoplasmic borders are not sharp. The two smaller adjacent cells are also histiocytic.

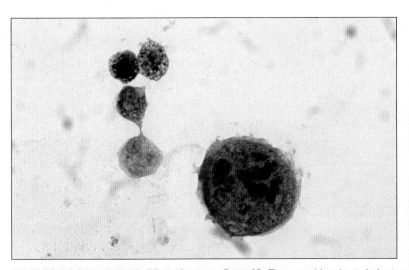

Fig. 7.32 Multinucleated siderophages – Pap x40. These multinucleated giant histiocytic cells act as scavengers, phagocytosing haemosiderin after haemorrhage has occurred. The pigment is also seen in the adjacent small foamy histiocytes.

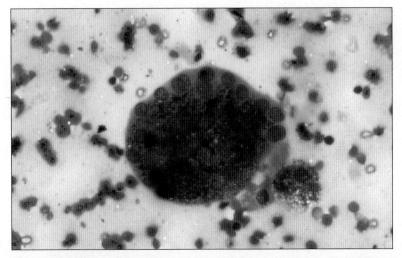

Fig. 7.33 Multinucleated siderophages – MGG x40. Only those nuclei which are at the periphery of the cell are visible, the others being obscured by the heavy load of greenish black pigment.

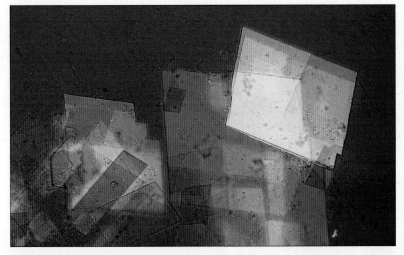

Fig. 7.34 Cholesterol crystals – unstained cyst fluid x40. Examination of thyroid cyst fluid under polarized light is a simple procedure which reveals cholesterol crystals in the event of previous haemorrhage. These are large crystals which are square or envelope-shaped with one missing corner.

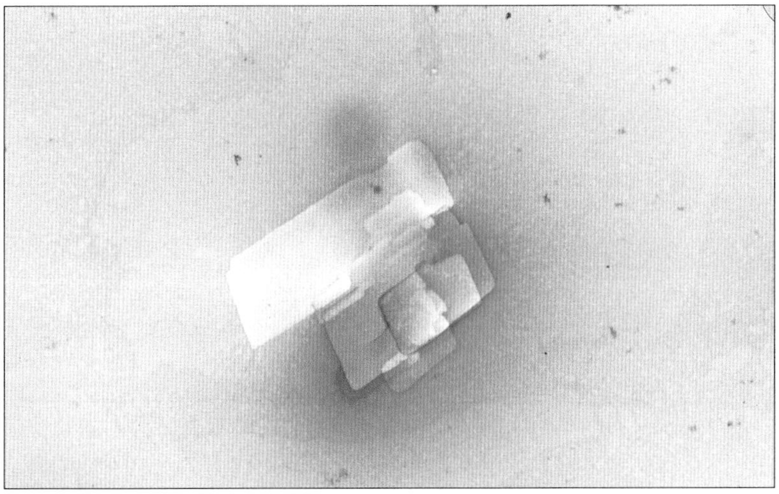

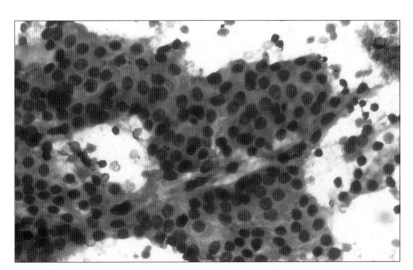

Fig. 7.35 Cholesterol crystals – MGG x40. Cholesterol crystals leave empty spaces corresponding to their shapes in air-dried, May Grunwald Giemsa stained smears. They are usually seen at the edges of the smear, where the material is more thinly spread.

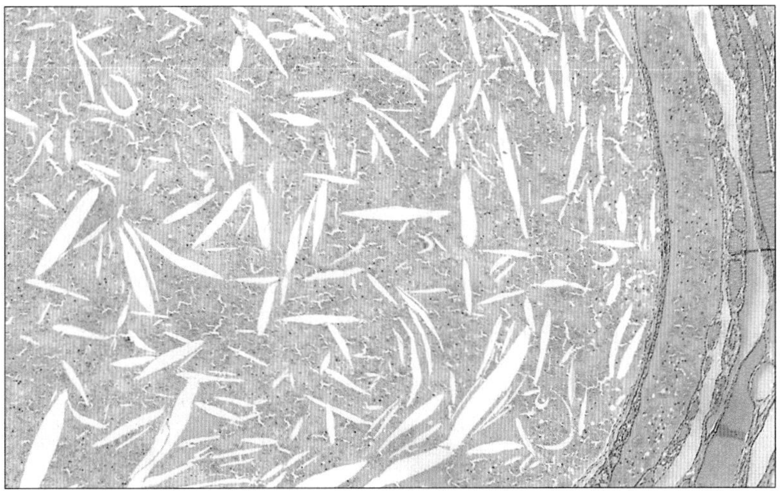

HYPERPLASIA

Hyperplasia of the thyroid can be difficult to diagnose in an aspirate, even when the clinical diagnosis of Graves' disease is known. The epithelial cells are seen in large sheets (**Fig. 7.38**), some of the nuclei showing marked enlargement (**Figs 7.39, 7.40**). A feature often visible is cytoplasmic vacuoles in cells at the periphery of clusters. These appear pale with a pink margin with the May Grunwald Giemsa stain (**Figs 7.41, 7.42**), but are barely perceptible with the Papanicolaou staining technique (**Fig. 7.43**). Psammoma bodies have been noted in aspirates from hyperplastic nodular goitres and care must be taken not to mistake these for papillary carcinoma.

Hyperplastic areas are not infrequently seen in histological sections of thyroid with colloid goitres, and these may also show oncocytic change simulating an oncocytic (Hurthle cell) adenoma (**Fig. 7.44**). This can lead to diagnostic problems with the fine needle aspirate if the predominant cell is the Hurthle cell and the other features of colloid goitre are not well-represented (**Fig. 7.45**).

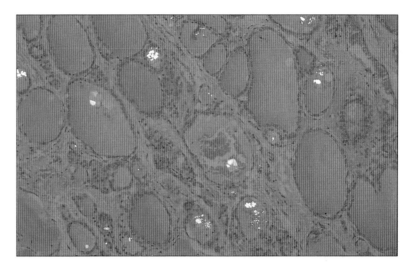

Fig. 7.36 Histology showing cholesterol crystals – H&E x4. Surprisingly, cholesterol crystals seen in histological sections have a totally different shape to those seen in cytological preparations. In the former, they are represented by the large cholesterol clefts left when the crystals are dissolved out during processing.

Fig. 7.37 Histology showing oxalate crystals – H&E x10. Oxalate crystals can be demonstrated in colloid in histological sections, as seen here, but are not as easy to find in cytological preparations, possibly being lost during staining of the smears.

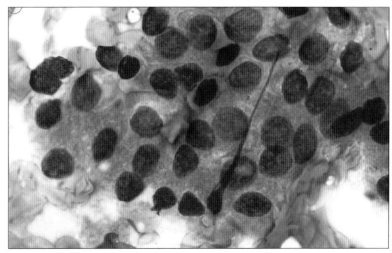

Fig. 7.38 Hyperplasia – MGG x40. The large sheet of epithelial cells seen here is from an aspirate of a thyroid which showed hyperplasia on histology. The features are not diagnostic, but two of the cells at the periphery show vacuolation, an uncommon finding in colloid goitre.

Fig. 7.39 Hyperplasia – MGG x100. In this field is a sheet of hyperplastic thyroid epithelium exhibiting nuclear enlargement and irregularity of nuclear outline. There is a hint of vacuolation in the cytoplasm of some of the cells.

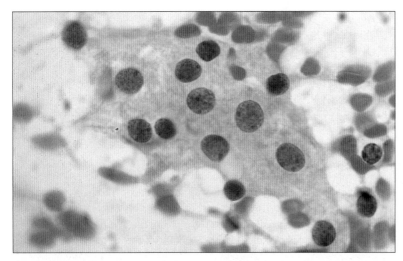

Fig. 7.40 Hyperplasia – Pap x100. The group of epithelial cells pictured here shows enlargement of some of their nuclei with a hint of vacuolation in the cytoplasm.

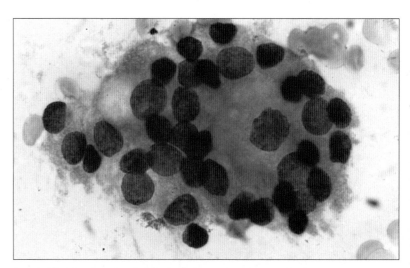

Fig. 7.41 'Fire flares' – MGG x100. Demonstrated here is a cluster of hyperplastic epithelial cells showing a peripheral vacuole bounded by a red margin – the so-called 'fire flare' appearance. The individual nuclei exhibit some variation in size.

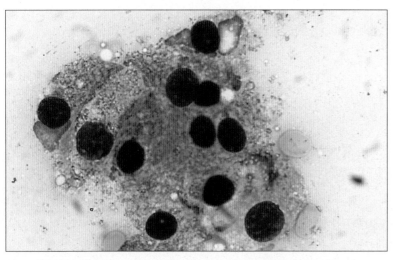

Fig. 7.42 'Fire flares' – MGG x100. This is another example of cells showing vacuoles bounded by red granular margins, indicative of hyperplasia.

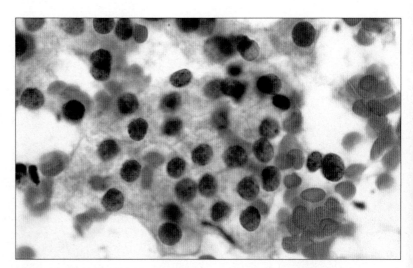

Fig. 7.43 Hyperplasia – Pap x100. These hyperplastic epithelial cells show a hint of vacuolation in their cytoplasm, but no definite 'fire flares'.

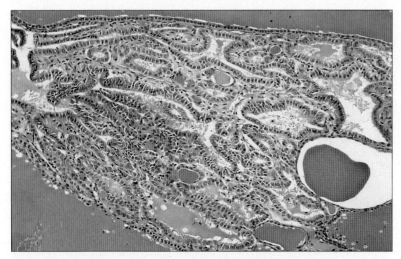

Fig. 7.44 Histology of oncocytic change in colloid goitre – H&E x10. This histological section of a colloid goitre demonstrates an area of oncocytic or Hurthle cell change. If this is the only area sampled by the needle during aspiration, the cytological appearances would be suggestive of a Hurthle cell neoplasm.

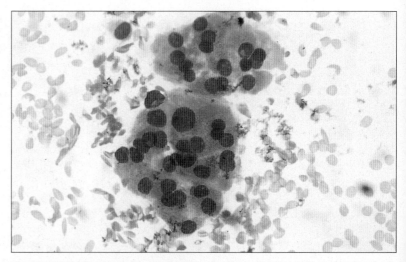

Fig. 7.45 Hurthle cells in colloid goitre – MGG x40. This field shows sheets of Hurthle cells with abundant cytoplasm and nuclei of variable size. There is no evidence of the colloid goitre from which the cells were aspirated. Such smears need to be carefully examined to prevent an incorrect diagnosis of Hurthle cell neoplasia.

LYMPHOCYTIC THYROIDITIS, HASHIMOTO'S THYROIDITIS

In **lymphocytic thyroiditis** the aspirate contains a large number of mixed lymphoid cells. These should not be mistaken for bare thyroid epithelial cell nuclei. Foci of lymphocytic thyroiditis are not infrequently associated with colloid goitres and the cytological features of both conditions are usually apparent in this case.

Hashimoto's thyroiditis shows several typical features. Histological sections show infiltration of the thyroid by lymphocytes, sometimes with fully formed lymphoid follicles, and also multinucleated histiocytes with many Hurthle cells **(Fig. 7.46)**. Very little normal thyroid tissue may be seen, a feature which is reflected in the aspirate because it often contains very little epithelium. There are numerous lymphocytes **(Figs 7.47, 7.48)** and plasma cells, multinucleated histiocytic giant cells **(Figs 7.49, 7.50)**, and, sometimes, epithelioid histiocytes **(Figs 7.51, 7.52)**. A notable feature is the presence of Askanazy cells with their

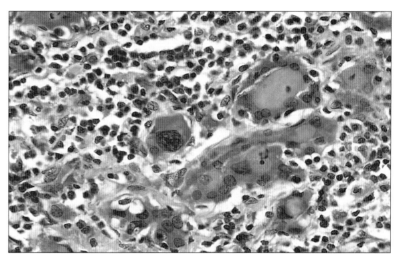

Fig. 7.46 Histology of Hashimoto's thyroiditis – H&E x10. This section shows a few remaining thyroid follicles with many lymphocytes and occasional Askanazy cells with very abnormal nuclei. Fully formed lymphoid follicles are not seen here.

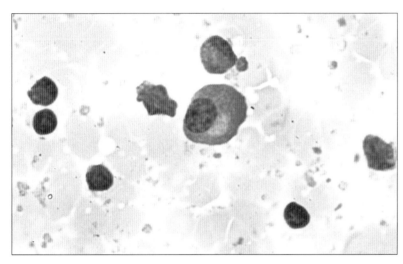

Fig. 7.47 Lymphoid cells in Hashimoto's disease – MGG x40. Normal lymphocytes and a plasma cell are seen in this aspirate from a case of Hashimoto's thyroiditis. One would expect to see the full range of follicle centre cells if lymphoid follicles were aspirated. The lymphocytes show no features to suggest a lymphoma in this case.

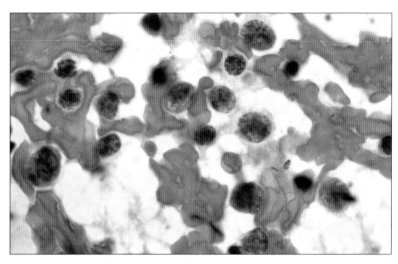

Fig. 7.48 Lymphoid cells in Hashimoto's disease – Pap x100. A range of small and large lymphoid cells occur in this aspirate, suggesting that formed lymphoid follicles were aspirated from this lesion.

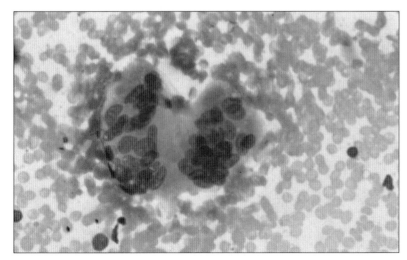

Fig. 7.49 Multinucleated giant cell in Hashimoto's disease – MGG x40. Giant histiocytes are not uncommon in aspirates from Hashimoto's thyroiditis. They show the same features as the multinucleated giant histiocytes seen in colloid goitre. The two cells pictured here have many overlapping nuclei and the cytoplasm is not particularly foamy.

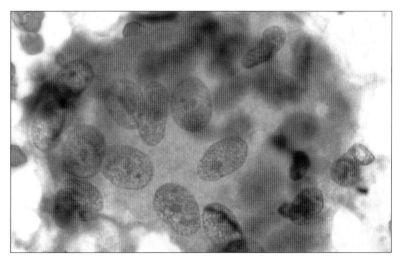

Fig. 7.50 Multinucleated giant cell in Hashimoto's disease – Pap x100. This wet-fixed smear shows a multinucleated histiocyte with sharp nuclear margins and visible nucleoli. The cytoplasm is translucent, rather than foamy.

distinctive cytoplasm and enlarged nuclei (**Figs 7.53, 7.54**). It is important to search for these cells as the abundance of lymphocytes may arouse the suspicion of lymphoma (**Fig. 7.55**).

Reidel's thyroiditis is usually diagnosed clinically and invariably produces an insufficient amount of aspirate for cytological diagnosis.

SUBACUTE (GRANULOMATOUS, DE QUERVAIN'S) THYROIDITIS

The cytological features of this lesion are characteristic. Even under low power, huge multinucleated histiocytes are evident (**Figs 7.56, 7.57**). Under higher magnification these cells are seen to contain tens and occasionally hundreds of nuclei (**Figs 7.58, 7.59**). Inflammatory cells are seen in the background with blobs of thick abundant colloid (**Figs 7.60, 7.61**). Epithelioid histiocytes are more common in this condition than in Hashimoto's disease. These cells have elongated, footprint-shaped nuclei with the delicate cytoplasm of histiocytes and tend to be

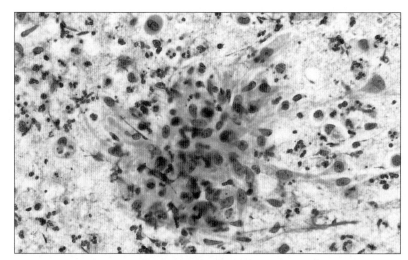

Fig. 7.51 Epithelioid histiocytes – Pap x40. The centre of this field shows a group of epithelioid histiocytes with elongated, footprint-shaped nuclei and delicate cytoplasm. These are easy to miss as they are very pale with the Papanicolaou stain. Note the lymphocytes in the background.

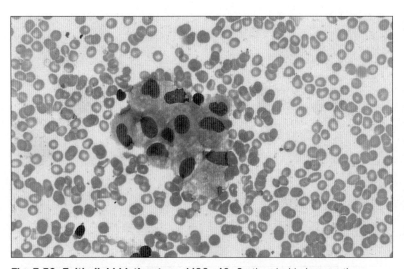

Fig. 7.52 Epithelioid histiocytes – MGG x40. On the air-dried smear the footprint-shape of the nuclei is not as obvious in epithelioid histiocytes. Here they appear slightly elongated and in a small group, suggestive of a granuloma.

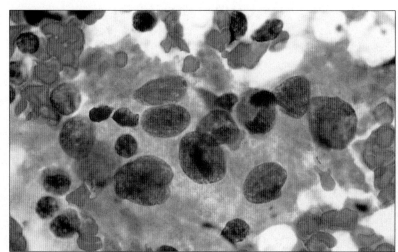

Fig. 7.53 Hurthle cells – Pap x100. The Hurthle cells illustrated here have enormous nuclei and abundant granular pink cytoplasm. There are a few lymphocytes in the background in this aspirate from Hashimoto's thyroiditis.

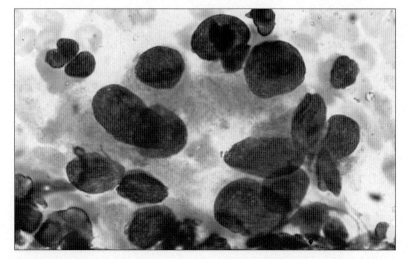

Fig. 7.54 Hurthle cells – MGG x100. The May Grunwald Giemsa stain enhances the enlarged nuclear size of the Hurthle cells seen in **Figure 7.53**. A few lymphocytes are also present.

FEATURES	HASHIMOTO'S THYROIDITIS	LYMPHOMA
Cellularity	Mixture of lympho-cytes and epithelial cells	Mainly lymphoid cells
Askanazy cells	Usually abundant	Not seen
Lymphoid cells	Mixed population	Monomorphic popu-lation
Lymphocytes	Normal	Abnormal
Multinucleated histiocytes	Common	Not seen
Epithelioid histiocytes	Common	Not seen
Colloid	May be seen	Uncommon

Fig. 7.55 Lymphocytic aspirates.

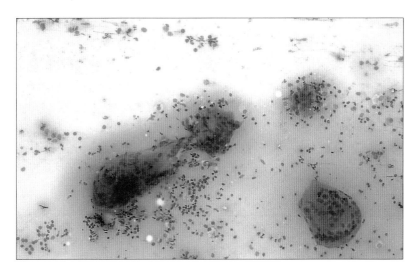

Fig. 7.56 De Quervain's thyroiditis – Pap x10. This low-power view of an aspirate from De Quervain's thyroiditis shows the characteristic messy background and huge multinucleated giant histiocytes seen in this disease. Colloid is not easy to identify under low power with the Papanicolaou stain.

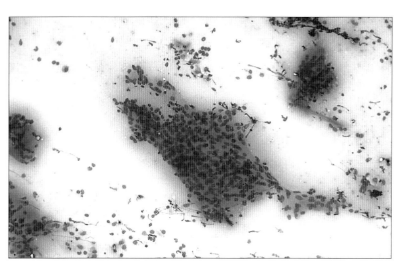

Fig. 7.57 De Quervain's thyroiditis – MGG x10. The enormous multinucleated histiocytes characteristic of this disease are evident even at low power. There are several smaller cells in the background.

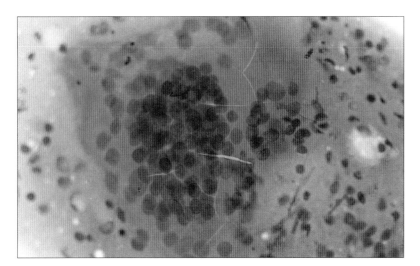

Fig. 7.58 De Quervain's thyroiditis – Pap x40. This poorly fixed smear stained by the Papanicolaou technique shows a huge multinucleated giant cell surrounded by inflammatory cells in the background.

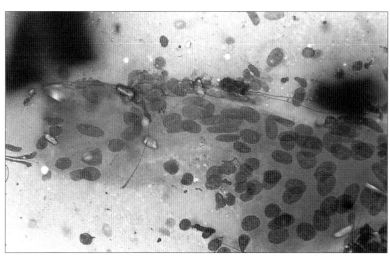

Fig. 7.59 De Quervain's thyroiditis – MGG x40. In this field there are large multinucleated histiocytes and clumps of thick, dark blue colloid. The bare nuclei in the background represent epithelial and inflammatory cells.

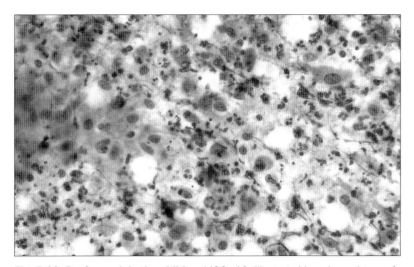

Fig. 7.60 De Quervain's thyroiditis – MGG x10. Illustrated here is a mixture of thick and fluffy colloid in an aspirate from De Quervain's thyroiditis.

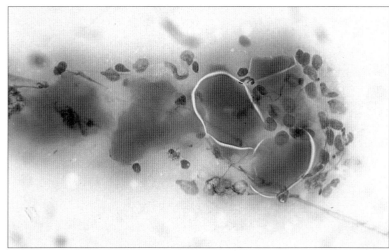

Fig. 7.61 De Quervain's thyroiditis – Pap x40. The clumps of thick colloid stain pinkish orange with the Papanicolaou stain; in the background are poorly preserved epithelial and inflammatory cells.

seen in clusters (**Figs 7.62, 7.63**), producing a granulomatous appearance.

The epithelial cells in De Quervain's thyroiditis often exhibit degenerative changes. These include poor nuclear and cytoplasmic preservation with granular intracytoplasmic pigment, which stains dark blue with May Grunwald Giemsa and golden yellow with the Papanicolaou stain (**Figs 7.64, 7.65**). Bare epithelial cell nuclei are often seen in the background.

THYROGLOSSAL DUCT CYST

Aspirates from thyroglossal duct cysts usually exhibit scanty cellularity. They may contain benign columnar or squamous cells derived from respiratory epithelium, some colloid, and occasionally foamy macrophages (**Fig. 7.66**).

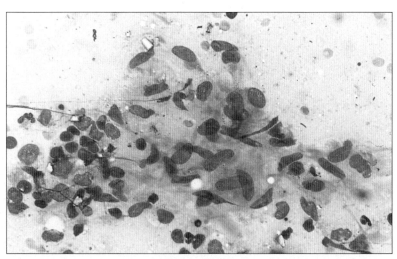

Fig. 7.62 De Quervain's thyroiditis – MGG x40. Pictured here are a group of epithelioid histiocytes with their typical elongated nuclei forming a granuloma, hence the other name for this disease – granulomatous thyroiditis. There are also some lymphocytes and debris in the background.

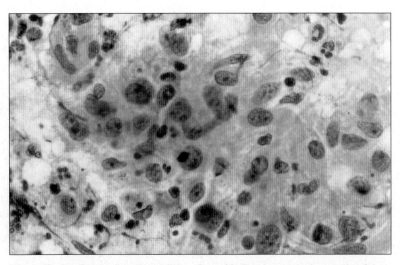

Fig. 7.63 De Quervain's thyroiditis – Pap x40. This is a typical example of the mixture of inflammatory cells, foamy histiocytes, debris, and epithelioid histiocytes seen in De Quervain's thyroiditis.

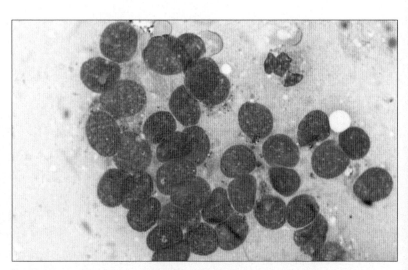

Fig. 7.64 De Quervain's thyroiditis – MGG x100. This cluster of epithelial cells shows the dark blue granular intracytoplasmic pigment supposed to indicate degenerative changes.

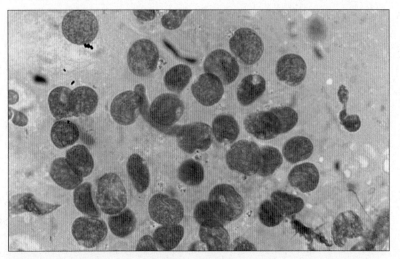

Fig. 7.65 De Quervain's thyroiditis – Pap x100. These poorly preserved epithelial cells show fine granular yellow pigment within their cytoplasm. Debris and occasional inflammatory cells are also seen.

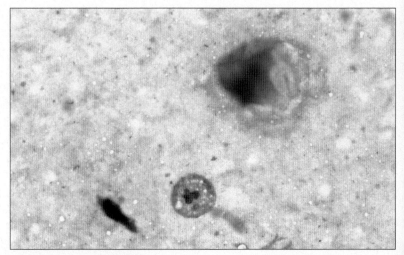

Fig. 7.66 Thyroglossal cyst – MGG x40. These cysts are poorly cellular. This fluid showed some colloid, anucleate squames, and foamy macrophages, all three of which are seen in this field.

FOLLICULAR NEOPLASMS OF THE THYROID

The distinction between a benign adenoma and a follicular carcinoma of the thyroid on histology is dependent upon the identification of invasion of either the capsule or blood vessels (**Fig. 7.67**). The morphology of the epithelial cells does not provide the diagnosis, hence it is impossible to differentiate between a benign and a malignant neoplasm on cytological preparations. The smears show striking cellularity. A common feature is the abundance of small, microfollicular clusters of epithelial cells, which are usually quite uniform (**Figs 7.68–7.70**) and closely resemble the histological pattern (**Fig. 7.71**). Large sheets of epithelial cells may also be seen (**Fig. 7.72**), which can lead to an erroneous diagnosis of hyperplasia or colloid goitre. The diagnostic features are shown in **Figure 7.73**. Variable amounts of colloid and Askanazy cells may also be present.

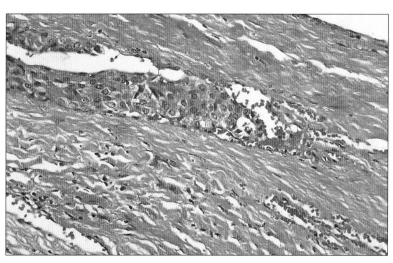

Fig. 7.67 Histology of follicular carcinoma – H&E x10. This section shows the capsule of a follicular thyroid neoplasm infiltrated by tumour cells, making it a follicular carcinoma rather than an adenoma. The cellular morphology is not used to make the diagnosis.

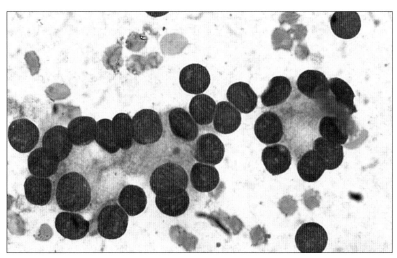

Fig. 7.68 Follicular neoplasm – MGG x100. In this field are two microfollicular structures or acini which are highly suggestive of a follicular neoplasm. There is no obvious cytological atypia.

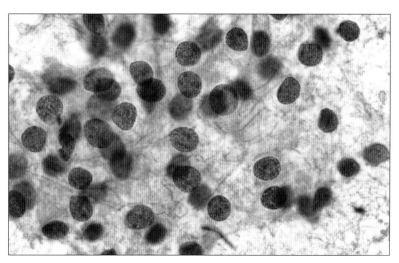

Fig. 7.69 Follicular neoplasm – Pap x100. This wet-fixed smear shows groups of bland epithelial cells arranged in a microfollicular pattern. No atypical features are seen in the cells.

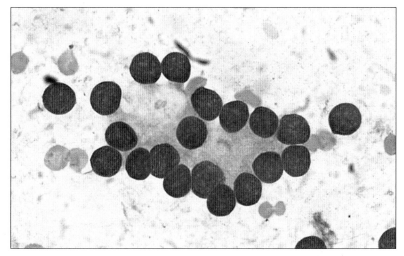

Fig. 7.70 Follicular neoplasm – MGG x100. Illustrated here are two small acinar structures composed of apparently benign epithelial cells. There are no cytological features that can be used to distinguish between an adenoma and a follicular carcinoma.

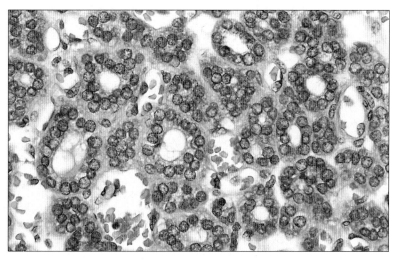

Fig. 7.71 Histology of follicular adenoma – H&E x40. This section shows the same microfollicular structure that is seen in aspirates from follicular neoplasms. No cytological atypia is seen.

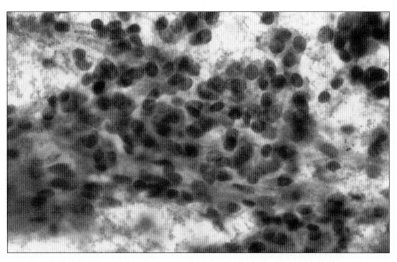

Fig. 7.72 Follicular neoplasm – Pap x63. This aspirate from a follicular neoplasm shows a large cluster of epithelial cells which may mislead, resulting in a diagnosis of colloid goitre or hyperplasia.

A distinctive variant of follicular neoplasm is the Hurthle cell or oxyphil adenoma. This is easily identified on histological sections by the abundant pink granular cytoplasm of the epithelial cells **(Fig. 7.74)**. The aspirate from a Hurthle cell adenoma is very cellular, composed almost entirely of fairly uniform oncocytic cells **(Figs 7.75, 7.76)**, unlike the variable Hurthle cells in Hashimoto's thyroiditis and in colloid goitre **(Fig. 7.77)**.

As there is as yet no absolutely foolproof method of distinguishing between follicular adenomas and carcinomas cytologically, such aspirates should be reported as follicular neoplasms and biopsy recommended.

Fig. 7.73 Diagnostic features of colloid goitre and follicular neoplasm.

FEATURES	COLLOID GOITRE	FOLLICULAR NEOPLASM
Cellularity	Variable	Usually cellular
Colloid	Abundant	Small amounts
Cell groups	Large sheets	Microfollicular clusters
Intact follicles	Present	Acini with lumina seen
Bare nuclei	Common	Uncommon
Epithelial cells	Uncommon	May be seen
Hurthle cells	Common, appear pleomorphic	Seen in Hurthle cell adenoma, monomorphic
Stromal strands	Not uncommon	Uncommon
Histiocytes	Abundant	Very occasional
Siderophages	Abundant	Uncommon
Multinucleated histiocytes	Common	Uncommon
Cholesterol crystals	Not uncommon	Uncommon

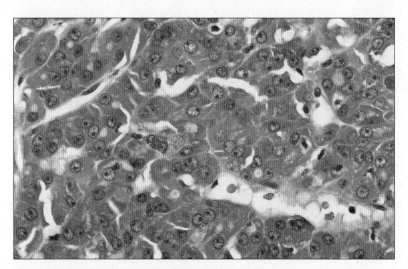

Fig. 7.74 Histology of oxyphil adenoma – H&E x40. In this section the cells are all oncocytic with abundant pink cytoplasm, sharply defined nuclei, and prominent nucleoli.

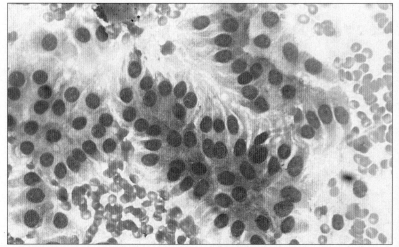

Fig. 7.75 Oxyphil adenoma – MGG x40. In this air-dried aspirate from an oxyphil adenoma some of the epithelial cells have a columnar shape, while others have the typical abundant cytoplasm of Hurthle cells.

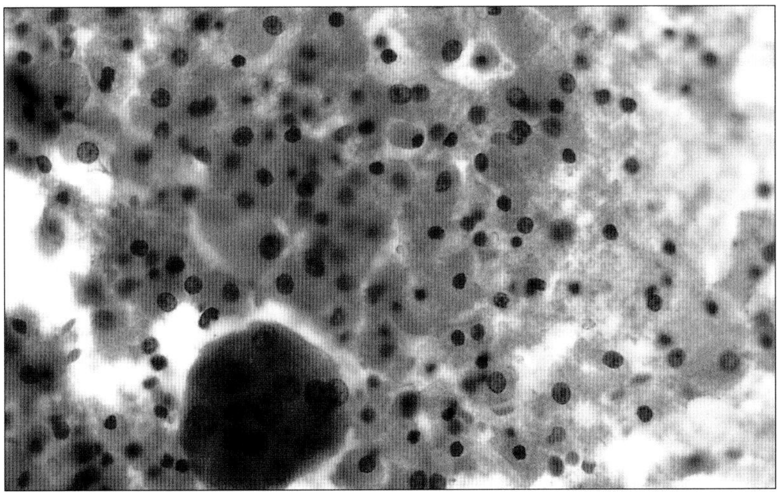

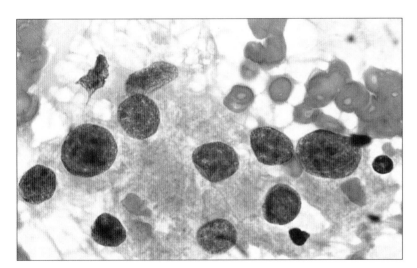

Fig. 7.76 Oxyphil adenoma – Pap x40. The wet-fixed smear from an oxyphil adenoma shows sheets of cells with abundant pink cytoplasm and rounded nuclei. There is a follicular structure composed of similar cells at the bottom of the field.

PAPILLARY CARCINOMA

Papillary carcinoma of the thyroid can sometimes present as a cystic lesion in the thyroid and occasionally as an enlarged lymph node with no obvious thyroid abnormality. The histological features are identical in both the primary and metastatic lesions (**Figs 7.78, 7.79**). The papillary pattern of the tumour is striking, but is not as important for the diagnosis as the nuclear features, which are essential, for example, in making the diagnosis of 'follicular variant of papillary carcinoma' (**Fig. 7.80**). Characteristic features are the watery 'Orphan Annie' nuclei (**Fig. 7.81**) and the nuclear grooves and inclusions (**Fig. 7.82**), which are clearly seen on histological sections.

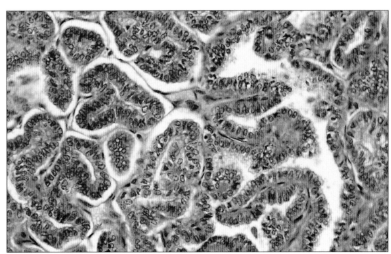

Fig. 7.78 Histology of papillary carcinoma – H&E x25. This section shows the papillary structures, composed of a vascular connective-tissue core surrounded by epithelial cells, which constitute this neoplasm. (Slide courtesy of Dr PH McKee, St Thomas' Hospital, London.)

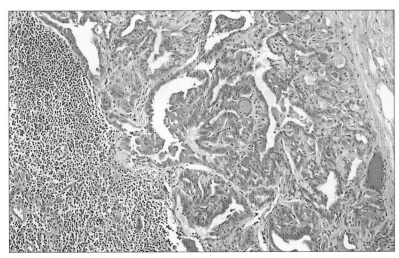

Fig. 7.77 Hurthle cells in Hashimoto's disease – Pap x100. Hurthle cells in Hashimoto's thyroiditis show marked variability in cell and nuclear size. They have abundant granular pink cytoplasm and can appear quite pleomorphic.

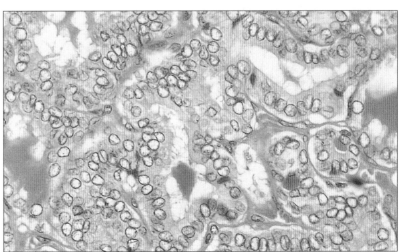

Fig. 7.79 Histology of metastatic papillary carcinoma of thyroid – H&E x10. In this lymph node section there is a focus of metastatic papillary carcinoma of thyroid, identical to the primary tumour.

Fig. 7.80 Histology of follicular variant of papillary carcinoma – H&E x40. Although this section shows follicular structures, the diagnosis is that of papillary carcinoma, follicular variant, because of the cytological features of the nuclei.

The cytological specimen does not always show all of the above characteristics. The smears are usually cellular with large papillary fragments of tissue (**Figs 7.83–7.85**), sometimes containing rounded aggregates of colloid and psammoma bodies. The tissue fragments may also exhibit vascular cores (**Fig. 7.86**) and sometimes have blunt, rounded papillary shapes, instead of the usual papillary fronds (**Fig. 7.87**). Psammoma bodies are frequently noted (**Figs 7.88, 7.89**). Under higher magnification the cells may appear bland, without the watery nuclei seen in histological sections. However, careful examination reveals nuclear grooves and inclusions (**Figs 7.90, 7.91**). Intranuclear inclusions have been noted in 91% of papillary carcinomas and grooves in 100% of these tumours. The cell clusters may show some of the typical features of adenocarcinoma, such as abnormally enlarged, irregular nuclei with prominent nucleoli (**Fig. 7.92**). The lesions are not infrequently cystic, in which case the aspirate may not be diagnostic, containing only debris, colloid, and some foamy macrophages. Aspirates from metastatic lesions in lymph nodes show exactly the same features as those of the

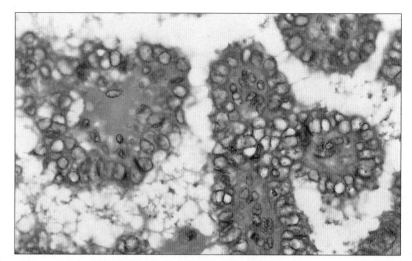

Fig. 7.81 Histology of papillary carcinoma – H&E x63. This section shows the typical clear or 'Orphan Annie' nuclei seen in papillary carcinoma of the thyroid. This characteristic is not reproduced in cytological preparations and is believed to be artefactual.

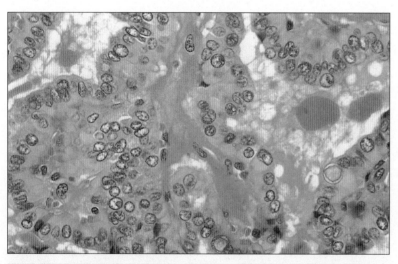

Fig. 7.82 Histology of papillary carcinoma – H&E x40. In this section the typical nuclear grooves and intranuclear inclusions of papillary carcinoma are well-illustrated.

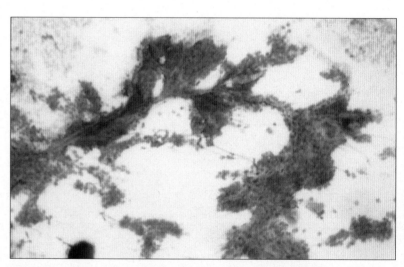

Fig. 7.83 Papillary carcinoma – MGG x4. This low-power view of an air-dried aspirate shows the large branching tissue fragments characteristic of papillary carcinoma of the thyroid.

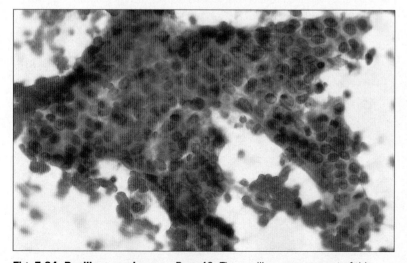

Fig. 7.84 Papillary carcinoma – Pap x40. The papillary arrangement of this cluster of cells is clearly shown in this wet-fixed smear, although no connective tissue cores are demonstrated.

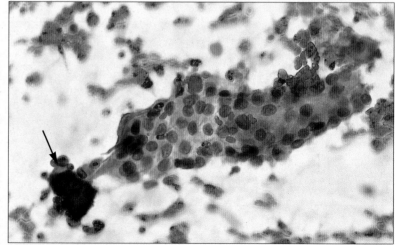

Fig. 7.85 Papillary carcinoma – Pap x40. At the tip of the frond of epithelial cells lie two adjacent psammoma bodies (arrowed). These are typically seen in papillary carcinoma, although they may occasionally be present in papillary hyperplasia and in colloid goitre.

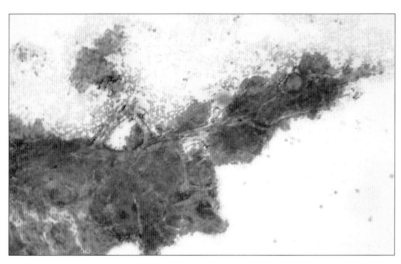

Fig. 7.86 Papillary carcinoma – Pap x4. Illustrated here under low power is a papillary cluster of carcinoma cells exhibiting vascular cores.

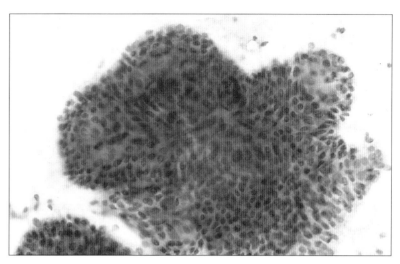

Fig. 7.87 Papillary carcinoma – Pap x40. This aspirate shows the blunted papillae sometimes seen in papillary carcinoma.

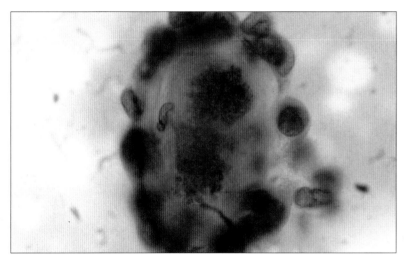

Fig. 7.88 Psammoma bodies – Pap x100. Carcinoma cells with grooved nuclei are seen encircling two psammoma bodies in this wet-fixed smear from papillary carcinoma of the thyroid.

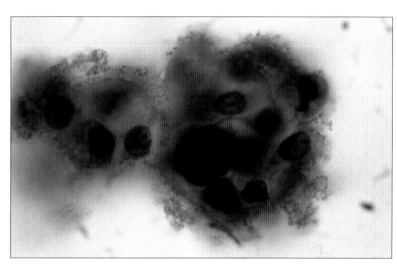

Fig. 7.89 Psammoma bodies – Pap x100. Psammoma bodies may be missed if the aspirate is not carefully examined, if necessary under oil immersion. Delicate laminations can be detected in this psammoma body.

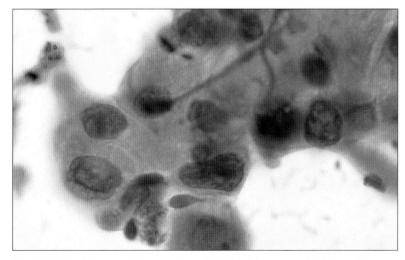

Fig. 7.90 Papillary carcinoma – Pap x100. This high-power field shows large irregular nuclei with well-defined grooves. Again, oil immersion may be necessary for the grooves to be visualized.

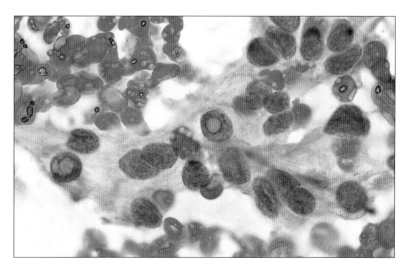

Fig. 7.91 Papillary carcinoma – Pap x100. In this group of carcinoma cells with irregular nuclei there are two with distinct nuclear inclusions.

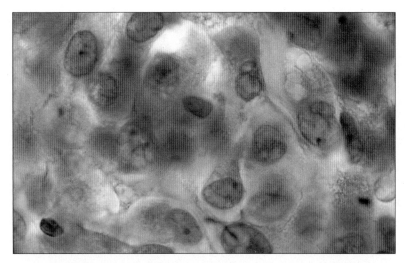

Fig. 7.92 Papillary carcinoma – Pap x100. This high-power view of cells from an aspirate of papillary carcinoma shows irregular pleomorphic hypochromatic nuclei, most of which also contain grooves.

primary tumour, namely cellular papillary fragments, psammoma bodies (**Fig. 7.93**), and, occasionally, colloid. The epithelial cells may contain the grooves and inclusions seen in the primary tumour (**Figs 7.94, 7.95**).

MEDULLARY CARCINOMA OF THE THYROID

The calcitonin-producing C cells of the thyroid, which are responsible for this neoplasm, are not readily seen on histological sections or aspirates of the normal thyroid. Medullary carcinoma may show variable appearances, with the solid cell (**Fig. 7.96**) and spindle forms usually being more common. The presence of spindle cells may be an important clue in making the diagnosis of medullary carcinoma.

The cytological appearances are readily recognizable. The smears are cellular with scattered or dispersed cells (**Figs 7.97, 7.98**), which are plasmacytoid in appearance because of their eccentric nuclei (**Figs 7.99, 7.100**). Much pleomorphism is noted, with some binucleation of cells (**Figs 7.101, 7.102**). Granularity of the cytoplasm is readily seen, both in the wet-fixed and

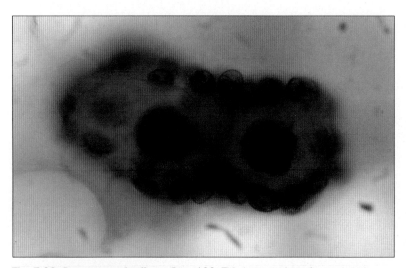

Fig. 7.93 Psammoma bodies – Pap x100. This is an aspirate from a lymph node containing metastatic papillary carcinoma. Two psammoma bodies are surrounded by cells, identical to the appearance in the primary lesion (**Fig. 7.88**).

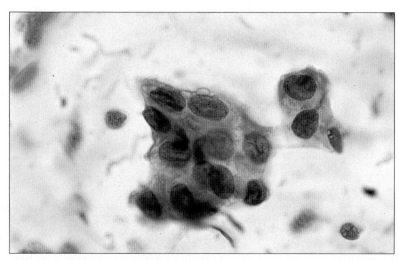

Fig. 7.94 Metastatic carcinoma – Pap x100. The cells seen here are in an aspirate from metastatic papillary carcinoma in a neck node. Note the nuclear grooves.

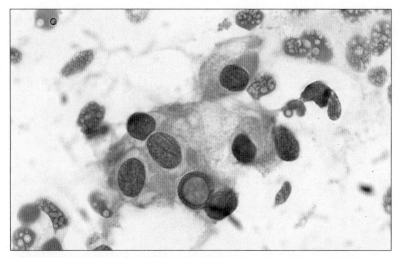

Fig. 7.95 Metastatic carcinoma – Pap x100. This is another field from the lymph node aspirate seen in **Figure 7.94**. One of the carcinoma cells contains a huge intranuclear inclusion.

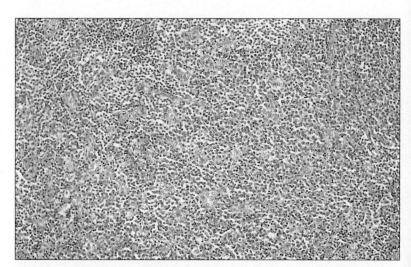

Fig. 7.96 Histology of medullary carcinoma – H&E x10. Illustrated here is a low-power view of the solid variant of medullary carcinoma of the thyroid. No amyloid is visible in this section.

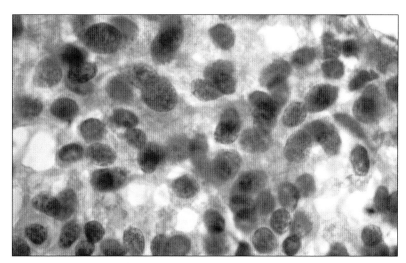

Fig. 7.97 Medullary carcinoma – Pap x100. This field shows the marked cellularity seen in medullary carcinoma. There is a fair amount of variability in cell and nuclear size.

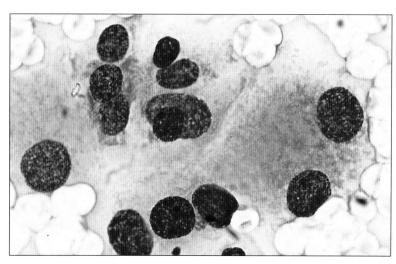

Fig. 7.98 Medullary carcinoma – MGG x100. A high-power view of medullary carcinoma shows dispersed cells which are pleomorphic. (Specimen courtesy of Dr N Derias, St Thomas' Hospital, London, UK.)

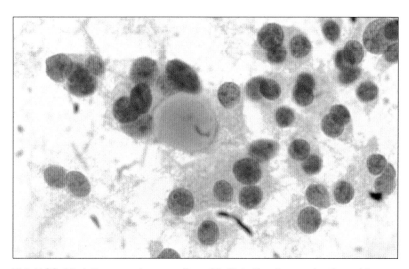

Fig. 7.99 Medullary carcinoma – Pap x40. Note the dispersed cells and the eccentric nuclei giving this aspirate a plasmacytoid appearance. (Specimen courtesy of Dr N Derias, St Thomas' Hospital, London, UK.)

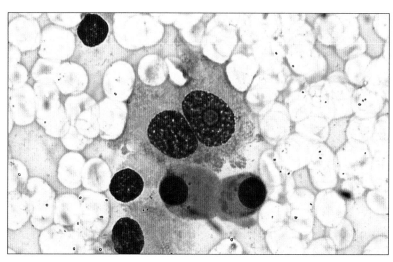

Fig. 7.100 Medullary carcinoma – MGG x100. In this field the plasmacytoid appearance of the tumour cells is well-illustrated. One of the larger nuclei has a huge nucleolus. (Specimen courtesy of Dr N Derias, St Thomas' Hospital, London, UK.)

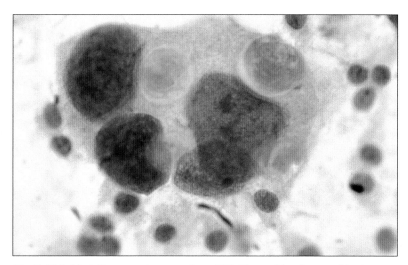

Fig. 7.101 Medullary carcinoma – Pap x100. The multinucleate cell in the centre of the field is enormous compared with the smaller tumour cells in the periphery, demonstrating marked pleomorphism. (Specimen courtesy of Dr N Derias, St Thomas' Hospital, London, UK.)

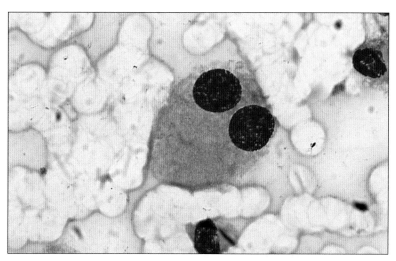

Fig. 7.102 Medullary carcinoma – MGG x100. In this air-dried smear a large binucleate cell is seen with some small cells in the background. (Specimen courtesy of Dr N Derias, St Thomas' Hospital, London, UK.)

the air-dried smears (**Figs 7.103, 7.104**). Intranuclear inclusions are not uncommon in medullary carcinoma (**Figs 7.105, 7.106**). The spindle-cell variety of medullary carcinoma can be mistaken for papillary carcinoma if care is not exercised because of the pattern of the cell clusters. The cells are spindle-shaped (**Fig. 7.107**), but may retain a degree of cohesiveness; the red granularity of the cytoplasm should provide a clue to the diagnosis (**Fig. 7.108**).

Amyloid is a characteristic feature of medullary carcinoma, but it may be mistaken for colloid. It appears as masses of purplish blue material in air-dried smears, often intimately associated with the neoplastic cells (**Fig. 7.109**). It stains a pale blue on the wet-fixed smear (**Fig. 7.110**). Amyloid shows typical Congo-red birefringence on histological sections, but special stains are unnecessary on cytological material as birefringence is easily demonstrated on Papanicolaou-stained smears (**Figs 7.111–7.113**) and on air-dried material (**Fig. 7.114**).

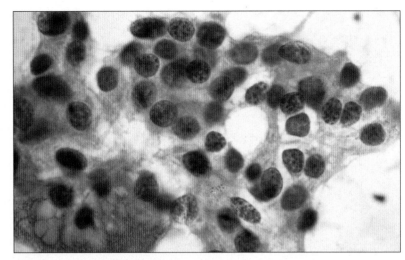

Fig. 7.103 Medullary carcinoma – Pap x100. The clusters of cells seen here show clumped chromatin, which resembles that of plasma cells. In addition, the cells have distinctive pink granular cytoplasm.

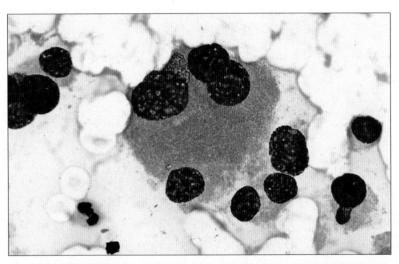

Fig. 7.104 Medullary carcinoma – MGG x100. The air-dried smear shows the pink granularity of the cytoplasm of the carcinoma cells much more clearly than in the wet-fixed smear. (Specimen courtesy of Dr N Derias, St Thomas' Hospital, London, UK.)

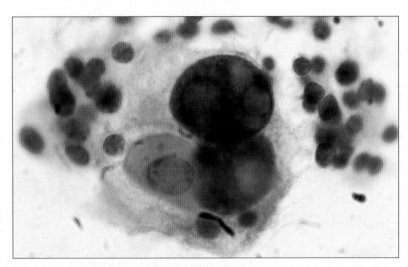

Fig. 7.105 Medullary carcinoma – Pap x100. Intranuclear inclusions are prominent in one of the nuclei of the large binucleate cell seen in this field. Although similar inclusions are seen in papillary carcinoma, these cells are much more pleomorphic. (Specimen courtesy of Dr N Derias, St Thomas' Hospital, London, UK.)

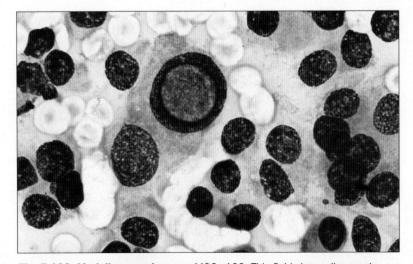

Fig. 7.106 Medullary carcinoma – MGG x100. This field shows dispersed pleomorphic cells and a large intranuclear inclusion. (Specimen courtesy of Dr N Derias, St Thomas' Hospital, London, UK.)

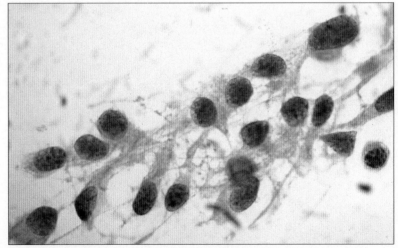

Fig. 7.107 Medullary carcinoma – Pap x100. These spindle cells are often seen in medullary carcinomas and provide a clue to the diagnosis in difficult cases.

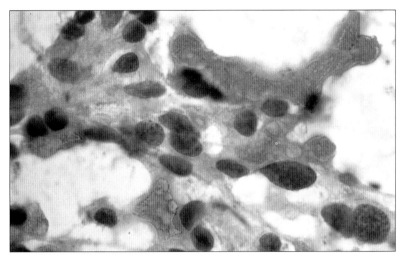

Fig. 7.108 Medullary carcinoma – Pap x100. In this field the spindle-shaped malignant cells exhibit the prominent red granularity typical of medullary carcinoma.

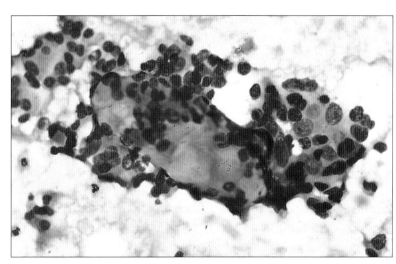

Fig. 7.109 Amyloid – MGG x40. Amyloid is a feature of medullary carcinoma which may be overlooked on the air-dried smear, being blue and often intimately associated with the tumour cells. (Specimen courtesy of Dr N Derias, St Thomas' Hospital, London, UK.)

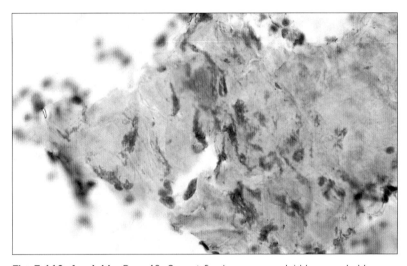

Fig. 7.110 Amyloid – Pap x40. On wet-fixed smears amyloid has a pale blue translucent appearance.

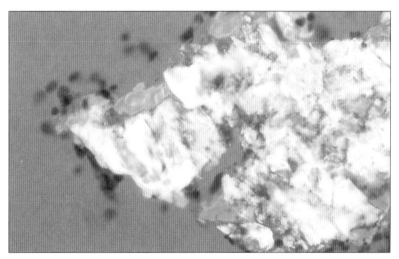

Fig. 7.111 Amyloid under polarized light – Pap x40. Birefringence can be demonstrated on Papanicolaou-stained material without the need for a Congo red stain.

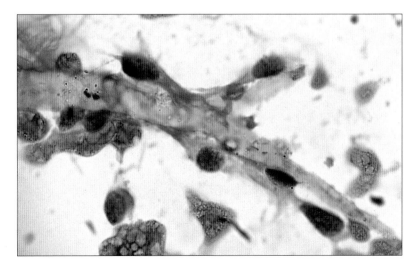

Fig. 7.112 Amyloid – Pap x100. Demonstrated here is amyloid associated with spindle cells.

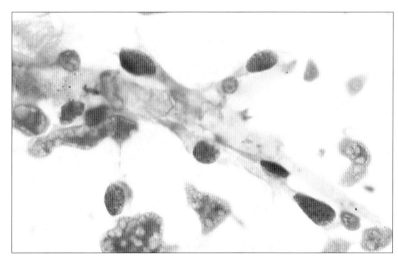

Fig. 7.113 Amyloid under polarized light – Pap x100. This is the same case and same field as that illustrated in **Figure 7.112**. The amyloid is birefringent under polarized light.

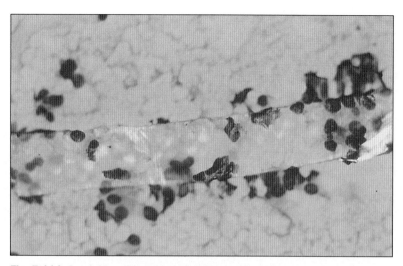

Fig. 7.114 Amyloid under polarized light – MGG x40. Amyloid in air-dried smears is not as clearly birefringent under polarized light as it is in wet-fixed material.

ANAPLASTIC CARCINOMA OF THE THYROID

The cells seen in this variant of malignancy are pleomorphic, sometimes spindle-shaped (**Fig. 7.115**), sometimes multinucleated (**Figs 7.116, 7.117**). Multinucleated giant cells may accompany the pleomorphic tumour cells (**Fig. 7.118**).

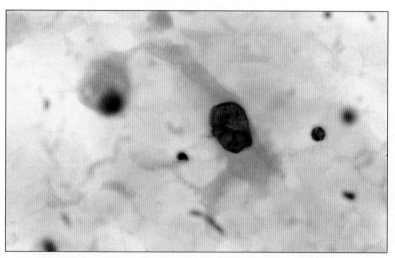

Fig. 7.115 Anaplastic carcinoma – Pap x100. A large tumour cell is seen in this field, with delicate cytoplasm showing a spindle-shaped distribution. Nuclear grooves are prominent.

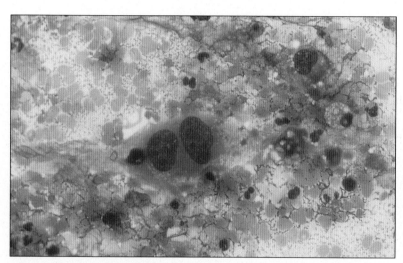

Fig. 7.116 Anaplastic carcinoma – MGG x40. This air-dried smear shows a large binucleate malignant cell with prominent multiple nucleoli, and blood and debris in the background.

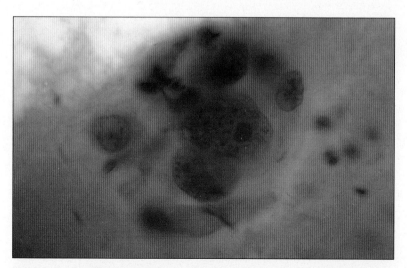

Fig. 7.117 Anaplastic carcinoma – Pap x100. This heavily blood-stained wet-fixed smear shows pleomorphic carcinoma cells with enormous red nucleoli and clumped chromatin.

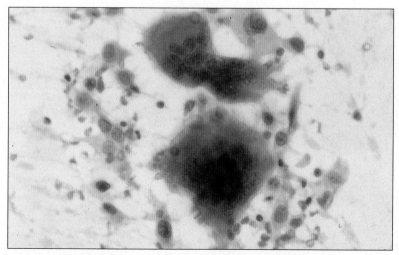

Fig. 7.118 Anaplastic carcinoma with osteoclast-type giant cells – Pap x40. Illustrated here are two large osteoclast-type giant cells with anaplastic carcinoma cells in the background.

LYMPHOMA OF THE THYROID

Both **Hodgkin's** and **non-Hodgkin's lymphoma** can occur in the thyroid. The histological appearance is characteristic (**Fig. 7.119**), but the cytological features have to be distinguished from lymphocytic thyroiditis and Hashimoto's disease. The aspirate shows the usual monotonous appearance of uniform lymphoid cells in non-Hodgkin's lymphoma (**Figs 7.120, 7.121**), while Hodgkin's disease typically demonstrates either Reed–Sternberg or Hodgkin's cells (**Figs 7.122, 7.123**).

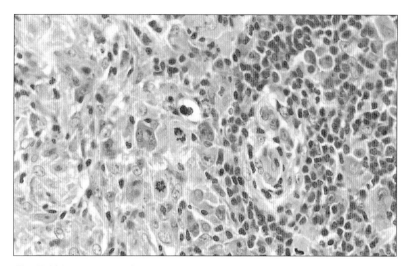

Fig. 7.119 Histology of lymphoma of the thyroid – H&E x10. This section of thyroid reveals extensive infiltration by a high-grade lymphoma.

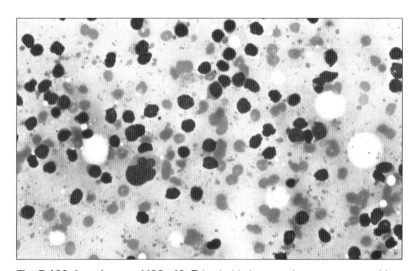

Fig. 7.120 Lymphoma – MGG x40. This air-dried smear shows a monomorphic population of lymphoid cells from a low-grade lymphoma of the thyroid, but distinguishing this from Hashimoto's thyroiditis can be very difficult and immunocytochemistry may be necessary.

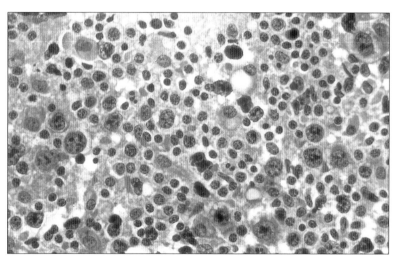

Fig. 7.121 Lymphoma – Pap x40. This wet-fixed smear shows a high-grade lymphoma of the thyroid with large abnormal lymphoid cells. These tumours are easily distinguished from lymphocytic thyroiditis on aspirates.

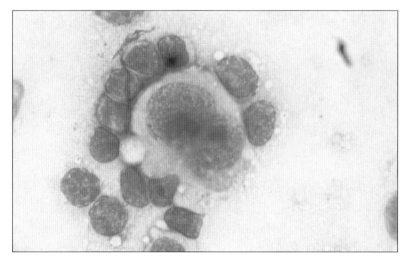

Fig. 7.122 Reed–Sternberg cell – MGG x100. This field illustrates a Reed–Sternberg cell with huge nucleoli, surrounded by smaller lymphoid cells. Histology showed Hodgkin's disease.

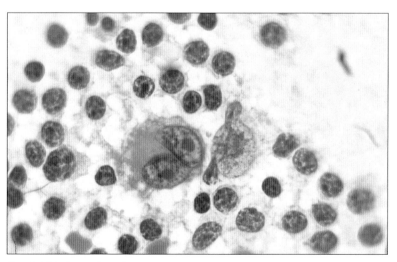

Fig. 7.123 Reed–Sternberg cell – Pap x100. In the centre of this field is a binucleated Reed–Sternberg cell with prominent red nucleoli, from the wet-fixed smear of the same case as in **Figure 7.122**.

METASTATIC TUMOURS TO THE THYROID

The thyroid is a fairly common site for metastatic tumours, such as adenocarcinoma of the breast (**Fig. 7.124**), lymphoma, renal cell carcinoma (**Fig. 7.125**), malignant melanoma (**Fig. 7.126**), and a squamous primary elsewhere (**Fig. 7.127**). The cytological features of these neoplasms are usually recognizable with Papanicolaou and May Grunwald Giemsa stains, but recourse may have to be made to immunocytochemical stains in difficult cases.

PARATHYROID ADENOMA

Aspirates from an adenoma of the parathyroid may be mistaken for thyroid aspirates. In the case of a chief-cell adenoma of the parathyroid (**Fig. 7.128**), the secretory material in the aspirate is delicate and granular, quite unlike the well-defined colloid seen in thyroid aspirates. The epithelial cells are small and often dispersed (**Figs 7.129, 7.130**), occasionally exhibiting an alarming degree of pleomorphism.

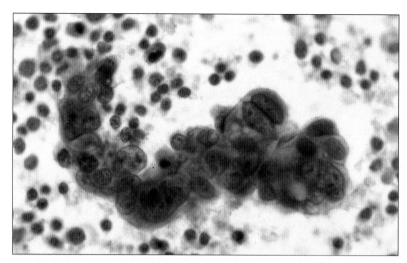

Fig. 7.124 Metastatic adenocarcinoma of the breast – Pap x63. This aspirate of the thyroid from a woman with carcinoma of the breast shows a papillary cluster of adenocarcinoma cells, demonstrating vacuolation, pleomorphism, and prominent nucleoli.

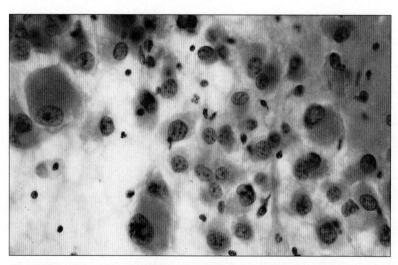

Fig. 7.125 Metastatic renal cell carcinoma – Pap x40. In this field pleomorphic carcinoma cells are visible, some with abundant cytoplasm and prominent red nucleoli. The patient had a primary renal cell carcinoma.

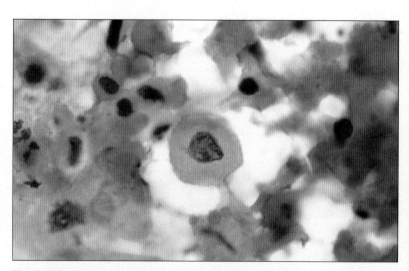

Fig. 7.126 Metastatic squamous cell carcinoma – Pap x40. This wet-fixed smear shows a keratinized squamous carcinoma cell surrounded by anucleate and degenerate squamous cells.

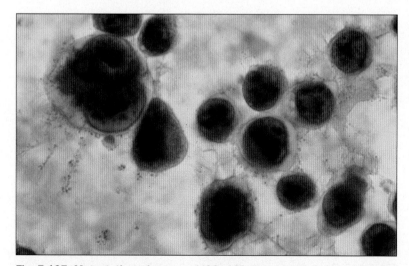

Fig. 7.127 Metastatic melanoma – MGG x100. This aspirate is from a thyroid involved by metastatic melanoma. The cells are pleomorphic and pigment is not present, so the history of melanoma is essential for diagnosis.

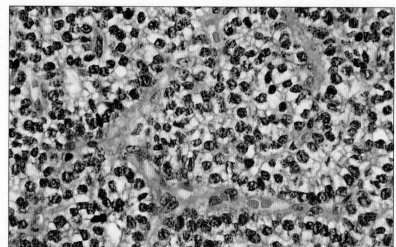

Fig. 7.128 Histology of chief-cell adenoma of the parathyroid – H&E x25. This section shows the typical bland features seen in a chief-cell adenoma of the parathyroid (same case as in **Figures 7.129** and **7.130**).

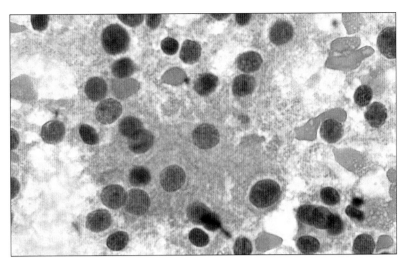

Fig. 7.129 Parathyroid adenoma – Pap x100. The parathyroid gland may sometimes be aspirated instead of the thyroid. Note the absence of colloid and the presence of finely granular secretory material, delicate pink granular cytoplasm in some cells, and small round nuclei.

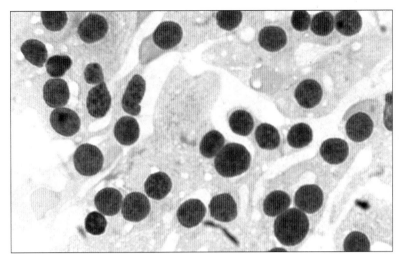

Fig. 7.130 Parathyroid adenoma – MGG x100. The air-dried smear from a parathyroid adenoma shows small epithelial cells. These may be indistinguishable from thyroid follicle cells because the secretory material in the background is pale blue and ill-defined. The lack of colloid is a clue to the correct diagnosis.

SUGGESTED READING

Anderson JB, Webb AJ. Fine needle aspiration biopsy and the diagnosis of thyroid cancer. *Br J Surg* 1987; **74**: 292–296.

Christ ML, Haja J. Intranuclear cytoplasmic inclusions (invaginations) in thyroid aspirations. *Acta Cytol* 1979; **23**: 327–331.

Fiorella RM, Isley W, Miller LK, Kragel PJ. Multinodular goiter of the thyroid mimicking malignancy: Diagnostic pitfalls in fine needle aspiration biopsy. *Diagn Cytopathol* 1993; **9**: 351–357.

Geddie WR, Bedard YC, Strawbridge HTG. Medullary carcinoma of the thyroid in fine needle aspiration biopsies. *Am J Clin Pathol* 1984; **82**: 552–558.

Gould E, Walzak L, Chamizo W, Albores-Saavedra J. Nuclear grooves in cytologic preparations. *Acta Cytol* 1989; **23**: 16–20.

Lowhagen T, Willems JS, Lundell G, *et al*. Aspiration biopsy cytology in the diagnosis of thyroid cancer. *World J Surg* 1981; **5**: 61–73.

Riazmontazer N, Bedayat G. Psammoma bodies in fine needle aspirates from thyroids containing nontoxic hyperplastic nodular goitres. *Acta Cytol* 1991; **35**: 563–566.

Rupp M, Ehya H. Nuclear grooves in the aspiration cytology of papillary carcinoma of the thyroid. *Acta Cytol* 1989; **33**: 21–26.

Santos JEC, Leiman G. Non aspiration fine needle cytology. Application of a new technique to nodular thyroid disease. *Acta Cytol* 1988; **32**: 353–356.

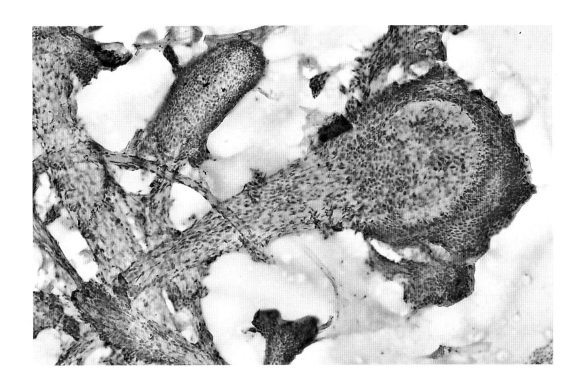

BENIGN BREAST CYTOLOGY

8

BENIGN BREAST CYTOLOGY

The breast is composed of varying proportions of fat, stroma, and epithelium (**Fig. 8.1**). The epithelium consists of small acinar structures, called lobules, continuous with small ducts (these two comprising the terminal ductulo-lobular units) and larger ducts which join to form the lactiferous ducts. These terminate in the lactiferous sinuses which open onto the nipple. The lobules are supported by delicate connective tissue stroma, the ducts are surrounded by somewhat denser stroma, and fat surrounds the breast tissue. The relationship of these components is seen clearly in histological sections (**Fig. 8.2**). In young women the proportion of epithelium is higher than in old women, whose breasts are composed largely of fat and connective tissue. An aspirate of normal breast is never very cellular, consisting mainly of stromal connective tissue, fat, and some small sheets of benign ductal epithelial cells. During pregnancy and lactation the acinar epithelium proliferates, so an aspirate taken at this time is much more cellular.

Benign ductal cells in aspirates are seen in the form of small sheets of cohesive cells with very little cytoplasm and uniform round-to-ovoid nuclei, each of which is approximately the size of an erythrocyte (**Figs 8.3, 8.4**). It is important to remember that benign cells in air-dried smears tend to show some loss of cohesion, so this should not be used as an indicator of malignancy. The nuclear margins are smooth and the chromatin pattern is vesicular with a delicate reticular network, better visualized on wet-fixed, Papanicolaou-stained material (**Figs 8.5, 8.6**). Benign ductal cells may show small nucleoli (**Fig. 8.7**). The histological structure of a duct, consisting of a layer of cuboidal cells supported by a layer of myoepithelial cells (**Fig. 8.8**), is well-illustrated in cytological material (**Fig. 8.9**).

Lobules are frequently aspirated intact, especially in stereotactic aspirates, and retain their three-dimensional structure that resembles clusters of mulberries (**Figs 8.10, 8.11**). These tight clusters of small epithelial cells contain small nuclei and little cytoplasm and, like ducts, are surrounded by a layer of supporting myoepithelial cells. In benign aspirates, numerous bare nuclei are seen in the background. Many of these are ovoid or bipolar, sometimes referred to as torpedo-shaped, and represent **myoepithelial cells**. However, others are more elongated and spindle-shaped with delicate wisps of cytoplasm at either end – these are **stromal** in origin (**Figs 8.12, 8.13**). The former stain positively with anti-actin and anti-S100, which are immunocytochemical markers for myoepithelial cells, while the latter stain with desmin markers.

Connective tissue stromal fragments are common in aspirates, and vary in size. They stain pale blue or pink with the Papanicolaou stain and contain a few spindle-shaped nuclei (**Fig. 8.14**), and are bright pink on the air-dried May Grunwald Giemsa stained smear with purple nuclei (**Fig. 8.15**). **Capillaries** are occasionally noted within stromal fragments. Clusters of fat cells are commonly seen, the cells being large and clear with inconspicuous nuclei, resembling soap suds (**Figs 8.16, 8.17**). It is not unusual to see delicate capillaries traversing fragments of fat (**Fig. 8.18**) or on their own (**Fig. 8.19**). **Fat cells** may also be seen attached to stroma. **Sebaceous glands** are plentiful in the dermis beneath the areola (**Fig. 8.20**), but are infrequently noted in aspirates. The cells contain small nuclei and abundant finely vacuolated cytoplasm (**Fig. 8.21**).

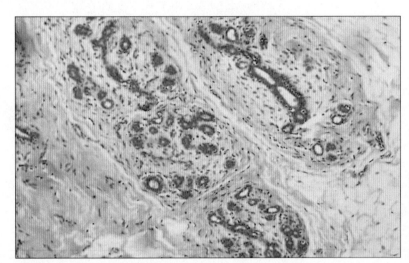

Fig. 8.2 Section of normal breast – H&E x10. This section of normal breast shows lobules and small ducts surrounded by delicate stroma, with denser connective tissue in the background.

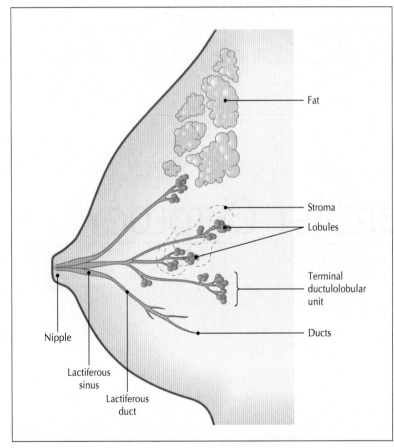

Fig. 8.1 Diagram showing structure of the normal breast.

Fat

Stroma

Lobules

Terminal ductulolobular unit

Ducts

Nipple

Lactiferous sinus

Lactiferous duct

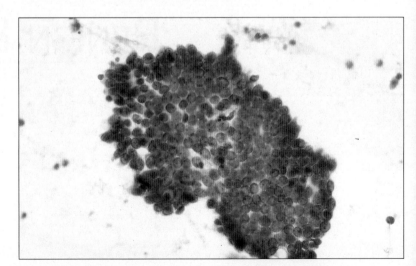

Fig. 8.3 Benign ductal cells – Pap x40. This field shows a cohesive sheet of benign ductal cells with uniform small nuclei, which are slightly larger than the erythrocytes in the background.

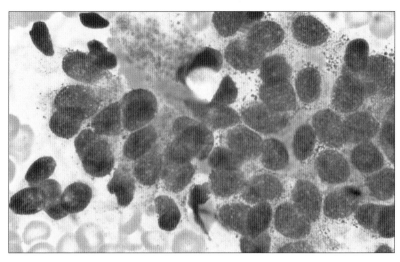

Fig. 8.4 Benign ductal cells – MGG x100. These air-dried ductal cells are in flat sheets and have small rounded nuclei. Note the slight dissociation of some of the cells . The nuclei are about the size of the erythrocytes seen in this field.

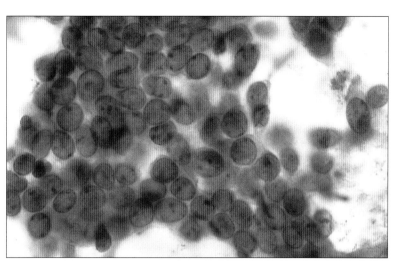

Fig. 8.5 Benign ductal cells – Pap x100. The vesicular nuclei are well-demonstrated in this flat, cohesive sheet of benign ductal cells.

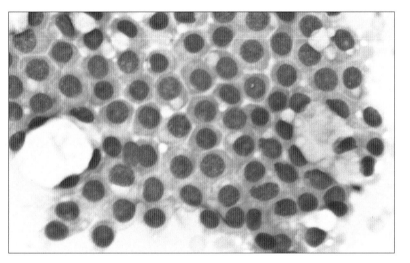

Fig. 8.6 Benign ductal cells – MGG x40. This sheet of benign ductal cells shows uniform nuclear and cell size, but the vesicular nature of the chromatin pattern is difficult to identify. Note the honeycombing pattern.

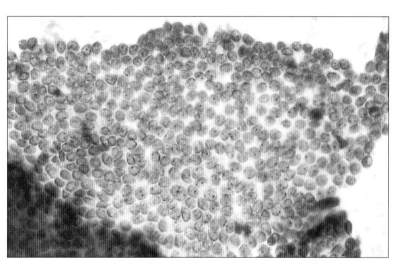

Fig. 8.7 Benign ductal cells – Pap x40. This large sheet of benign ductal cells displays nuclei with vesicular chromatin and small, but clearly visible, nucleoli.

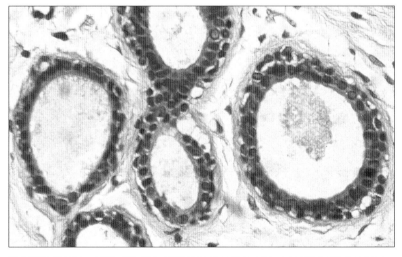

Fig. 8.8 Ducts – H&E x40. This histological section shows small ducts lined by two layers of cells – the inner cuboidal ductal cells and the outer layer of myoepithelial cells, some of which appear vacuolated. In the background are spindle-shaped stromal cells.

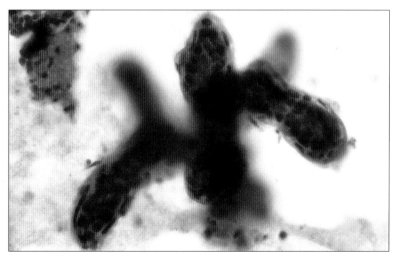

Fig. 8.9 Ducts – Pap x40. This aspirate demonstrates interconnecting intact ducts composed of small cuboidal cells with an outer layer of flattened myoepithelial cells. In the top left corner there is part of a flat sheet of benign ductal cells.

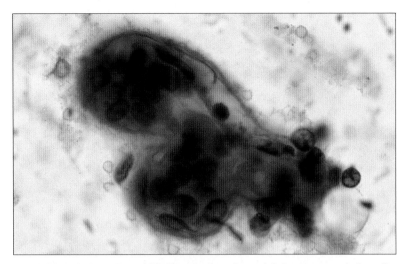

Fig. 8.10 Lobules – Pap x100. Illustrated are intact lobules composed of small epithelial cells surrounded by a layer of myoepithelial cells.

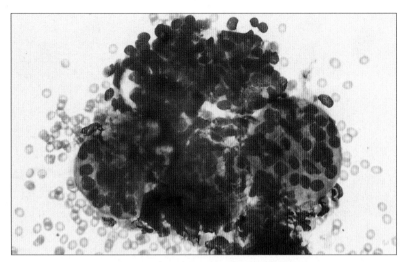

Fig. 8.11 Lobules – MGG x40. This cluster of intact lobules is seen to contain small cuboidal cells. The myoepithelial cells are difficult to identify in air-dried smears.

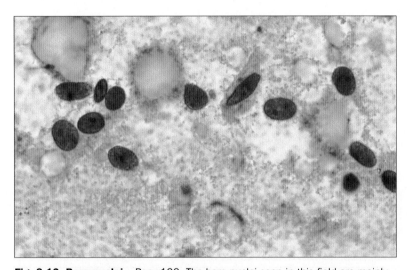

Fig. 8.12 Bare nuclei – Pap x100. The bare nuclei seen in this field are mainly ovoid or torpedo-shaped with no evident cytoplasm, representing myoepithelial cells. In the centre of the field is a spindle-shaped cell with apparent wisps of cytoplasm indicating its stromal origin.

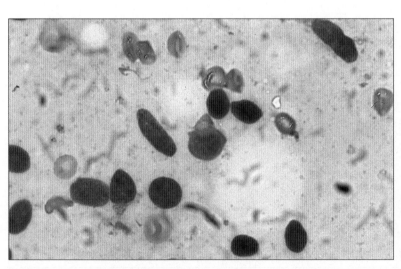

Fig. 8.13 Bare nuclei – MGG x100. Illustrated here are the two types of bare nuclei – the ovoid myoepithelial cells and spindle-shaped stromal cells.

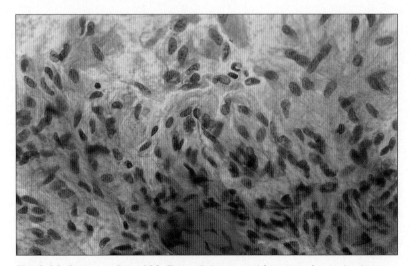

Fig. 8.14 Stroma – Pap x100. This cellular stromal fragment, from a benign breast aspirate, contains spindle-shaped vesicular nuclei that resemble those often seen in the background (see **Figure 8.12**).

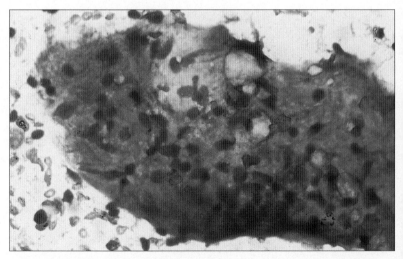

Fig. 8.15 Stroma – MGG x100. Stroma stains bright pink with the May Grunwald Giemsa stain, as illustrated here. The nuclei are rather poorly preserved, unlike those in the wet-fixed smear in **Figure 8.14**.

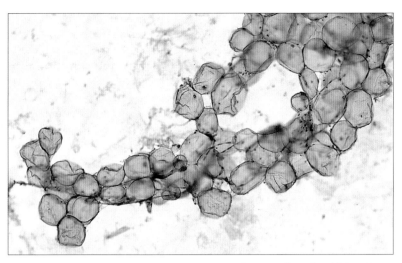

Fig. 8.16 Fat cells – Pap x10. This is a cluster of mature fat cells which stain pale blue with the Papanicolaou stain, contain inconspicuous nuclei, and are all of the same size. Occasionally, the proteinaceous material in the background of an aspirate shows rounded spaces of varying sizes, which may be mistaken for fat cells.

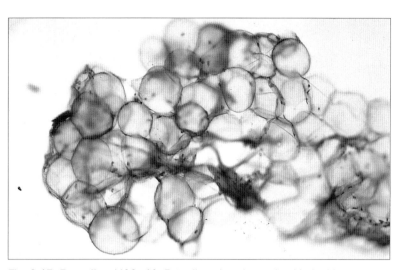

Fig. 8.17 Fat cells – MGG x10. Fat cells stain pale purple with the May Grunwald Giemsa stain. They have sharp clear outlines and similar in size.

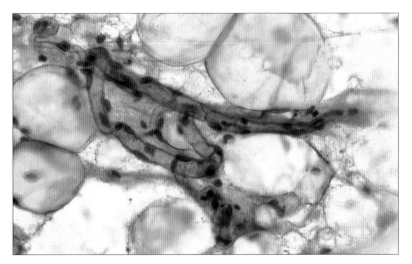

Fig. 8.18 Fat cells – Pap x100. Capillaries are often seen attached to fat cells. Note the flattened endothelial lining of the capillary in this field.

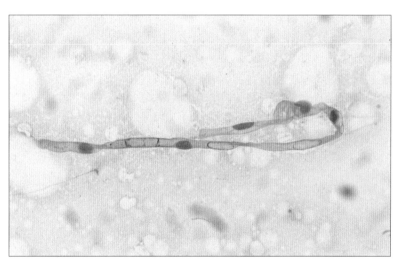

Fig. 8.19 Capillary – Pap x100. This detached capillary contains flattened erythrocytes and is lined by endothelial cells.

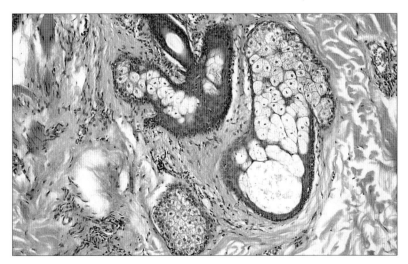

Fig. 8.20 Sebaceous glands – H&E x10. This section from the subareolar region of a normal breast includes sebaceous glands surrounded by stroma.

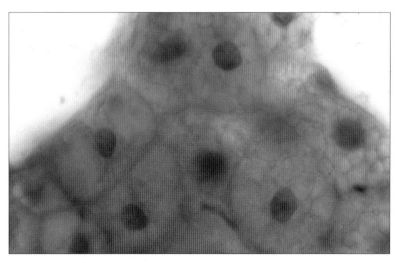

Fig. 8.21 Sebaceous glands – Pap x40. Seen here is a group of cells from a sebaceous gland, showing relatively small nuclei and abundant vacuolated cytoplasm. These cells are sometimes mistaken for apocrine cells.

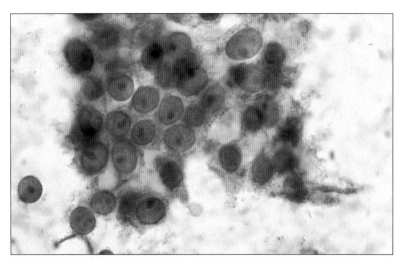

Fig. 8.22 Lactational changes – Pap x100. The cluster of loosely cohesive epithelial cells pictured here contains enlarged, but round, nuclei with prominent red nucleoli and vacuolated, disintegrating cytoplasm. These secretory changes are common in aspirates taken in late pregnancy and during lactation.

PREGNANCY AND LACTATIONAL CHANGES

It is important that the cytopathologist is made aware when an aspirate is taken from a pregnant woman, as the cellular features can mimic malignancy. The acinar cells are plentiful and show secretory changes, namely slight nuclear enlargement, abundant vacuolated cytoplasm, and active nucleoli (**Figs 8.22, 8.23**). Distended intact lobules are frequently seen (**Fig. 8.24**). Numerous single epithelial cells are seen in the background, many with prominent nucleoli, and also bare epithelial nuclei, raising the suspicion of malignancy (**Fig. 8.25**). However, there are also many myoepithelial cells and the secretory background confirms pregnancy changes. In some

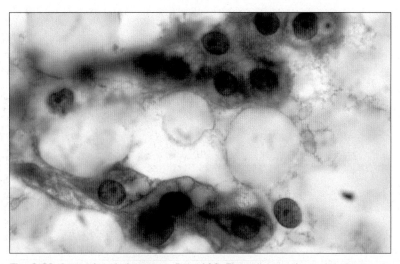

Fig. 8.23 Lactational changes – Pap x100. The cells seen here also show lactational changes, including nuclear enlargement, prominent nucleoli, secretory vacuolation, and some dissociation. The background appears to contain rounded spaces, which should not be mistaken for fat cells as they have no structure and are of varying sizes.

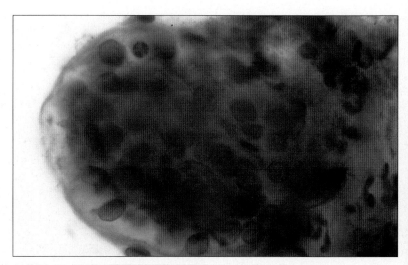

Fig. 8.24 Lobule, lactational changes – Pap x100. This field shows a distended lobule (compare its size with the normal lobules in **Figure 8.10**) which is very cellular. Myoepithelial cells are not clearly seen in this lobule.

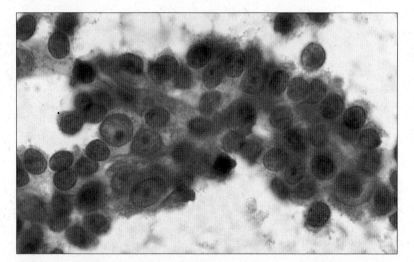

Fig. 8.25 Lactational changes – Pap x100. The cluster of cells pictured here looks abnormal because of the variable nuclear size and large red nucleoli. There are also single epithelial cells in the background. However, the history of lactation and the secretory changes in the cells provide a clue to the correct diagnosis of lactational change.

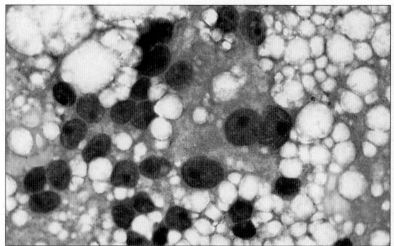

Fig. 8.26 Lactational changes – MGG x40. The cells in this cluster show dissociation, prominent nucleoli, and some vacuolation of the cytoplasm, which is otherwise granular. Note the lipid-rich vacuolar secretory background.

needle aspirates from lactating breasts there is a lipid-rich vacuolar appearance to the background, best seen on the May Grunwald Giemsa stained specimen (**Fig. 8.26**).

The cytological appearances of **lactational adenomas** are very similar to those of the histology (**Fig. 8.27**). The aspirate is cellular, containing many distended lobular structures composed of acinar epithelial cells showing secretory changes (**Figs 8.28–8.30**). The background is composed of secretory material with scattered epithelial and myoepithelial cells. Fibroadenomas in pregnancy may show secretory changes (**Figs 8.31, 8.32**), in addition to their usual cytological features (see **Figures 8.92–8.97**).

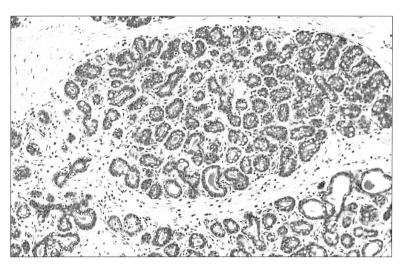

Fig. 8.27 Lactational adenoma – H&E x10. This histological section of a lactational adenoma shows lobules composed of acini lined by vacuolated epithelial cells and containing secretion.

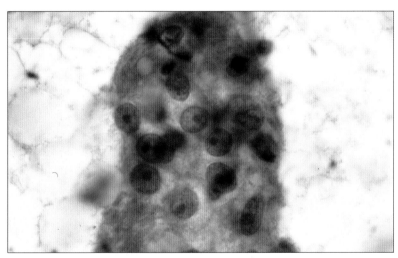

Fig. 8.28 Lactational adenoma – Pap x100. The distended lobule illustrated here, from a lactational adenoma, is composed of cells with enlarged nuclei, prominent red nucleoli, and vacuolated cytoplasm.

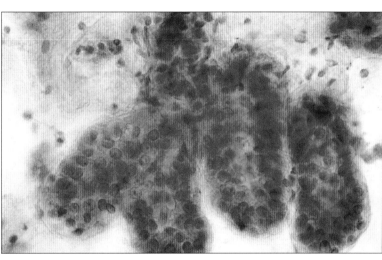

Fig. 8.29 Lactational adenoma – Pap x40. Several acinar structures are seen here, composed of cells showing secretory changes, closely resembling the histological picture (see **Figure 8.27**).

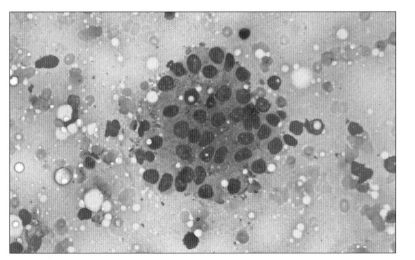

Fig. 8.30 Lactational adenoma – MGG x40. The distended lobule illustrated here does not show the marked secretory changes noted in the wet-fixed smear (see **Figure 8.28**).

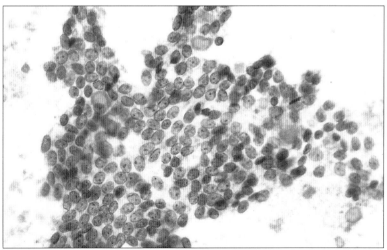

Fig. 8.31 Lactational changes in fibroadenoma – Pap x40. The sheet of benign ductal cells seen in this field displays secretory changes and prominent nucleoli related to pregnancy, but also the sesame-seed type of scattered myoepithelial cells on the surface.

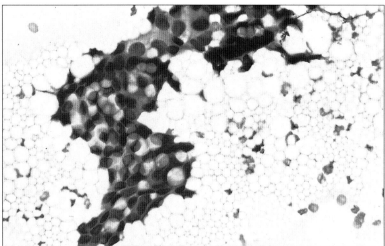

Fig. 8.32 Lactational changes in fibroadenoma – MGG x40. This air-dried smear, from the same case as in **Figure 8.31**, contains a sheet of loosely cohesive ductal cells showing secretory changes. Myoepithelial cells are not evident.

INFLAMMATORY LESIONS

Mastitis is an inflammatory process seen more commonly in young women, especially in relation to breast-feeding. Clinically, the diagnosis is obvious with the presenting symptom of a tender, reddened mass in the breast. An aspirate shows numerous, acute inflammatory cells, mostly neutrophil polymorphs with some histiocytes and multinucleated giant histiocytes (**Figs 8.33, 8.34**). Some epithelial cells may also be seen which invariably show reactive changes, consisting mainly of nuclear enlargement and visible nucleoli. At a later stage, chronic inflammatory cells, including lymphocytes, are seen and the epithelial cells lose their reactive appearance.

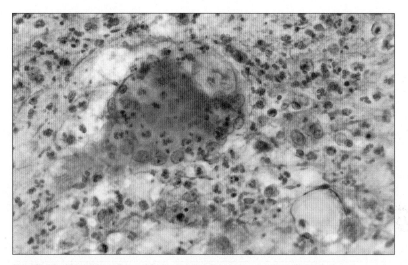

Fig. 8.33 Mastitis – Pap x40. Illustrated is a large multinucleated giant histiocyte surrounded by foamy macrophages, polymorphs, and debris characteristic of mastitis.

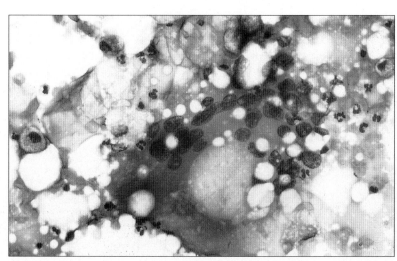

Fig. 8.34 Mastitis – MGG x40. This air-dried smear, prepared from an aspirate of mastitis, shows a multinucleated giant histiocyte with foamy macrophages and some neutrophils in the background.

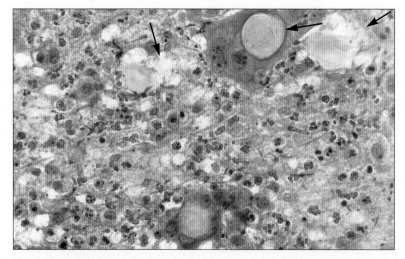

Fig. 8.35 Subareolar abscess – Pap x40. The cytological features of a subareolar abscess, as seen here, are the same as those of mastitis, except for the presence of anucleate, sometimes keratinized, squames (arrowed).

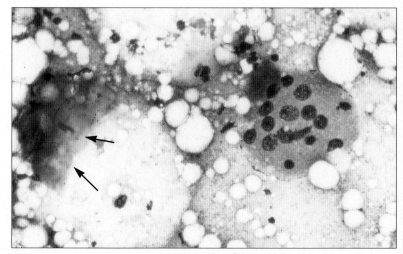

Fig. 8.36 Subareolar abscess – MGG x40. This field shows a multinucleated giant histiocyte on the right with azure blue, keratinized, anucleate squames on the left (arrowed). There are a few polymorphs in the background.

Cytology of a subareolar abscess has an identical appearance to mastitis, except for the presence of anucleate squames. These cells, when keratinized, stain a refractile orange in wet-fixed smears, but otherwise are pale pink and may be missed **(Fig. 8.35)**. On the air-dried smear, anucleate squames are pale blue or even colourless, but are a bright azure blue when keratinized **(Fig. 8.36)**.

Granulomatous mastitis **(Fig. 8.37)** has a typical cytological appearance. The smears are often blood-stained and cellular, containing proliferating blood vessels **(Figs 8.38, 8.39)** and numerous inflammatory cells, including plasma cells and lymphocytes **(Fig. 8.40)** and multinucleated histiocytes **(Fig. 8.41)**, which may resemble Langhans' giant cells **(Figs 8.42)**. Collections of epithelioid histiocytes may be seen **(Fig. 8.43)**.

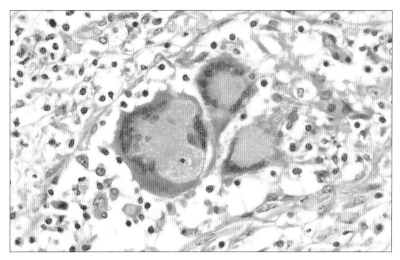

Fig. 8.37 Granulomatous mastitis – H&E x10. This histological section of granulomatous mastitis shows multinucleated giant histiocytes, resembling Langhans' giant cells, and a chronic inflammatory infiltrate.

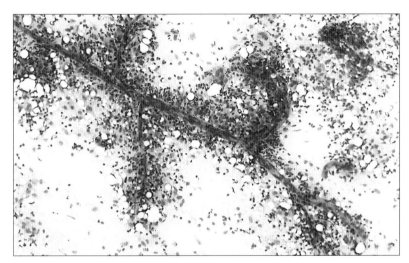

Fig. 8.38 Granulomatous mastitis – MGG x4.5. Under low power the proliferating blood vessels in this lesion look spectacular, with scattered acute and chronic inflammatory cells in the background.

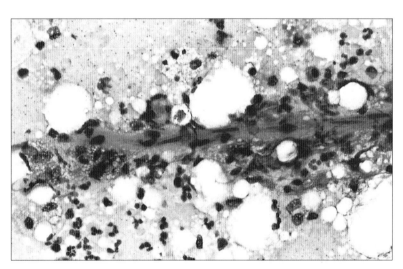

Fig. 8.39 Granulomatous mastitis – MGG x10. This field shows a thickened capillary surrounded by neutrophils, lymphocytes, and foamy macrophages, consistent with granulomatous mastitis.

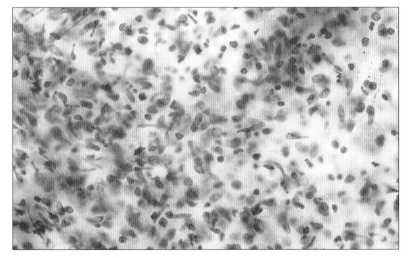

Fig. 8.40 Granulomatous mastitis – Pap x40. This rather thickly spread smear from a case of granulomatous mastitis shows a mixture of inflammatory cells, including plasma cells, lymphocytes, and occasional macrophages.

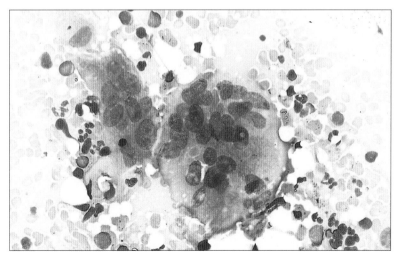

Fig. 8.41 Granulomatous mastitis – MGG x40. Two multinucleated histiocytes are seen here with nuclei scattered throughout the cytoplasm, rather than around the periphery. There are inflammatory cells in the background.

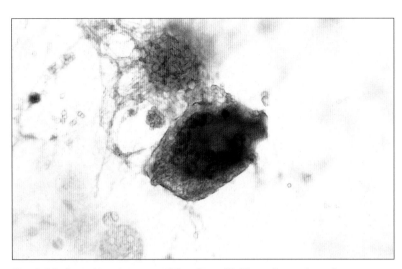

Fig. 8.42 Granulomatous mastitis – Pap x40. The cell seen here, in an aspirate from granulomatous mastitis, is a multinucleated giant histiocyte with its nuclei around the periphery, resembling a Langhans' giant cell.

Fat necrosis mimics carcinoma of the breast clinically and mammographically, especially if the patient does not recall any history of trauma. A fine needle aspirate is one of the simplest and quickest ways of arriving at a diagnosis and reflects the underlying histology (**Fig. 8.44**). The features are characteristic, with abundant clusters of degenerate fat cells (**Figs 8.45, 8.46**) and cells with foamy cytoplasm, which appear to be foamy macrophages, but may be another form of degenerate fat cells (**Figs 8.47**). Multinucleated giant histiocytes are usually present (**Fig. 8.48**). Inflammatory cells may also be seen in the early stages. Epithelial cells are rarely noted in aspirates from fat necrosis.

BREAST CYSTS

Epidermal cysts can occur in the breast (**Fig. 8.49**). Aspirates from these lesions contain anucleate squames (**Figs 8.50, 8.51**) and inflammatory cells, including multinucleated histiocytes (**Fig. 8.52**).

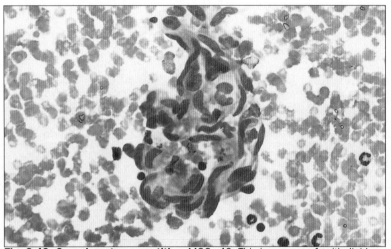

Fig. 8.43 Granulomatous mastitis – MGG x40. This is a group of epithelioid histiocytes with elongated nuclei and cytoplasmic margins, seen in granulomatous mastitis.

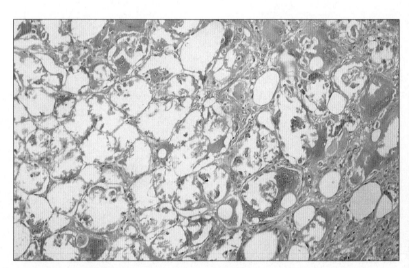

Fig. 8.44 Fat necrosis – H&E x10. This histological section of fat necrosis shows degenerate fat cells.

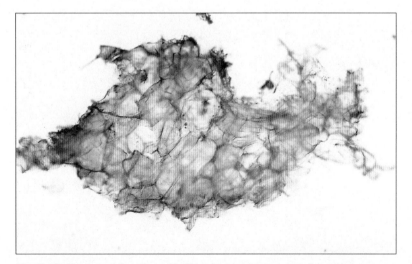

Fig. 8.45 Fat necrosis – Pap x40. This cluster of degenerate fat cells shows hazy cell borders and pink instead of blue staining. The nuclei are not visible. Compare these degenerate cells with the viable fat cells in **Figure 8.16**.

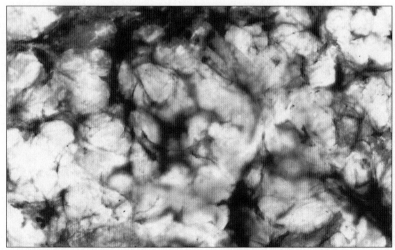

Fig. 8.46 Fat necrosis – MGG x40. The degenerate fat cells in this cluster represent fat necrosis in an air-dried aspirate. Individual fat cells are not clearly defined.

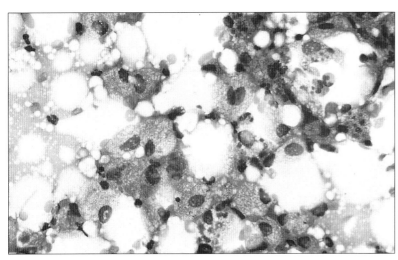

Fig. 8.47 Fat necrosis – MGG x40. A particular feature of fat necrosis is the presence of cells with foamy cytoplasm, which resemble foamy macrophages, but may be degenerate fat cells.

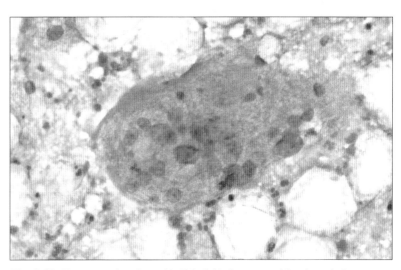

Fig. 8.48 Fat necrosis – Pap x40. This field shows a multinucleated giant histiocyte surrounded by degenerate fat cells and some foamy cells, which could be either degenerate fat cells or foamy macrophages.

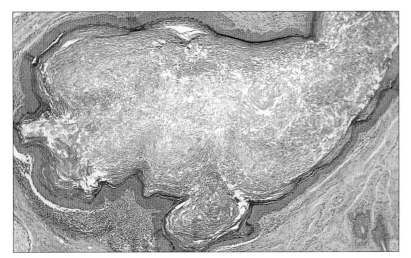

Fig. 8.49 Epidermal cyst – H&E x10. This section shows a cyst lined by squamous epithelium, including a granular cell layer and containing keratinous debris. (Courtesy of Dr PH McKee, St Thomas' Hospital, London, UK).

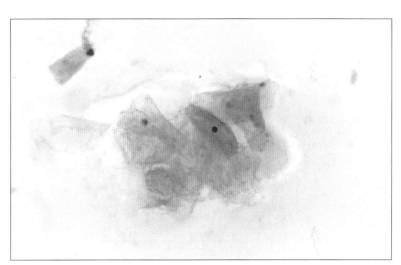

Fig. 8.50 Epidermal cyst – Pap x40. This field shows the contents of an epidermal cyst, namely anucleate squames, many of which are keratinized.

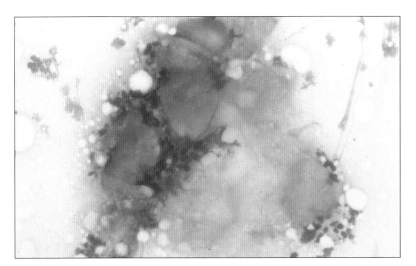

Fig. 8.51 Epidermal cyst – MGG x40. Epidermal cysts may become infected, as seen in this example where the anucleate keratinized squamous cells are accompanied by neutrophils.

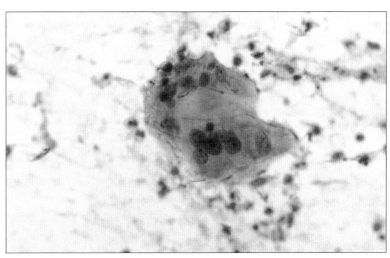

Fig. 8.52 Epidermal cyst – Pap x40. Infected epidermal cysts may contain multinucleated giant histiocytes and neutrophils, as illustrated here, as well as anucleate squames.

Cysts of the breast are almost always benign. They are palpable and easily visualized on mammograms and on ultrasound examination. Cyst fluid is discarded if it is colourless and clear, but is sent for cytological examination if blood-stained, coloured, or has residual thickening after aspiration, or if the cyst is recurrent. The fluid is sent to the laboratory in a universal container, where it is spun down and smears prepared. The most noticeable feature is the presence of abundant granular cyst debris with scattered foamy macrophages (**Figs 8.53, 8.54**); usually, there are abundant sheets and clusters of apocrine cells, which may show degenerative changes (**Figs 8.55, 8.56**). Cyst debris is formed partly of cytoplasmic granular material derived from apocrine cells. Apocrine cells have abundant granular cytoplasm, which stains pinkish orange with the Papanicolaou stain and purple with May Grunwald Giemsa (**Figs 8.57, 8.58**). The cells may be in flat sheets with a palisaded edge (**Fig. 8.59**) or in the form of papillary clusters. Benign ductal cells are occasionally seen, which may display degenerative changes in the form of cytoplasmic vacuolation or reactive atypia (**Fig. 8.60**). Inflamed cysts show histiocytes as well as numerous polymorphs (**Fig. 8.61**). If bleeding has occurred into a cyst, the fluid is often dark brown or green and the smear shows altered blood (**Figs 8.62, 8.63**), as well as

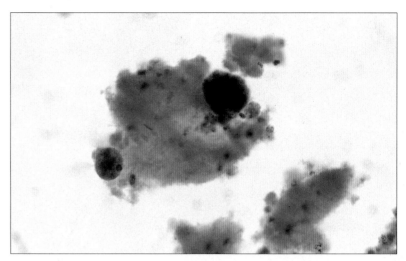

Fig. 8.53 Cyst – Pap x40. Breast cysts contain abundant debris and often not much else. This field shows cyst debris and some degenerate foamy macrophages.

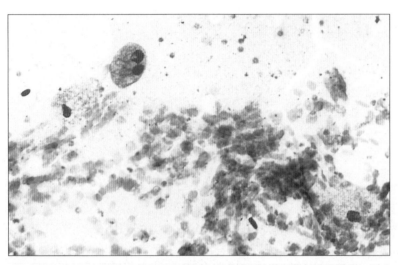

Fig. 8.54 Cyst – MGG x40. This air-dried smear shows foamy macrophages, grey erythrocytes, and pale purple cyst debris.

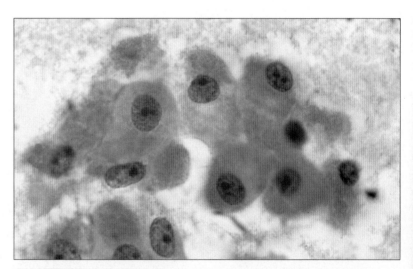

Fig. 8.55 Cyst, apocrine cells – Pap x140. The apocrine cells in this field contain abundant pinkish orange granular cytoplasm, which appears to be disintegrating in some of the cells. This granular material forms the debris seen in cysts. Note the large round or oval nuclei and prominent nucleoli in these cells.

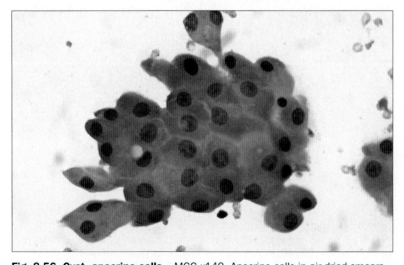

Fig. 8.56 Cyst, apocrine cells – MGG x140. Apocrine cells in air-dried smears have bluish purple granular cytoplasm and clear-cut cytoplasmic borders.

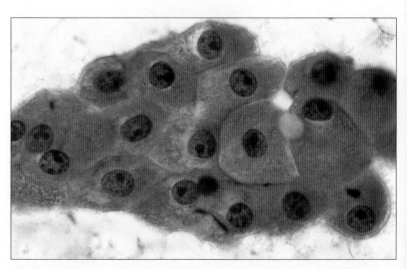

Fig. 8.57 Apocrine cells – Pap x100. Under high magnification the sharp cytoplasmic border, abundant cytoplasm, and prominent red nucleoli of apocrine cells are evident.

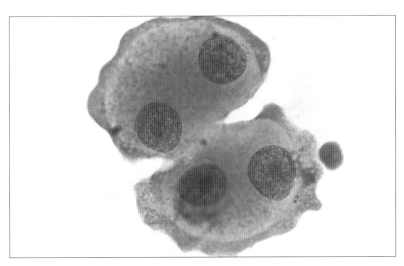

Fig. 8.58 Apocrine cells – MGG x100. These apocrine cells show binucleation and granular cytoplasm, but the nucleoli are not as prominent as in the wet-fixed preparation **(Fig. 8.57)**.

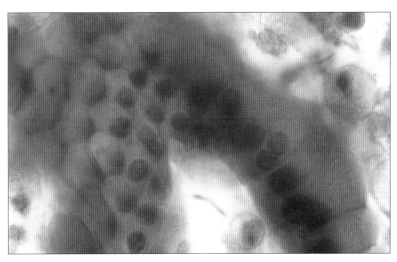

Fig. 8.59 Apocrine cells – Pap x100. Sheets of apocrine cells often have a palisaded edge, as demonstrated here.

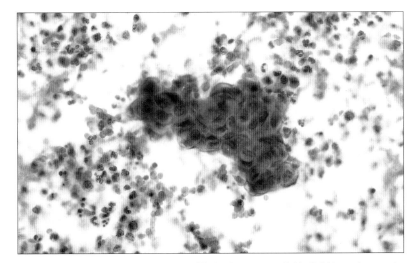

Fig. 8.60 Cyst, ductal cells – Pap x40. In the centre of this field is a cluster of degenerate ductal cells showing vacuolation. These should not be interpreted as being suggestive of malignancy. Note the neutrophils surrounding the ductal cells. These inflammatory cells are not infrequent in a breast-cyst aspirate.

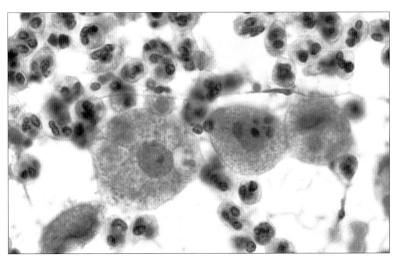

Fig. 8.61 Cyst, inflamed – MGG x40. This field contains foamy macrophages. There are also many neutrophil polymorphs, indicative of inflammatory changes in a cyst.

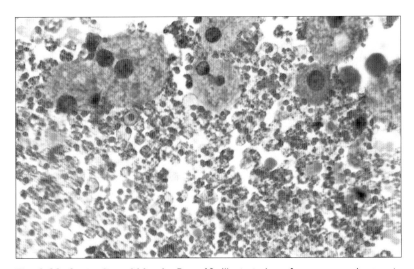

Fig. 8.62 Cyst, altered blood – Pap x40. Illustrated are foamy macrophages at the top of the field, blue cyst debris, orange erythrocytes and red granular material, which is altered blood.

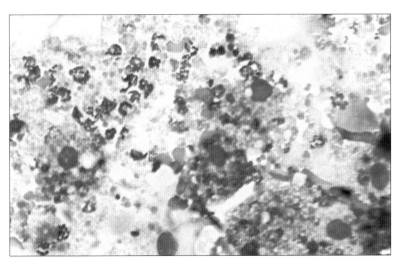

Fig. 8.63 Cyst, altered blood – MGG x40. This air-dried smear contains foamy macrophages, brownish orange erythrocytes, and altered blood in the form of blue granular material.

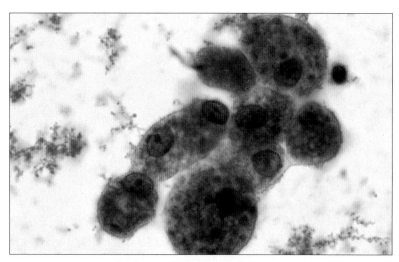

haemosiderin-filled foamy macrophages (**Figs 8.64, 8.65**) and multinucleated histiocytes of varying sizes (**Fig. 8.66**). Occasionally, large cells with abundant, fairly dense cytoplasm, almost spindle-shaped, are seen in breast-cyst aspirates (**Figs 8.67, 8.68**). These are believed to arise from granulation tissue at the edge of an inflamed cyst. Calcium may be seen in cyst fluid, either as loose particles or within macrophages (**Fig. 8.69**).

The mammogram and ultrasound film of some cysts show a solid area projecting from the cyst wall into the lumen. This usually represents an intracystic papilloma, an aspirate of which contains papillary clusters of epithelial cells, both ductal and apocrine, as well as myoepithelial cells (**Figs 8.70, 8.71**). Small papillary clusters of mildly atypical ductal cells may also be seen in aspirates from benign cysts which do not contain intracystic papillomas. Varying degrees of cellular atypia may be present, but definite features of malignancy must be present for the diagnosis of intracystic carcinoma (**Figs 8.72–8.74**).

Fig. 8.64 Cyst, siderophages – Pap x100. The foamy macrophages pictured here contain abundant greenish yellow haemosiderin, indicative of previous haemorrhage.

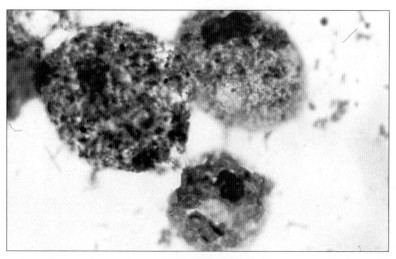

Fig. 8.65 Cyst, siderophages – MGG x100. Haemosiderin-laden macrophages in air-dried smears have purple nuclei and dark blue–black intracytoplasmic granules.

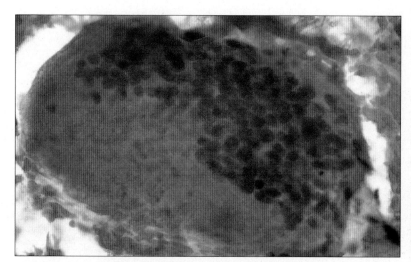

Fig. 8.66 Cyst, multinucleated histiocyte – Pap x100. This multinucleated histiocyte has over 100 nuclei and a hazy cytoplasmic margin.

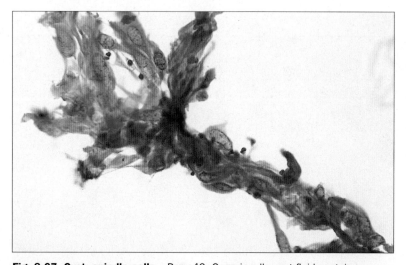

Fig. 8.67 Cyst, spindle cells – Pap x40. Occasionally, cyst fluid contains spindle-shaped cells with vesicular nuclei, resembling fibroblasts, as seen here. This cells are thought to be derived from the granulation tissue at the edge of an inflamed cyst.

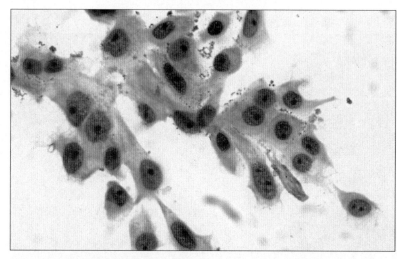

Fig. 8.68 Cyst, spindle cells – MGG x40. The air-dried smear from the same case as in **Figure 8.67** shows similar spindle-shaped cells, which are probably fibroblasts. The nucleoli are clearly visible in these cells.

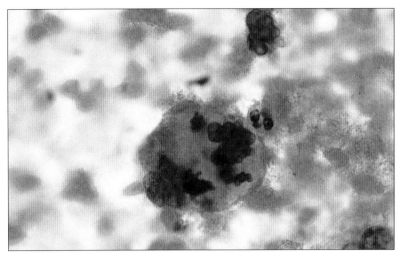

Fig. 8.69 Cyst, calcium – Pap x40. Illustrated here is a macrophage containing calcium, and also loose particles of calcium in the background.

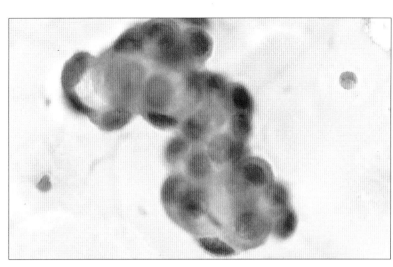

Fig. 8.70 Intracystic papilloma – Pap x100. These degenerate, mildly pleomorphic ductal cells contain vacuoles, but show no evidence of malignancy. A certain degree of atypia is permitted in benign epithelial cells in cyst fluids.

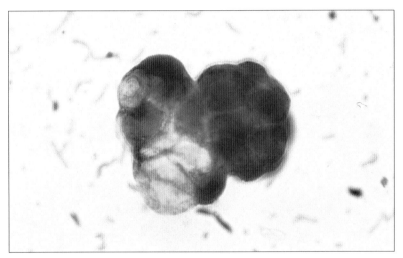

Fig. 8.71 Intracystic papilloma – MGG x100. This rounded cluster of slightly enlarged ductal cells shows some vacuolation, probably a degenerative feature.

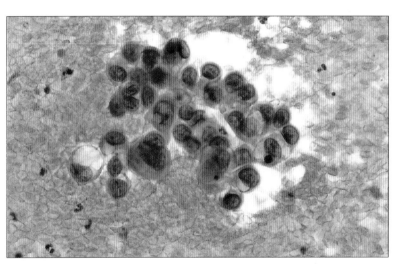

Fig. 8.72 Intracystic carcinoma – Pap x40. In contrast to the cells in **Figures 8.69–8.71**, these epithelial cells, although small, are pleomorphic, have irregular nuclear margins, and abnormal chromatin, consistent with carcinoma.

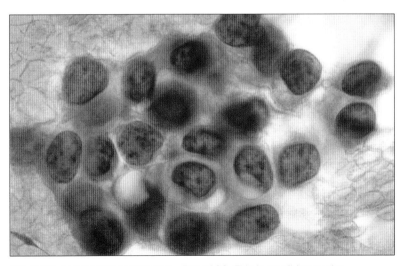

Fig. 8.73 Intracystic carcinoma – Pap x100. This is an oil-immersion photomicrograph of another group of carcinoma cells from the same case as in **Figure 8.72**. The cells have very irregular nuclear margins and an abnormal chromatin pattern.

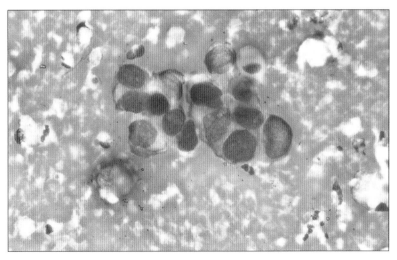

Fig. 8.74 Intracystic carcinoma – MGG x40. This air-dried sample from the same case as in **Figures 8.72** and **8.73** contains pleomorphic carcinoma cells, but the chromatin details are not well visualized.

BENIGN PROLIFERATIVE BREAST CHANGES

Benign proliferative breast changes, **fibrocystic disease**, and **cystic mastopathy** are various terms used to describe the proliferative and involutional changes that occur in older women **(Fig. 8.75)**. Clinically, the lesion may present as an ill-defined thickening or ridge of tissue. Aspiration may produce a drop of fluid if cystic changes predominate. The smears are often cellular, with sheets and groups of benign ductal cells showing some crowding **(Figs 8.76, 8.77)**, apocrine cells, foamy macrophages, and myoepithelial cells. The appearances differ from those of a fibroadenoma in that the sheets of cells are smaller, they do not show honey-combing [as the nuclei often overlap, suggesting simple hyperplasia **(Fig. 8.78)**], and there are usually no large stromal fragments. Apocrine cells often constitute a large proportion of the epithelial cells in benign proliferative breast disease.

Ductal hyperplasia in cytological material contains clusters of ductal cells showing overlapping nuclei, slight nuclear pleomorphism, and crowding. Epithelial proliferation **(Fig. 8.79)**, including papillary changes, is accurately reflected in the aspirate **(Fig. 8.80)**. In **atypical ductal hyperplasia (ADH)** the feature of ductal hyperplasia are exaggerated, producing clusters of epithelial cells which are three-dimensional and show atypia in the form of nuclear enlargement, hyperchroma-

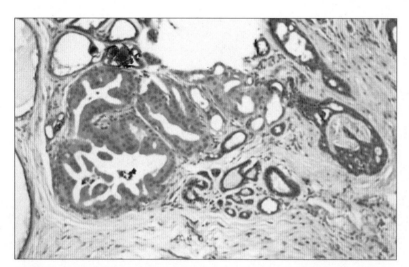

Fig. 8.75 Benign proliferative breast changes – H&E x10. This section of breast shows proliferative changes, including apocrine metaplasia, cystic changes, and epitheliosis. Note the calcium present.

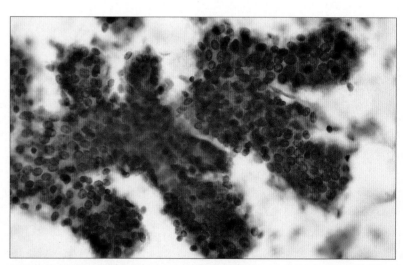

Fig. 8.76 Benign proliferative breast changes – Pap x40. The cells illustrated are in the form of branching clusters with some overlapping of nuclei. A few scattered myoepithelial cells are seen.

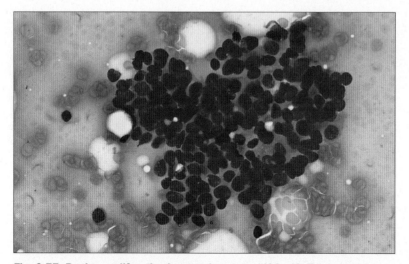

Fig. 8.77 Benign proliferative breast changes – MGG x40. This group of ductal cells exhibits some nuclear overlapping and a few myoepithelial cells.

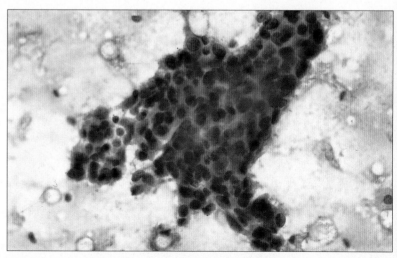

Fig. 8.78 Benign proliferative breast changes – Pap x40. Mild pleomorphism and nuclear overlapping are obvious in this cluster of ductal cells.

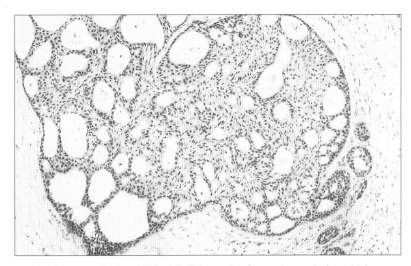

Fig. 8.79 Epitheliosis – H&E x4.5. This section from a breast lesion which contained widespread proliferative alterations shows changes reported as epitheliosis, with epithelial cells lining connective tissue bridges.

sia, and visible nucleoli (**Figs 8.81, 8.82**). In some instances, especially with stereotactic aspirates of impalpable radial lesions, the cells show malignant features such as markedly enlarged nuclei, irregular nuclear margins, and prominent nucleoli (**Fig. 8.83**). However, these cytological changes, if seen in only one duct on the histological section, are diagnosed as ADH. Such cases of apparent false positive cytological diagnoses must be carefully correlated with histology and additional levels of the sections should be examined for features that may change the diagnosis to ductal carcinoma-in-situ. The cytological features, however, remain identical, with the cells showing malignant features in both.

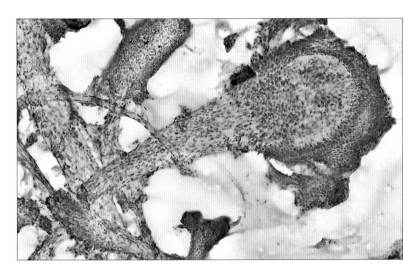

Fig. 8.80 Epitheliosis – Pap x10. An aspirate from the lesion in **Figure 8.79** showed strange papillary structures, with connective tissue cores covered by several layers of benign epithelial cells.

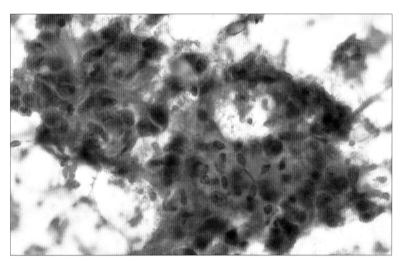

Fig. 8.81 ADH – Pap x40. This field displays irregular three-dimensional clusters of cells which are moderately pleomorphic and have irregular outlines. A few myoepithelial cells are also seen. Although the features are not diagnostic of malignancy, they are highly suspicious and such an aspirate would fall into the C4 category, (see Chapter 6).

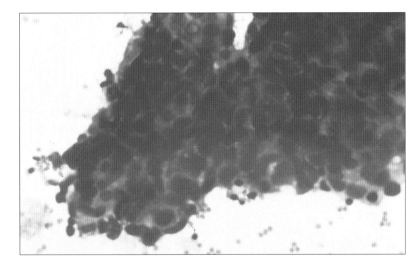

Fig. 8.82 ADH – MGG x40. This air-dried smear from the same lesion as in **Figure 8.81** shows similar cytological findings, with crowding and overlapping of nuclei and hyperchromasia. Myoepithelial cells are difficult to identify.

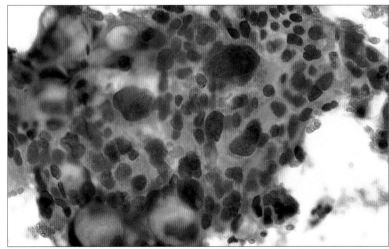

Fig. 8.83 ADH/DCIS – Pap x100. This aspirate of a radial lesion, taken under stereotactic guidance, contains markedly pleomorphic and hyperchromatic large carcinoma cells. The initial histological diagnosis was ADH. However, further levels revealed more ductal involvement by the same process and the diagnosis was revised to DCIS.

Atypical lobular hyperplasia is difficult to diagnose on cytology. The features are similar to those of lobular carcinoma-in-situ (see Chapter 9.).

Sclerosing adenosis (Fig. 8.84) produces aspirates which contain thick fragments of tissue composed of a mixture of epithelial and myoepithelial cells **(Fig. 8.85)**, sometimes accompanied by atypical apocrine cells **(Fig. 8.86)** and sometimes by calcium **(Fig. 8.87)**. As with frozen sections the features may suggest malignancy, but the presence of myoepithelial cells is a clue to the correct diagnosis.

Radial scars are impalpable spiculate or stellate lesions detected on mammograms; they may be benign or malignant. There may be only one small area of malignant change in such lesions; as this may not be sampled on stereotactic aspiration, current practice is to excise all radial scars. These lesions have a dense sclerotic centre with trapped ducts and show varying degrees of proliferative change in the radial portions, including those mentioned above – namely fibrocystic changes, ductal and lobular hyperplasia, atypical hyperplasia, sclerosing adenosis, and apocrine adenosis. The carcinoma usually associated with radial scars is the tubular type (see Chapter 9).

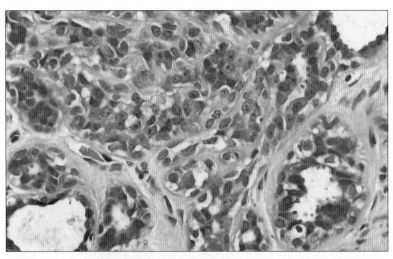

Fig. 8.84 Sclerosing adenosis – H&E x40. This histological section shows sclerosing adenosis in a lesion demonstrating a variety of proliferative changes. This lesion can be mistaken for malignancy in frozen sections as well as in cytological preparations.

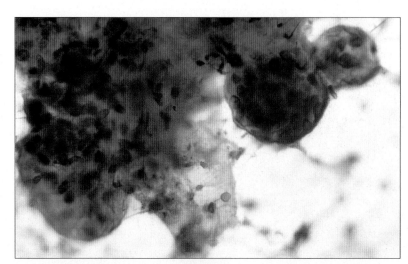

Fig. 8.85 Sclerosing adenosis – Pap x100. This smear shows a thick fragment of tissue composed of lobules, connective tissue, and myoepithelial cells. The diagnosis of sclerosing adenosis is arrived at by eliminating other possible entities, such as lobular carcinoma producing distended lobules and infiltrating carcinoma within the stroma. The presence of myoepithelial cells is a pointer to the correct diagnosis.

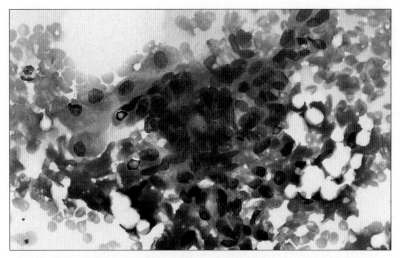

Fig. 8.86 Sclerosing adenosis – MGG x40. Illustrated here is a small, thick cluster of epithelial cells with overlying myoepithelial cells and closely associated apocrine cells. Occasionally, the apocrine cells show atypia, mimicking carcinoma.

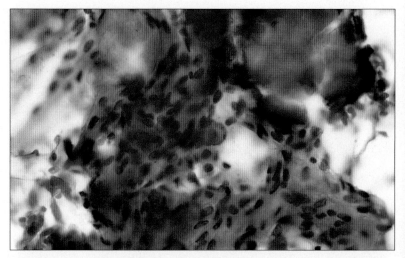

Fig. 8.87 Sclerosing adenosis – Pap x40. Sclerosing adenosis is commonly associated with calcium, which is reflected in the aspirate, as demonstrated in this field. The thick, swirling clusters of epithelial and myoepithelial cells are seen adjacent to the calcium in the top right corner.

FIBROADENOMA

Fibroadenomas typically present as rounded firm masses in the breast, which are sometimes referred to as 'breast mice' because of their mobility. A fibroadenoma has to be well-immobilized for a fine needle aspirate or the needle just pushes it forwards. The lesion has a rubbery feel to the tip of the needle and, if very fibrotic, it feels as though the needle is being inserted into a rubber tyre. The amount of material aspirated often seems very scanty, but usually contains plenty of cells. The histological appearance is that of a well-demarcated lesion composed of ducts and stroma (**Fig. 8.88**). The cytological features of fibroadenoma may overlap, to some extent, with those of benign proliferative breast changes, but there are specific criteria which help in their distinction (**Fig. 8.89**).

The most common feature is the presence of large, flat sheets of ductal cells (**Figs 8.90, 8.91**), with uniform nuclei and little cytoplasm. Many of the sheets show either staghorn (**Fig. 8.92**) or club-shaped branching (**Fig. 8.93**). A characteristic feature is the presence of myoepithelial cells on the surface of the sheets, resembling sesame seeds on a bun (**Fig. 8.94**), and many more in the background (**Fig. 8.45**), often with scattered stromal cells (**Figs 8.96, 8.97**).

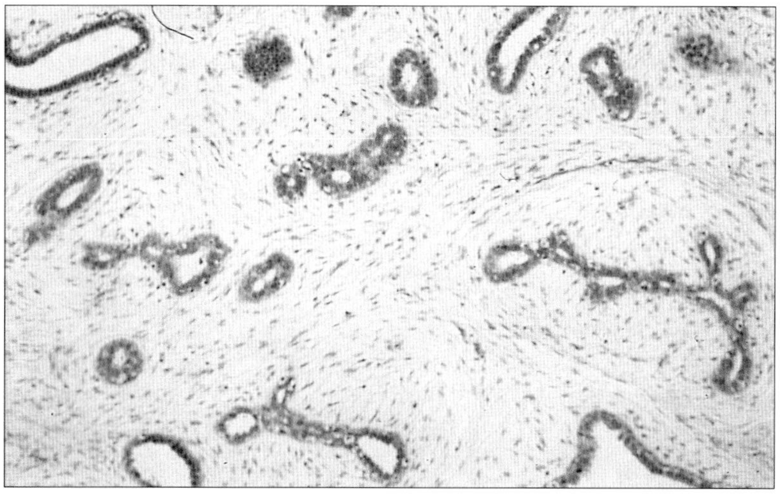

FEATURES	FIBROADENOMA	BENIGN PROLIFERATIVE CHANGES
Clinical	Rounded, clearly defined Mobile lump Rubbery to needle tip	Not well-defined, nodular Not mobile Not rubbery
Cellularity	Very cellular	Cellular
Pattern	Large flat sheets of cells Honeycombing may be seen Cribriform holes occasionally Staghorn or club-shaped branches	Smaller sheets and groups Not usual Not seen No particular branching pattern
'Sesame seed' myoepithelial cells	Typical on the large sheets	May be seen
Bare nuclei	Present in large numbers	Present
Stromal fragments	Usually present	Not common
Apocrine cells	Occasionally seen	Common
Foamy macrophages	Occasionally seen	Common

Fig. 8.88 Fibroadenoma – H&E x10. This section of a fibroadenoma shows the two components of this lesion – stromal and glandular. Although there appears to be much stroma, the aspirates are usually very cellular with the duct lining cells being aspirated in sheets.

Fig. 8.89 Fibroadenoma versus benign proliferative breast changes.

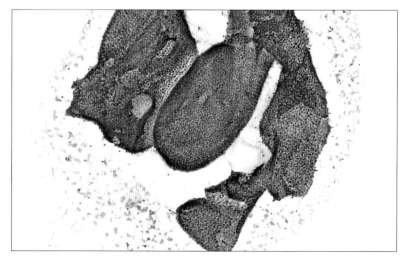

Fig. 8.90 Fibroadenoma – Pap x10. This low-power view of an aspirate from a fibroadenoma shows huge sheets of benign ductal cells, which are folded over in areas. Neat palisaded edges are obvious, even at this low magnification.

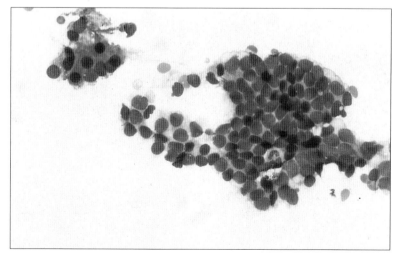

Fig. 8.91 Fibroadenoma – MGG x40. The benign ductal cells seen in this aspirate from a fibroadenoma are in the form of flat sheets.

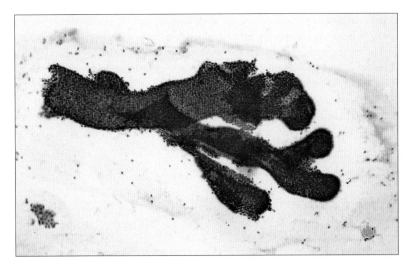

Fig. 8.92 Fibroadenoma – Pap x10. A typical pattern seen with fibroadenomas is the large branched sheet of benign ductal cells that resembles a staghorn (also called antler horn). Note the scattered, small bare nuclei in the background, which are myoepithelial cells.

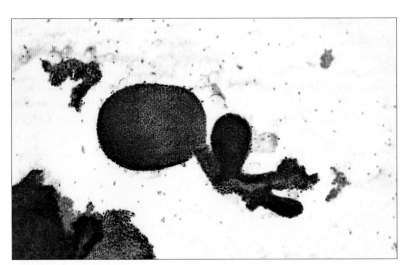

Fig. 8.93 Fibroadenoma – Pap x10. Another pattern often seen in aspirates from fibroadenomas is the club-shaped branching of sheets of ductal cells, as illustrated here. Adjacent to this example is a large, folded, flat sheet of benign ductal cells.

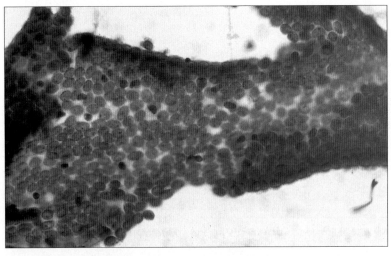

Fig. 8.94 Fibroadenoma – Pap x40. This sheet of benign ductal cells has a scattering of darker smaller cells on the surface, resembling sesame seeds on a bun. Note the palisaded upper edge of the sheet and the other folded edges.

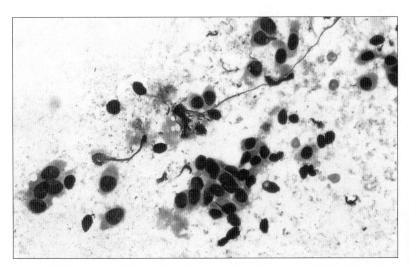

Fig. 8.95 Fibroadenoma – MGG x40. Adjacent to the ductal cells in the small sheets illustrated here are small, dark myoepithelial cells. The ductal cells show apparent loss of cohesion, but this is a common finding with air-dried aspirates.

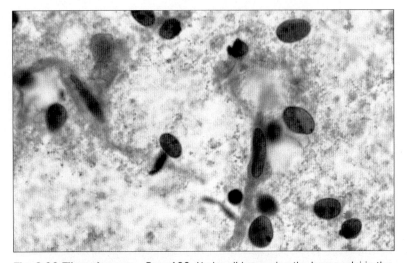

Fig. 8.96 Fibroadenoma – Pap x100. Under oil immersion the bare nuclei in the background of aspirates are seen to consist of two types of cells – small ovoid cells with no cytoplasm, which are myoepithelial, and spindle-shaped cells with wisps of delicate pale blue cytoplasm, which are identical to stromal cells.

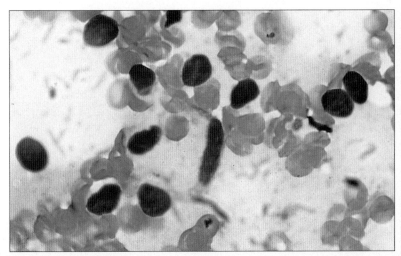

Fig. 8.97 Fibroadenoma – MGG x100. The air-dried smear examined under oil immersion reveals two types of bare nuclei, the ovoid myoepithelial cells and the spindle-shaped stromal nuclei. The cytoplasm of the stromal cells is not seen in this preparation.

Occasionally, the sheets show a cribriform pattern with holes (**Figs 8.98, 8.99**), a feature normally associated with cribriform ductal carcinoma (see **Figure 9.66.**). Small acinar groups of benign ductal cells may be seen (**Fig. 8.100**). The nuclear chromatin is usually vesicular (**Fig. 8.101**), but may be granular and nucleoli may be prominent (**Fig. 8.102**). Stromal fragments of varying sizes are often noted. They are pale pink or blue on wet-fixed smears (**Fig. 8.103**) and bright pink on air-dried material (**Fig. 8.104**). The stromal fragments tend to display ill-defined edges and contain a few thin wavy nuclei, but occasionally the fragments are leaf-shaped with the sharp, well-defined margins that are usually associated with benign phyllodes tumours. Foamy macrophages and apocrine cells may be seen. Occasionally, sheets and clusters of enlarged epithelial cells with hyperchromatic nuclei and nucleoli may be seen in an otherwise typical fibroadenoma aspirate (**Figs 8.105, 8.106**), representing atypia in a fibroadenoma .These can be mistaken for malignancy if the associated myoepithelial cells are not noticed. On the other hand, carcinomas can arise in fibroadenomas and should be reported as such if there are definite cellular features of malignancy. Mucin-like material derived from stroma may be seen in small amounts in aspirates from a fibroadenoma (**Fig. 8.107**), and the picture may be interpreted as a low-grade mucinous carcinoma if the myoepithelial cells are ignored.

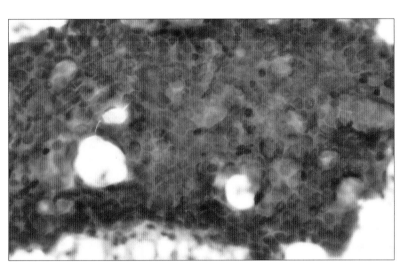

Fig. 8.98 Fibroadenoma – Pap x40. This sheet of benign ductal cells shows several cribriform spaces of varying size. Note the scattered myoepithelial cells on the surface of the ductal sheet. The differential diagnosis is cribriform ductal carcinoma-in-situ.

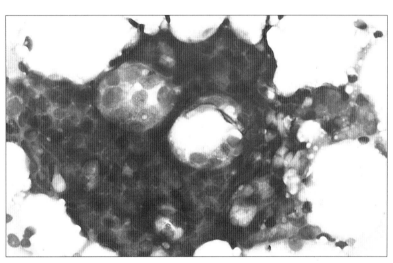

Fig. 8.99 Fibroadenoma – MGG x40. This air-dried smear contains a benign ductal sheet which exhibits a cribriform pattern.The myoepithelial cells on the surface are not as clearly visible as those in the background.

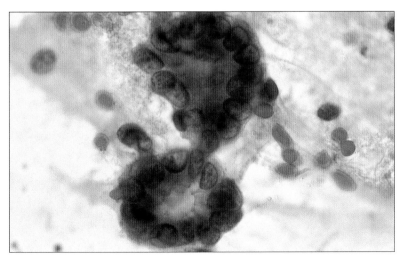

Fig. 8.100 Fibroadenoma – Pap x100. In this field there are two acinar structures composed of benign epithelial cells, a feature not very common in aspirates from fibroadenomas. Myoepithelial cells are also seen.

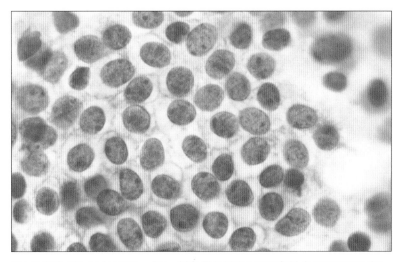

Fig. 8.101 Fibroadenoma – Pap x100. This high-power field demonstrates the vesicular chromatin pattern commonly observed in fibroadenomas. Good fixation is necessary to appreciate the subtle variation in chromatin.

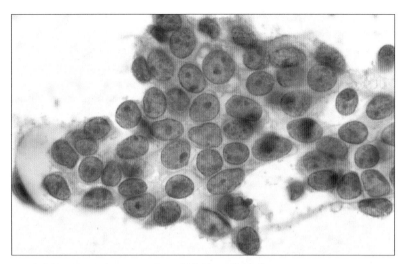

Fig. 8.102 Fibroadenoma – Pap x100. This sheet of benign ductal cells shows reactive changes with granular chromatin and visible nucleoli. No features of malignancy are present. Note the indistinct myoepithelial cells on the surface of the ductal group.

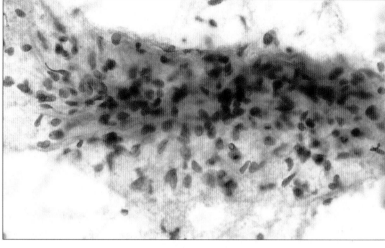

Fig. 8.103 Fibroadenoma – Pap x40. The stromal fragment seen here is a common feature of fibroadenomas. The cellularity is variable, this fragment being more cellular than usual. However, the edge of the fragment is indistinct, unlike the sharp border of the fragments in phyllodes tumours (see **Figures 8.108–8.110**).

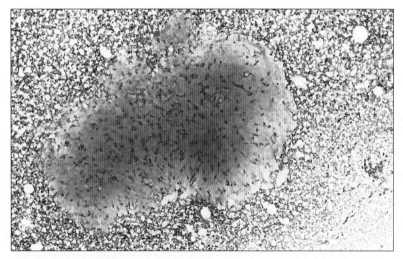

Fig. 8.104 Fibroadenoma – MGG x10. The air-dried smear also demonstrates the ill-defined border of stromal fragments. The deep purple, spindle-shaped nuclei are clearly seen within the bright pink stroma.

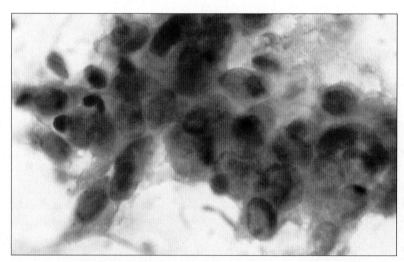

Fig. 8.105 Fibroadenoma showing atypia – Pap x40. The cells in this field show marked nuclear enlargement. This could be mistaken for malignancy if the adjacent myoepithelial cells are not noticed.

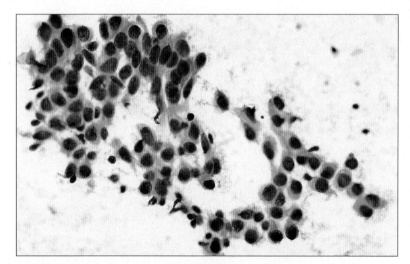

Fig. 8.106 Fibroadenoma showing atypia – Pap x40. This aspirate is from a similar case to that shown in **Figure 8.105** and demonstrates loosely cohesive, mildly pleomorphic cells, which would be of concern if the myoepithelial cells scattered around were absent.

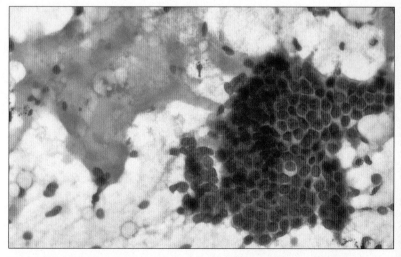

Fig. 8.107 Fibroadenoma – Pap x40. In this field there is a small sheet of benign ductal cells, some mucin, and scattered myoepithelial cells. Only small amounts of mucin are seen in fibroadenomas, unlike the large mucin pools of colloid carcinoma.

Benign **phyllodes tumours (Fig. 8.108)** can be very difficult to distinguish from fibroadenomas if the aspirate does not contain much stromal connective tissue. There are similar features with sheets of benign ductal cells and myoepithelial cells, but the stromal fragments tend to be larger, hypercellular, and leaf-shaped with sharply defined margins usually. They contain plump spindle-shaped nuclei **(Figs 8.109–8.111)**. Single stromal cells are seen occasionally in little collections **(Fig. 8.112)**. Apocrine cells are not usually seen in phyllodes tumours. If the cells within the stromal fragments show marked variability and atypia with numerous mitoses, malignant phyllodes tumour must be considered (see Chapter 9).

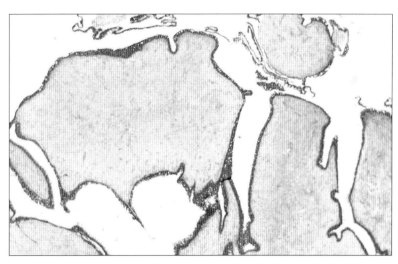

Fig. 8.108 Phyllodes tumour – H&E x10. This histological section shows the characteristic features of a benign phyllodes tumour, with stromal fragments covered by hyperplastic epithelium.

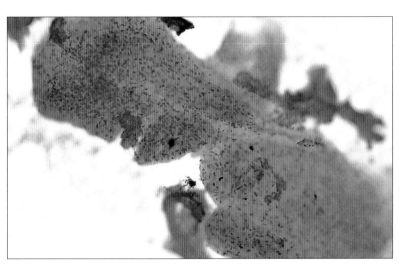

Fig. 8.109 Phyllodes tumour – Pap x10. In this field there are well-defined, leaf-shaped fragments of cellular stroma. In the absence of this feature it is very difficult to distinguish between a fibroadenoma and a phyllodes tumour.

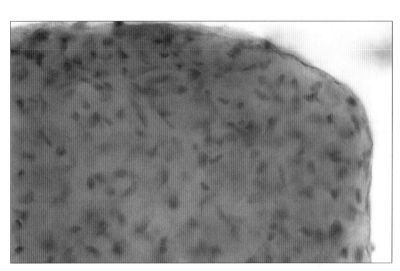

Fig. 8.110 Phyllodes tumour – Pap x100. This oil-immersion magnification view of a stromal fragment from a phyllodes tumour shows its sharp margins and increased cellularity.

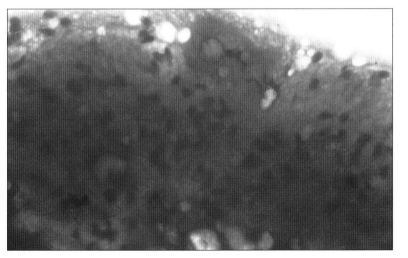

Fig. 8.111 Phyllodes tumour – MGG x100. The air-dried aspirate shows the increased cellularity of a fragment of phyllodes stroma, but the margin is not as well-defined as in a wet-fixed smear.

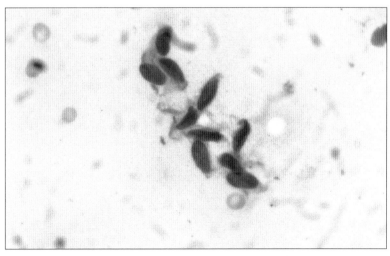

Fig. 8.112 Phyllodes tumour – MGG x100. Illustrated here is a group of single stromal cells. These are commonly seen in aspirates from phyllodes tumours.

OTHER BENIGN LESIONS

Duct ectasia is a common benign condition in which ducts become distended with secretion and foamy macrophages, and the ductal cell lining may become inflamed and then attenuated **(Fig. 8.113)**. Chronic inflammatory cells may be seen outside the wall of the duct, giving the condition its former name of plasma-cell mastitis. The cytological appearances are non-specific, with numerous foamy macrophages and granular debris, multinucleated histiocytes, and, occasionally, inflammatory cells **(Figs 8.114, 8.115)**. Secretory material is sometimes seen in breast aspirates in the form of delicate laminated structures known as Liesegang rings **(Figs 8.116, 8.117)**. Their significance is unknown.

Collagenous spherulosis is a benign entity which is seen in association with ductal and lobular hyperplasia. Its importance lies in the fact that it can be confused with adenoid cystic carcinoma on fine needle aspiration cytology. The smears show globules of hyaline material, pale pink or blue on the wet-fixed smear and bright pink on the air-dried sample **(Figs 8.118, 8.119)**. The

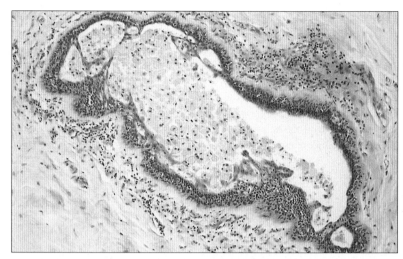

Fig. 8.113 Duct ectasia – H&E x10. This section of breast shows duct ectasia, with foamy macrophages within the duct lumen and inflammatory cells encircling the duct.

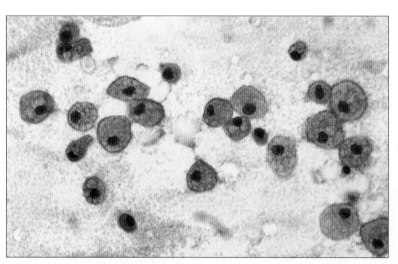

Fig. 8.114 Duct ectasia – Pap x40. Abundant foamy macrophages are common in duct ectasia. Ductal cells and inflammatory cells are rarely seen.

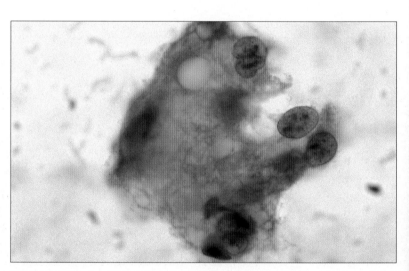

Fig. 8.115 Duct ectasia – Pap x100. Multinucleated histiocytes are also often seen in duct ectasia.

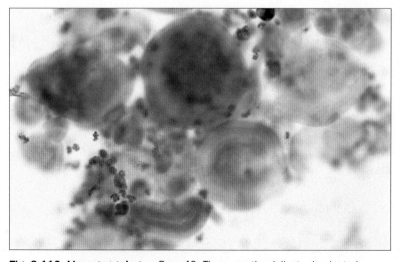

Fig. 8.116 Liesegang rings – Pap x40. These are the delicate, laminated structures seen among the secretory material in this aspirate. Their significance is not known.

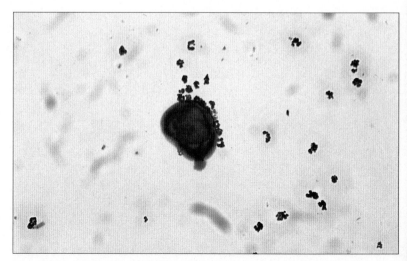

Fig. 8.117 Liesegang ring – MGG x40. Liesegang rings are not usually well-defined on air-dried material. This field shows a ring with indistinct laminations.

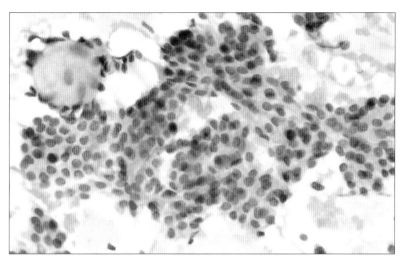

Fig. 8.118 Collagenous spherulosis – Pap x40. Illustrated here are a globule of hyaline material surrounded by benign epithelial cells and adjacent sheets of benign ductal cells. The hyaline material is pale pink to blue and may be mistaken for the basement–membrane globules of adenoid cystic carcinoma.

epithelial cells present show no atypia and there are myoepithelial cells in the background. The cylinders of basement membrane-like material seen in adenoid cystic carcinoma are not present in collagenous spherulosis (see **Figure 9.145**).

Intramammary lymph nodes are not uncommon. They are easily discernible on mammograms, but cannot be reliably distinguished from fibroadenomas. Aspirates are usually cellular, containing a mixed population of lymphoid cells (**Figs 8.120**), reflecting the structure of a normal node. They should not be mistaken for lymphoma.

Granular cell tumour of the breast is relatively uncommon. It may present as a discrete mass or as a thickening in the breast. The histological section shows typical large cells with granular cytoplasm which is PAS and S100 positive (**Figs 8.121, 8.122**); similar features are seen on the aspirate The cells have abundant granular cytoplasm with ovoid vesicular nuclei and are seen in sheets as well as singly (**Figs 8.123, 8.124**).

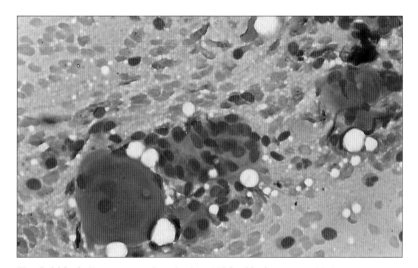

Fig. 8.119 Collagenous spherulosis – MGG x40. On the air-dried smear the secretory globules are pink. There are also small groups of benign ductal cells and several myoepithelial cells in this field.

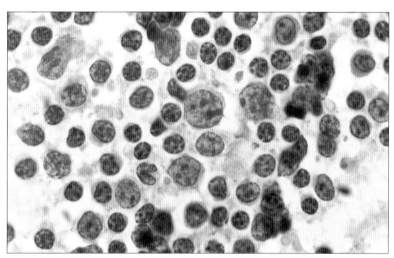

Fig. 8.120 Intramammary lymph node – Pap x100. This field shows a mixed population of lymphoid cells, including follicle centre cells.

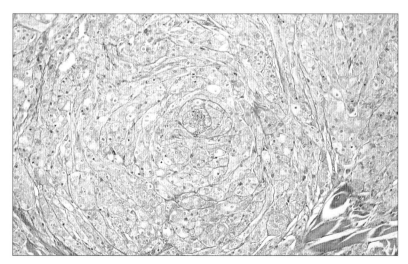

Fig. 8.121 Granular cell tumour – H&E x10. This histological section shows the abundant, pink granular cytoplasm of the cells comprising this neoplasm.

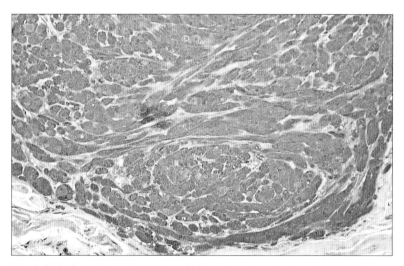

Fig. 8.122 Granular cell tumour – S100 x10. This tumour is S100 positive, as demonstrated in this histological section.

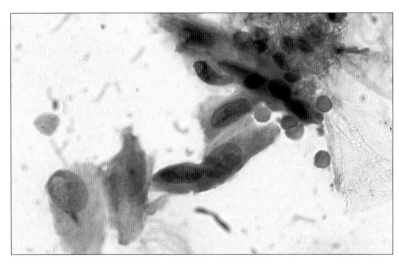

Fig. 8.123 Granular cell tumour – Pap x100. In this field there are loosely cohesive cells with large nuclei and abundant cytoplasm. Some of the cells have just visible nucleoli.

Pleomorphic adenoma is a rare tumour in the breast. The features are similar to those in the salivary gland, with abundant fibrillary myxoid material and epithelial cells with moderate amounts of cytoplasm (see **Figures 14.8–14.13**).

Myoepithelioma is an uncommon benign tumour of the breast, identical with that in the salivary gland; it is composed of small cells with minimal cytoplasm and ovoid nuclei (see **Figures 14.17, 14.18**). No ductal cells are seen usually.

Myofibroblastoma is a rare benign neoplasm which clinically mimics a fibroadenoma. Histologically, it is composed of swirling and interweaving groups of spindle cells which are desmin positive (**Figs 8.125, 8.126**). The aspirate is cellular, composed of loose clusters of cells which appear to be mesenchymal, with spindle-to-ovoid nuclei and inconspicuous nucleoli (**Figs 8.127, 8.128**).

Nodular fasciitis and **fibromatosis** of the breast are difficult diagnoses to make on cytological material, as the features are not specific. The aspirates are often acellular, but may contain a few stromal fragments or spindle-shaped mesenchymal cells in groups and lying singly (**Fig. 8.129**).

Gynaecomastia is a benign proliferative process of the male breast with

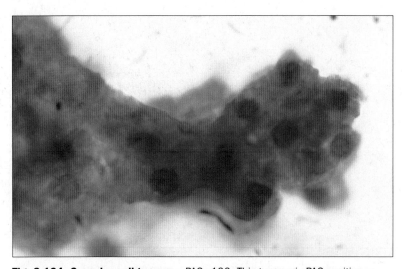

Fig. 8.124 Granular cell tumour – PAS x100. This tumour is PAS positive as demonstrated in this aspirate. The abundant cytoplasm is clearly seen and the nucleoli are visible in the neoplastic cells.

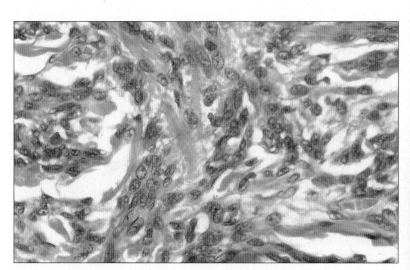

Fig. 8.125 Myofibroblastoma – H&E x40. This uncommon tumour is composed of swirling groups of plump spindle cells. Mitoses are not seen in this field.

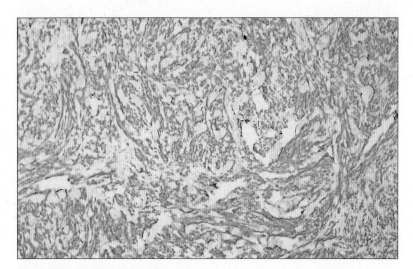

Fig. 8.126 Myofibroblastoma – Desmin x10. This histological section demonstrates strong positivity for desmin.

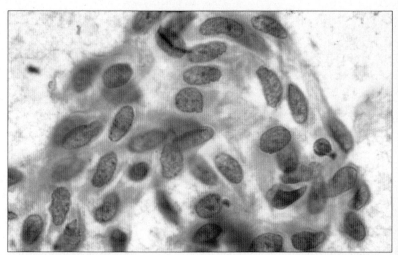

Fig. 8.127 Myofibroblastoma – Pap x100. The aspirate from this tumour is composed entirely of plump spindle-shaped cells with ovoid nuclei and speckled chromatin. Nucleoli are not prominent.

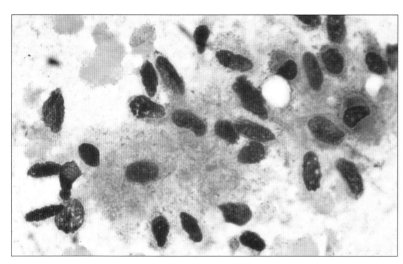

Fig. 8.128 Myofibroblastoma – MGG x40. This air-dried smear from a myofibroblastoma shows poorly preserved spindle-to-ovoid nuclei without well-defined cytoplasm. These features are non-specific.

similar cytological features to those of a fibroadenoma. In the early stages, the lesion is cellular and the aspirate contains sheets or clusters of cohesive benign ductal cells, with associated myoepithelial cells and scattered bare nuclei in the background (**Figs 8.130, 8.131**). Small fragments of poorly cellular stroma may also be seen. The epithelial cells may, on occasion, show some atypia with enlarged and hyperchromatic nuclei, but not enough to be suspicious of malignancy.

RADIATION CHANGES

Radiotherapy is a commonly used form of treatment for carcinoma of the breast. The woman may develop a thickened or nodular area in the same breast several months after cessation of treatment and fine needle aspiration cytology is performed to determine whether she has a recurrence or radiation fibrosis. The latter can mimic malignancy, so great care must be taken in assessing the sample. Often the smears are scanty, with a few fragments of stroma and some blood only. The stromal fragments may be composed of plump fibroblasts (**Figs 8.132, 133**),

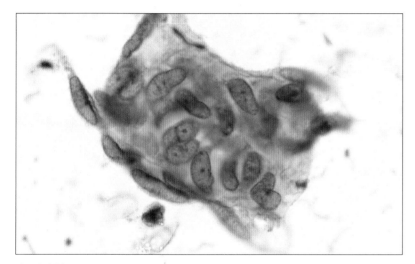

Fig. 8.129 Fibromatosis – Pap x100. This aspirate from fibromatosis of the breast shows a small group of spindle-shaped cells with elongated nuclei and unremarkable chromatin. The features are very similar to those of the case of myofibroblastoma illustrated above (**Figs 8.125–8.128**), except that the cells in fibromatosis are more ovoid and appear to contain more cytoplasm although the aspirate is usually scanty. Histological examination is necessary to distinguish between the two lesions.

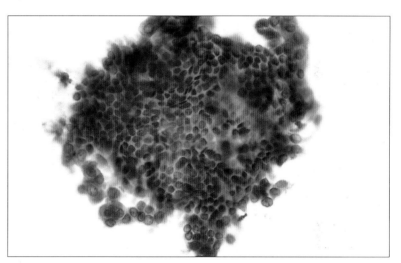

Fig. 8.130 Gynaecomastia – Pap x40. Illustrated is a sheet of benign ductal cells aspirated from gynaecomastia. The sheets are similar to those seen in fibroadenoma, but are smaller and do not appear to have many myoepithelial cells on the surface.

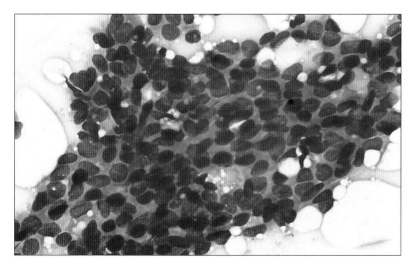

Fig. 8.131 Gynaecomastia – MGG x40. This sheet of cells in the air-dried smear of a case of gynaecomastia shows features identical to those of a fibroadenoma, with uniform ductal cells and a sprinkling of darker myoepithelial cells on the surface.

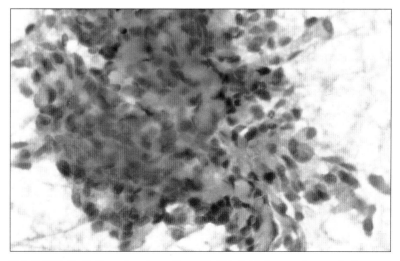

Fig. 8.132 Radiation changes – Pap x40. This field shows a fragment of cellular stroma composed of plump fibroblasts. This is occasionally seen in radiation fibrosis, although in most cases the aspirate is acellular.

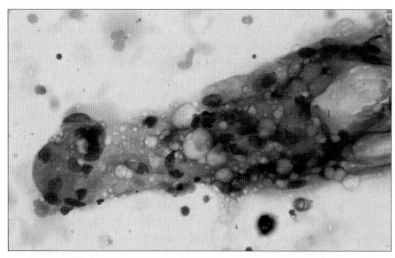

Fig. 8.133 Radiation changes – MGG x40. This small fragment of stroma in an aspirate from a breast with radiation fibrosis contains plump fibroblasts. These may be accompanied by foamy macrophages.

accompanied by bizarre multinucleated histiocytes (**Fig. 8.134**) and epithelial cells showing nuclear enlargement and hyperchromasia (**Fig. 8.135**). However, closer inspection of the nuclei reveals vacuolar degeneration and a bland chromatin pattern, possibly even pyknosis, ruling out recurrent tumour.

NIPPLE DISCHARGE CYTOLOGY

There is often a small amount of discharge during compression of the breast on mammography; this should be sent to the cytology laboratory in the form of an air-dried smear. A clean glass slide is applied to the discharge on the nipple, and the material allowed to dry. Examination of nipple discharge material can provide clues to changes within the breast without the need for invasive techniques. Most nipple discharges are benign, especially when they are bilateral or from several ducts. Unilateral nipple discharge from a single duct may be an indicator of a more sinister process, even more so if blood-stained. It is easier to prepare

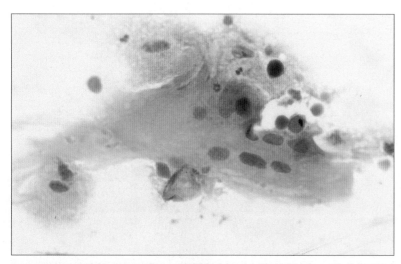

Fig. 8.134 Radiation changes – Pap x40. Illustrated here is a multinucleated giant histiocyte in an aspirate from a previously irradiated breast. The cytoplasmic outline is irregular and the cytoplasm appears to be more dense than usual in a histiocyte. Some small foamy macrophages are also visible in this field.

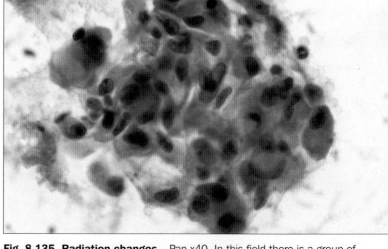

Fig. 8.135 Radiation changes – Pap x40. In this field there is a group of loosely cohesive epithelial cells with varying amounts of cytoplasm, displaying pleomorphism. This type of change is difficult to distinguish from recurrent carcinoma without examination of the nuclei under higher magnification to determine whether the cells are viable rather than degenerate.

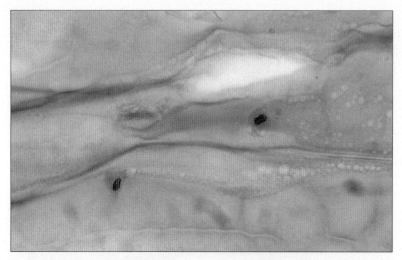

Fig. 8.136 Proteinaceous material – Pap x40. Nipple discharges often contain proteinaceous material, as illustrated here, staining pink or blue. Note the histiocytes within the material.

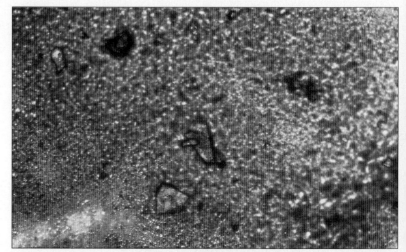

Fig. 8.137 Proteinaceous material – MGG x40. The proteinaceous material seen in this air-dried smear is pink in colour and contains some anucleate squames.

air-dried smears if discharge is noted during mammograms, but if there is plenty of material both wet-fixed and air-dried smears should be dispatched to the laboratory.

Duct ectasia is the most common cause of nipple discharge. The discharge may be serous and the smear shows proteinaceous material (**Figs 8.136, 8.137**), with numerous foamy macrophages (**Fig. 8.138**), and occasional multinucleated giant histiocytes (**Fig. 8.139**). Anucleate squames are frequently seen (**Figs 8.140, 8.141**).

With **mastitis** there may be a thick, sometimes blood-stained nipple discharge, which contains acute inflammatory cells and foamy macrophages.

Duct papilloma is a common cause of blood-stained nipple discharge. The histological appearances are well-demonstrated in the nipple discharge smear, with papillary clusters of benign ductal cells (**Figs 8.142, 8.143**) in a background of foamy macrophages, siderophages, and erythrocytes. The macrophages may be seen to contain phagocytosed erythrocytes (**Fig. 8.144**). The epithelial cells

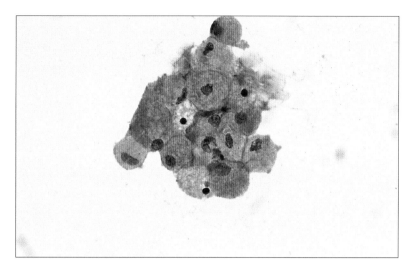

Fig. 8.138 Foamy macrophages – Pap x40. Foamy macrophages are often seen in duct ectasia, both in aspirates and in nipple discharge specimens. Epithelial cells are rarely seen.

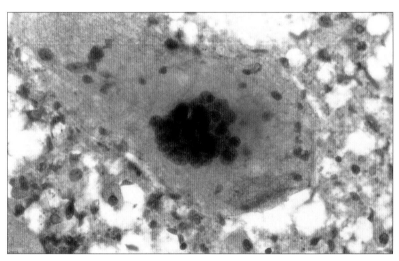

Fig. 8.139 Multinucleated giant histiocyte – Pap x40. This huge multinucleated histiocyte is in a nipple discharge specimen from a case of duct ectasia. It appears to be engulfing foamy histiocytes at intervals along its cytoplasmic border.

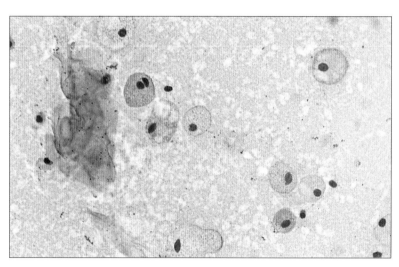

Fig. 8.140 Anucleate squames – Pap x40. These are often seen in nipple discharge specimens. Here they are accompanied by foamy macrophages, suggesting duct ectasia.

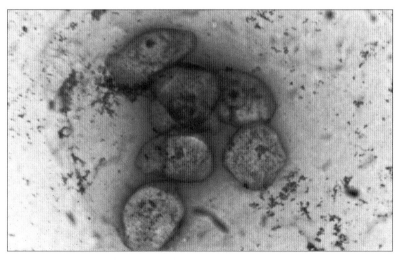

Fig. 8.141 Anucleate squames – MGG x40. Anucleate squames stain various shades, from colourless to pale blue to azure blue when keratinized. Here they are pink.

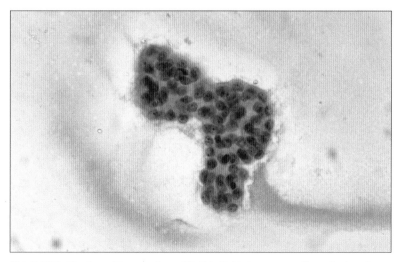

Fig. 8.142 Duct papilloma – Pap x40. This field shows a papillary cluster of small uniform ductal cells. Nipple discharge specimens do not contain benign epithelial cells, except in duct papilloma.

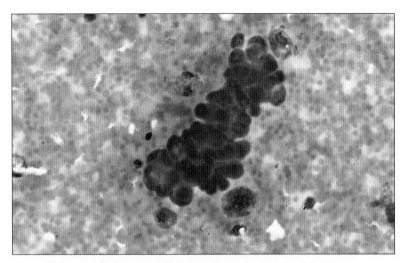

Fig. 8.143 Duct papilloma – MGG x40. The corresponding air-dried smear from the same case as shown in **Figure 8.142** displays a similar papillary cluster of small benign ductal cells. Note also the foamy macrophage and siderophage present.

frequently show a minor degree of atypia with vacuolation and nuclear enlargement, but these changes are usually related to degeneration (**Fig. 8.145**).

Eczema may be difficult to distinguish clinically from Paget's disease of the nipple. The nipple-scrape smear contains anucleate squames, some inflamed squamous cells (**Fig. 8.146**), and inflammatory cells.

Nipple adenoma is a lesion that can mimic carcinoma clinically with a reddened inflamed, abnormal nipple. Histology shows a papillomatous but benign appearance (**Fig. 8.147**), and smears show marked cellularity (**Figs 8.148, 8.149**) with clusters of benign ductal cells.

Ductal carcinoma-in-situ (DCIS) may, on occasion, present as a nipple discharge with no corresponding mammographic or clinical abnormality. The nipple discharge is blood-stained and smears show, in addition to the usual foamy macrophages, numerous clusters of large pleomorphic carcinoma cells, and also single malignant cells (**Figs 8.150, 8.151, 9.167– 9.169**). A fine needle aspirate deep to the nipple will produce similar carcinoma cells to confirm the diagnosis, if there is any doubt.

Fine needle aspiration cytology is an exceptionally useful diagnostic tool in differentiating between benign and malignant lesions (**Fig. 8.152**). It prevents unnecessary surgery on benign lesions and, with experience, can be used to differentiate between the various types of benign conditions rather than to just provide a report of 'no malignant cells seen'.

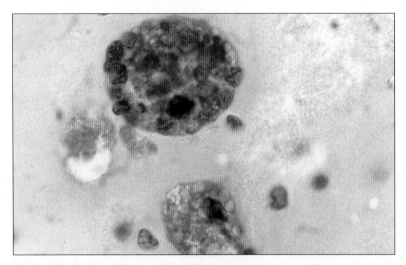

Fig. 8.144 Duct papilloma – Pap x100. Illustrated here are a foamy macrophage and a larger macrophage which has ingested erythrocytes. Note the erythrocytes in the background of this nipple discharge smear from a case of duct papilloma.

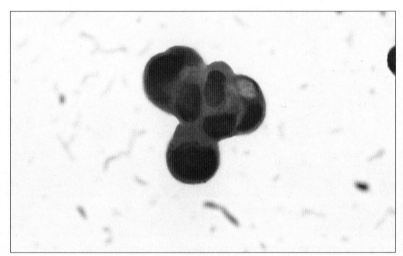

Fig. 8.145 Duct papilloma – MGG x100. This cluster of epithelial cells seen in a nipple discharge smear shows some pleomorphism. Mild atypia is permissible in ductal cells in a duct papilloma.

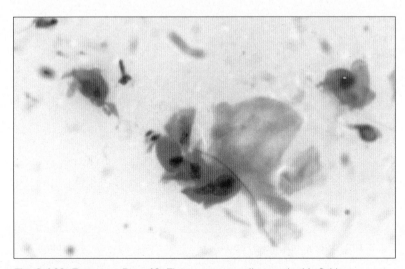

Fig. 8.146 Eczema – Pap x40. The squamous cells seen in this field are keratinized and inflamed with enlarged hyperchromatic nuclei. There are also anucleate squamous cells present. The picture in eczema is a purely inflammatory one, unlike the mixture of inflammation and malignant cells seen in Paget's disease (see **Figure 9.165**).

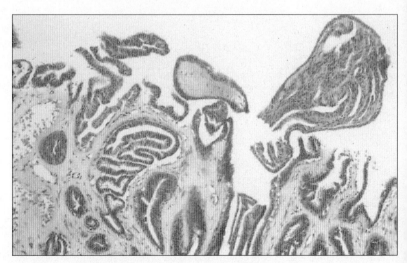

Fig. 8.147 Nipple adenoma – H&E x10. This section of a nipple shows the papillomatous appearance of this lesion with benign covering epithelial cells.

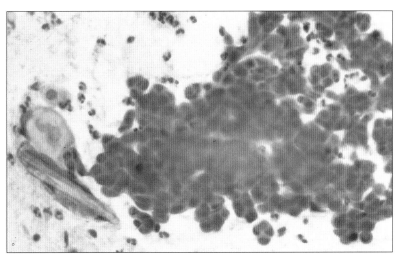

Fig. 8.148 Nipple adenoma – Pap x40. Smears from nipple adenomas are very cellular, as illustrated here, with clusters of benign ductal cells similar to those seen in a duct papilloma, but in greater numbers.

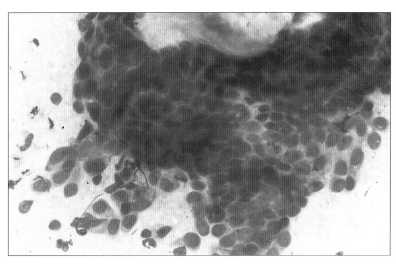

Fig. 8.149 Nipple adenoma – MGG x40. This field displays the marked cellularity of this lesion. This large cluster of benign ductal cells shows no features of malignancy.

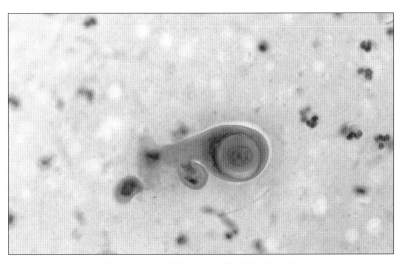

Fig. 8.150 Nipple discharge, DCIS – Pap x40. This field shows a cluster of abnormal epithelial cells displaying a 'cell-in-cell' appearance. The nuclear pleomorphism makes these cells suspicious of malignancy.

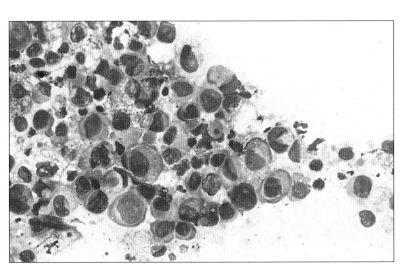

Fig. 8.151 Nipple discharge, DCIS – MGG x40. This is a very cellular smear composed of pleomorphic carcinoma cells. Malignant cells in the nipple discharge may be the first sign of DCIS.

FEATURES	BENIGN	MALIGNANT
Cellularity	Poor to moderate (fibroadenomas are cellular)	Cellular
Cell dissociation	Cohesive sheets or clusters	Single cells common
Cell clusters	Smooth or palisaded edges	Ragged edges
Cell size	Small	Usually large
Nuclear size	The size of an erythrocyte	Large
Pleomorphism	None	Common
Nucleus	Smooth margin	Irregular margin
Chromatin	Vesicular or finely granular	Clumping and clearing
Necrosis	Absent	May be present
Myoepithelial cells	Plentiful	Rare
Single stromal cells	Common	Rare
Stromal fragments	Common	Rare
Cytoplasmic vacuoles	Uncommon	May be seen
Intranuclear inclusions	Uncommon	May be seen
Mucin	Rare (sometimes in fibroadenoma)	Common in mucoid carcinoma
Inflammatory cells	May be present	May be present
Foamy macrophages	Often present	Sometimes present
Tumour giant cells	Absent	May be present
Calcium	May be present	May be present
Apocrine cells	Common	Rare
Mitoses	Uncommon	Common
Cribriform pattern	Occasionally in fibroadenoma	Seen in cribriform DCIS

Fig. 8.152 Benign versus malignant criteria in breast aspirates.

SUGGESTED READING

Dahl I, Akerman M. Nodular fasciitis. A correlative, cytologic and histologic study of 13 cases. *Acta Cytol* 1981; **25**: 215–222.

Dusenbery D, Frable WJ. Fine needle aspiration cytology of phyllodes tumour, potential diagnostic pitfalls. *Acta Cytol* 1992; **36**: 215–221.

Page DL, Anderson TJ, Rogers LW. Epithelial hyperplasia. In: Page DL, Anderson TJ, eds. *Diagnostic Histopathology of the Breast*. Edinburgh: Churchill Livingstone; 1987: 120–156

Peterse JL, Koolma–Schellekens MA. Atypia in fine needle aspiration cytology of the breast: A histologic follow-up study of 301 cases. *Semin Diagn Pathol* 1989; **6**: 126–134.

Novotny DB, Maygarden SJ, Shermer RW, Frable WJ. Fine needle aspiration of benign and malignant breast masses associated with pregnancy. *Acta Cytol* 1991; **35**: 676–686.

Rosen PP, Caicco JA. Florid papillomatosis of the nipple. A study of 51 patients, including nine with mammary carcinoma. *Am J Surg Pathol* 1986; **10**: 87–101.

Silverman JF, Lannin DR, Unverferth M, Norris HT. Fine needle aspiration cyto-logy of subareolar abscess of the breast: Spectrum of cytomorphologic findings and potential diagnostic pitfalls. *Acta Cytol* 1986; **30**: 413–419.

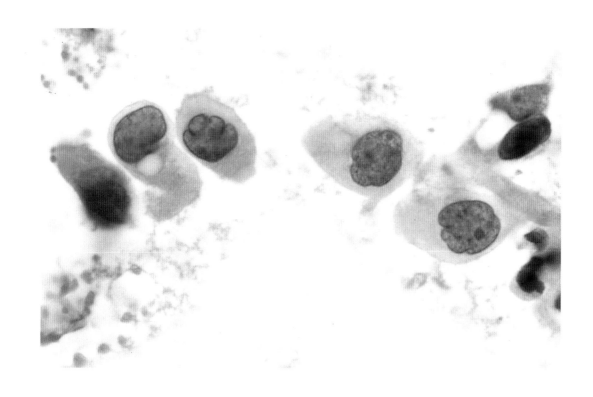

CARCINOMA OF THE BREAST

9

Breast cancer is one of the commonest causes of death in women in the US and Britain. The incidence in Western countries is much higher than that in the Far East and in underdeveloped countries.

Early detection of breast carcinoma is the rationale behind the screening programmes which have been set up in various countries. In the UK, the National Breast Screening Programme was set up in 1987 with women aged 50 to 64 years being invited for 3-yearly mammography screening. Mammographic lesions, such as masses, spiculate or stellate distortion, and microcalcification, require further investigation to exclude carcinoma. This is done by stereotactic fine needle aspiration cytology, which can sample lesions even smaller than 5 mm in size. In the past, only palpable abnormalities have been aspirated for cytological examination. Although patients with palpable masses are usually referred to the surgical breast clinic, some do attend mammography screening centres. Some lesions are more easily aspirated by using ultrasound-guided techniques, but this is of no use for microcalcification. Cytology plays a very important role not only in the diagnosis of mammographic lesions, but also in assisting to keep the benign-to-malignant biopsy ratio low, so that unnecessary surgery is not performed.

As with benign breast cytology, reliable diagnosis requires a properly sampled, well-spread, and well-fixed smear. In the US and in many laboratories in Britain, wet fixation of material followed by the Papanicolaou staining technique is favoured, with air-dried smears stained with May Grunwald Giemsa being examined for additional information. In Scandinavian countries the preference is for air-dried smears. Where instant reporting is required an air-dried smear stained with DiffQuik is useful. For those who prefer wet-fixed material a modification of this method has been described.

Stereotactic aspirates are performed more commonly now as a result of the breast screening programmes being set up in many countries. Many smaller cancers are being sampled, as well as early lesions, such as atypical hyperplasias and radial scars, some of which prove to be diagnostic dilemmas for both the cytopathologist and the histopathologist. Correlation of cytology and histol-ogy is of the utmost importance, especially in cases where there is doubt as to whether a lesion represents atypical ductal hyperplasia or ductal carcinoma-in-situ (DCIS). In certain centres core biopsies are being performed either with or instead of fine needle aspirates.

CYTOLOGICAL FEATURES

There are several cytological features which are assessed in making the diagnosis of malignancy (**Fig. 9.1**). These are **cellularity, cell dissociation, nuclear and cell size, cell pleomorphism, nuclear margin, chromatin pattern, nucleoli,** and the presence of **abnormal mitoses**. Other criteria of lesser importance include necrosis, absence of myoepithelial cells and intranuclear inclusions. However, cancers do not always show every feature of malignancy. The well-differentiated or low-grade carcinomas are often difficult to differentiate from benign cells and may have to be reported as C4, namely highly suspicious, rather than a definite carcinoma C5 (see Chapter 6 for the categories).

Cellularity

Normal breast aspirates and most benign lesions are notorious for their scanty cellularity. Carcinomas, on the other hand, are usually extremely cellular, although this depends partially on the expertise of the aspirator (**Figs 9.2, 9.3**). On the other hand, some carcinomas may be hypocellular, especially those with a scirrhous component (**Figs 9.4, 9.5**). A tradition that has been upheld for many years is that lobular carcinoma aspirates are often acellular or scanty, but in our experience their cellularity does not significantly differ from that of ductal carcinomas.

Cell dissociation

On aspirates benign epithelial cells tend to stay together in sheets or clusters (**Figs 9.6, 9.7**), whereas malignant cells lose this feature and appear singly (**Figs 9.8, 9.9**). A word of warning: ductal cells from benign aspirates, although cohesive in the wet-fixed smear, tend to show dissociation in air-dried smears which can

FEATURES	BENIGN	MALIGNANT
Cellularity	Sparse	Cellular
Cell cohesiveness	Cohesive	Loss of cohesion
Nuclear size	Equals that of an erythrocyte	Usually larger
Cell uniformity	Monomorphic	Pleomorphic
Nucleoli	Not visible or small	Often abnormal
Nuclear margin	Smooth	Irregular
Chromatin pattern	Vesicular	Abnormal
Mitoses	Rare but normal	Abnormal
Necrosis	Absent	May be present
Myoepithelial cells	Plentiful	Rare
Apocrine cells	Often seen	Rare
Foamy macrophages	Common	May be present
Intranuclear inclusions	Rare	May be present
Calcium	Not common	May be present

Fig. 9.1 Diagnostic criteria of malignancy.

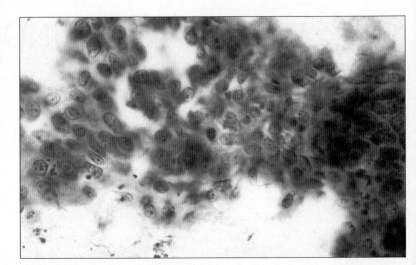

Fig. 9.2 Cellularity – Pap x40. This is a large cluster of ductal carcinoma cells which show pleomorphism and prominent nucleoli.

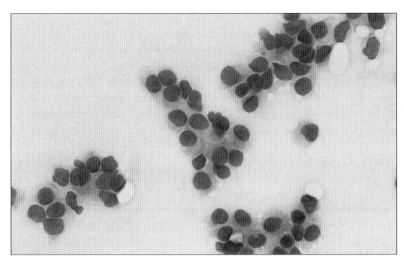

Fig. 9.3 Cellularity – MGG x40. This air-dried smear shows several clusters of mildly pleomorphic carcinoma cells with some single cells. No myoepithelial cells are seen.

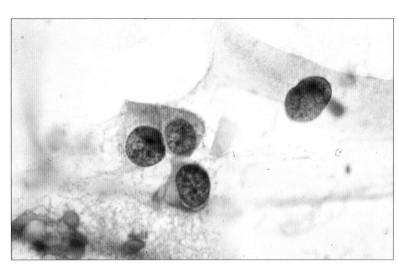

Fig. 9.4 Scanty cellularity – Pap x100. This poorly cellular aspirate shows four large carcinoma cells (the nuclei being at least 4–5 times the size of an erythrocyte). The nuclear margin is round and smooth, but the chromatin pattern is abnormally granular.

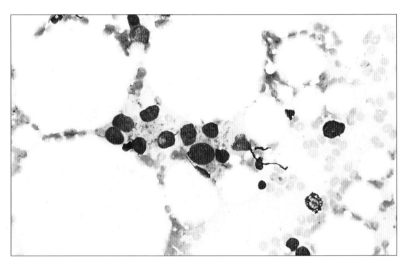

Fig. 9.5 Scanty cellularity – MGG x40. In this field there are some loosely cohesive irregular carcinoma cells, much larger than the erythrocytes in the background.

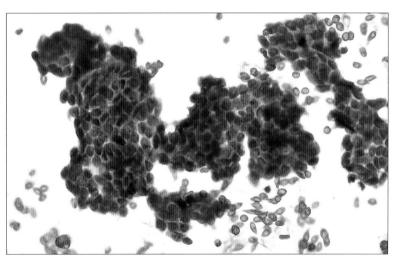

Fig. 9.6 Cell cohesion, benign ductal cells – Pap x40. Illustrated here are sheets of cohesive benign ductal cells with nuclei that are just slightly larger than the surrounding erythrocytes. A few myoepithelial cells are seen on the surface of the ductal sheets.

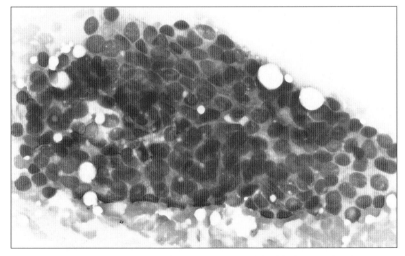

Fig. 9.7 Cell cohesion, benign ductal cells – MGG x40. This air-dried smear shows a sheet of uniform, cohesive benign ductal cells.

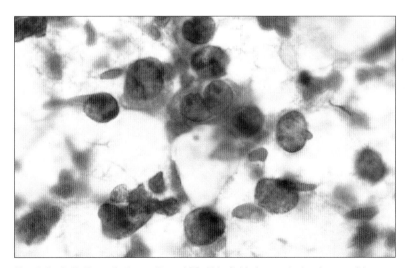

Fig. 9.8 Cell dissociation – Pap x100. This field shows single pleomorphic carcinoma cells with irregular nuclear margins and prominent nucleoli. The chromatin pattern is pale.

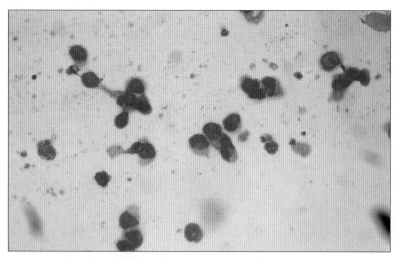

Fig. 9.9 Cell dissociation – MGG x40. In this air-dried smear there are single pleomorphic carcinoma cells.

lead to a false suspicion of malignancy (see **Figure 8.4**). There are exceptions to the rule that carcinoma cells are usually dyshesive: *in situ* ductal and lobular carcinomas, as well as low-grade invasive carcinomas, produce aspirates with cohesive sheets and clusters of cells (**Figs 9.10, 9.11**). Another type of carcinoma which has sheets of cohesive cells is the mucoid or mucinous variety, also known as colloid carcinoma (**Fig. 9.12**). A feature which points to a malignant rather than a benign diagnosis is the presence of three-dimensional clusters, rather than flat sheets of cells.

Nuclear and cell size

The size of carcinoma cells tends to be larger than that of benign ductal cells (**Figs 9.13, 9.14**). There are exceptions, as some carcinomas are composed of very small cells, such as lobular cancers, some low-grade ductal cancers (**Figs 9.15, 9.16**), and cribriform carcinomas (**Figs 9.17, 9.18**). The nuclear size is also increased, often quite out of proportion to the size of the cell, thus producing an increased nuclear–cytoplasmic ratio (**Figs 9.19, 9.20**).

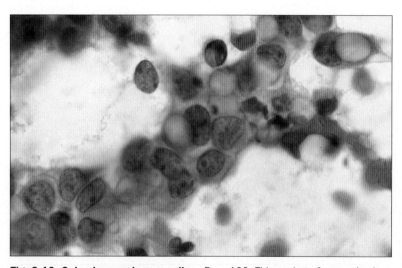

Fig. 9.10 Cohesive carcinoma cells – Pap x100. This aspirate from an *in situ* lobular carcinoma shows a cohesive group of small carcinoma cells with vesicular, mildly pleomorphic nuclei and some intracytoplasmic vacuoles.

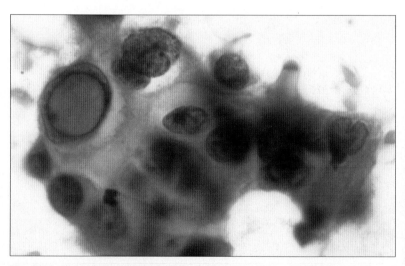

Fig. 9.11 Cohesive carcinoma cells – Pap x100. This cluster of large pleomorphic carcinoma cells from a comedo-type DCIS contains nuclei which are much larger than the erythrocytes in the field. The nuclei are irregular and one contains an enormous intranuclear inclusion.

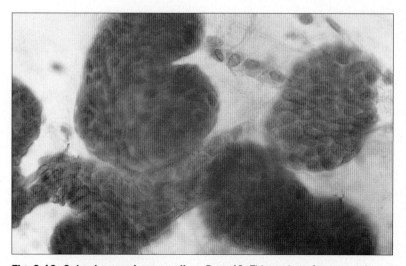

Fig. 9.12 Cohesive carcinoma cells – Pap x40. This aspirate from a mucinous carcinoma is composed of clusters of small uniform cohesive cells. A few single cells are seen. At low power the clusters appear benign, especially as the mucin in the background is very pale.

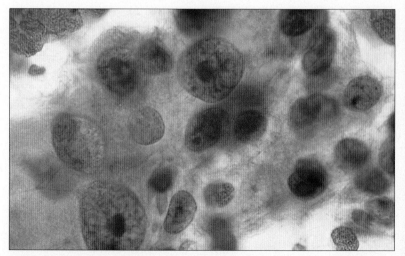

Fig. 9.13 Cell size – Pap x100. The carcinoma cells seen in this cluster are greatly enlarged, some cells more so than others. Benign cells do not enlarge to this extent. Note also the large red nucleoli and granular chromatin.

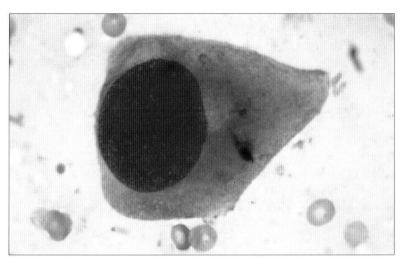

Fig. 9.14 Cell size – MGG x100. The enormous carcinoma cell pictured dwarfs the erythrocytes around it. Benign ductal cells have nuclei that are approximately the size of erythrocytes.

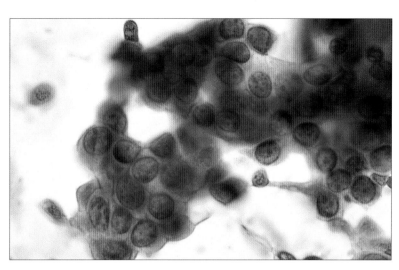

Fig. 9.15 Cell size – Pap x100. Illustrated is a cluster of small ductal carcinoma cells with nuclei just slightly larger than the surrounding erythrocytes. Although the cluster is cohesive, the cells show abnormal chromatin.

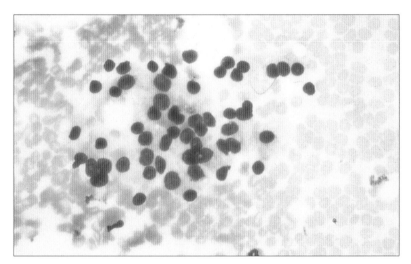

Fig. 9.16 Cell size – MGG x40. The dyshesive group of small ductal carcinoma cells shown contains nuclei which are approximately the size of erythrocytes.

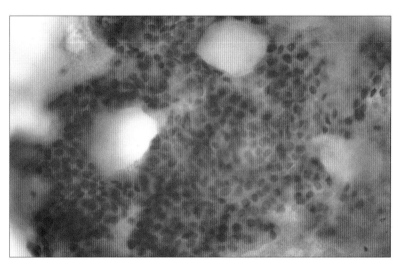

Fig. 9.17 Cell size – Pap x40. This aspirate is from a cribriform carcinoma of the breast, and shows an irregular sheet of small, but mildly pleomorphic, carcinoma cells which displays a cribriform pattern. The differential diagnosis here is a benign proliferative process with cribriform sheets of cells, but in this case myoepithelial cells would be plentiful.

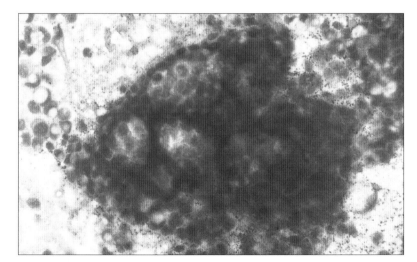

Fig. 9.18 Cell size – MGG x40. This field shows the air-dried smear from the same case as in **Figure 9.17**. There is a large sheet of small cells in which cribriform spaces are seen. However, in the background are single epithelial cells, suggesting a diagnosis of malignancy.

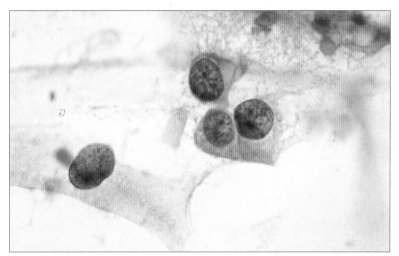

Fig. 9.19 Nuclear size – Pap x100. These carcinoma cells contain large nuclei which occupy almost the whole cell. It must be remembered that benign ductal cells also have a relatively high nuclear–cytoplasmic ratio; however, the nuclei of the carcinoma cells seen here are at least ten times the size of erythrocytes.

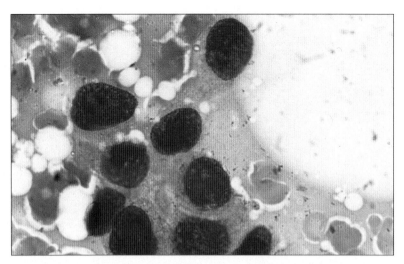

Fig. 9.20. Nuclear size – MGG x100. In this air-dried smear the carcinoma cells display enlarged nuclei with a narrow rim of greyish blue cytoplasm.

Pleomorphism

This variation in the morphology of the cells is a typical feature of carcinomas (**Figs 9.21, 9.22**), although there are some tumours which appear monomorphic, such as tubular carcinomas (**Figs 9.23, 9.24**), in which case other features of malignancy must be sought to determine the diagnosis.

Irregularity of the nuclear margin

Benign cells have smooth nuclear margins, even when they are reactive. Carcinoma cells show irregular margins, varying from slight indentations (**Figs 9.25, 9.26**), to folds or grooves (**Figs 9.27, 9.28**), and to more obvious abnormalities, such as buds or clefts (**Figs 9.29, 9.30**). Some cancers, however, have smooth nuclear margins (**Figs 9.31, 9.32**), so other features of malignancy need to be evident for a correct diagnosis to be made.

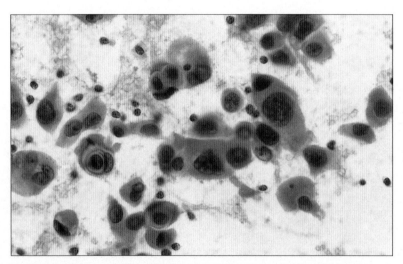

Fig. 9.21 Pleomorphism – Pap x40. This photomicrograph of a high-grade ductal carcinoma aspirate shows marked variation in cell and nuclear size and shape – an undisputed feature of malignancy.

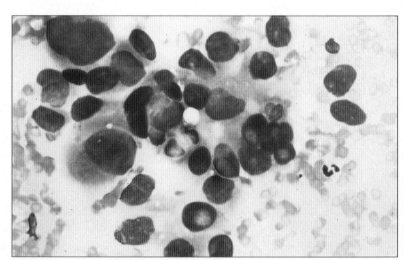

Fig. 9.22 Pleomorphism – MGG x40. In this field there are many pleomorphic carcinoma cells, some very large. The nuclei are many times larger than the surrounding erythrocytes.

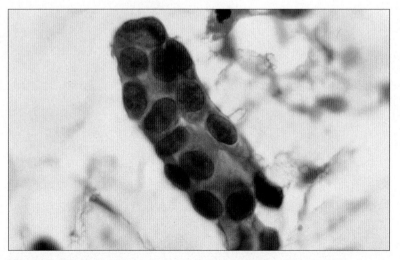

Fig. 9.23 Monomorphism – Pap x40. This is an aspirate from a tubular carcinoma showing a tubular cluster of small carcinoma cells which are uniform in size and shape.

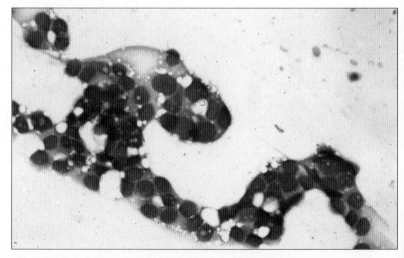

Fig. 9.24 Monomorphism – MGG x40. In the air-dried smear from the same case as shown in **Figure 9.23**, similar monomorphic cells are seen in an ill-defined tubular pattern.

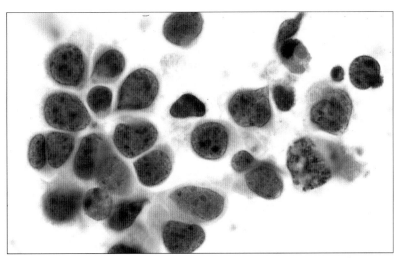

Fig. 9.25 Nuclear margin – Pap x100. This group of carcinoma cells shows slight indentation and occasional sharp projections of the nuclear margins. Note the abnormal clumped chromatin.

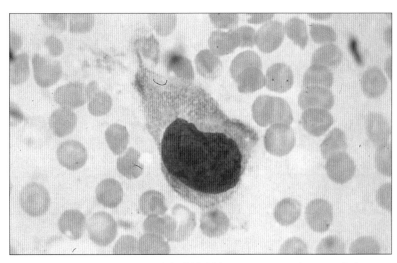

Fig. 9.26 Nuclear margin – MGG x100. This enormous carcinoma cell shows indentation of its nuclear margin. A large nucleolus is just visible.

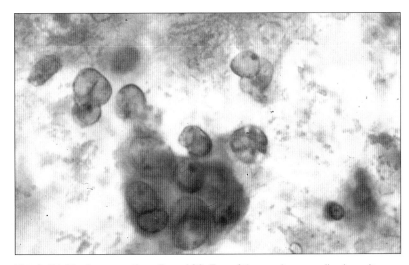

Fig. 9.27 Nuclear margin – Pap x100. Two of the carcinoma cells show deep grooves in their nuclei. The chromatin pattern is abnormally colourless, consisting predominantly of euchromatin.

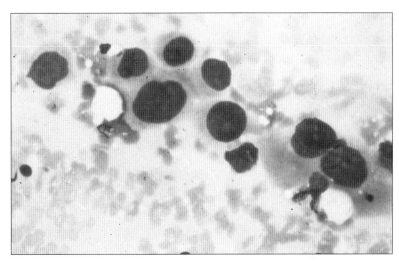

Fig. 9.28 Nuclear margin – MGG x40. This feature is not as easily assessable on the air-dried smear. These cells have indented nuclear margins, but the subtler features within the nucleus are not obvious.

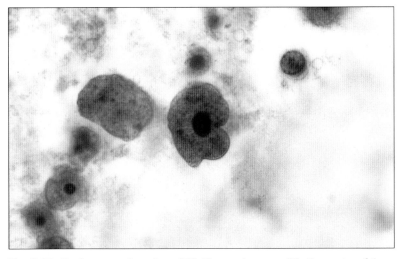

Fig. 9.29 Nuclear margin – Pap x100. The carcinoma cell in the centre of the field contains a huge red nucleolus and exhibits marked budding of the nuclear margin. This is a feature of high-grade carcinomas.

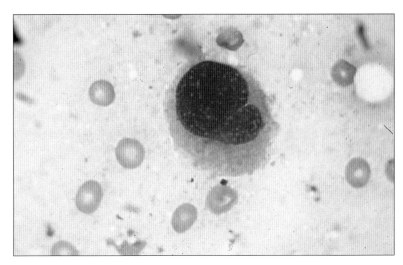

Fig. 9.30 Nuclear margin – MGG x100. This single carcinoma cell contains an enormous hyperchromatic nucleus with a deep cleft in the margin.

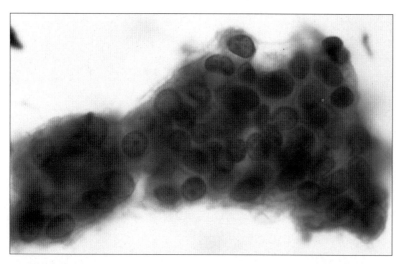

Fig. 9.31 Nuclear margin – Pap x100. This cluster is composed of small carcinoma cells with smooth, rounded nuclei. A few nucleoli are present.

Abnormal chromatin pattern

Benign epithelial cells have a vesicular or 'open' chromatin pattern (see **Figure 8.5**), which is not easily identifiable on the air-dried, May Grunwald Giemsa stained smear (see **Figure 8. 6**). Carcinomas may display a normal vesicular chromatin pattern, but more frequently it is abnormal, varying from simple hyperchromasia (**Figs 9.33, 9.34**), to granularity, which is more clearly seen on the wet-fixed smear (**Fig. 9.35**), and to more obvious abnormalities, such as clumping and clearing of chromatin (**Figs 9.36, 9.37**). An interesting feature to note is that the areas of clumping and clearing are unevenly placed within the nucleus

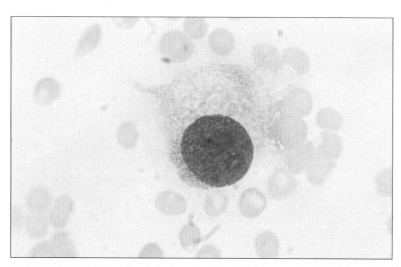

Fig. 9.32 Nuclear margin – MGG x100. This field shows a single carcinoma cell with a perfectly round, smooth nuclear margin. The chromatin pattern is finely granular and the nuclear–cytoplasmic ratio is increased.

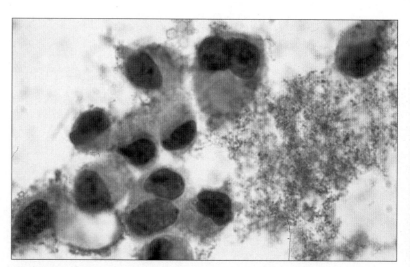

Fig. 9.33 Chromatin pattern – Pap x100. In this field the carcinoma cells display hyperchromasia and somewhat irregular nuclear margins. Several of the cells have eccentric nuclei and one is binucleate.

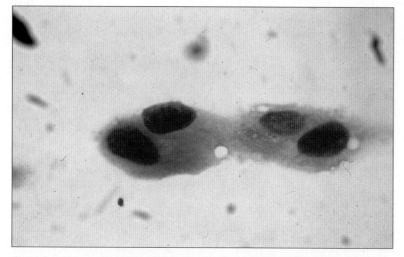

Fig. 9.34 Chromatin pattern – MGG x40. Illustrated are single carcinoma cells which have irregular nuclear margins and are hyperchromatic. Sometimes overstaining can give an impression of hyperchromasia on the air-dried smear.

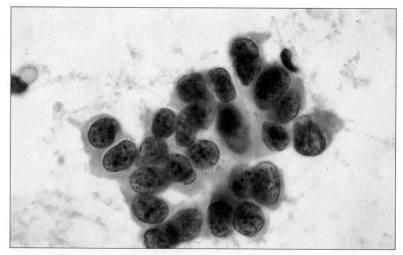

Fig. 9.35 Chromatin pattern – Pap x100. In this group of small carcinoma cells the nuclear features of granular or speckled chromatin and irregular margins are demonstrated clearly.

(**Fig. 9.38**). There are some carcinomas which have pale hypochromic nuclei, composed predominantly of the active form of chromatin, euchromatin (**Fig. 9.39**). This feature is not evident on air-dried smears.

Abnormal nucleoli

Nucleoli, which are present (although not always visible) in all cells, are a sign of activity. Most benign ductal cells do not have noticeable nucleoli, except when they are reactive. Even fibroadenomas may have visible nucleoli (**Fig. 9.40**), but these are single and stain blue with the Papanicoloau stain. Carcinomas tend to

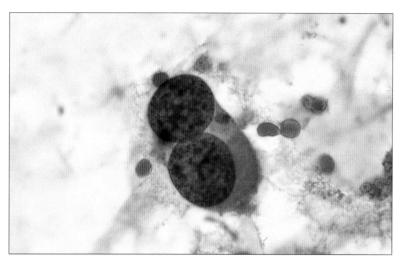

Fig. 9.36 Chromatin pattern – Pap x100. This binucleate carcinoma cell has two very large round nuclei which contain coarsely clumped, hyperchromatic heterochromatin with interspersed clear areas composed of pale euchromatin. The erythrocytes in the background give an idea of how large these nuclei are, as benign ductal nuclei are about the size of 1–2 erythrocytes.

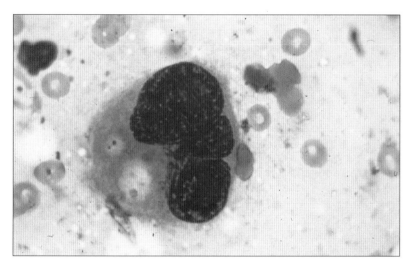

Fig. 9.37 Chromatin pattern – MGG x100. The large multinucleated carcinoma cell in this field displays chromatin clumping and clearing, and darker areas within the nuclei which may represent nucleoli.

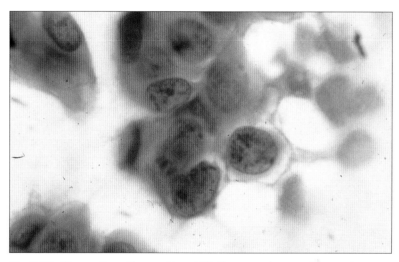

Fig. 9.38 Chromatin pattern – Pap x100. These carcinoma cells contain chromatin in the form of irregularly distributed clumps. The nuclear margins are sharply delineated by the peripheral condensation of chromatin.

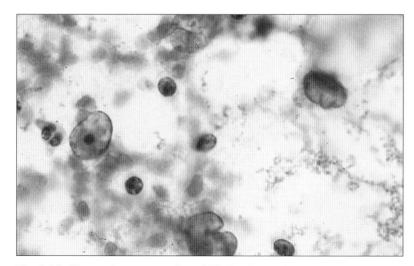

Fig. 9.39 Chromatin pattern – Pap x100. The four carcinoma cells in this field have nuclei which are colourless, being composed of active euchromatin. The nuclear margins, which are crisply defined, are markedly irregular in three of the cells, and the fourth cell has an abnormal red nucleolus.

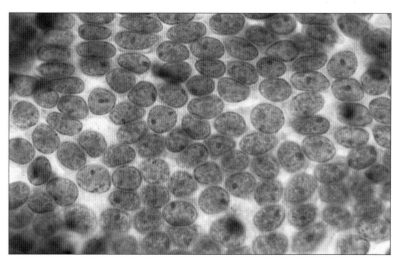

Fig. 9.40 Nucleoli – Pap x100. This sheet of benign ductal cells is from an aspirate of a fibroadenoma. The cells are cohesive, small, and uniform, but contain noticeable small nucleoli, which indicates that they are active.

have large nucleoli, occasionally single, staining blue (**Fig. 9.41**), sometimes red (**Fig. 9.42**), occasionally multiple (**Fig. 9.43**), and sometimes very abnormal in size and shape (**Fig. 9.44**). Nucleoli may be seen on air-dried smears (**Fig. 9.45**), but the subtler changes are not as obvious.

Abnormal mitoses

Normal mitotic figures are occasionally found in aspirates from active benign lesions, such as epithelial hyperplasia and fibroadenomas showing atypia. They are also noted in carcinomas (**Figs 9.46, 9.47**). However, the presence of abnormal mitoses is a feature seen only in malignant lesions.

Necrosis

Cellular necrosis is rarely a faeture of benign conditions. Debris is often seen in cyst aspirates, especially when many apocrine cells are present (**Fig. 9.48**). True necrosis is a feature of certain types of carcinoma, namely large cell, pleomorphic comedo-type DCIS (**Fig. 9.49**), intracystic carcinomas (**Fig. 9.50**), and

squamous carcinoma of the breast (**Fig. 9.51**). Occasionally, lobular carcinomas may show necrosis in the histological section (**Fig. 9.52**), but this feature is rarely seen in the cytological preparation.

Absence of myoepithelial cells

Benign aspirates, especially those from fibroadenomas, contain many scattered bare nuclei in the background. As has been described in Chapter 8, these are composed of two types of cells – myoepithelial cells, which are ovoid, torpedo-shaped, or bipolar, and single stromal cells, which are more spindle-shaped with wisps of cytoplasm at either end. Aspirates from carcinomas normally do not show any bare benign background nuclei, with the exception of some *in situ* carcinomas. It must be borne in mind, however, that when a lesion is being aspirated the needle may pass through benign tissue and thus may aspirate benign epithelial cells and myoepithelial cells as well as malignant cells. If an aspirate contains relatively few carcinoma cells and numerous myoepithelial cells, it is wiser to make a diagnosis of C4 (highly suspicious of malignancy) than of C5 (definite carcinoma).

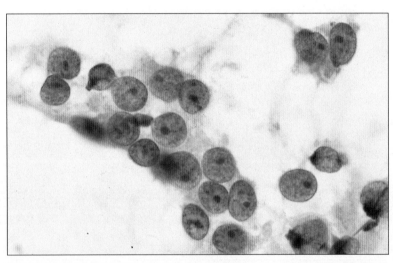

Fig. 9.41 Nucleoli – Pap x100. In this field there are several loosely aggregated carcinoma cells with smooth, round nuclei, each with a fairly prominent, single blue nucleolus. The chromatin pattern is granular.

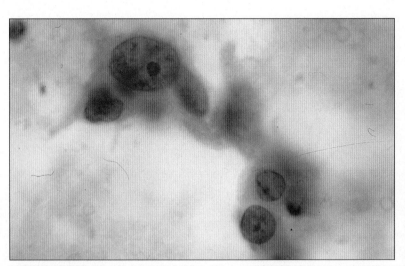

Fig. 9.42 Nucleoli – Pap x100. These carcinoma cells display single large red nucleoli. Note the predominantly colourless euchromatin with specks of heterochromatin.

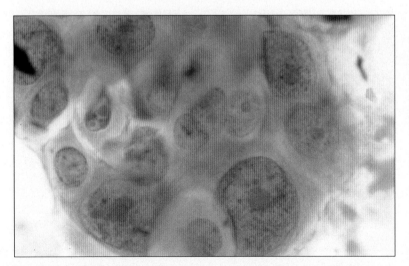

Fig. 9.43 Nucleoli – Pap x100. These carcinoma cells contain large red nucleoli, the smaller ones containing more than one nucleolus. The cells are pleomorphic, with much clumping and clearing of chromatin.

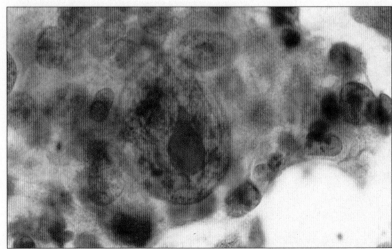

Fig. 9.44 Nucleoli – Pap x100. Within this cluster of pleomorphic malignant cells there is a huge cell with an enormous teardrop-shaped nucleolus. Abnormally shaped nucleoli are always associated with malignancy.

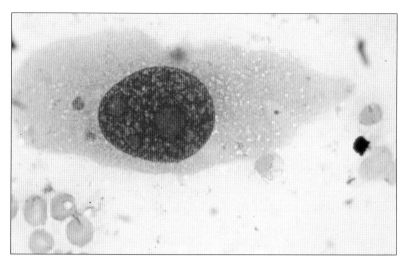

Fig. 9.45 Nucleoli – MGG x100. This air-dried smear shows a large carcinoma cell with at least three just visible nucleoli. Nucleoli are seen much more clearly in wet-fixed smears.

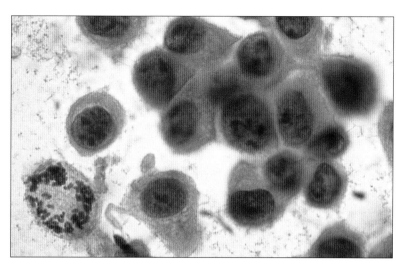

Fig. 9.46 Mitosis – Pap x100. There is an abnormal mitotic figure in this cluster of carcinoma cells, with chromosomes at the periphery of the nucleus rather than in the centre (see Chapter 1). The neoplastic cells contain granular chromatin and irregular multiple nucleoli.

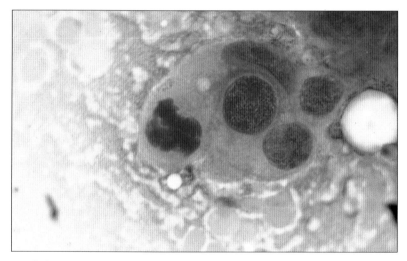

Fig. 9.47 Mitosis – MGG x100. The air-dried smear of the same case as shown in **Figure 9.46** shows a mitotic figure in the centre of the field. Mitoses are seen frequently in aspirates from high-grade breast carcinomas, as well as in medullary carcinoma and comedo-type DCIS.

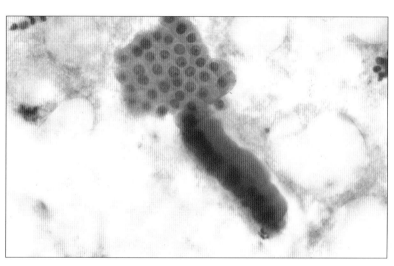

Fig. 9.48 Debris – Pap x40. This photomicrograph illustrates a flat sheet of benign apocrine cells with an adjacent strip of similar cells arranged in a picket-fence manner. There is cyst debris in the background, which is partly derived from the granular cytoplasm of apocrine cells.

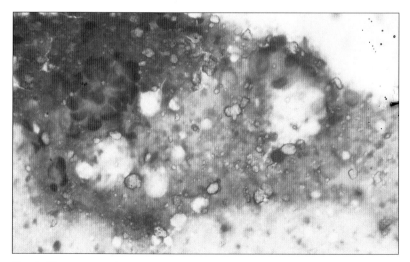

Fig. 9.49 Necrotic debris – MGG x40. In this air-dried smear from a comedo-type DCIS there are groups of poorly preserved large carcinoma cells, occasional single cells, and much necrotic cellular debris.

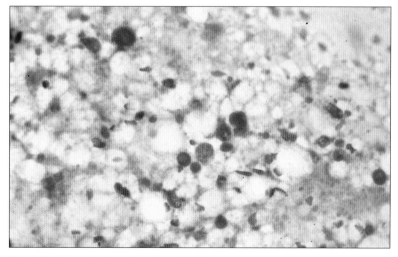

Fig. 9.50 Necrotic debris – Pap x40. This aspirate is from an intracystic carcinoma. There is much necrotic cellular debris, with some erythrocytes but no intact cells. In such cases it should not be assumed that this is a benign cyst, especially if apocrine cells are not seen.

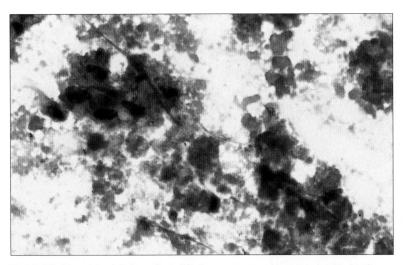

Fig. 9.51 Necrotic debris – Pap x40. Squamous carcinomas are notoriously associated with cellular necrosis and cavitation. This aspirate from a primary squamous carcinoma of the breast shows necrotic cellular debris and hyperchromatic, degenerate, but keratinized, squamous carcinoma cells.

Intranuclear inclusions

Under the light microscope, these are apparent as rounded, clear areas within the nucleus, but in reality are invaginations of the cytoplasm. They are occasionally noted in benign ductal cells (**Fig. 9.53**), but are more commonly seen in certain types of neoplasm, for example, in papillary carcinomas of the thyroid (see **Figure 7.91**), in aspirates from malignant melanomas (see **Figures 10.73, 10.74**), and in some breast cancers. They are easily visible in the Papanicolaou-stained preparation (**Fig. 9.54**), but may also be seen in the air-dried smear (**Fig. 9.55**).

CLASSIFICATION OF CARCINOMAS

The simplest method of classifying carcinomas is into two categories: **ductal** or **lobular**, each of which may be *in situ* or **invasive**. Ductal cancers can be further subdivided into various types: **NOS** (not otherwise specified) and special types such as **cribriform, papillary, mucinous, apocrine, medullary,** and **tubular**. These different types of carcinomas can be reliably diagnosed only on histology, in which the whole tumour can be examined, as there is often more than one type in a single tumour. However, the cytopathologist is often able to indicate the probability of a particular type of carcinoma from the nature of the aspirate.

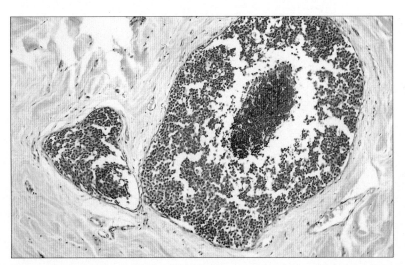

Fig. 9.52 Necrosis – H&E x4. This histological section shows lobular carcinoma-in-situ with central necrosis, an uncommon finding which is not represented in the aspirate.

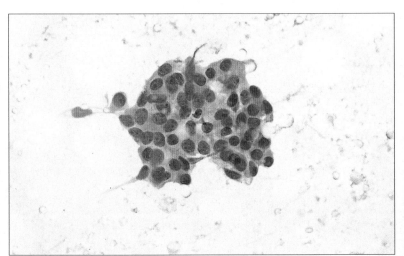

Fig. 9.53 Intranuclear inclusions – Pap x40. In this sheet of benign ductal cells there are two that show small intranuclear inclusions.

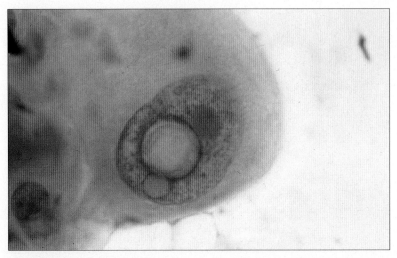

Fig. 9.54 Intranuclear inclusions – Pap x100. The huge carcinoma cell in the centre of the field contains two intranuclear inclusions, as well as a large red nucleolus and granular chromatin.

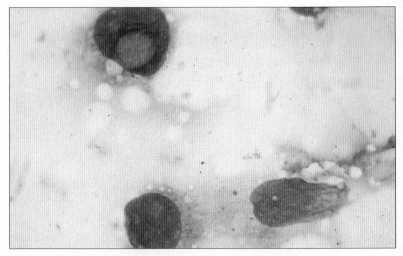

Fig. 9.55 Intranuclear inclusions – MGG x100. In this air-dried smear the cell at the top of the field contains a large intranuclear inclusion.

DUCTAL CARCINOMA-IN-SITU

The present trend is to classify DCIS according to cell type rather than by architectural pattern. Thus, it is now reported as either **large cell, pleomorphic DCIS** (formerly known as **comedo carcinoma-in-situ**), including the solid type, **small cell DCIS**, including the former **clinging, cribriform**, and **micropapillary** types, and **intermediate cell DCIS**. It is not possible to accurately differentiate *in situ* from invasive carcinomas on cytology.

In some instances where the mammogram shows irregular, coarse branching microcalcification, radiologists are able to predict **comedo-type DCIS**. In these cases the histological picture (**Fig. 9.56**) is reflected in the cytological findings – large pleomorphic carcinoma cells (**Figs 9.57, 9.58**), necrosis with foamy macrophages (**Figs 9.59, 9.60**), and calcium (**Figs 9.61, 9.62**). The calcium particles seen in aspirates are occasionally laminated (**Figs 9.63, 9.64**). It must be remembered that calcium may also be seen in benign aspirates, in association with proliferative conditions.

Cribriform and small cell DCIS are readily identifiable on histology by their architectural patterns. However, they are not easily distinguishable from benign aspirates on cytology, as the cells are small and usually cohesive (**Figs 9.65. 9.66**).

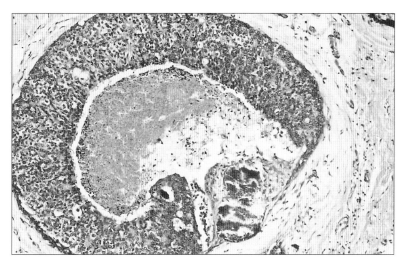

Fig. 9.56 Comedo-type DCIS – H&E x4. This section of large cell or comedo-type DCIS shows a duct composed of large malignant cells, filled with necrotic debris. Note the calcium in the wall of the duct.

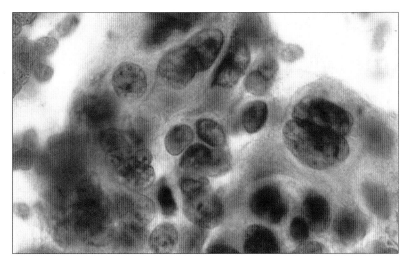

Fig. 9.57 Comedo-type DCIS – Pap x100. This cluster of carcinoma cells displays marked pleomorphism. Cells tend to be large and usually in cohesive groups in this variety of DCIS. Cytological grading would place these cells in the high-grade category.

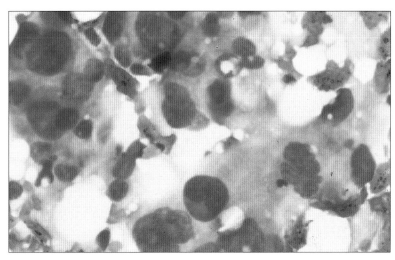

Fig. 9.58 Comedo-type DCIS – MGG x100. Air-dried smears also show pleomorphic, mostly cohesive clusters of large carcinoma cells in this lesion.

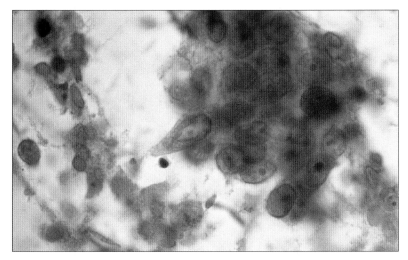

Fig. 9.59 Comedo-type DCIS – Pap x100. In this field there is a cluster of carcinoma cells with prominent nucleoli and in the background there is much pale-blue necrotic cellular debris. Myoepithelial cells are not seen.

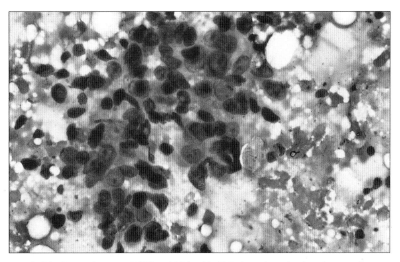

Fig. 9.60 Comedo-type DCIS – MGG x40. This loosely cohesive cluster of malignant cells is accompanied by necrotic cellular debris, which stains light purple.

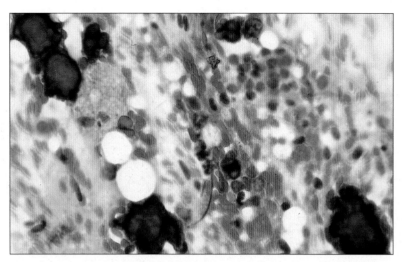

Fig. 9.61 Comedo-type DCIS – Pap x40. This field shows irregular red chunks of calcium, with some smaller blue particles at the top. Carcinoma cells and an occasional foamy macrophage are also visible.

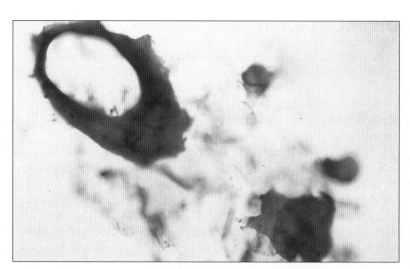

Fig. 9.62 Comedo-type DCIS – MGG x40. The two fragments of calcium seen here illustrate the varied appearances that may occur.

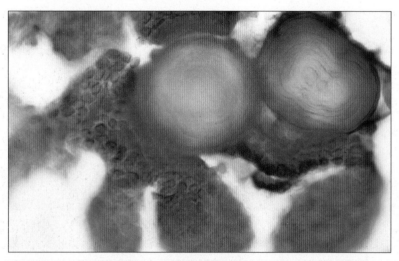

Fig. 9.63 Calcium – Pap x40. The reddish laminated calcium seen here is associated with small carcinoma cells, which are quite different from the large pleomorphic malignant cells seen in comedo-type DCIS. However, laminated calcium can occur in any type of malignant or benign lesion.

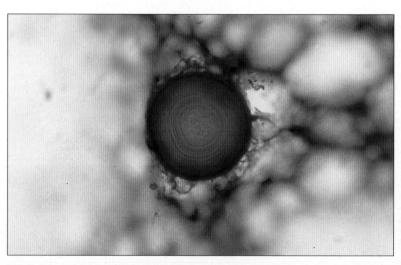

Fig. 9.64 Calcium – MGG x40. Laminated calcium is detected more easily than irregular particles in air-dried smears. Both varieties stain blue and may be found in both benign and malignant disease.

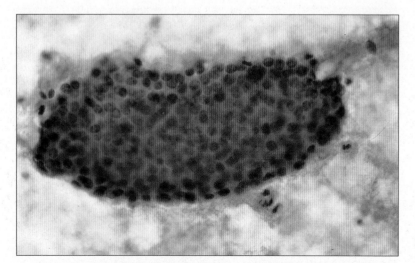

Fig. 9.65 Small cell DCIS – Pap x40. This aspirate from a small cell DCIS contains three-dimensional clusters of small cohesive cells with rounded nuclei. The darker, smaller cells at the edges of the cluster may represent myoepithelial cells. These aspirates are difficult to classify as malignant with certainty unless single epithelial cells and some degree of pleomorphism are evident.

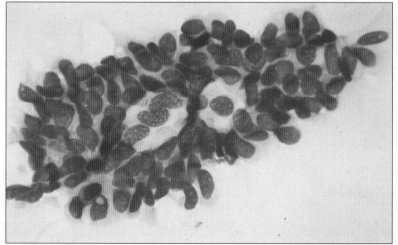

Fig. 9.66 Cribriform DCIS – MGG x40. The air-dried aspirate from a case of cribriform DCIS shows a cluster of small epithelial cells with ovoid nuclei and a number of smaller, darker myoepithelial cells on the surface. Note the two small holes in the cluster. This was classified as suspicious of malignancy (C4) rather than C5 as there are no definite features of malignancy.

A feature that is often seen is the presence of cribriform spaces in the sheets of small carcinoma cells (see **Figures 9.17, 9.18**). A search must be made for single epithelial cells to distinguish carcinoma from a benign proliferative lesion. Myoepithelial cells may be noted in close association with the cell clusters in the aspirates from these tumours, which often leads to a 'suspicious' (C4) rather than a C5 diagnosis (**9.67, 9.68**).

INVASIVE DUCTAL CARCINOMA NOS

Invasive ductal carcinoma NOS shows several of the features of malignancy described above, including dissociation of cells, pleomorphism, abnormal nucleoli, and chromatin, also irregular nuclear outlines. These tumours are now routinely graded cytologically, in our department, at the time of diagnosis, with the grade forming part of the cytology report (see **Figure 9.170**).

LOBULAR CARCINOMA-IN-SITU

Lobular carcinoma-in-situ (LCIS) on histology is composed of small carcinoma cells which fill and distend the lobules (**Fig. 9.69**). They are uniform and often contain intracytoplasmic lumina (**Fig. 9.70**). Aspirates from such tumours may show distended lobular structures (**Figs 9.71, 9.72**), but also, surprisingly, single

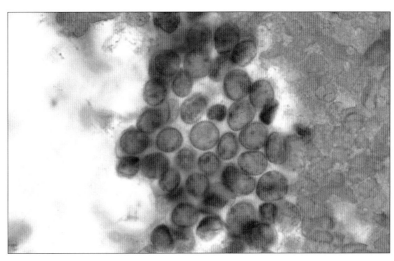

Fig. 9.67 Small cell DCIS – Pap x100. The cells in this cluster are mildly pleomorphic with vesicular nuclei. A few cells have small nucleoli. Some myoepithelial cells, in the form of small dark nuclei, are seen between the epithelial cells. These cells mimic benign ductal cells, but are in a three-dimensional cluster rather than in a flat sheet, and are therefore suspicious of malignancy.

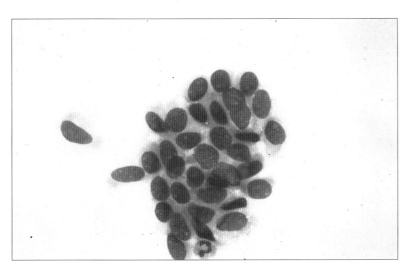

Fig. 9.68 Small cell DCIS – MGG x40. This cluster of small cells (the nuclei are just slightly larger than the neutrophil at the bottom of the cluster) shows darker, elongated myoepithelial cells among the epithelial cells. There is some dissociation, with cells falling off the edge of the cluster. Because there is no pleomorphism and myoepithelial cells are present, this aspirate was reported as suspicious rather than malignant.

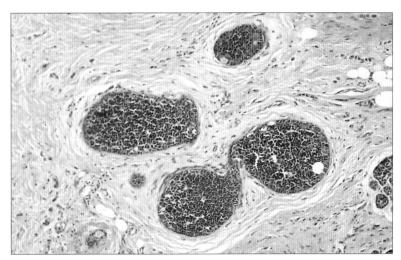

Fig. 9.69 LCIS – H&E x4. This section shows the features of LCIS, with small carcinoma cells filling the lobules.

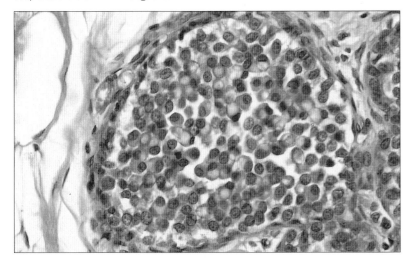

Fig. 9.70 LCIS – H&E x40. Illustrated is a section of LCIS under high magnification. The neoplastic cells are very small and many of them contain intracytoplasmic vacuoles. This is an important feature which is often seen in the aspirate.

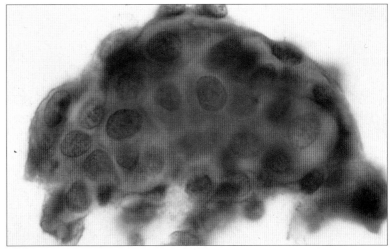

Fig. 9.71 LCIS – Pap x100. This is a distended lobular structure composed of small cells in an aspirate from a case of LCIS confirmed histologically. A few vacuoles are seen within the group.

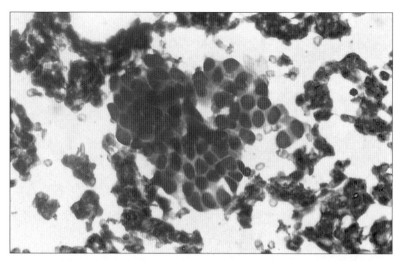

Fig. 9.72 LCIS – MGG x40. The cells in this air-dried smear are from the same case as shown in **Figure 9.71**. The distended lobules lose their three-dimensional appearance due to air-drying. The cells are slightly larger than the surrounding erythrocytes.

carcinoma cells, some containing intracytoplasmic vacuoles (**Figs 9.73, 9.74**). This may be due to forced cell separation during smear preparation. The cells are occasionally more pleomorphic than they appear in the histological section and may contain secretions within acinar structures (**Fig. 9.75**). An interesting feature to note is that small tumour cells are often seen, apparently infiltrating fragments of fat or stroma, even in cases which are pure LCIS on histology. This may reflect the effects of the spreading technique used for the aspirate. The cells in LCIS show features of malignancy, such as irregular nuclear margins, which are absent in atypical lobular hyperplasia. Small holes may also be visible in the distended lobular structures seen in the latter condition (**Fig. 9.76**).

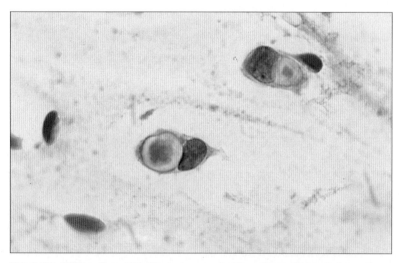

Fig. 9.73 LCIS – Pap x100. These two small cells, with nuclei barely larger than erythrocytes, contain intracytoplasmic vacuoles, both with targetoid mucin. Special stains are unnecessary for the central dot of mucin, as it is well-demonstrated with the Papanicolaou stain.

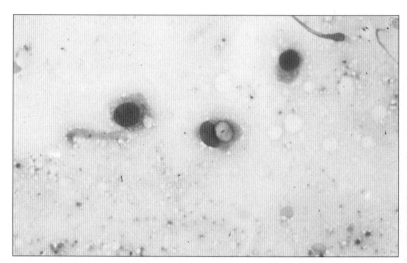

Fig. 9.74 LCIS – MGG x40. Illustrated are three small carcinoma cells, one of which contains an intracytoplasmic vacuole. Elsewhere in this smear there were distended lobules that contained small malignant cells.

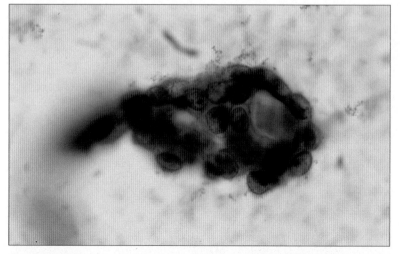

Fig. 9.75 LCIS – Pap x100. An unusual finding in LCIS is the presence of small acinar structures that contain secretions. The cells are slightly pleomorphic and contain small nucleoli. Similar features may be seen in fibroadenomas (see **Figure 8.100**).

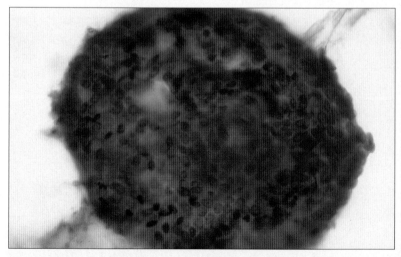

Fig. 9.76 Lobular hyperplasia – Pap x40. This huge, distended lobular structure is filled with small epithelial cells and studded with myoepithelial cells on the surface. Note the small holes in the sphere of cells. No intracytoplasmic vacuoles are seen and there is no pleomorphism.

INVASIVE LOBULAR CARCINOMA

This tumour on histological examination is composed of small cells which infiltrate in a targetoid (**Fig. 9.77**) or Indian-file fashion (**Fig. 9.78**). Unfortunately, cytological preparations do not reflect architectural patterns, only cellular features. The aspirates are usually cellular in our experience (**Fig. 9.79**), contrary to the many published reports of scanty cellularity. Large clusters of small cells (**Figs 9.80, 9.81**) and distended lobules (**Fig. 9.82**) are often seen, while many single small cells, including signet ring forms, are common (**Fig. 9.83**).

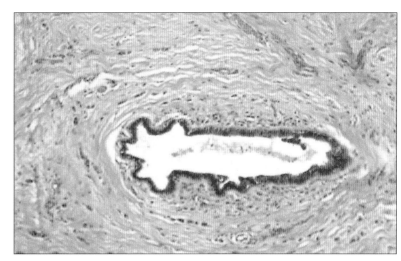

Fig. 9.77 Invasive lobular carcinoma – H&E x10. This histological section shows the characteristic targetoid pattern of infiltration by small carcinoma cells around a duct.

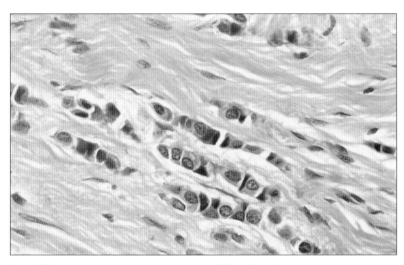

Fig. 9.78 Invasive lobular carcinoma – H&E x40. In this section another typical feature of infiltrating lobular carcinoma is demonstrated – Indian filing. The small cells are in single files; some cells have squared-off nuclei, others contain intracytoplasmic vacuoles.

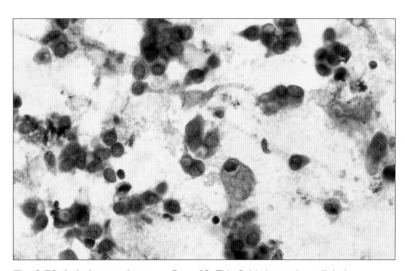

Fig. 9.79 Lobular carcinoma – Pap x40. This field shows the cellularity commonly noted in lobular carcinoma. There are small groups and single carcinoma cells, several with intracytoplasmic vacuoles. In this aspirate the nuclei are rounded, whereas they are often irregular and eccentric.

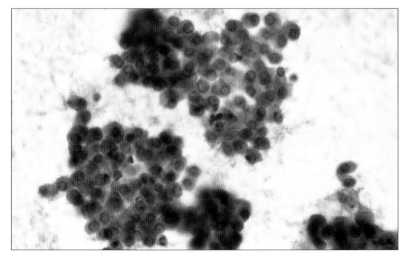

Fig. 9.80 Lobular carcinoma – Pap x40. Large clusters of small cells are visible in this field, with the edges of the clusters being irregular, rather than smooth as seen in benign ductal sheets. This is a common finding, contrary to the traditional idea that lobular carcinomas are poorly cellular.

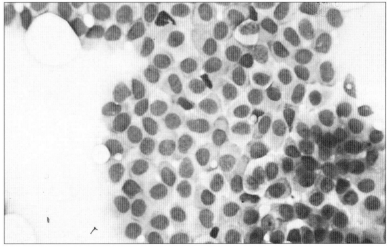

Fig. 9.81 Lobular carcinoma – MGG x40. The cell clusters in air-dried smears flatten out and the edges are not as ragged as in the wet-fixed preparation. The nuclei appear quite bland, but there are scattered intracytoplasmic vacuoles.

A feature noted in the majority of cases studied by the author is the presence of intracytoplasmic lumina, sometimes clear and sometimes containing a speck of mucin, visible with both the Papanicolaou and the May Grunwald Giemsa stain (**Figs 9.84, 9.85**), without the aid of special stains such as Alcian blue or PAS. Sometimes, clusters of these small carcinoma cells are arranged in an acinar fashion, with small lumina seen centrally (**Figs 9.86, 9.87**).

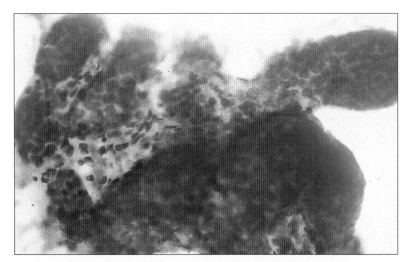

Fig. 9.82 Lobular carcinoma – Pap x40. This field displays a collection of distended lobules from a case of lobular carcinoma. The cells are small and not pleomorphic. Distended lobules are seen in invasive as well as in *in situ* lobular carcinoma.

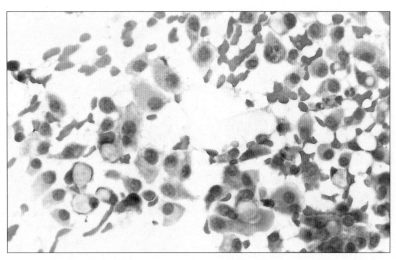

Fig. 9.83 Lobular carcinoma – Pap x40. In this aspirate from an invasive lobular carcinoma there are many single carcinoma cells, with a few signet ring types. Other cells have smaller vacuoles.

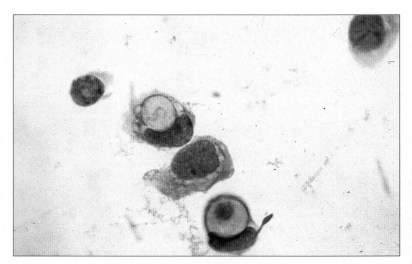

Fig. 9.84 Lobular carcinoma – Pap x100. Illustrated here are a few lobular carcinoma cells, one with a clear vacuole, another with a vacuole containing targetoid mucin. Note the eccentric and pleomorphic nuclei, and the vacuole pushing the nucleus to the periphery.

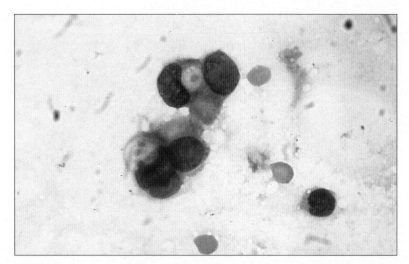

Fig. 9.85 Lobular carcinoma – MGG x100. This field shows a small cluster of lobular carcinoma cells. Two cells contain targetoid intracytoplasmic vacuoles, one of which is indenting the nucleus.

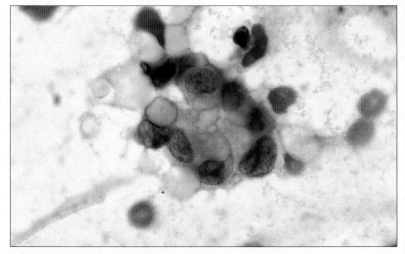

Fig. 9.86 Lobular carcinoma – Pap x100. The acinus in the centre of this field is composed of carcinoma cells with eccentric, irregular nuclei and intracytoplasmic vacuoles arranged towards the lumen of the acinus. The nuclei are about the size of erythrocytes.

Indian file arrangements of cells may be seen, both with and without intracytoplasmic lumina (**Figs 9.88–9.91**). The individual cells are small with irregular nuclei (**Figs 9.92–9.94**), but may have round, less pleomorphic nuclei (**Fig. 9.95**). Often the cells have substantial amounts of cytoplasm with eccentric nuclei, giving them a plasmacytoid appearance (**Fig. 9.96**).

A feature which is occasionally seen is the presence of fairly prominent nucleoli in some lobular carcinomas (**Fig. 9.97**), but most of these tumours are composed of cells with twisted irregular nuclei without visible nucleoli.

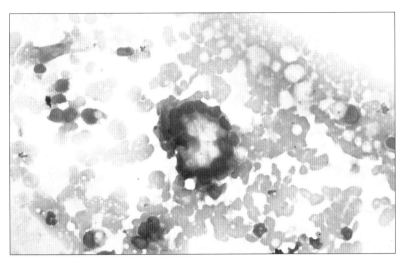

Fig. 9.87 Lobular carcinoma – MGG x40. Illustrated in this air-dried smear is an acinus composed of small cells with intracytoplasmic vacuoles towards the lumen. Note the single, small malignant cells in the background, several of which also contain vacuoles.

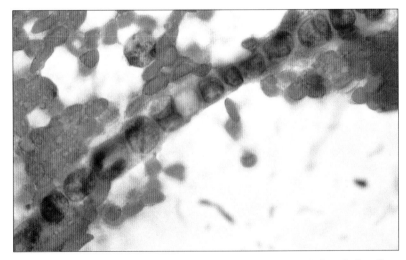

Fig. 9.88 Lobular carcinoma – Pap x100. This is a remarkably long Indian file of lobular carcinoma cells (perhaps a train rather than a file), composed of mildly pleomorphic cells with one containing an intracytoplasmic vacuole.

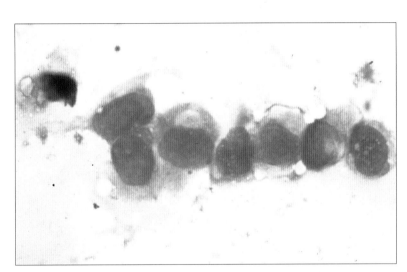

Fig. 9.89 Lobular carcinoma – MGG x100. An Indian file is seen in this air-dried preparation, with two cells containing intracytoplasmic vacuoles.

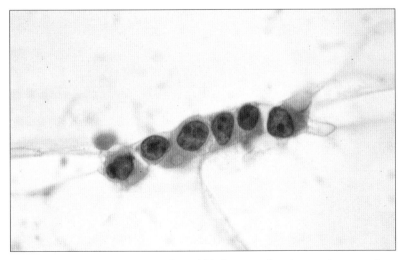

Fig. 9.90 Lobular carcinoma – Pap x100. Intracytoplasmic vacuoles are not as obvious in this Indian file as in the examples in **Figures 9.88** and **9.89**. The cells are small, with irregular nuclei and small nucleoli.

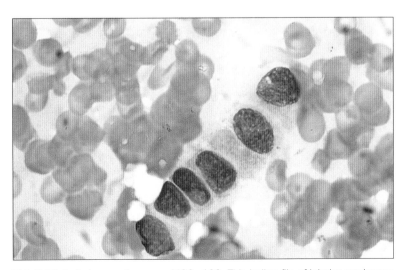

Fig. 9.91 Lobular carcinoma – MGG x100. This Indian file of lobular carcinoma cells displays the almost moulded appearance sometimes seen in these neoplasms. No vacuoles are visible.

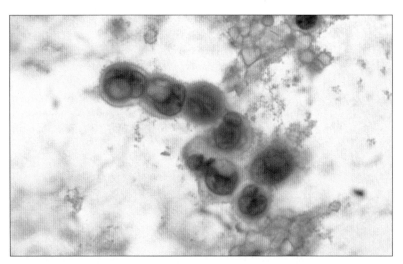

Fig. 9.92 Lobular carcinoma – Pap x100. This little group of small cells demonstrates the extremely irregular and pleomorphic nuclei often seen in lobular carcinomas. Some of the nuclei appear to show buds. Vacuoles are present.

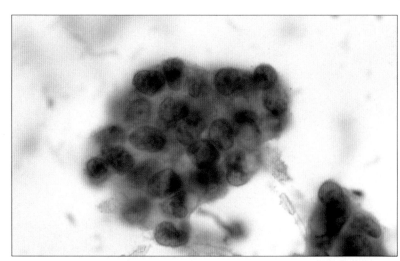

Fig. 9.93 Lobular carcinoma – Pap x100. In this field there is a rounded cluster of small cells with very irregular nuclei and some vacuoles, resembling a distended lobule.

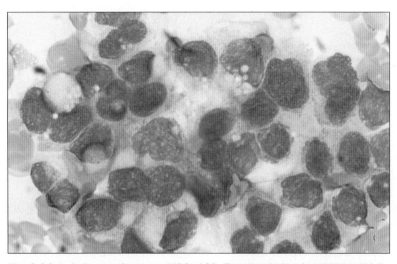

Fig. 9.94 Lobular carcinoma – MGG x100. The irregularity of nuclear outline in lobular carcinoma cells is here unusually well-illustrated for an air-dried aspirate.

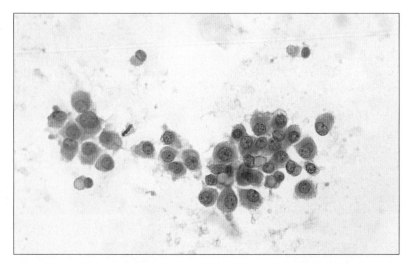

Fig. 9.95 Lobular carcinoma – Pap x40. This loosely cohesive cluster of lobular carcinoma cells contains rounded, rather than the more common irregular, nuclei. Several vacuoles are present.

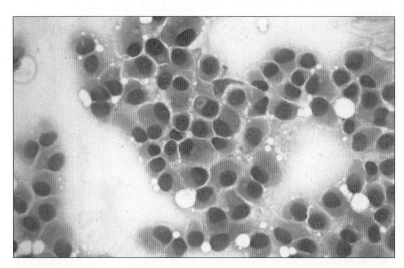

Fig. 9.96 Lobular carcinoma – Pap x40. Most of the carcinoma cells seen here are single with eccentric nuclei, giving them a plasmacytoid appearance. Note also the targetoid intracytoplasmic vacuoles.

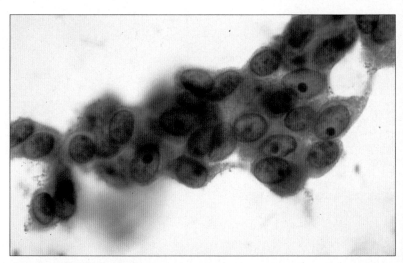

Fig. 9.97 Lobular carcinoma – Pap x100. An uncommon feature seen here is the presence of prominent nucleoli. They are much more common in ductal than in lobular carcinoma.

Another feature of note in aspirates from lobular carcinomas is the infiltration of clusters of fat cells and stromal fragments by small tumour cells (**Fig. 9.98**). In our series of lobular carcinomas we found infiltration by tumour cells of fragments of fat and stroma in both invasive and *in situ* lobular carcinomas; therefore, this criterion cannot be used reliably to diagnose invasion. We also noted that single malignant cells are seen frequently in LCIS, and that distended lobular structures are seen in both forms of the tumour, but more frequently in pure LCIS.

The diagnosis of lobular carcinoma, particularly the classic histological type, can be very difficult, especially when the cells are small but not pleomorphic and also when they do not have prominent nucleoli. The various histological types, such as solid and mixed, cannot be confidently diagnosed on cytology. Pleomorphic lobular carcinomas also have readily discernible intracytoplasmic lumina, and the cells are often larger and have more cytoplasm than in the class-ic type (**Fig. 9.99**).

There are criteria which help to distinguish between ductal and lobular carcinomas (**Fig. 9.100**), but the distinction is not always clear-cut.

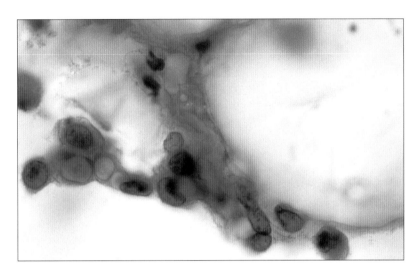

Fig. 9.98 Lobular carcinoma – Pap x100. This photomicrograph shows small vacuolated lobular carcinoma cells infiltrating between and around fat cells. Interestingly, this feature is also seen in some aspirates of pure LCIS.

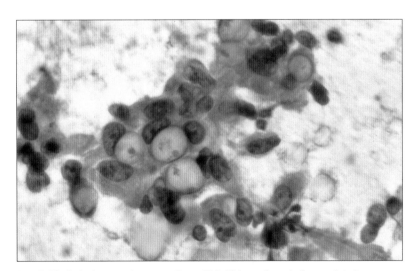

Fig. 9.99 Lobular carcinoma – Pap x100. This aspirate is from a lobular carcinoma which was subclassified as of pleomorphic type on histology. The cells are slightly larger than in the classical type and contain more cytoplasm. Irregular nuclei and large intracytoplasmic vacuoles are prominent features.

FEATURES	DUCTAL CARCINOMA NOS	LOBULAR CARCINOMA
Cellularity	Cellular	Cellular
Cell cohesiveness	Clusters and single cells	Clusters and single cells
Clusters	Sharp outlines	Irregular outlines
Distended lobules	Absent	Present
Indian files	Absent	Present
Cytoplasmic vacuoles	Rarely present	Usually present
Cell uniformity	Varies with grade	Usually uniform
Nucleus	Central	Eccentric
Nuclear pleomorphism	Variable	Usually marked
Nuclear size	Large	Small
Nucleoli	Usually abnormal	Small/not visible
Nuclear margin	Irregular	Irregular
Chromatin pattern	Abnormal	Vesicular
Myoepithelial cells	Absent	May be present
Necrosis	May be present (in DCIS)	Absent
Calcium	May be present	Not common
Mitoses	May be present	Rarely seen
Clinical features	Definite mass	Vague thickening
Mammogram	Usually characteristic	No characteristic features

Fig. 9.100 Criteria for distinguishing between ductal and lobular carcinomas.

TUBULAR CARCINOMA

This special type of breast cancer is seen more frequently in breast screening centres where early lesions are aspirated using stereotactic equipment. The histological features are easily recognizable as the tumour consists of well-differentiated carcinoma cells arranged predominantly in tubules (**Fig. 9.101**). The diagnosis of this type from cytological preparations is much more difficult as the cells show very few of the criteria of malignancy. The aspirates are usually cellular, containing sheets of uniform epithelial cells, often with no visible nucleoli, and with neat, almost palisaded edges (**Fig. 9.102**). Associated with these sheets of cells are test-tube like structures, which are three-dimensional, enabling the cells at the bottom of the 'tubule' to be examined by carefully focusing on the wet-fixed smear (**Fig. 9.103**). The cells in the air-dried smear are flattened, so it is not possible to see the cells beneath those in the upper layer (**Fig. 9.104**). Occasionally, bowl-like arrangements of cells are seen (**Fig. 9.105**) and acinar structures may be noted (**Figs 9.106, 9.107**). The cells may show some pleomorphism (**Fig. 9.108**), but, if not, the presence of single uniform epithelial cells is a pointer to the

diagnosis. In many cases these tumours are diagnosed as highly suspicious (C4) rather than as definite carcinomas.

Tubulo-lobular carcinomas, which show a combination of both tubular and lobular features, may sometimes be recognized on aspirates. The smears show a mixture of small single cells containing intracytoplasmic vacuoles, distended lobules, and acini or tubular structures similar to those seen in tubular cancers (**Fig. 9.109**).

MUCINOUS (MUCOID, COLLOID) CARCINOMA

This variety of carcinoma of the breast, which has a good prognosis, presents a lobulated, fairly well-circumscribed appearance on mammograms. The clinician often has an idea of the type of tumour, as the aspirate may be thick and gelatinous. Histological sections show islands of fairly uniform carcinoma cells floating in lakes of mucin (**Fig. 9.110**). The cytological features are typical – the background shows streaks and pools of mucin, which is often pale pink or blue on the wet-fixed smear and therefore may be missed (**Fig. 9.111**). Mucin is much more obvious with the May Grunwald Giemsa stain, showing a bright, pinkish purple hue (**Fig. 9.112**).

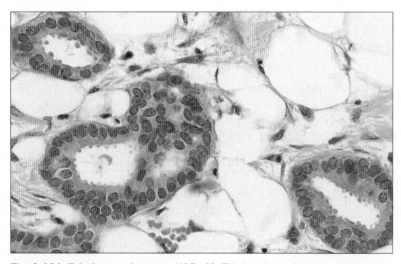

Fig. 9.101 Tubular carcinoma – H&E x40. This histological section shows a tubular carcinoma with tubules infiltrating fat. The cells have small, bland nuclei with no evidence of pleomorphism.

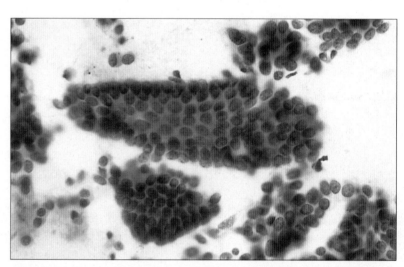

Fig. 9.102 Tubular carcinoma – Pap x40. These sheets of cohesive cells are from a tubular carcinoma. The cells are small and uniform, with apparent palisading of the edges of the groups. However, the single cells in the background are an indicator of malignancy.

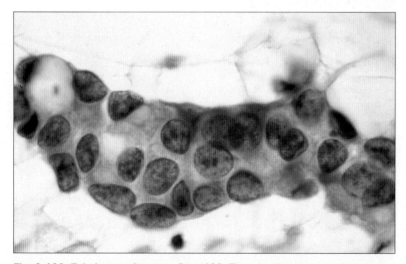

Fig. 9.103 Tubular carcinoma – Pap x100. The tube-like structure displayed here is typical of tubular carcinoma. It is three-dimensional rather than flat and the cells at the bottom of the tube can be observed by changing the focus. The cells are mildly pleomorphic, but cohesive, and may be interpreted as benign.

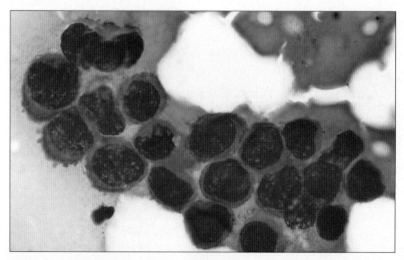

Fig. 9.104 Tubular carcinoma – MGG x100. This group of carcinoma cells displays more hyperchromasia and pleomorphism than is usually seen in tubular carcinomas. Air-drying precludes the observation of cells at the bottom of the tubular structure.

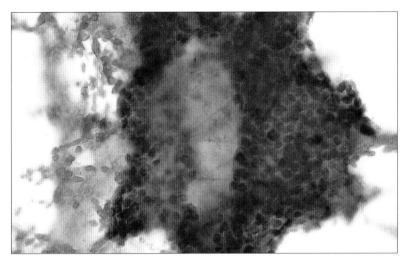

Fig. 9.105 Tubular carcinoma – Pap x40. A rare finding in tubular carcinoma is the presence of bowl-shaped structures composed of well-differentiated small carcinoma cells, as illustrated here. This feature can sometimes be seen in benign aspirates, so single carcinoma cells must be found before such an aspirate can be reported as malignant.

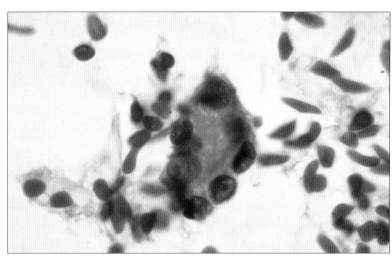

Fig. 9.106 Tubular carcinoma – Pap x100. Illustrated is an acinar arrangement of small, mildly pleomorphic carcinoma cells, some with prominent nucleoli. This is a common finding in aspirates from tubular carcinoma.

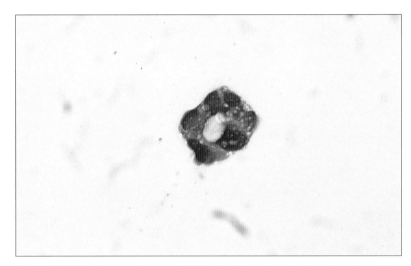

Fig. 9.107 Tubular carcinoma – MGG x40. This acinar cluster of small, variably sized carcinoma cells is from an aspirate of the same case as shown in **Figure 9.106.**

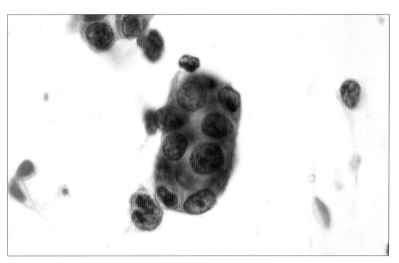

Fig. 9.108 Tubular carcinoma – Pap x100. The small tubular structure in the centre of the field is composed of mildly pleomorphic cells, with prominent nucleoli and granular chromatin. There are also single similar cells in the background, which are a pointer to malignancy when the cells in clusters are very well differentiated.

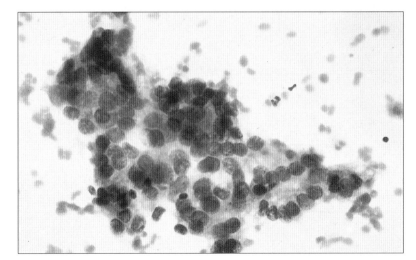

Fig. 9.109 Tubulo-lobular carcinoma – Pap x40. This field shows two distended lobules composed of small carcinoma cells, two acinar structures composed of similar cells, and some erythrocytes. Elsewhere in the aspirate there were cells containing intracytoplasmic vacuoles.

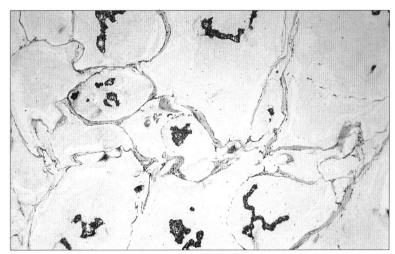

Fig. 9.110 Mucinous carcinoma – H&E x10. This section shows small groups of carcinoma cells floating in lakes of mucin. (Slide courtesy of Dr PH McKee, St Thomas' Hospital, London.)

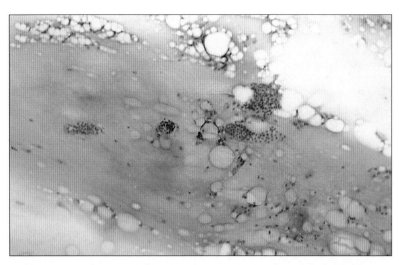

Fig. 9.111 Mucinous carcinoma – Pap x10. The background of this smear is composed of pale pink mucin with a few scattered islands of small cells. The mucin is often missed on wet-fixed smears because of the pale staining.

The carcinoma cells, which are often small, may be seen in small tightly cohesive groups and may be mistaken for benign ductal cells if the mucin is not noticed (**Fig. 9.113**). Care must be taken to search for single malignant cells, which may be seen around the mucin pools. Interesting features sometimes noted are the presence of blood vessels that apparently traverse the mucin (**Figs 9.114, 9.115**) and the single, almost spindle-shaped, cells occasionally seen within the mucinous material (**Fig. 9.116**). Rarely, colloid carcinoma aspirates contain cells which are pleomorphic (**Fig. 9.117**) or contain prominent nucleoli (**Fig. 9.118**).

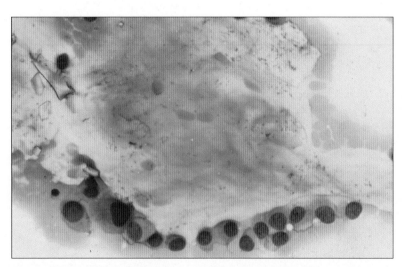

Fig. 9.112 Mucinous carcinoma – MGG x40. This aspirate from a mucinous carcinoma shows pinkish purple mucin with some mildly pleomorphic carcinoma cells.

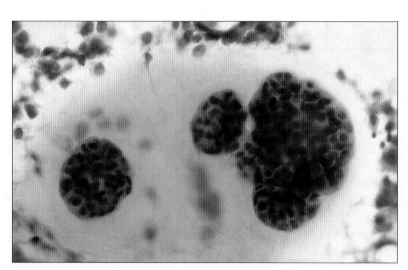

Fig. 9.113 Mucinous carcinoma – Pap x40. In this wet-fixed smear the neoplastic cells are in round, cohesive groups with pink mucin in the background.

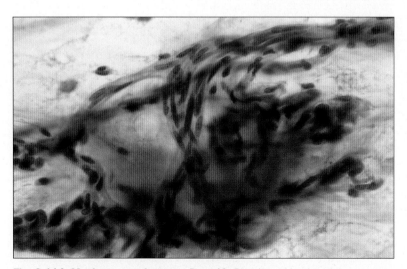

Fig. 9.114 Mucinous carcinoma – Pap x40. Prominent blood vessels are seen traversing the pale pink mucin in this field. This is a common finding in mucinous carcinomas.

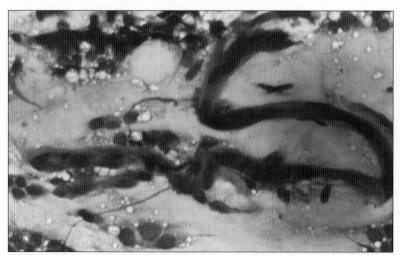

Fig. 9.115 Mucinous carcinoma – MGG x40. This air-dried smear shows blood vessels surrounded by pinkish purple mucin. Note the carcinoma cells at the edges of the field.

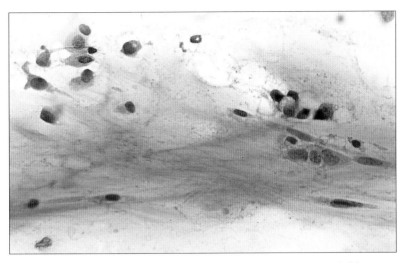

Fig. 9.116 Mucinous carcinoma – Pap x40. In this field there is pale blue mucin in which are lying some foamy macrophages and spindle cells. A few single carcinoma cells are seen in the top left corner.

MEDULLARY CARCINOMA

These tumours are composed of pleomorphic carcinoma cells in syncytial sheets or groups with a typical histological pattern of lymphocytic infiltration (**Fig. 9.119**). The fine needle aspirate shows large, pleomorphic tumour cells with abnormal nucleoli and chromatin in syncytial groups (**Figs 9.120, 9.121**), and also scattered lymphocytes and plasma cells (**Fig. 9.122**). The cells may be mistaken for a high-grade carcinoma if the lymphocytes are not observed. Another cytological problem is that the presence of lymphocytes is not diagnostic of medullary carcinoma of the breast; it may simply denote lymphocytic infiltration. Atypical medullary carcinoma cannot be distinguished from medullary carcinoma on cytological appearances alone. The cytology report should describe the types of cells seen and raise the possibility of a medullary carcinoma.

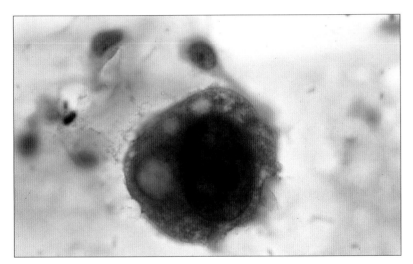

Fig. 9.117 Mucinous carcinoma – Pap x100. Although the cells in mucinous carcinoma are usually small and well-differentiated, occasionally the neoplasm is composed of large, pleomorphic cells, such as the one illustrated here. Note the huge nucleus and abnormal chromatin pattern.

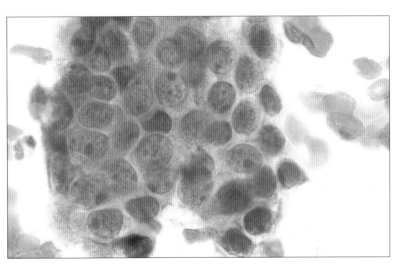

Fig. 9.118 Mucinous carcinoma – Pap x100. This cluster of carcinoma cells shows variation in nuclear size, and pronounced red nucleoli with granular chromatin, features which are unusual for mucinous neoplasms.

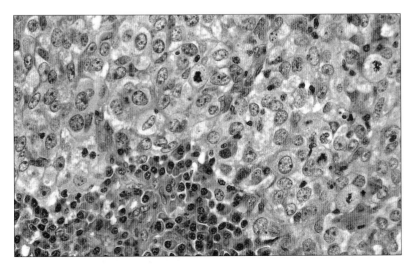

Fig. 9.119 Medullary carcinoma – H&E x40. This section shows a medullary carcinoma composed of pleomorphic large cells, mitotic figures, and a characteristic lymphocytic infiltrate. (Slide courtesy of Dr PH McKee, St Thomas' Hospital, London.)

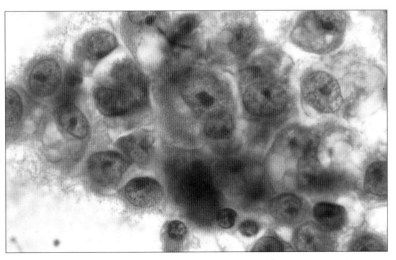

Fig. 9.120 Medullary carcinoma – Pap x100. Illustrated are large malignant cells with delicate cytoplasm and ill-defined cytoplasmic borders. Note the large red nucleoli, and the lymphocytes and plasma cell at the bottom of the cluster.

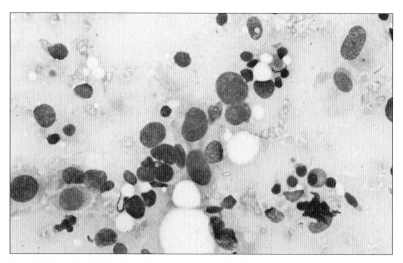

Fig. 9.121 Medullary carcinoma – MGG x40. The tumour cells seen here are large with pale blue nucleoli. Their cytoplasm is indistinct. There are also several lymphocytes and a plasma cell with a well-defined 'hof'.

APOCRINE CARCINOMA

The incidence of this type of carcinoma varies from centre to centre. The histological features are those of invasive ductal carcinoma, with large apocrine-type cells displaying typical abundant eosinophilic cytoplasm (**Fig. 9.123**). Aspirates from apocrine carcinomas show similar cytological characteristics to benign apocrine cells – the malignant cells have abundant granular cytoplasm and large round nuclei with enormous red nucleoli on the Papanicolaou stain (**Fig. 9.124**). On the air-dried smear the cytoplasmic granularity and nucleoli are not always evident (**Fig. 9.125**). The cells are usually in clusters, but occasionally are single. Great care must be taken to establish that the cells, although apocrine, are malignant and not benign. Sometimes, foamy macrophages spread thinly on a smear can mimic apocrine cells.

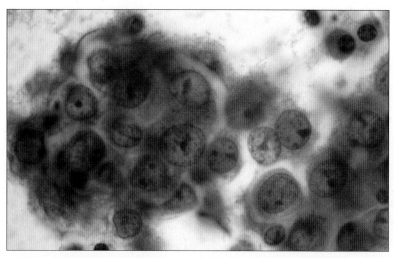

Fig. 9.122 Medullary carcinoma – Pap x100. This is a syncytial group of carcinoma cells with abnormally shaped red nucleoli and clearing and clumping of chromatin. There are two plasma cells in the top right corner and a few lymphocytes elsewhere in the cluster. These carcinomas invariably score a high grade with the cytological grading system (see **Figure 9.170**) and may not be diagnosed as medullary in type.

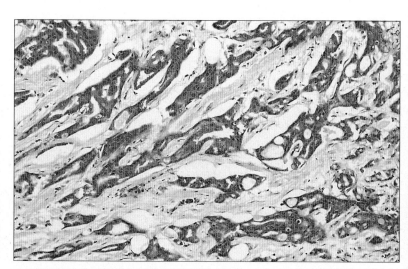

Fig. 9.123 Apocrine carcinoma – H&E x4. This section shows an apocrine carcinoma with infiltrating islands of cells containing abundant pink cytoplasm.

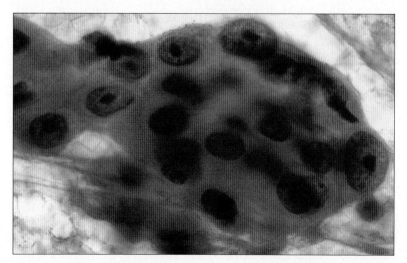

Fig. 9.124 Apocrine carcinoma – Pap x100. This cluster of large cells combines the features of apocrine cells, namely large nucleoli and abundant granular cytoplasm, with the features of carcinoma – pleomorphism and an abnormal chromatin pattern.

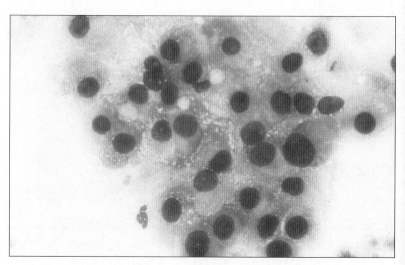

Fig. 9.125 Apocrine carcinoma – MGG x40. These apocrine carcinoma cells show nuclear pleomorphism and abundant cytoplasm, but nucleoli are not well visualized.

INTRACYSTIC PAPILLARY CARCINOMA

This type of malignancy may present as a well-defined, palpable cystic lesion clinically, and can be confirmed mammographically. The history given may be of a long-standing breast lump. Histologically, the lesion shows papillary architecture with lining cells that vary from bland to mildly pleomorphic (**Fig. 9.126**). The aspirate is usually heavily blood-stained and cellular, with cohesive flat sheets (**Figs 9.127, 9.128**) and clusters (**Figs 9.129, 9.130**) of uniform epithelial cells, some showing palisading (**Fig. 9.131**). Many single, columnar-type cells are seen in the background, suggesting a benign lesion (**Fig. 9.132**), but there are usually other cells which are more pleomorphic that would provide the diagnosis (**Fig. 9.133**).

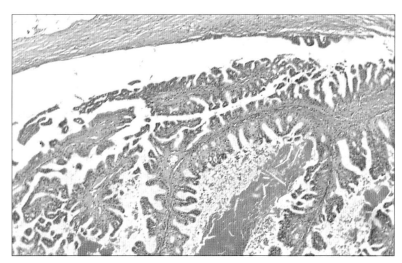

Fig. 9.126 Papillary carcinoma – H&E x4. This section shows an intracystic papillary carcinoma.

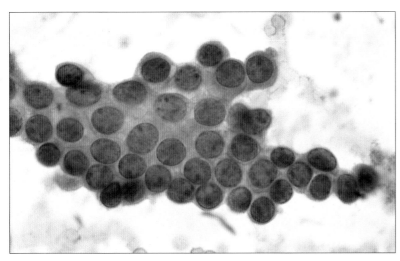

Fig. 9.127 Intracystic papillary carcinoma – Pap x100. The sheet of cohesive epithelial cells illustrated here displays rounded nuclei and vesicular chromatin. The cells look benign, but there are no myoepithelial cells. Papillary carcinomas are often composed of bland cells.

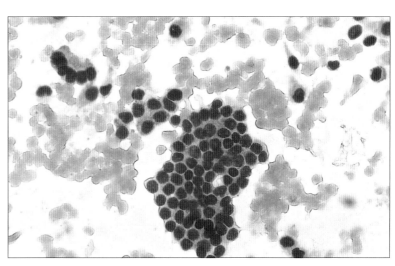

Fig. 9.128 Intracystic papillary carcinoma – MGG x40. In this field there is a flat sheet of uniform cells with rounded nuclei, a smaller, less cohesive group, a few cells in a row, and some single cells which are slightly pleomorphic. No myoepithelial cells are seen.

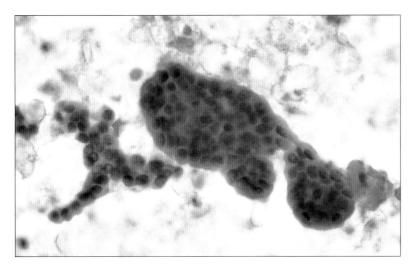

Fig. 9.129 Intracystic papillary carcinoma – Pap x40. Here the cells are in clusters with some cyst debris in the background. No single cells are seen.

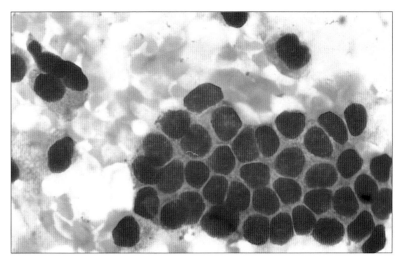

Fig. 9.130 Intracystic papillary carcinoma – MGG x100. The epithelial cells in this field are monomorphic, but there are some single epithelial cells which should raise the suspicion of malignancy.

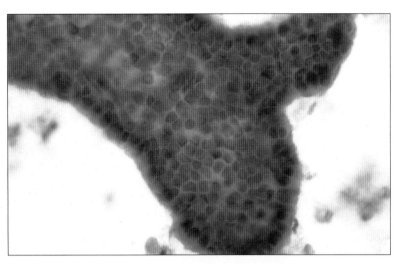

Fig. 9.131 Intracystic papillary carcinoma – Pap x40. This large sheet of small uniform epithelial cells shows palisading of nuclei around the edges, similar to the palisading seen in benign endocervical cells.

CARCINOMA WITH NEUROENDOCRINE FEATURES

It is not uncommon for areas of breast carcinomas to show neuroendocrine features. Occasionally, the whole of the tumour is composed of such cells and the aspirate shows clusters of small cells which may have eccentric nuclei, delicate ill-defined cytoplasm, and speckled chromatin similar to that of oat cell carcinomas (**Figs 9.134, 9.135**). Rosettes may be seen (**Figs 9.136, 9.13**7) and a Grimelius stain is usually positive (**Fig. 9.138**).

METAPLASTIC CARCINOMA

Carcinoma of the breast can exhibit features suggestive of other tissues, in the form of osseous or sarcomatous metaplasia. A fine needle aspirate from the case illustrated below contained a cellular spread of uniform spindle cells with abnormal chromatin (**Fig. 9.139**) and mitotic figures (**Fig. 9.140**). The nucleoli were not grossly enlarged. The air-dried smear contained unremarkable spindle cells (**Fig. 9.141**), which showed the features of a sarcoma NOS (not otherwise specified); the histology also showed the features of a mesenchymal neoplasm. Only immunocytochemical stains performed on the excision specimen revealed the true epithelial nature of the neoplasm.

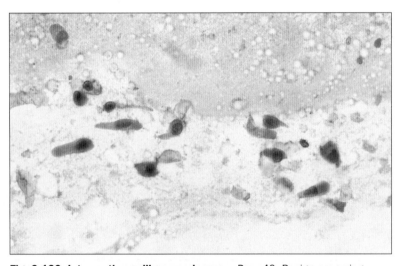

Fig. 9.132 Intracystic papillary carcinoma – Pap x40. Benign-appearing columnar cells are frequently seen lying singly in the background in these aspirates. No features of malignancy are noted in this field.

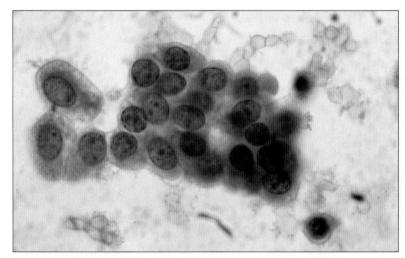

Fig. 9.133 Intracystic papillary carcinoma – Pap x100. Usually in the aspirate there are at least a few clusters of cells which show mild pleomorphism. Here, nucleoli are visible, but not abnormally enlarged.

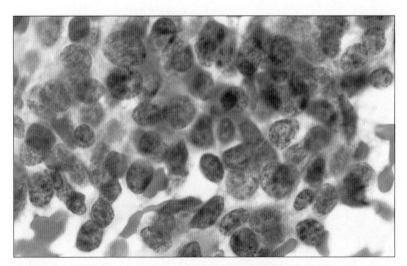

Fig. 9.134 Carcinoma with neuroendocrine features – Pap x100. This field is composed of cells with round to ovoid nuclei and distinctly speckled chromatin. Cytoplasm is not evident.

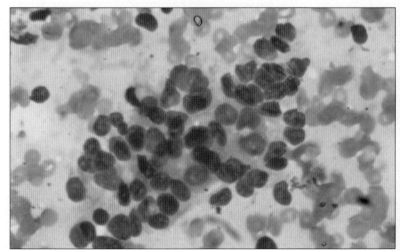

Fig. 9.135 Carcinoma with neuroendocrine features – MGG x40. The cluster of cells seen in this field does not display the speckled chromatin that is obvious in the wet-fixed smear. The cells are small, the nuclei being slightly larger than erythrocytes. Air-dried smears do not show the subtle nuclear changes that are present in wet-fixed material.

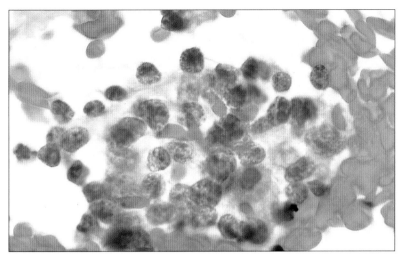

Fig. 9.136 Carcinoma with neuroendocrine features – Pap x100. The cluster of cells seen here contains two ill-defined rosettes or acinar structures. The cells show speckled chromatin and some irregularity of nuclear outline.

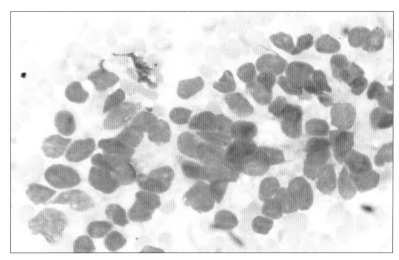

Fig. 9.137 Carcinoma with neuroendocrine features – MGG x40. Vague rosettes are seen in this field from an aspirate of a carcinoma with neuroendocrine features. No nuclear details are discernible with this method of smear preparation.

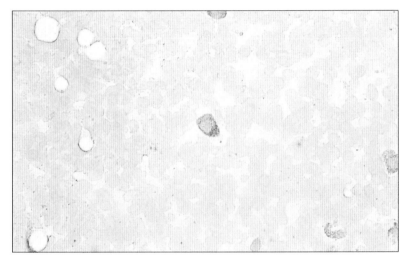

Fig. 9.138 Carcinoma with neuroendocrine features – Grimelius stain x40. This field contains a few epithelial cells which show positive granular staining.

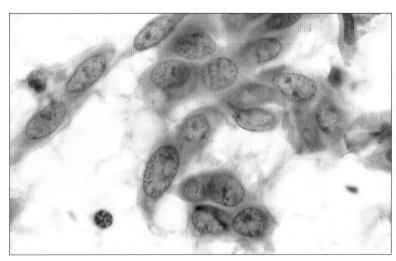

Fig. 9.139 Carcinoma with metaplastic features – Pap x100. This cellular aspirate contains spindle-shaped cells and ovoid nuclei with abnormal chromatin, comprising mostly euchromatin with irregular specks of heterochromatin. Pleomorphism is evident, but no mitotic figures or epithelial cells are seen. This resembles a mesenchymal neoplasm, as did the histological specimen, but immunocytochemical stains on the latter showed the neoplasm to be a carcinoma with sarcomatous metaplasia.

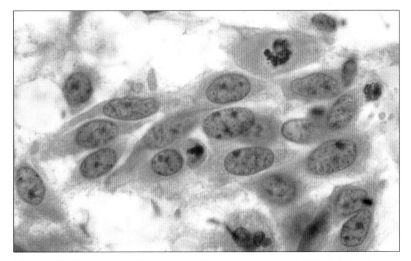

Fig. 9.140 Carcinoma with metaplastic features – Pap x100. This field contains similar cells to those shown in **Figure 9.139**, but it also shows a mitotic figure.

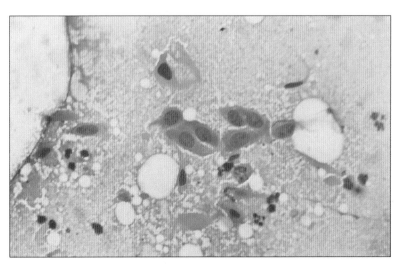

Fig. 9.141 Carcinoma with metaplastic features – MGG x40. The air-dried aspirate for the same case as in **Figure 9.140** is disappointingly bland, as no abnormal nuclear features can be seen.

ADENOID CYSTIC CARCINOMA

This is an uncommon neoplasm in the breast, but should not be missed as the features are quite typical. Histologically, the picture is similar to the appearances seen in adenoid cystic carcinoma of the salivary gland (**Fig. 9.142**). Aspirates are usually cellular with a fairly uniform population of small, bland cells. The identifying features are the small globular or cylindrical hyaline structures that stain pale blue or pink with the Papanicolaou stain and bright purple or pink with the May Grunwald Giemsa stain (**Figs 9.143–9.145**).

The differential diagnoses of this condition include collagenous spherulosis and pleomorphic adenoma (see Chapter 8 on benign breast lesions). The globules in collagenous spherulosis are identical to those in adenoid cystic carcinoma, therefore the cells in the background need to be scrutinized to make a diagnosis of malignancy. Single epithelial cells may be seen, and the large, flat sheets of benign cells, commonly associated with collagenous spherulosis, are absent in this carcinoma. With pleomorphic adenoma the hyaline material is fibrillary or finger-shaped, rather than in the form of globules or cylinders; in addition, the cells are typically benign.

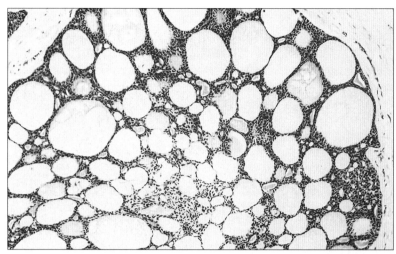

Fig. 9.142 Adenoid cystic carcinoma – H&E x10. This is a histological section showing adenoid cystic carcinoma of the breast, with features similar to those seen in the salivary gland neoplasm of the same name (see **Figure 14.26**).

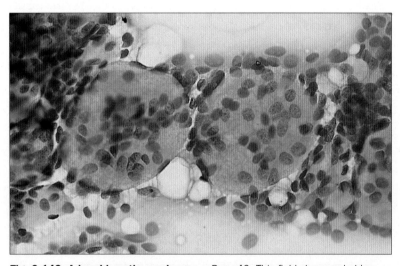

Fig. 9.143 Adenoid cystic carcinoma – Pap x40. This field shows pale blue globular structures covered by small epithelial cells with vesicular nuclei. If the staining is very pale the globules of basement membrane material are not seen clearly. This is one of the very few disadvantages of wet fixation.

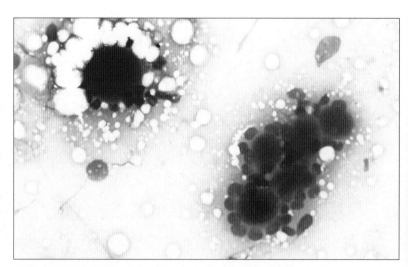

Fig. 9.144 Adenoid cystic carcinoma – MGG x40. Demonstrated here are magenta-coloured globules of basement membrane material surrounded by small epithelial cells.

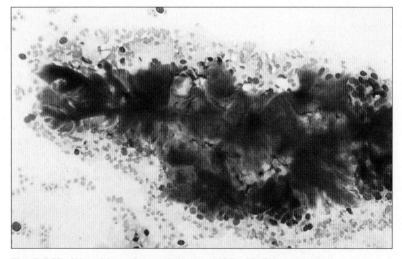

Fig. 9.145 Adenoid cystic carcinoma – MGG x40. This is another characteristic appearance of basement membrane material in adenoid cystic carcinoma, this time in the form of cylinders.

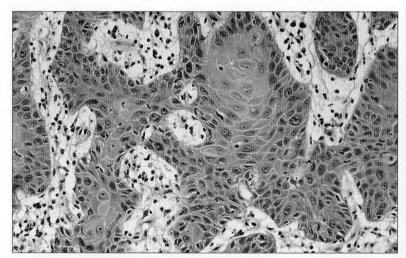

Fig. 9.146 Squamous carcinoma – H&E x10. This histological section shows a well-differentiated squamous cell carcinoma of the breast.

SQUAMOUS CARCINOMA

Primary squamous carcinoma of the breast is very rare. Squamous differentiation may be seen in areas of otherwise typical adenocarcinomas. Histologically, the squamous cell nest and keratinization make identification of this tumour simple (**Fig. 9.146**). On cytological material the distinguishing features include keratinized squamous carcinoma cells, which stain a bright refractile orange on the wet-fixed smear (**Fig. 9.147**) and a typical azure blue on the air-dried smear (**Fig. 9.148**). A common feature is the presence of cellular necrosis and debris in the background. A most helpful procedure is to examine a fine needle aspirate of an involved lymph node, which will show keratin debris, foamy macrophages, and multinucleated giant histiocytes containing engulfed keratinized squamous carcinoma cells (**Fig. 9.149**). Pyknotic degenerate squamous malignant cells may be seen in the background. Adenosquamous carcinomas of the breast do occur (**Figs 9.150, 9.151**), with the aspirate showing a mixture of adenocarcinoma and squamous carcinoma cells.

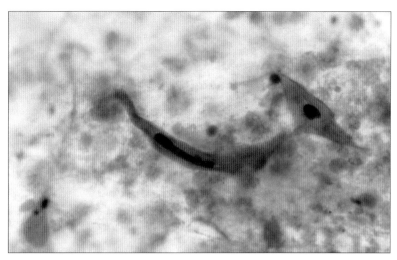

Fig. 9.147 Squamous carcinoma – Pap x63. Illustrated are the characteristic features of keratinizing squamous carcinoma – bright refractile orange cytoplasm and hyperchromatic, sometimes pyknotic nuclei, and also the necrotic cellular debris in the background. It is not possible to differentiate between a primary and a metastatic neoplasm.

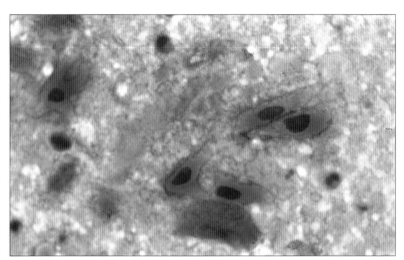

Fig. 9.148 Squamous carcinoma – MGG x63. Keratinizing squamous carcinoma cells exhibit a particular shade of azure blue with the May Grunwald Giemsa stain, as illustrated. Note the necrotic debris in the background.

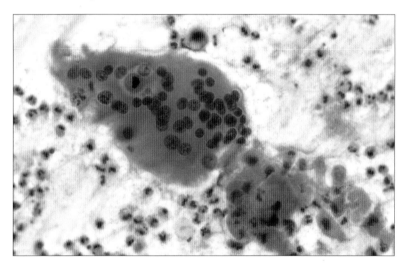

Fig. 9.149 Metastatic squamous carcinoma in lymph node – Pap x40. This aspirate from a lymph node with metastatic squamous carcinoma shows multinucleated giant histiocytes with phagocytosed squamous carcinoma cells.

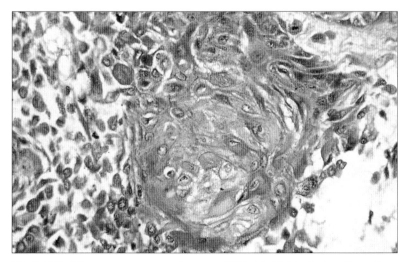

Fig. 9.150 Adenosquamous carcinoma – H&E x10. Histological sections show areas of tumour containing squamous carcinoma in the form of cell nests, along with other areas of adenocarcinoma.

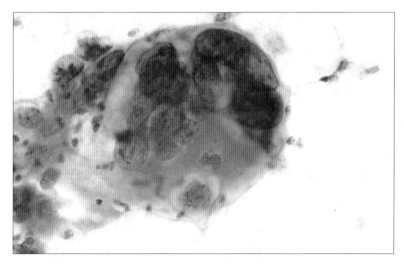

Fig. 9.151 Adenosquamous carcinoma – Pap x40. This aspirate contained many clusters of adenocarcinoma cells, as well as larger cells such as the ones illustrated. The multinucleated cell in the centre contains pinkish orange keratin in the cytoplasm.

PRIMARY LYMPHOMA OF THE BREAST

Both Hodgkin's and non-Hodgkin's lymphoma can occur as primary lesions in the breast. The fine needle aspirate is usually cellular in both cases. In non-Hodgkin's lymphoma, abnormal lymphoid cells are seen, producing a monomorphic picture (**Fig. 9.152**). The differential diagnosis is a reactive intramammary lymph node, but here the aspirate shows mixed cellularity with a variety of follicle-centre cells and often plasma cells. In Hodgkin's disease it is necessary to identify either Reed–Sternberg cells or Hodgkin's cells to make the diagnosis with certainty (see Chapter 10).

MALIGNANT PHYLLODES TUMOUR

Phyllodes tumours are not invariably benign. They may show borderline changes or be frankly malignant (**Fig. 9.153**). The aspirate is usually cellular and shows a mixture of pleomorphic spindle cells (**Fig. 9.154**) and rounded malignant cells showing marked pleomorphism (**Figs 9.155, 9.156**), with mitotic figures (**Fig. 9.157**).

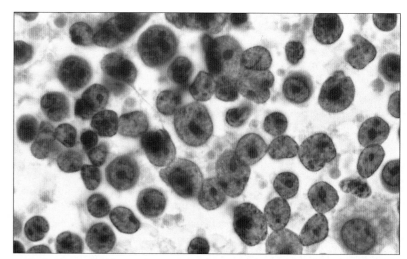

Fig. 9.152 Lymphoma – Pap x100. Illustrated are single abnormal lymphoid cells resembling immunoblasts with large central nucleoli, in a breast aspirate. It is not possible cytologically to determine whether this is a primary or metastatic tumour.

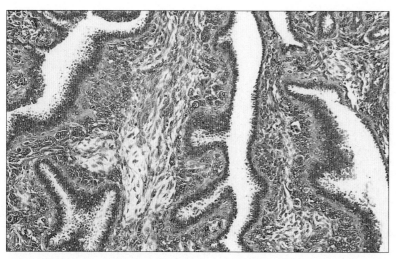

Fig. 9.153 Malignant phyllodes tumour – H&E x10. This is a histological section of a malignant phyllodes tumour showing malignant proliferation of the stroma with glandular hyperplasia.

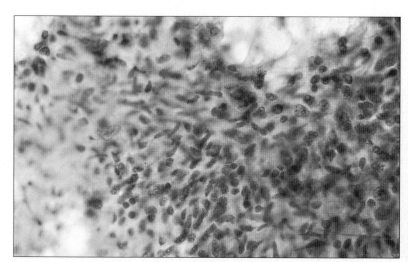

Fig. 9.154 Malignant phyllodes tumour – Pap x40. This field contains a fragment of cellular stroma composed of hyperchromatic spindle cells.

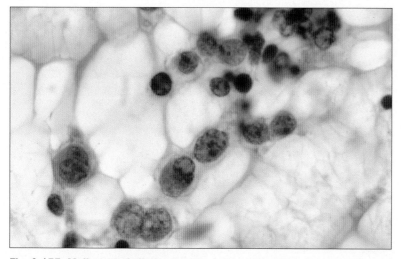

Fig. 9.155 Malignant phyllodes tumour – Pap x100. Elsewhere in the aspirate from the same case as shown in **Figures 9.153** and **9.154** there were rounded cells of varying sizes with abnormal clumped chromatin.

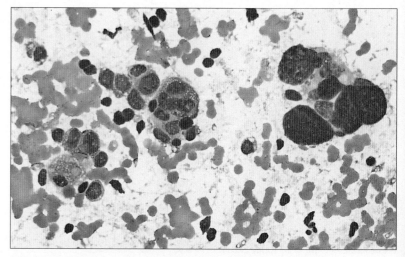

Fig. 9.156 Malignant phyllodes tumour – MGG x10. The extreme pleomorphism of this tumour is evident in this field.

SARCOMA OF THE BREAST

Sarcomas of the breast are rare and of various types. They can be difficult to diagnose on cytology as the aspirates are often scanty in cellularity. Sarcoma cells are usually spindle-shaped, with plump ovoid or spindle-shaped nuclei and prominent nucleoli (**Fig. 9.158**). Mitoses are often seen. Angiosarcomas are notoriously heavily blood-stained and may contain small cells which are bland. and not diagnostic.

METASTATIC TUMOURS

The breast is a fairly common site for tumour metastases. Some of the more frequent ones are small-cell anaplastic carcinoma of the lung (oat cell carcinoma), lymphoma, squamous carcinoma, melanoma, and renal cell carcinoma. Small-cell anaplastic carcinoma is associated with a cellular aspirate composed of small cells with minimal cytoplasm, sharp nuclear margins, speckled 'salt and pepper' chromatin, inconspicuous nuclei, and moulding of adjacent nuclei (**Fig. 9.159**). Lymphomas, which are secondary, are indistinguishable from the primary lesions described above. Squamous cell carcinoma metastases are also identical to the primary lesions. Metastatic malignant melanoma has typical features – the cells are often large, single, and show abundant cytoplasm, with or without pigment granules (**Fig. 9.160**). Many cells are binucleate and a typical feature is the presence of intranuclear inclusions (see Chapter 10). Renal cell carcinoma metastases may reflect the typical cytological appearances of renal cell tumours, with abundant vacuolated cytoplasm and variable nuclei with prominent nucleoli. On occasion, the secondary tumour may be quite anaplastic, and only the history of a similar cancer in the surgically removed kidney provides a clue to the diagnosis. Carcinoid tumours have been known to metastasize to the breast. The features are similar to those of neuroendocrine tumours described above (see **Figure 9.134**).

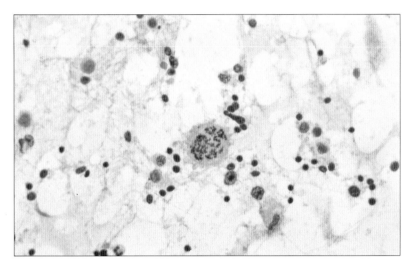

Fig. 9.157 Malignant phyllodes tumour – Pap x40. Mitotic figures are seen commonly.

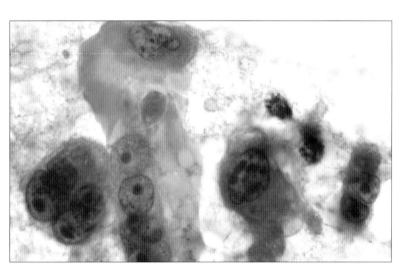

Fig. 9.158 Sarcoma – Pap x100. This field contains pleomorphic multinucleated sarcoma cells with huge red nucleoli. Elsewhere in the aspirate there were some spindle cells. The combination of spindle and pleomorphic cells points to a diagnosis of sarcoma.

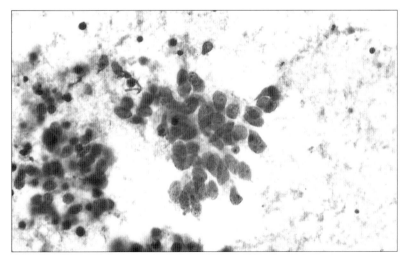

Fig. 9.159 Metastatic oat cell carcinoma – Pap x40. This field shows a cluster of small cells with very little cytoplasm and speckled chromatin. There are degenerate nuclei adjacent to the well-preserved cluster. The features are consistent with metastatic small cell carcinoma (the patient had primary small cell carcinoma of the lung).

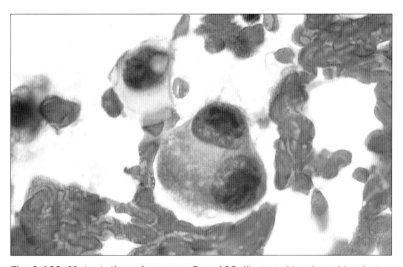

Fig. 9.160 Metastatic melanoma – Pap x100. Illustrated is a large binucleate cell with abundant cytoplasm and huge red nucleoli. This is characteristic of malignant melanoma, although neither pigment nor intranuclear inclusions can be seen in this case.

PAGET'S DISEASE OF THE NIPPLE

This neoplastic process presents as an itchy, sometimes red and inflamed area over the nipple, and can be mistaken for eczema. Most lesions are associated with underlying carcinoma of the breast, although the intramammary tumour may not become evident for some years, either mammographically or clinically. Histology reveals large malignant cells with clear cytoplasm infiltrating through the epidermis of the nipple (**Fig. 9.161**). A simple scrape of the affected area, dabbing the material on to a glass slide, can provide the diagnosis without the necessity of a formal surgical biopsy. The smears often contain anucleate squames (**Figs 9.162, 9.163**) and debris, sometimes accompanied by inflammatory cells. Typically, large, single malignant cells with abundant, often clear, cytoplasm are visible (**Figs 9.164, 9.165**).

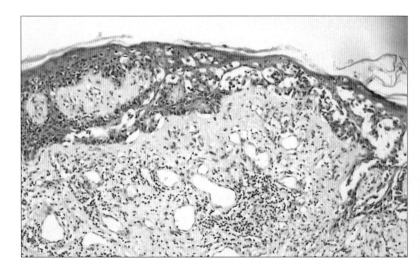

Fig. 9.161 Paget's disease of the nipple – H&E x10. This section of nipple shows infiltration of the epithelium by large clear cells, which are Paget's cells.

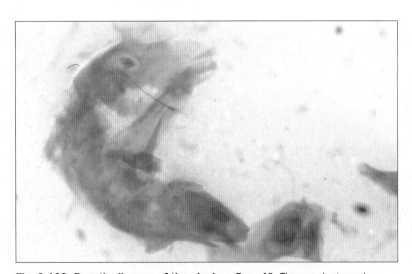

Fig. 9.162 Paget's disease of the nipple – Pap x40. The anucleate and inflamed keratinized squames illustrated often accompany eczema as well as Paget's disease of the nipple.

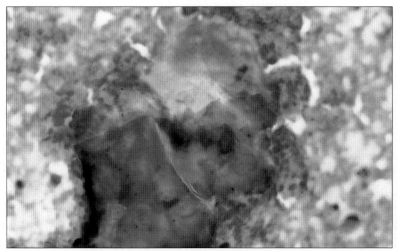

Fig. 9.163 Paget's disease of the nipple – MGG x40. Keratinized anucleate squames take on a bright blue appearance with this stain.

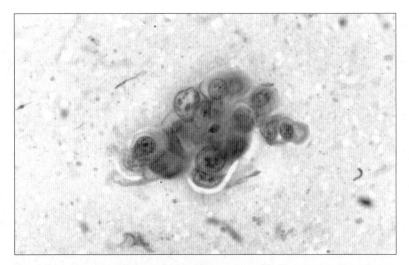

Fig. 9.164 Paget's disease of the nipple – Pap x63. The cluster of carcinoma cells shown here exhibits abnormal chromatin and clear cytoplasm.

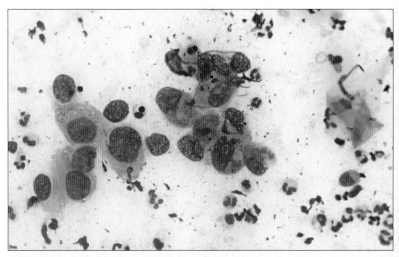

Fig. 9.165 Paget's disease of the nipple – MGG x40. The carcinoma cells seen in this field have abundant cytoplasm and prominent nucleoli. Note the inflammatory cells in the background.

NIPPLE DISCHARGE IN DCIS

DCIS may present as a nipple discharge. These specimens are easy to prepare by placing a slide over the discharge from the nipple and wet-fixing or air-drying the material. Rarely, this may be the only means of identifying a DCIS when it shows no clinical or mammographic abnormality. The smears are usually cellular, often blood-stained, and contain, in addition to siderophages (**Fig. 9.166**), clusters of pleomorphic carcinoma cells (**Figs 9.167–9.169**). Inflammatory cells are not usually a feature of DCIS, but are common in Paget's disease.

CYTOLOGICAL GRADING OF BREAST CARCINOMA

Grading of carcinoma of the breast is traditionally performed on the surgically excised specimen using either Elston's modification of the Bloom and Richardson grading or a version of Black's nuclear grading system. In the present climate of neoadjuvant therapy, it is helpful for the clinician to know what the grade of the carcinoma is likely to be before starting therapy. Tamoxifen and chemotherapy are often used pre-operatively and treatment regimes could be refined if the grade of the tumour is known. It is also useful information in planning the type and extent of surgery and lymph node clearance.

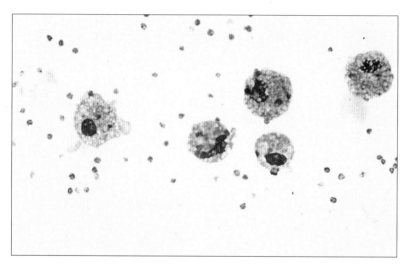

Fig. 9.166 DCIS, nipple discharge – Pap x40. The nipple discharge frequently contains siderophages, as illustrated. However, these are also seen with duct papillomas.

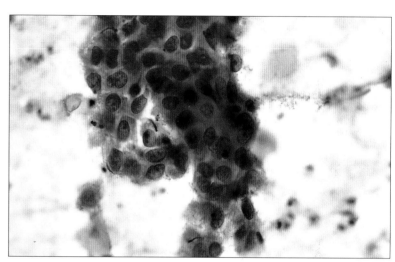

Fig. 9.167 DCIS, nipple discharge – Pap x40. This field shows a large cluster of loosely cohesive carcinoma cells with pleomorphic nuclei and visible nucleoli. These may appear similar to the carcinoma cells in Paget's disease, but the clinical appearance of the nipple is usually normal.

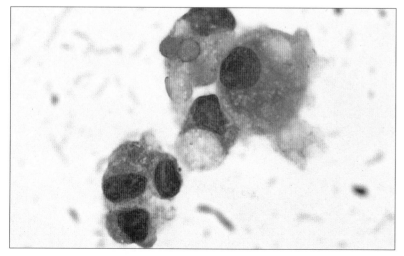

Fig. 9.168 DCIS, nipple discharge – MGG x100. These carcinoma cells contain vacuoles and have irregular nuclei. Note the ingested erythrocyte in one of the cells. This would not be seen in Paget's disease of the nipple, although the cells may be similar.

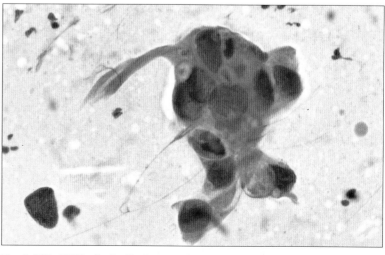

Fig. 9.169 DCIS, nipple discharge – Pap x63. This cluster of cells is not very well preserved, but displays pleomorphism, vacuolation, and ingested erythrocytes.

With these aims in mind we devised a new cytological grading system for breast carcinomas was devised in 1991 at the Royal County Hospital, Guildford, using cellular features that are assessed routinely when diagnosing fine needle aspirates. Six criteria were selected on the basis that they would provide a more refined system than if only three criteria were used. These are cell dissociation, nuclear size, cell uniformity, nucleolar characteristics, nuclear margin, and chromatin pattern (**Fig. 9.170**).

Wet-fixed material is necessary for grading, as many of the nuclear features assessed are too subtle to be graded on a smear stained with May Grunwald Giemsa. Tubule formation and mitoses are present in aspirates so infrequently that they are of no use in identifying grades of carcinoma. The three different total-score categories neatly divide carcinomas according to their cytology into grades which compare favourably with the subsequent histological grade of the surgically excised specimen.

This method of grading is simple to use and can be performed during routine reporting without any additional time being taken. It is essential that wet-fixed areas of the smear are assessed, as air-drying can produce errors in grading.

Cell dissociation

Low-grade tumours tend to retain their cohesive qualities (**Fig. 9.171**) and are awarded a score of 1. Most of the cells are in clusters (75% or more). Tumours which show an equal mixture of cell clusters and single cells are given a score of 2 (**Fig. 9.172**) and those which show dissociation of 75% or more of the cells a score of 3 (**Fig. 9.173**).

CRITERION	SCORE 1	SCORE 2	SCORE 3
Cell clusters	Mostly clusters	Single cells and clusters	Mostly single cells
Nuclear size	1–2 times size of an erythrocyte	3–4 times size of an erythrocyte	5 or >5 times size of an erythrocyte
Cell uniformity	Monomorphic	Mildly pleomorphic	Pleomorphic
Nucleoli	Indistinct/small	Noticeable	Abnormal
Nuclear margin	Smooth	Slightly irregular/folds or grooves	Buds and clefts
Chromatin pattern	Vesicular/reticular	Granular	Clumping and clearing

Score 6–11	Grade 1
Score 12–14	Grade 2
Score 15–18	Grade 3

Fig. 9.170 Protocol for cytological grading of breast carcinomas.

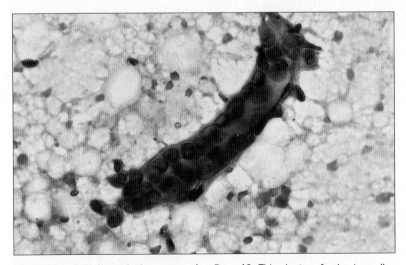

Fig. 9.171 Cell dissociation, score 1 – Pap x40. This cluster of cohesive cells represents most of the aspirate, which scores 1 for dissociation.

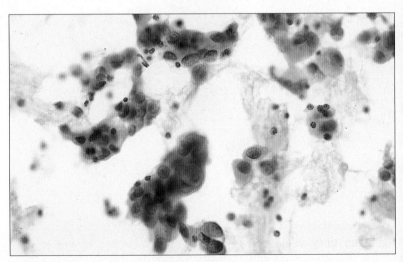

Fig. 9.172 Cell dissociation, score 2 – Pap x40. This field shows an equal mixture of single carcinoma cells and clusters, and therefore scores 2 for dissociation.

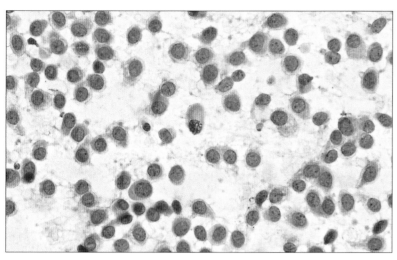

Nuclear size

The best method of assesssing nuclear size is by using a built-in unit of measurement, such as an erythrocyte. Most aspirates contain erythrocytes in varying numbers. The largest cells are assessed, a score of 1 being allocated to nuclei which are approximately the size of 1–2 erythrocytes (**Fig. 9.174**), a score of 2 to nuclei which are about the size of 3–4 erythrocytes (**Fig. 9.175**), and a score of 3 to nuclei which are 5 times the size of an erythrocyte, or more (**Fig. 9.176**).

Cell uniformity

Again, the most pleomorphic or worst cells are assessed. Aspirates with a monomorphic appearance score 1 (**Fig. 9.177**), those exhibiting mild pleomorphism score 2 (**Fig. 9.178**), and those that are pleomorphic score 3 (**Fig. 9.179**).

Fig. 9.173 Cell dissociation, score 3 – Pap x40. As all the cells in this field are single, the score for dissociation is 3.

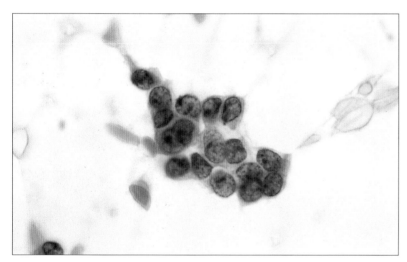

Fig. 9.174 Nuclear size, score 1 – Pap x100. The carcinoma cells in this field have nuclei which are approximately the size of the erythrocytes nearby, and therefore are allotted a score of 1.

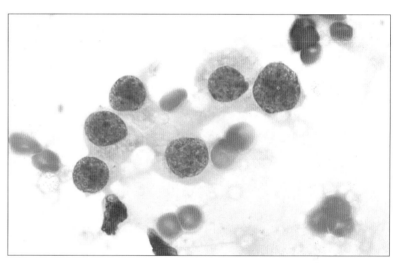

Fig. 9.175 Nuclear size, score 2 – Pap x100. These carcinoma cells have nuclei which are 3–4 times the size of the surrounding erythrocytes and therefore score 2 for nuclear size.

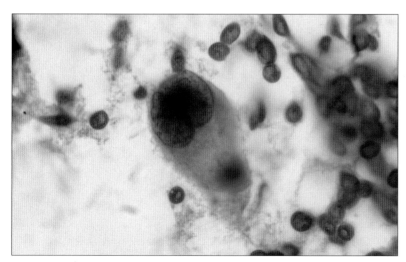

Fig. 9.176 Nuclear size, score 3 – Pap x100. The large cell in this field has a nucleus which is more than 5 times the size of the erythrocytes seen and so scores 3 for nuclear size.

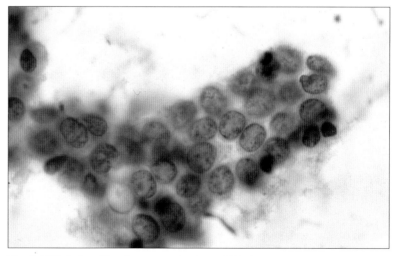

Fig. 9.177 Cell uniformity, score 1 – Pap x100. These small carcinoma cells are well-differentiated and monomorphic, scoring 1 for uniformity.

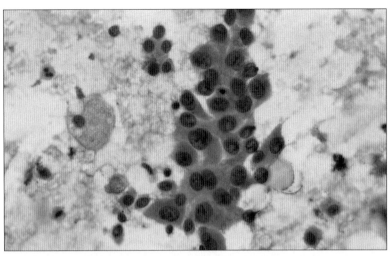

Fig. 9.178 Cell uniformity, score 2 – Pap x40. The cells in this field show moderate pleomorphism, warranting a score of 2 for uniformity.

Nucleoli

If nucleoli are not seen or are just visible a score of 1 is allocated (**Fig. 9.180**). Nucleoli that are prominent, but single, score 2 (**Fig. 9.181**) and those that are multiple or variable in size and shape score 3 (**Fig. 9.182**). The cells with the most abnormal nucleoli are graded when this criterion is used.

Nuclear margin

The worst cells are again assessed for accurate grading, in this case the ones with the most irregular margins. A score of 1 is given to nuclei which have smooth, round or oval margins (**Fig. 9.183**), 2 to nuclei which show some slight irregularities or depressions (**Fig. 9.184**), and a score of 3 to nuclei which exhibit deep clefts or protruding buds (**Fig. 9.185**).

Chromatin pattern

Once again the most abnormal cells should be assessed. Chromatin that resembles that of benign cells, i.e. is vesicular or bland, scores 1 (**Fig. 9.186**), a granular chromatin pattern scores 2 (**Fig. 9.187**), and irregular clumping and clearing of chromatin scores 3 (**Fig. 9.188**).

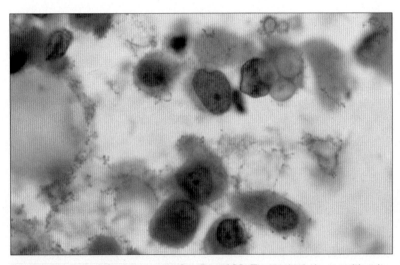

Fig. 9.179 Cell uniformity, score 3 – Pap x100. The marked pleomorphism in these cells warrants a score of 3 for uniformity.

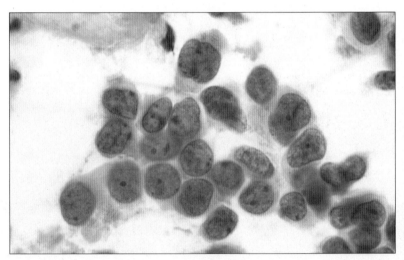

Fig. 9.180 Nucleoli, score 1 – Pap x100. These carcinoma cells have small blue nucleoli which are just visible, so score 1 for nucleoli.

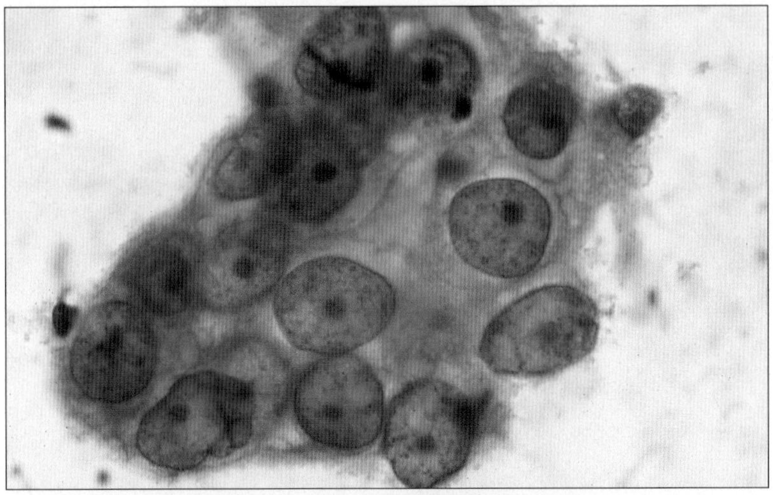

Fig. 9.181 Nucleoli, score 2 – Pap x100. In this field the carcinoma cells contain prominent red nucleoli, scoring 2 for nucleoli.

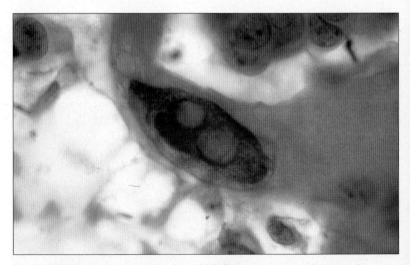

Fig. 9.182 Nucleoli, score 3 – Pap x100. This enormous malignant cell contains a large, red irregular nucleolus, thus scoring 3 for nucleoli.

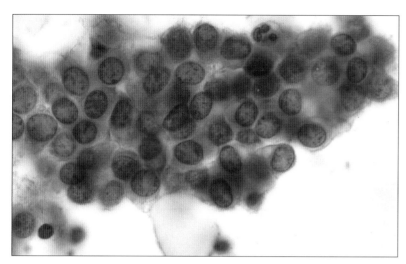

Fig. 9.183 Nuclear margin, score 1 – Pap x100. The cells in this field have smooth, round or oval nuclear margins, and so score 1 for nuclear margin.

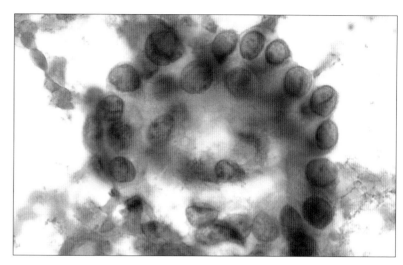

Fig. 9.184 Nuclear margin, score 2 – Pap x100. Note the grooves and slight indentations in some of the nuclei seen in this field. This scores 2 for nuclear margin.

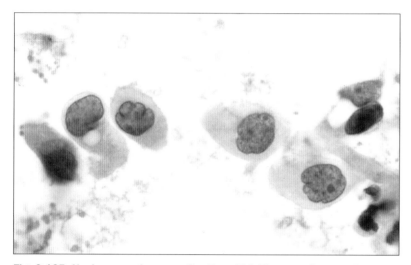

Fig. 9.185 Nuclear margin, score 3 – Pap x100. These carcinoma cells have definite budding of the nuclear margin, scoring 3.

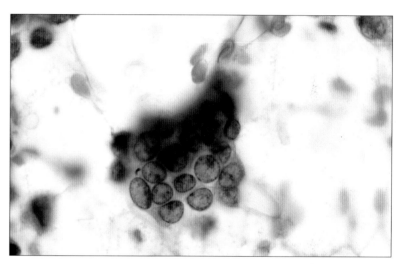

Fig. 9.186 Chromatin pattern, score 1 – Pap x100. These cells display vesicular chromatin, thus scoring 1 for chromatin pattern.

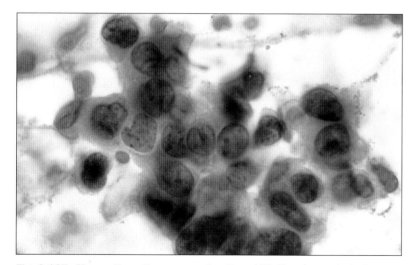

Fig. 9.187 Chromatin pattern, score 2 – Pap x100. The chromatin in these cells is granular, scoring 2 for chromatin pattern.

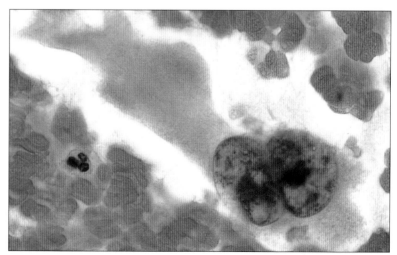

Fig. 9.188 Chromatin pattern, score 3 – Pap x100. This large malignant cell shows irregular clumping and clearing of chromatin, warranting a score of 3 for chromatin pattern.

Total score

A total score between 6 and 11 indicates a grade 1 carcinoma, that between 12 and 14 a grade 2, and that between 15 and 18 a grade 3 carcinoma. Although these grades correspond roughly to well, moderately, and poorly differentiated tumours as diagnosed by a cursory glance, it is a more refined process of grading which correlates well with histological grades. This protocol is easy to use and rapid to perform and provides much more information to the clinician than just a 'malignant cells present' diagnosis.

SUGGESTED READING

Bloom H, Richardson W. Histological grading and prognosis in breast cancer. *Br J Cancer* 1957; **11**: 359–377.

Domfield JM, Thompson SK, Shurbaji M. Radiation-induced changes in the breast: A potential pitfall on fine-needle aspiration. *Diagn Cytopathol* 1992; **8**: 79–81.

Kline T, Kannan V, Kline I. Appraisal and cytomorphological analysis of common carcinomas of the breast. *Diagn Cytopathol* 1985; **1**: 188–193.

Nguyen G-K, Redburn J. Aspiration biopsy cytology of papillary carcinoma of the breast. *Diagn Cytopathol* 1992; 511–516. **8**:

NHS. Breast Screening Programme Guidelines for Cytopathology Procedures and Reporting in Breast Cancer Screening. Sheffield: NHS; 1993: NHSBSP publication no. 22.

Orell S, Sterrett G, Walters M, Whittaker D. *Manual and Atlas of Fine Needle Aspiration Cytology.* Edinburgh: Churchill Livingstone; 1992: 63–93.

Robinson IA, McKee G, Jackson PA, et al. Lobular carcinoma of the breast: Cytological features supporting the diagnosis of lobular cancer. *Diagn Cytopathol* 1995; **13**: 196–201.

Robinson IA, McKee G, Kissin MW. Typing and grading breast carcinoma on fine-needle aspiration: Is this clinically useful information? *Diagn Cytopathol* 1995; **13**: 260–265.

Robinson I, McKee G, Nicholson A, *et al*. Prognostic value of fine-needle aspirates from breast carcinomas. *Lancet* 1994; **343**: 947–949.

Zajdela A, Chossein NA, Pillerton JP. The value of aspiration cytology in the diagnosis of breast cancer. *Cancer* 1975; **35**: 499–506.

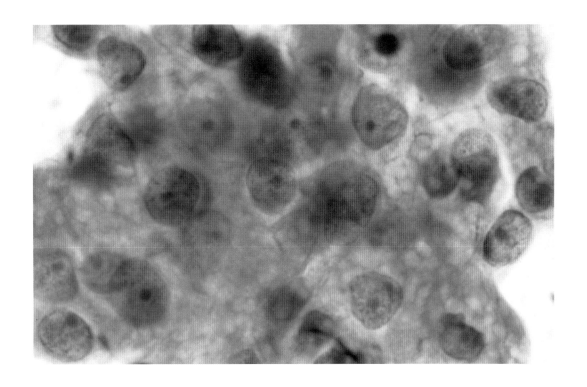

LYMPH NODES

10

LYMPH NODES

Fine needle aspiration cytology of lymph nodes is an extremely useful diagnostic procedure, not only in the detection of metastatic malignancy, but also in the diagnosis of inflammatory conditions and, with some caution, in the diagnosis of lymphomas.

Aspirates of lymph nodes are relatively easy to perform if the nodes are superficial and enlarged. Deep-seated nodes, such as the para-aortic and mediastinal nodes, are usually sampled by radiologists using ultrasound or computerized tomography. The technique is the same as for all fine needle aspirates, with both wet-fixed and air-dried smears being sent to the cytology laboratory together with the needle washings (see Chapter 6). The smears stained with Papanicolaou and May Grunwald Giemsa complement each other as they highlight different aspects of the same disease process, and the needle washings are useful for special stains or research purposes.

The normal lymph node is somewhat bean-shaped on cross-section, with a hilum in which the afferent and efferent lymphatics are situated and a thin capsule with a subcapsular sinus, which is the primary site of metastasis (Fig. 10.1). A histological section shows the normal structure, which consists of pale lymphoid follicles surrounded by a darker mantle zone of small lymphocytes (Fig. 10.2). A fine needle aspirate of a normal node shows a mixed population of

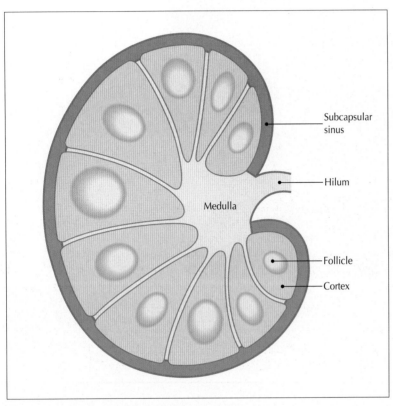

Fig. 10.1 Structure of normal lymph node.

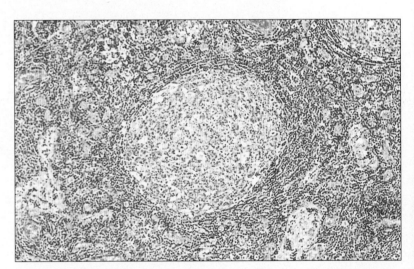

Fig. 10.2 Normal lymph node – H&E x10. This section of a normal lymph node shows rounded follicles composed of pale cells surrounded by a mantle of darker small lymphocytes. There are also some small blood vessels visible in this field.

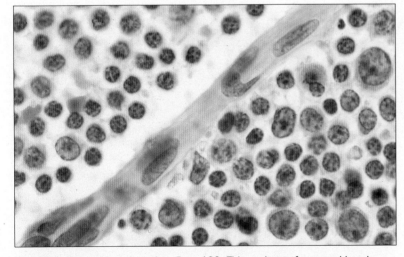

Fig. 10.3 Normal lymph node – Pap x100. This aspirate of a normal lymph node shows a mixture of lymphoid cells, mainly small lymphocytes with occasional centrocytes and centroblasts. Note also the small blood vessel crossing the field.

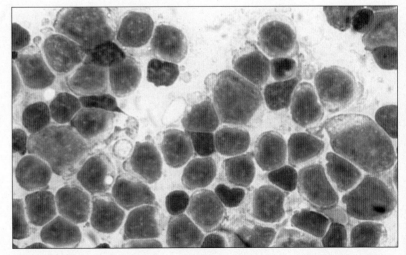

Fig. 10.4 Normal lymph node – MGG x100. This air-dried aspirate of a normal lymph node shows a mixture of small and larger lymphoid cells. Note the thin rim of cytoplasm around the cells.

lymphoid cells (**Figs 10.3, 10.4**). Follicle centre cells may appear quite alarming to the trainee cytopathologist, as the cells are large, irregular, and pleomorphic. They are of varying types: the **small centrocytes** or **small cleaved cells** are slightly larger than normal lymphocytes and are irregular in shape (**Figs 10.5, 10.6**). **Large centrocytes** or **cleaved cells** are larger than small centrocytes and also have irregular nuclear outlines (**Figs 10.7, 10.8**). **Centroblasts** are the size of large centrocytes and have more rounded nuclei that contain two or three nucleoli, some at the nuclear margin (**Figs 10.9, 10.10**). **Immunoblasts** are larger still and round with a thin rim of cytoplasm and a huge central nucleolus (**Figs 10.11, 10.12**). Histiocytic cells are also seen, including **tingible body macrophages**, which are histiocytes that have phagocytosed debris (**Figs 10.13, 10.14**) and are seen mainly in benign and reactive conditions. **Follicular dendritic cells** are difficult to recognize in aspirates (**Figs 10.15, 10.16**). The mantle zone around the lymphoid follicles contains small lymphocytes. **Plasma cells** may also be seen with their characteristic eccentric nuclei and pale 'hof' adjacent to the nucleus (**Figs 10.17, 10.18**).

Aspirates from **reactive nodes** are cellular and show a striking mixture of lymphoid cells, mainly follicle centre cells (**Fig. 10.19**). Tingible body macrophages are easily found. In conditions such as sinus histiocytosis numerous histiocytes may be seen in the aspirate (**Fig. 10.20**).

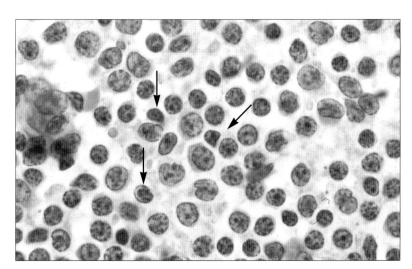

Fig. 10.5 Normal lymph node, small centrocytes – Pap x100. In this field there are small lymphocytes and small (arrowed) as well as large centrocytes with irregular, cleaved nuclei. The cytoplasm is very delicate and difficult to visualize with this stain.

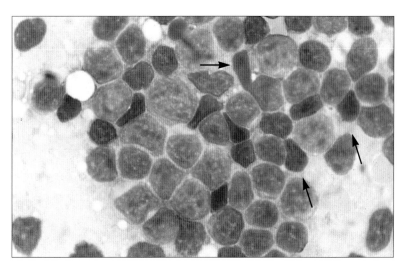

Fig. 10.6 Small centrocytes – MGG x100. The cells in this field are a mixture of small centrocytes with bent, irregular nuclei (arrowed) and larger paler centroblasts. (This aspirate is not from a normal lymph node, but from a lymphoma.)

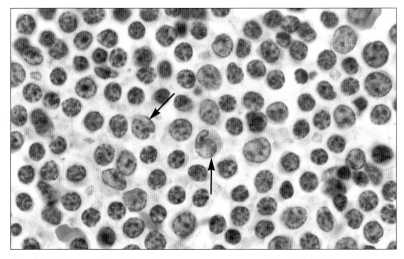

Fig. 10.7 Normal lymph node, large centrocytes – Pap x100. This aspirate shows larger centrocytes with cleaved nuclei in the centre of the field (arrowed), interspersed with small lymphocytes.

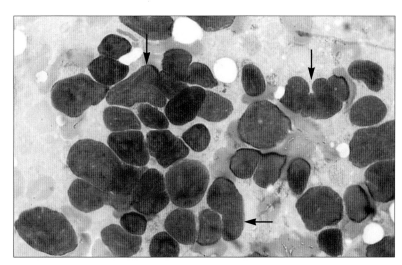

Fig. 10.8 Large centrocytes – MGG x100. The large cells (arrowed) with bent, irregular nuclei are large centrocytes. The more rounded large nuclei are those of centroblasts, while the small cells are small lymphocytes. (This aspirate is not from a normal lymph node, but from a lymphoma.)

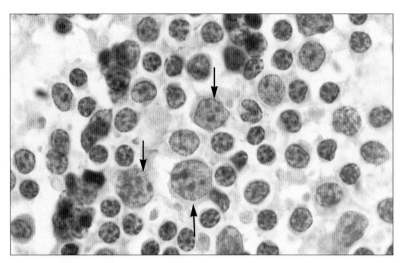

Fig. 10.9 Normal lymph node, centroblasts – Pap x100. In the centre of this field are several centroblasts with large nuclei and more than one nucleolus (arrowed). They are much larger than the small lymphocytes and small centrocytes which are also present.

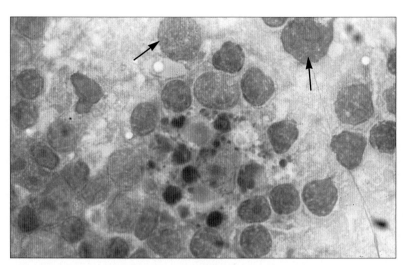

Fig. 10.10 Normal lymph node, centroblasts – MGG x100. The two larger cells (arrowed) at the top of field are centroblasts which are poorly preserved, so the nucleoli are not seen clearly. In the centre of the field is a tingible body macrophage.

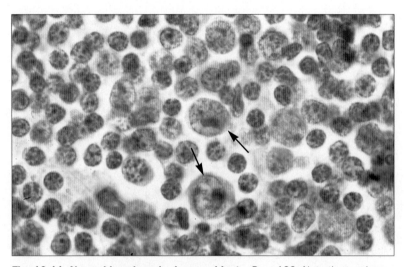

Fig. 10.11 Normal lymph node, immunoblast – Pap x100. Note the two large immunoblasts (arrowed), each with a big red central nucleolus in the centre of the field, surrounded by small lymphocytes, occasional small centrocytes, and centroblasts.

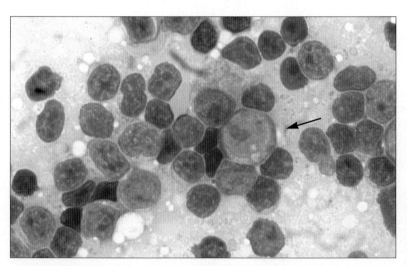

Fig. 10.12 Normal lymph node, immunoblast – MGG x100. In the centre of this field is a large cell with a big central nucleolus and a pale rim of cytoplasm; this is an immunoblast (arrowed).

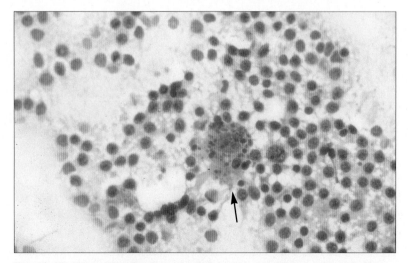

Fig. 10.13 Normal lymph node, tingible body macrophage – Pap x40. This field shows a large tingible body macrophage (arrowed) filled with debris and surrounded by small lymphoid cells. Although these histiocytes are commonly seen in benign conditions, they may also be noted occasionally in lymphomas.

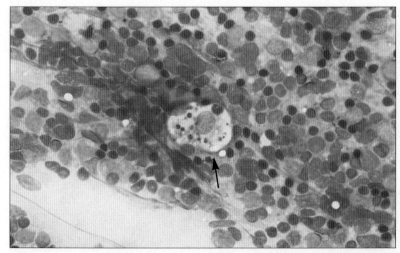

Fig. 10.14 Normal lymph node, tingible body macrophages – MGG x40. In this air-dried aspirate there is a mixture of small dark lymphocytes, larger paler lymphoid cells, and a large tingible body macrophage in the centre, containing intracytoplasmic debris (arrowed).

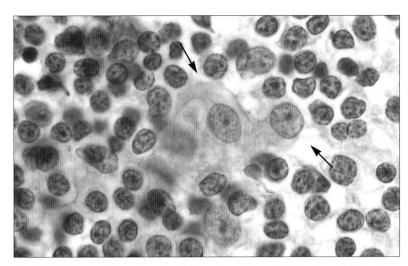

Fig. 10.15 Normal lymph node, histiocytes – Pap x100. The large histiocytic cells in the centre of the field, with abundant pale blue filmy cytoplasm, are probably follicular dendritic cells (arrowed). They are surrounded by a mixed population of lymphoid cells.

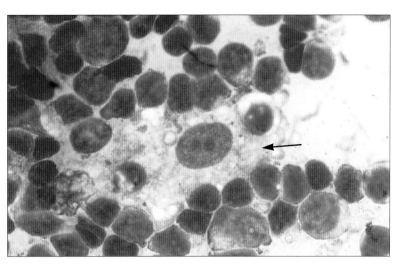

Fig. 10.16 Normal lymph node, histiocytes – MGG x100. In the centre of the field is a large histiocytic cell with abundant cytoplasm, which is probably a follicular dendritic cell (arrowed).

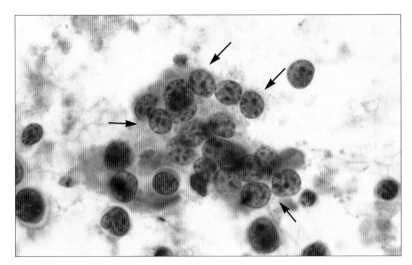

Fig. 10.17 Normal lymph node, plasma cell – Pap x100. This photomicrograph displays a group of plasma cells (arrowed) with eccentric nuclei and clock-face or cart-wheel chromatin pattern. The cytoplasm is very pale and not easily discernible.

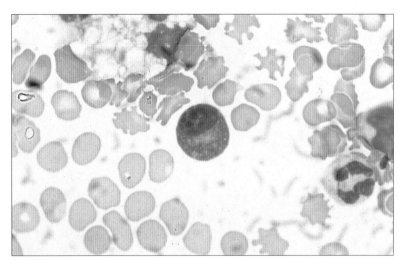

Fig. 10.18 Normal lymph node, plasma cell – MGG x100. The cell in the centre of the field shows the characteristic clock-face chromatin pattern and clear 'hof' of a plasma cell.

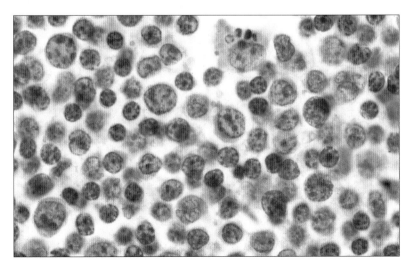

Fig. 10.19 Reactive lymph node – Pap x100. This field shows a mixture of lymphoid cells, including centroblasts, centrocytes, small lymphocytes, and a tingible body macrophage. The features overlap with those of a normal lymph node (see **Figures 10.5, 10.7**).

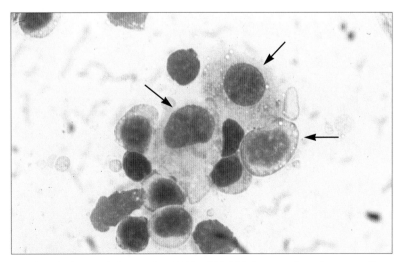

Fig. 10.20 Sinus histiocytosis – MGG x100. This is an aspirate from an axillary lymph node in a patient who had carcinoma of the breast. The node showed sinus histiocytosis on histology. The field seen here contains large histiocytic cells (arrowed) and a few small lymphocytes.

INFLAMMATORY CONDITIONS

Acute inflammatory processes, irrespective of the organisms involved, produce similar cytological features: a mixed population of lymphoid cells and acute inflammatory cells, mainly neutrophil polymorphs. Small amounts of necrotic cellular debris may also be visible. Bacteriological investigation is essential to identify and isolate the causative organism.

Granulomatous inflammatory processes are identifiable without difficulty from lymph node aspirates. Clusters of epithelioid histiocytes are seen, with their typical footprint- or carrot-shaped nuclei and delicate, often abundant, cytoplasm (**Figs 10.21, 10.22**). There are several causes of granulomatous inflammation, including sarcoid, toxoplasmosis, cat scratch disease, and tuberculosis; the incidence of the last is on the increase. The large areas of caseation necrosis characteristically seen in histological sections of a **tuberculous node (Fig. 10.23)** are represented by necrotic material on smears (**Figs 10.24, 10.25**).

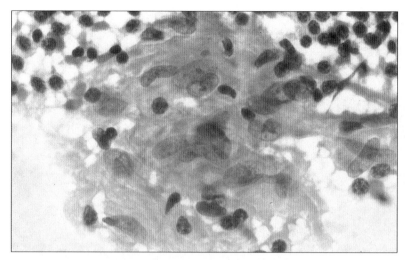

Fig. 10.21 Epithelioid histiocytes – Pap x40. Illustrated here are large histiocytic cells with elongated, footprint-shaped nuclei and abundant cytoplasm.

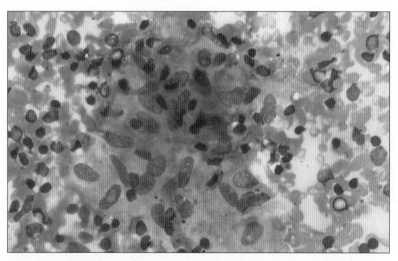

Fig. 10.22 Epithelioid histiocytes – MGG x40. The elongated nuclei of epithelioid histiocytes are well illustrated in this field. Note the abundant cytoplasm.

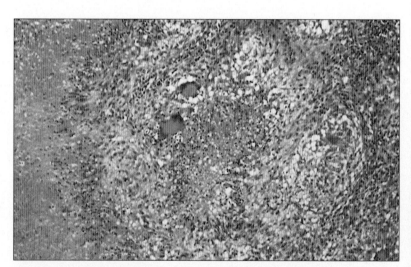

Fig. 10.23 Tuberculous node – H&E x4. This section shows areas of caseation necrosis surrounded by epithelioid histiocytes, granulomata, and Langhans'-type giant cells.

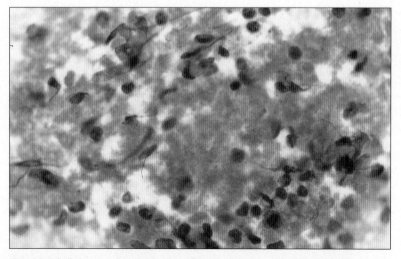

Fig. 10.24 Tuberculous node, caseation necrosis – Pap x40. This field displays necrotic material which stains pale blue to pale pink. Degenerate lymphocytes are also seen.

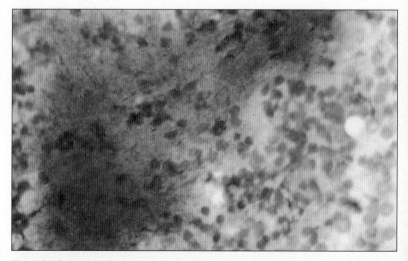

Fig. 10.25 Tuberculous node, caseation necrosis – MGG x40. In the air-dried smear caseation necrosis is represented by amorphous bright blue material. The lymphocytes surrounding the necrotic material are all degenerate.

Langhans' giant cells (**Fig. 10.26**) and granulomata are also recognizable (**Fig. 10.27**). Acid-fast bacilli may be demonstrable with a Ziehl–Neelsen stain (**Fig. 10.28**).

LYMPHOMA

The diagnosis of **lymphoma** is not always straightforward, even on histology. Cytology is beset with even more difficulties, except for high-grade lymphomas. Aspirates from follicular lymphomas resemble those from reactive lymph nodes. The most important feature in the cytological diagnosis of lymphoma is the monomorphic or monotonous population of lymphoid cells. A particular type of lymphoid cell usually predominates; this can be described in the report and a histological confirmation requested. For example, the aspirate may consist mostly of centrocytes (**Figs 10.29–10.31**).

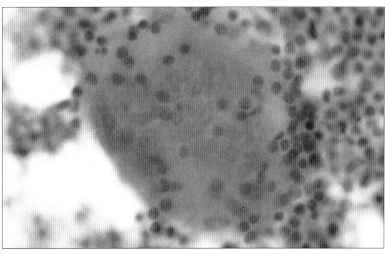

Fig. 10.26 Tuberculous node, Langhans'-type giant cell – Pap x63. This large multinucleated histiocytic cell differs from multinucleated foreign body histiocytes because its nuclei are arranged peripherally. Although these cells are characteristic of tuberculosis, they may also be seen in other granulomatous conditions, such as granulomatous mastitis.

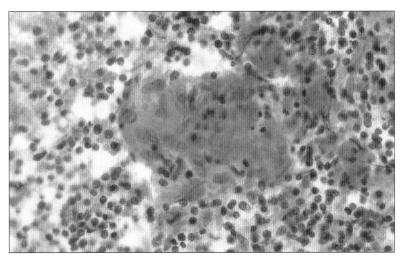

Fig. 10.27 Tuberculous node, granuloma – Pap x40. In the centre of this field is a large, ill-defined granuloma composed of epithelioid histiocytes. Small lymphocytes and some necrotic material are seen in the background.

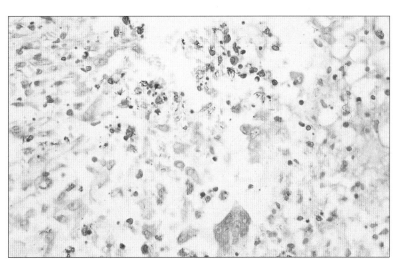

Fig. 10.28 Tuberculous lymph node – Ziehl–Neelsen stain x100. Illustrated are numerous, small, rod-shaped, bright pink tubercle bacilli. Their curved, beaded appearance is best demonstrated under oil immersion.

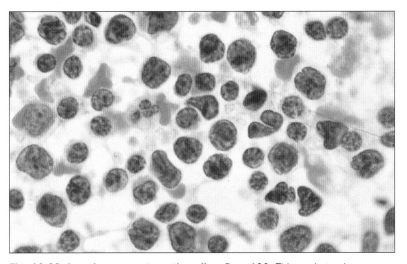

Fig. 10.29 Lymphoma, centrocytic cells – Pap x100. This aspirate shows a monomorphic picture, composed predominantly of centrocytes.

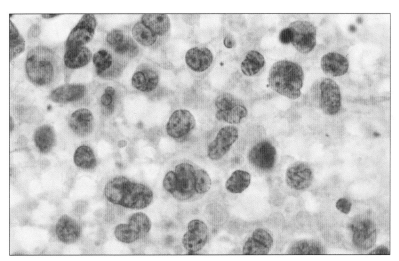

Fig. 10.30 Lymphoma, centrocytic cells – Pap x100. Illustrated is an aspirate composed of centrocytes from a lymphoma. This cell uniformity is the opposite of the mixed picture seen in aspirates from reactive nodes.

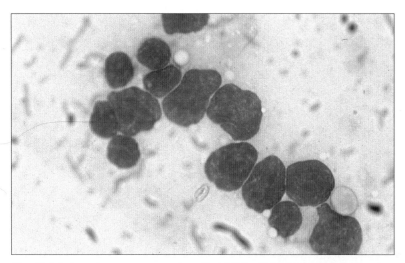

Fig. 10.31 Lymphoma, centrocytic cells – MGG x100. This air-dried smear is from a centrocytic lymphoma. The convoluted nuclear outlines are not as obvious as in the wet-fixed smear (see **Figure 10.30**).

In centroblastic–centrocytic lymphomas a mixture of centrocytes and centroblasts is apparent (**Figs 10.32, 10.33**). Aspirates from immunoblastic lymphomas show a predominance of immunoblasts (**Fig. 10.34**), others may show plasmacytoid features (**Fig. 10.35**), and yet others, such as T cell lymphomas, are composed mainly of convoluted lymphoid cells (**Fig. 10.36**). Aspirates from lymphomas often show smear artefact due to the destruction of delicate nuclear membranes when the smear is made (**Fig. 10.37**). The cells are disrup-ted and the chromatin pulled out in strands, often making identification of the cells impossible. However, this feature is also seen in small-cell anaplastic carcino-

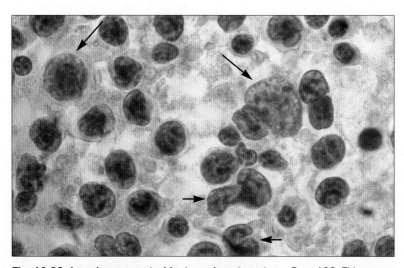

Fig. 10.32 Lymphoma, centroblasts and centrocytes – Pap x100. This aspirate from a centroblastic–centrocytic lymphoma clearly displays both these types of cells (centroblasts long arrows, centrocytes short arrows).

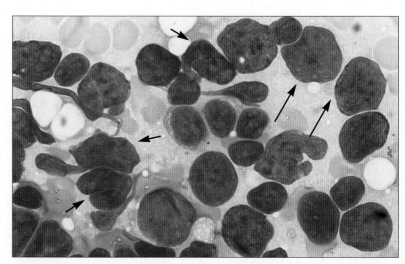

Fig. 10.33 Lymphoma, centroblasts and centrocytes – MGG x40. In this field there are two types of cells, centroblasts (long arrows) and centrocytes (short arrows).

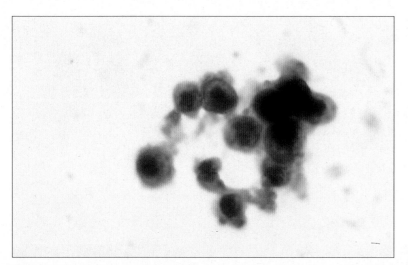

Fig. 10.34 Lymphoma, immunoblasts – Pap x100. This aspirate is composed predominantly of immunoblasts.

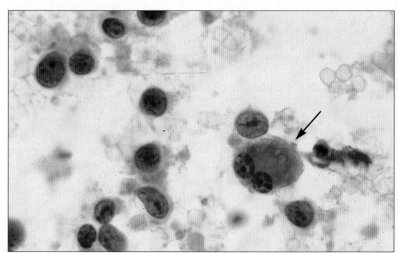

Fig. 10.35 Lymphoma, plasmacytoid features – Pap x100. Some aspirates from predominantly small-celled lymphomas contain cells with plasmacytoid features, such as the binucleate cell with clock-face chromatin (arrowed).

mas. Many lymphomas cannot be classified, except as low or high grade, on the cytological appearances alone – the high-grade tumours are very pleomorphic and display numerous mitotic figures (**Figs 10.38, 10.39**), and a histological examination should always be recommended when lymphoma is suspected or diagnosed on an aspirate.

Hodgkin's lymphoma cannot be diagnosed without the presence of Reed–Sternberg cells (**Figs 10.40, 10.41**) or Hodgkin's cells (**Figs 10.42, 10.43**) in the aspirate. Eosinophils are not difficult to find (**Figs 10.44, 10.45**). It is not possible to diagnose the type of Hodgkin's disease from cytological material.

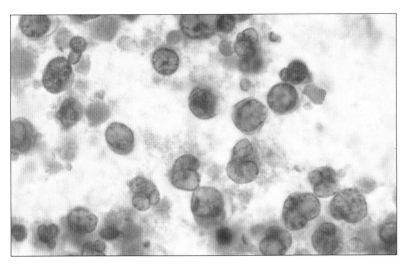

Fig. 10.36 Lymphoma, convoluted cells – Pap x100. This field contains markedly convoluted lymphoid cells with nuclear buds and protrusions. This was reported as being suggestive of a high-grade lymphoma. The biopsy specimen showed a T cell lymphoma.

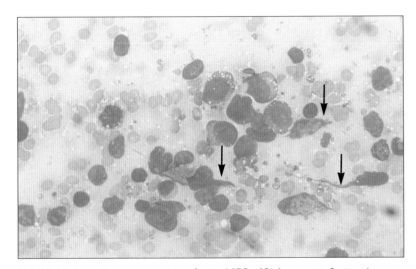

Fig. 10.37 Lymphoma, smear artefact – MGG x40. A common feature in aspirates from lymphomas is streak artefact caused by destruction of the delicate neoplastic cells during smearing. Note the pulled-out chromatin in some of the nuclei (arrowed).

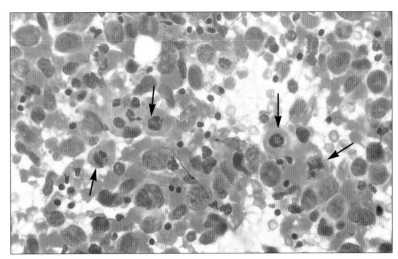

Fig. 10.38 Lymphoma, high grade – Pap x40. This high-grade tumour is composed of very large lymphoid cells with a few scattered normal lymphocytes which are much smaller. Many mitoses are present in this field (arrowed).

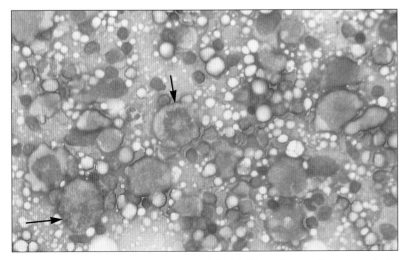

Fig. 10.39 Lymphoma, high grade – MGG x40. The rather poorly-preserved, air-dried smear from the same case as shown in **Figure 10.38** shows mitoses (arrowed) as well as pleomorphic neoplastic cells.

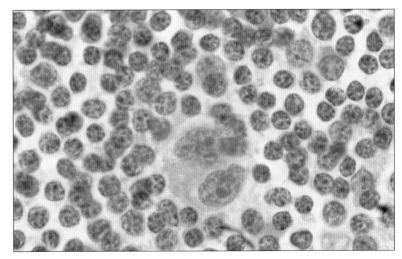

Fig. 10.40 Hodgkin's disease – Pap x100. In the centre of this field is a binucleate Reed–Sternberg cell with huge red nucleoli; there are small lymphocytes in the background. Eosinophils are not in evidence.

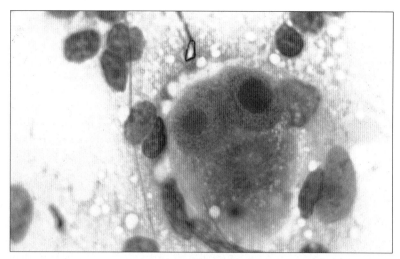

Fig. 10.41 Hodgkin's disease – MGG x100. This air-dried aspirate from a case of Hodgkin's disease shows large nucleoli and binucleation in a Reed–Sternberg cell, although the preservation of the sample is not perfect.

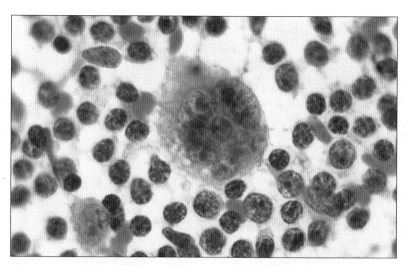

Fig. 10.42 Hodgkin's disease – Pap x100. In this aspirate from a lymph node affected by Hodgkin's disease, no typical Reed–Sternberg cells were found. However, there were numerous large multi- or poly-lobated Hodgkin's cells, such as the one illustrated here in the centre of the field. Note the large red nucleoli, and the mixed population of lymphoid cells in the background.

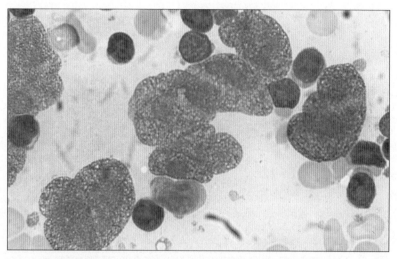

Fig. 10.43 Hodgkin's disease – MGG x100. Many Hodgkin's cells are illustrated here, with enormous nucleoli. The granularity of the chromatin is due to poor preservation rather than being a feature of the cells.

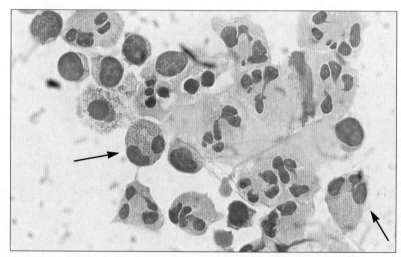

Fig. 10.44 Eosinophils – Pap x100. Eosinophils are bilobed with orange cytoplasmic granules (arrowed). Small lymphocytes and neutrophils are also present in this field. (This photomicrograph is not of an aspirate from Hodgkin's disease.)

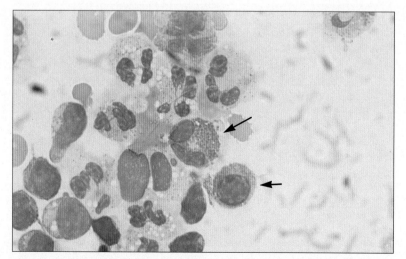

Fig. 10.45 Eosinophils – MGG x100. Eosinophils in air-dried preparations contain pink-staining cytoplasmic granules (long arrow). Note the plasma cell (short arrow) adjacent to the eosinophil in the centre of the field.

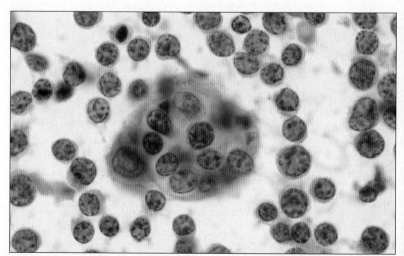

Fig. 10.46 Aggregates of lymphocytes – Pap x40. The small lymphocytes in this aspirate from a plasmacytoid lymphoma are aggregated together in the centre of the field, resembling a cluster of epithelial cells and so may be mistaken for metastatic carcinoma.

METASTATIC TUMOURS

Metastatic tumours in lymph nodes are easily identified in most cases. Care must be taken in interpreting aspirates where the spreading of the material has caused aggregation of lymphocytes and histiocytes, mimicking epithelial cells (**Figs 10.46, 10.47**). Benign epithelial rests also occur in nodes and should not be mistaken for metastatic deposits. Metastatic adenocarcinoma cells are seen in clusters, often resembling the primary tumour. **Lobular carcinoma** of the breast produces metastases composed of small cells containing intracytoplasmic lumina (**Figs 10.48, 10.49**). **Ductal carcinoma** metastases usually show similar pleomorphism to that of the original tumour – low or high grade (**Figs 10.50, 10.51**). Immunocytochemical stains can be used to confirm the nature of the cells in difficult cases (**Fig. 10. 52**). It is possible to state whether a tumour is high grade from its cytological appearance, even if the site of origin is unknown (**Fig. 10.53**). Metastatic deposits from **papillary carcinoma of the thyroid** look

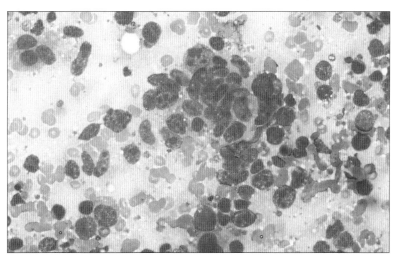

Fig. 10.47 Aggregates of lymphocytes – MGG x40. In this field the cells in the centre appear to be forming a cohesive cluster, almost simulating small-cell anaplastic carcinoma. However, careful examination shows that they are all lymphoid, identical to the single cells in the aspirate. This is an aspirate from a lymphoma, not from a metastatic neoplasm.

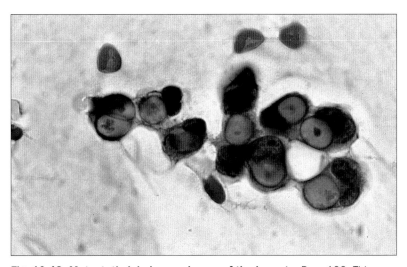

Fig. 10.48 Metastatic lobular carcinoma of the breast – Pap x100. This aspirate contains a group of very small epithelial cells with small pleomorphic, hyperchromatic nuclei, which are indented by round vacuoles containing a speck of mucin. The nuclei are about the size of erythrocytes. These are characteristic features of lobular carcinoma of the breast, seen in a metastatic deposit in the axillary lymph node.

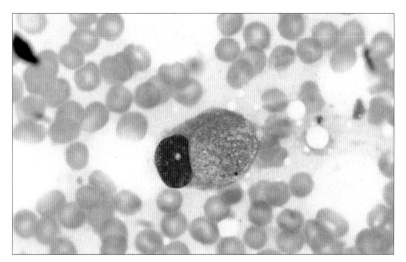

Fig. 10.49 Metastatic lobular carcinoma of the breast – MGG x100. This field shows a single carcinoma cell with a hyperchromatic nucleus slightly indented by a large intracytoplasmic vacuole. Air-drying renders the nucleus much larger than the erythrocytes; therefore, air-dried smears should not be used to estimate cell or nuclear size.

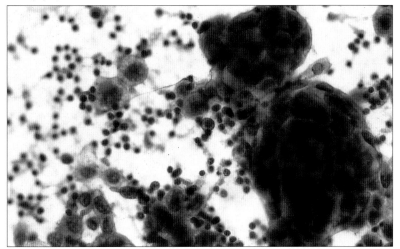

Fig. 10.50 Metastatic ductal carcinoma of the breast – Pap x40. In this field there are several clusters of adenocarcinoma cells, as well as single cells, surrounded by small lymphocytes. This aspirate is from an axillary node in a woman with carcinoma of the breast.

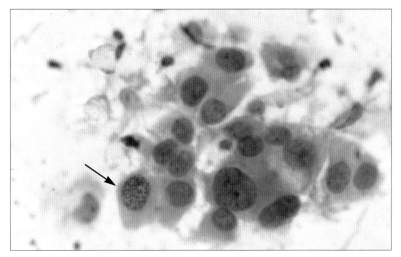

Fig. 10.51 Metastatic ductal carcinoma of the breast – Pap x63. The carcinoma cells in this aspirate are high grade, loosely cohesive, show marked variation in nuclear size and shape, and are much larger than the lymphocytes in the background. Note the mitotic figure (arrowed).

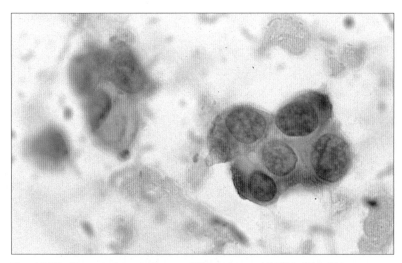

Fig. 10.52 Metastatic carcinoma of the breast – HMFG2 x100. This immunocytochemical stain shows positivity, confirming that there are metastatic adenocarcinoma cells in the aspirate. This is a very useful procedure when the epithelial cells are not clearly visible on the smears and when needle washings are available for special stains.

exactly like the original tumour, with psammoma bodies **(Fig. 10.54)** and intranuclear inclusions **(Fig. 10.55)**; in fact, these may be the first indication of a neoplasm in the thyroid. Similarly, metastatic adenocarcinoma in an axillary lymph node may be the first symptom of breast carcinoma.

Squamous carcinoma often metastasizes to local nodes. Metastatic tumour cells in the neck nodes may have spread from a primary neoplasm in the head, neck, or lung. Uncommonly, a urothelial tumour with squamous differentiation spreads to the para-aortic lymph nodes, then up into the neck, where the enlarged node is the first symptom of disease and may show only squamous carcinoma cells in the aspirate. Squamous metastases are often keratinized **(Figs 10.56, 10.57)**, the cells may be in whorls or nests **(Fig. 10.58)**, or they may be poorly differentiated (see below). They are often accompanied by necrotic cellular debris **(Figs 10.59, 10.60)**. Histiocytes are commonly seen, many with ingested keratin **(Fig. 10.61)**. Extracellular keratin is sometimes seen in the background. In some cases the necrosis produces a cystic feel to the node and the aspirate has the appearance of pus, with the smears containing numerous neutrophils **(Fig. 10.62)**.

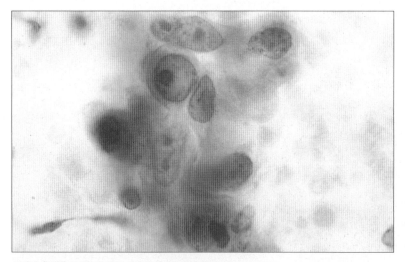

Fig. 10.53 Metastatic adenocarcinoma – Pap x100. It is not possible to be dogmatic about the primary site of metastatic adenocarcinoma from cytological material. This field shows pleomorphic adenocarcinoma cells with huge, irregular red nucleoli and an abnormal chromatin pattern, suggesting a high-grade adenocarcinoma.

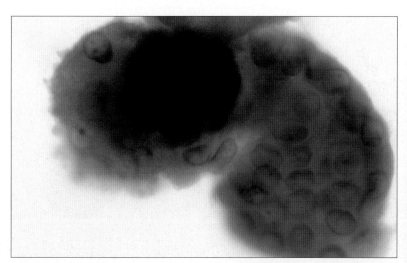

Fig. 10.54 Metastatic papillary carcinoma of the thyroid – Pap x100. This field shows a laminated psammoma body and a cluster of adenocarcinoma cells in an aspirate from a cervical node in a patient with no clinical thyroid lesion. A small papillary carcinoma was eventually detected in the thyroid.

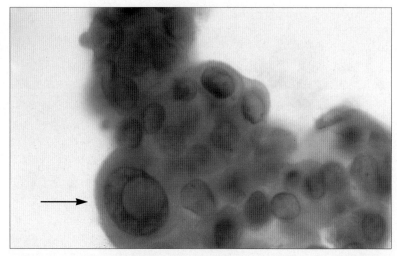

Fig. 10.55 Metastatic papillary carcinoma of the thyroid – Pap x100. This group of adenocarcinoma cells from the same case as shown in **Figure 10.54** shows adenocarcinoma cells with variably sized nuclei, the largest of which contains an intranuclear inclusion (arrowed), characteristic of papillary carcinoma of the thyroid (but also seen in melanomas and some ductal carcinomas of breast).

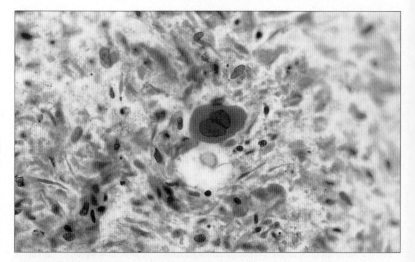

Fig. 10.56 Metastatic squamous carcinoma – Pap x40. This field shows a keratinized binucleate squamous carcinoma cell surrounded by necrotic cellular debris and some spindle-shaped neoplastic cells.

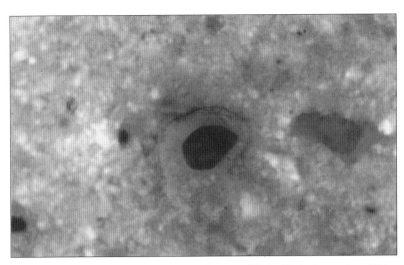

Fig. 10.57 Metastatic squamous carcinoma – MGG x40. In the centre of this field is a large keratinized squamous carcinoma cell with azure blue cytoplasm. Note the necrotic debris in the background.

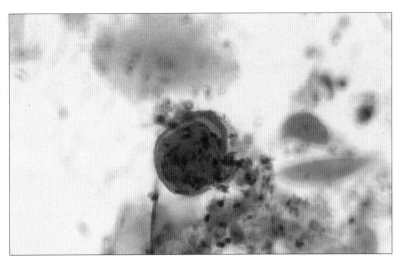

Fig. 10.58 Metastatic squamous carcinoma – Pap x40. The squamous pearl or whorl illustrated here is characteristic of well-differentiated squamous neoplasms. The cells in the pearl appear to be degenerate, with pyknotic nuclei.

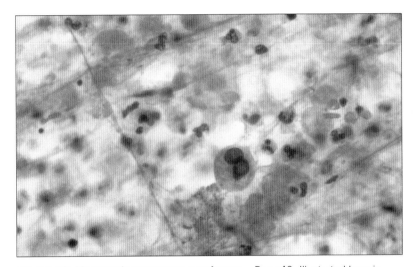

Fig. 10.59 Metastatic squamous carcinoma – Pap x40. Illustrated here is necrotic cellular debris, which is often a feature of squamous carcinoma, both primary and metastatic. There are also a few neutrophils in the background and a binucleate neoplastic cell in the centre of the field.

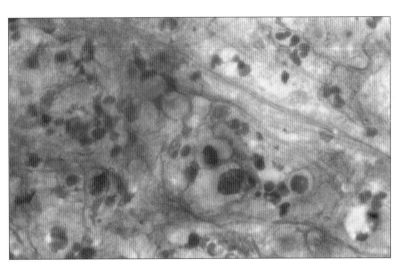

Fig. 10.60 Metastatic squamous carcinoma – MGG x40. In the air-dried smear from the same case as shown in **Figure 10.59** the cellular necrotic debris stains purple. Note the neutrophils and small carcinoma cells in the centre of the field.

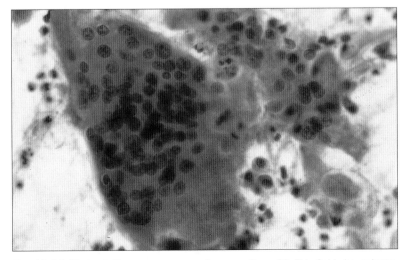

Fig. 10.61 Metastatic squamous carcinoma – Pap x40. This field shows large multinucleated histiocytes which contain phagocytosed keratin, seen as orange material within the pink cytoplasm of the histiocytes.

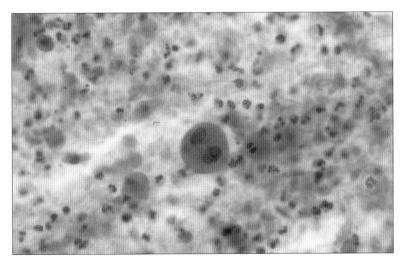

Fig. 10.62 Metastatic squamous carcinoma – Pap x40. This aspirate looked like pus macroscopically, but the smear shows keratinized squamous carcinoma cells as well as polymorphs and necrotic debris. Clinicians should be made aware of this type of gross appearance of aspirates from lymph nodes involved in metastatic squamous carcinoma.

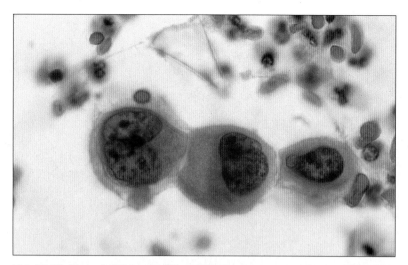

Fig. 10.63 Metastatic poorly differentiated squamous carcinoma – Pap x100. This field displays lymphocytes and erythrocytes, as well as a large carcinoma cell with red nucleoli. No keratinization is seen in this field. The patient had squamous carcinoma of the larynx with lymph node metastases.

The specimen may be sent for bacteriological examination alone if the clinician is not aware that metastatic squamous carcinomas often show this type of appearance. Poorly differentiated squamous carcinomas do not show keratinization. The cells are large with moderate amounts of cytoplasm and often contain prominent nucleoli (**Figs 10.63, 10.64**) – a feature not as commonly seen with well-differentiated squamous carcinoma.

Urothelial carcinoma also metastasizes to lymph nodes, the cells usually being present in clusters with moderate amounts of cytoplasm and abnormal nuclei (**Figs 10.65, 10.66**). They can be quite difficult to distinguish from metastatic poorly differentiated squamous carcinoma. **Renal cell carcinoma** metastases typically have relatively small nuclei and abundant foamy cytoplasm. Nucleoli are frequently prominent (**Figs 10.67, 10.68**).

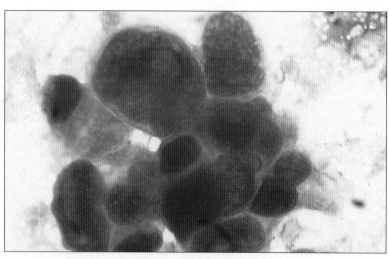

Fig. 10.64 Metastatic poorly differentiated squamous carcinoma – MGG x100. This air-dried smear contains large undifferentiated squamous carcinoma cells and a few lymphocytes.

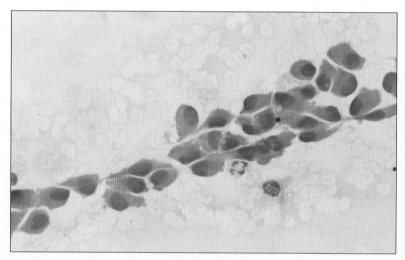

Fig. 10.65 Metastatic urothelial carcinoma – Pap x40. This is an aspirate from a para-aortic lymph node in a patient with a carcinoma of the bladder. The cells contain moderate amounts of fairly dense cytoplasm and large rounded nuclei. The differential diagnosis would be squamous carcinoma.

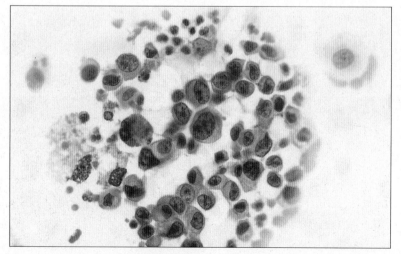

Fig. 10.66 Metastatic urothelial carcinoma – Pap x40. In this aspirate the urothelial cells are much more pleomorphic than those in **Figure 10.65**, with abnormal clumped and cleared chromatin. The bladder tumour in this case was an aggressive urothelial carcinoma.

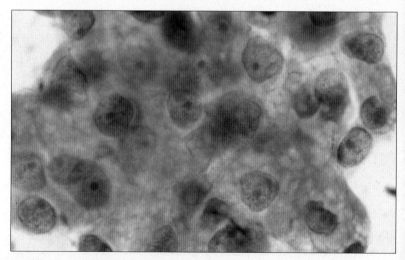

Fig. 10.67 Metastatic renal cell carcinoma – Pap x100. The cluster of adenocarcinoma cells illustrated here shows vacuolated cytoplasm, round nuclei, and prominent nucleoli, typical of renal cell carcinoma.

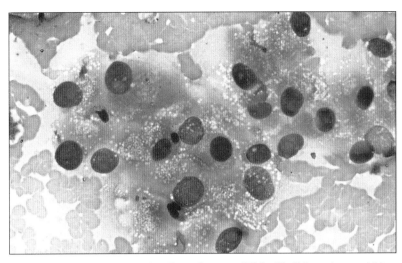

Fig. 10.68 Metastatic renal cell carcinoma – MGG x40. This aspirate exhibits the characteristics of renal cell carcinoma in the form of relatively small rounded nuclei, prominent nucleoli, and abundant vacuolated cytoplasm.

Metastatic **malignant melanoma** has a variable appearance. Melanin is not always seen in the aspirate, but it is very helpful when present **(Figs 10.69, 10.70)**. It appears as large, yellowish brown intracytoplasmic granules in the wet-fixed smear and as bluish black granules on the air-dried slide. Occasionally, only the histiocytes in the aspirate contain melanin and the tumour cells appear to have none. Characteristically, melanoma cells are large, usually single, with moderate amounts of cytoplasm and large nuclei with prominent nucleoli **(Figs 10.71, 10.72)**. Intranuclear inclusions (intranuclear cytoplasmic invaginations) are common **(Figs 10.73, 10.74)**. Binucleation is another feature frequently noted **(Figs 10.75, 10.76)**, as is multinucleation **(Fig. 10.77)**. The neoplastic cells are sometimes small, with ovoid nuclei, vesicular chromatin, and little cytoplasm **(Fig. 10.78)**. Nucleoli and intranuclear inclusions may be sparse in these aspi-

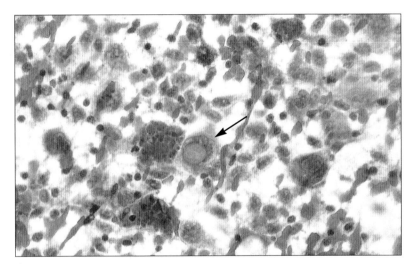

Fig. 10.69 Metastatic melanoma, pigment – Pap x40. In this field there are several cells which contain large granules of yellowish brown melanin pigment. In the centre of the field there is a neoplastic cell which displays a huge intranuclear inclusion (arrowed).

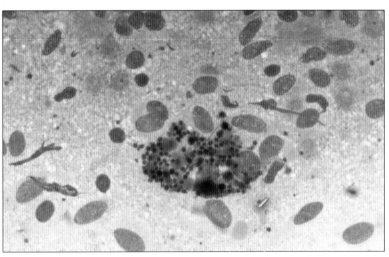

Fig. 10.70 Metastatic melanoma, pigment – MGG x40. The cell in the centre of this illustration contains large bluish black granules of melanin pigment, and is possibly a macrophage. The cells in the background are neoplastic melanoma cells.

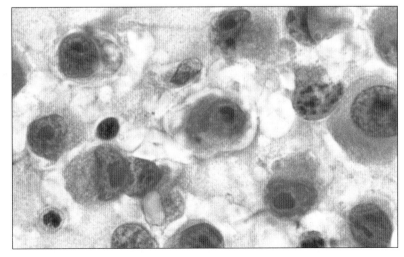

Fig. 10.71 Metastatic melanoma, nucleoli – Pap x100. This aspirate, from a groin node in a patient whose melanoma had been excised several months before, contains large cells with huge, irregular red nucleoli. The cytoplasm is not clearly visualized and no pigment is visible.

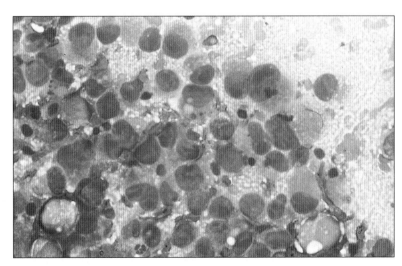

Fig. 10.72 Metastatic melanoma, nucleoli – MGG x40. This air-dried aspirate from a metastatic melanoma contains large, single neoplastic cells with abnormally shaped nucleoli. The lymphocytes in the background are an indicator of how large the melanoma cells are.

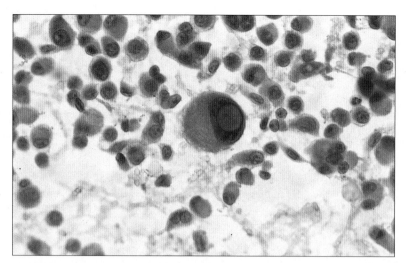

Fig. 10.73 Metastatic melanoma, intranuclear inclusions – Pap x40. In this field there are numerous small melanoma cells and a single huge cell with a large intranuclear inclusion.

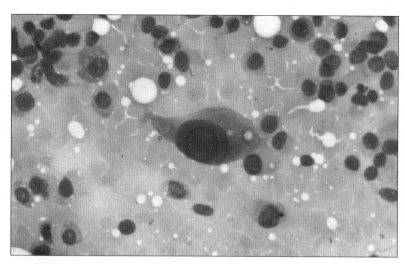

Fig. 10.74 Metastatic melanoma, intranuclear inclusion – MGG x40. This photomicrograph shows single small melanoma cells with a very large cell containing an enormous intranuclear inclusion.

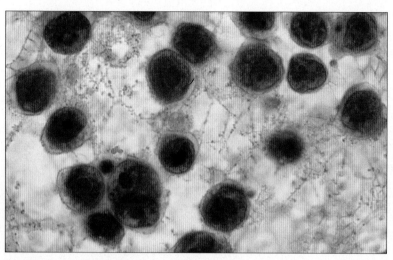

Fig. 10.75 Metastatic melanoma, binucleation – Pap x100. There is one binucleate cell in this field; all the rest have only one nucleus. Note the enormous red nucleoli. The amount of cytoplasm in the cells is variable.

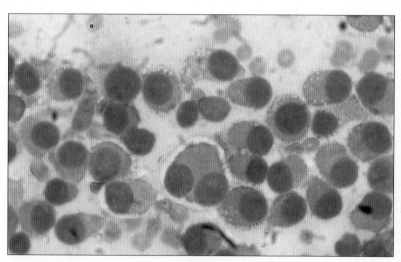

Fig. 10.76 Metastatic melanoma, binucleation – MGG x40. In the centre of this field is a binucleate cell; the others all have a single nucleus. No pigment is seen.

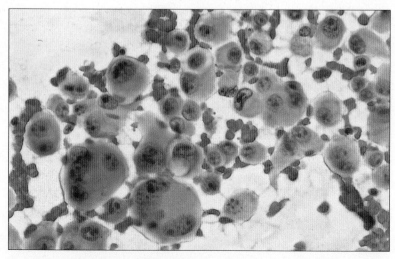

Fig. 10.77 Metastatic melanoma, multinucleation – Pap x40. Multinucleation is another common feature in aspirates from melanomas, as illustrated here. Note the prominent red nucleoli in all the cells.

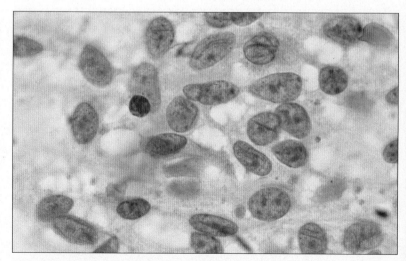

Fig. 10.78 Metastatic melanoma – Pap x100. This aspirate from a metastatic melanoma is composed of cells with ovoid nuclei and vesicular chromatin, with some of the nuclei exhibiting grooves. The nucleoli are small and red, and the cytoplasm is ill-defined. A few granules of yellowish brown extracellular pigment are visible. The cells are small when compared to the erythrocytes in the aspirate.

rates, but if no pigment can be found immunocytochemical staining for S100 will confirm the diagnosis (**Fig. 10.79**). The spindle-cell variety of malignant melanoma contains cells which are ovoid-to-spindle in shape and often, though not always, exhibit some of the features mentioned above (**Fig. 10.80**). The cells are usually not as extremely spindled as are sarcoma cells, although there are exceptions, and tissue fragments are not seen, unlike in an aspirate from a sarcoma. Immunocytochemical stains would help with the diagnosis in such cases. Melanomas may be composed of cells with a plasmacytoid appearance due to their eccentric nuclei (**Fig. 10.81**).

Small-cell anaplastic carcinomas (oat cell type) metastasize commonly to lymph nodes, but can be missed on an aspirate as the cells are about the same size as or slightly larger than lymphocytes (**Figs 10.82, 10.83**). The cytoplasm is barely discernible, the nuclei show moulding, and the chromatin has a speckled, 'salt and pepper' appearance (**Fig. 10.84**). The cells are in clusters, unlike lymphoid cells, and are slightly paler than lymphocytes. Streaks of tumour cells may be seen in metastases (**Fig. 10.85**), just as in sputum preparations.

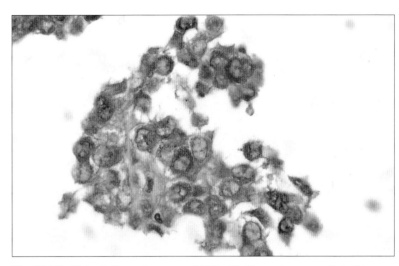

Fig. 10.79 Metastatic melanoma – S100 x40. The melanoma cells in this aspirate show strong positive staining with S100 markers.

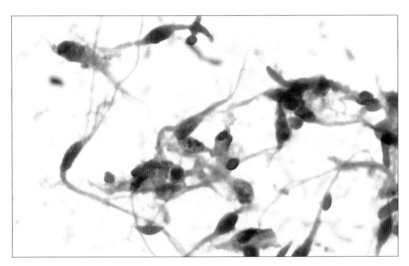

Fig. 10.80 Metastatic melanoma, spindle cells – Pap x63. The spindle cells seen in this illustration bear none of the usual features of melanoma. The history of a previous melanoma and a review of the original histology, which showed a spindle-cell melanoma, were essential for the diagnosis. Immunocytochemical stains are useful in such cases (see **Figure 10.79**).

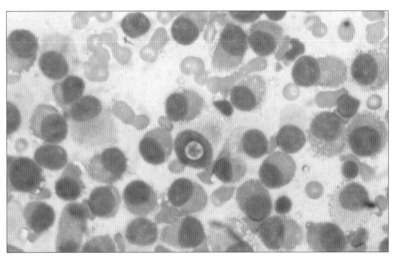

Fig. 10.81 Metastatic melanoma, plasmacytoid appearance – MGG x40. Occasionally melanoma cells display eccentric rounded nuclei, which give them a plasmacytoid appearance. The cells here also have prominent nucleoli.

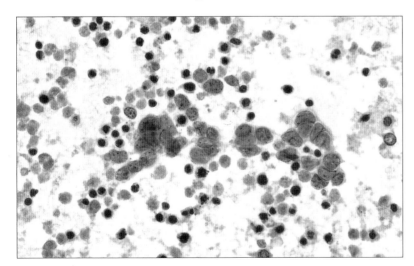

Fig. 10.82 Metastatic oat cell carcinoma – Pap x40. The small-cell anaplastic carcinoma cells in this field are larger than the surrounding lymphocytes and have paler nuclei, with some evidence of moulding.

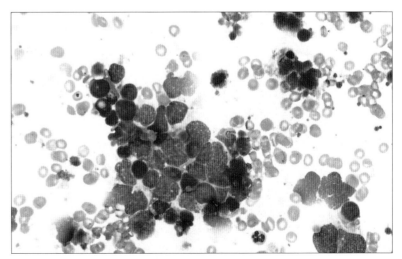

Fig. 10.83 Metastatic oat cell carcinoma – MGG x40. The neoplastic oat cells in this aspirate are much larger than the lymphocytes because of air-drying. They are paler than the lymphocytes and exhibit moulding.

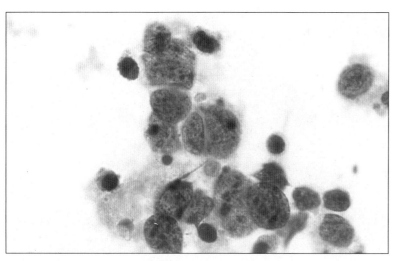

Fig. 10.84 Metastatic oat cell carcinoma – Pap x100. This field illustrates the moulding of nuclei which is characteristic of small-cell anaplastic carcinoma, along with speckled chromatin and imperceptible cytoplasm.

Carcinoid tumour metastases in nodes produce cellular aspirates. The cells have a plasmacytoid appearance due to their eccentric nuclei, clock-face chromatin pattern, and abundant cytoplasm (**Figs 10.86, 10.87**).

Seminomas may metastasize to nodes, but can be impossible to diagnose without a history if only epithelioid neoplastic cells are seen in the aspirate (**Fig. 10.88**). However, most seminoma metastases are composed of large neoplastic

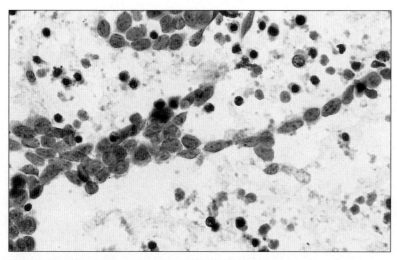

Fig. 10.85 Metastatic oat cell carcinoma – Pap x40. Clearly illustrated here is a streak of small anaplastic carcinoma cells merging into a larger cluster. The 'salt and pepper' chromatin is obvious, even at this magnification.

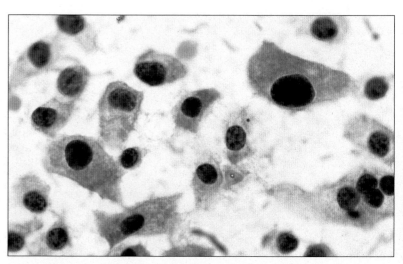

Fig. 10.86 Metastatic carcinoid tumour – Pap x63. In this field there are neoplastic cells which are very variable in size. Many of them have a plasmacytoid appearance with eccentric nuclei, but the two larger cells have central nuclei.

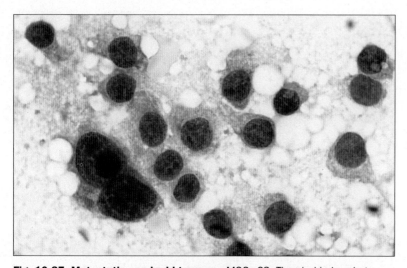

Fig. 10.87 Metastatic carcinoid tumour – MGG x63. The air-dried aspirate from the same case as shown in **Figure 10.86** displays a large binucleate cell and smaller tumour cells with a vaguely plasmacytoid appearance.

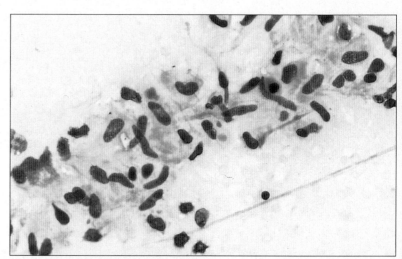

Fig. 10.88 Metastatic seminoma – MGG x40. This field shows epithelioid-type cells which would be impossible to diagnose correctly if there were no typical seminoma cells with prominent nucleoli elsewhere in the aspirate.

cells with huge central nucleoli (**Fig. 10.89**).

Merkel cell tumour deposits in lymph nodes cannot be diagnosed confidently, as the cells are usually small with round-to-ovoid nuclei, very little cytoplasm, and speckled chromatin. Scattered, larger multinucleated tumour cells may be seen (**Figs 10.90, 10.91**). The differential diagnosis includes oat cell carcinoma and lymphoma.

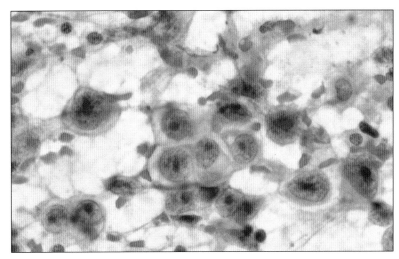

Fig. 10.89 Metastatic seminoma – Pap x100. The seminoma cells in this field are characteristically large with huge red nucleoli and very delicate cytoplasm.

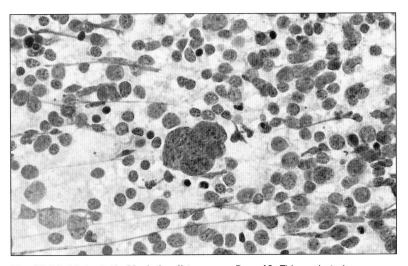

Fig. 10.90 Metastatic Merkel cell tumour – Pap x40. This aspirate is composed of small cells with rounded nuclei and speckled chromatin, similar to that of oat cell carcinoma and carcinoid tumours. No cytoplasm is visible in this smear.

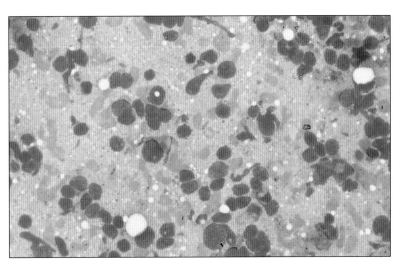

Fig. 10.91 Metastatic Merkel cell tumour – MGG x40. In an air-dried smear Merkel cells resemble lymphocytes. The speckled chromatin, obvious in wet-fixed smears, is not detectable and the diagnosis would not be possible without a history of a primary Merkel cell tumour.

SUGGESTED READING

Frable WJ, Kardos TF. Fine needle aspiration biopsy: Applications in the diagnosis of lymphoproliferative diseases. *Am J Surg Pathol* 1988; **12**: 62–72.

Moriarty AT, Banks ER, Bloch T. Cytological criteria for subclassification of Hodgkin's disease using fine needle aspiration. *Diagn Cytopathol* 1989; **5**: 122–125.

Oertel J, Oertel B, Kastner M, et al. The value of immunocytochemical staining of lymph node aspirates in diagnostic cytology. *Br J Haematol* 1988; **5**: 122–125.

Orell S, Sterrett G, Walters M, Whittaker D. *Manual and Atlas of Fine Needle Aspiration Cytology.* Edinburgh: Churchill Livingstone, 1992: 63–93.

Skoog L, Tani E. The role of fine needle aspiration cytology in the diagnosis of non-Hodgkin's lymphoma. *Diagn Cytopathol* 1991; **1**: 12–18.

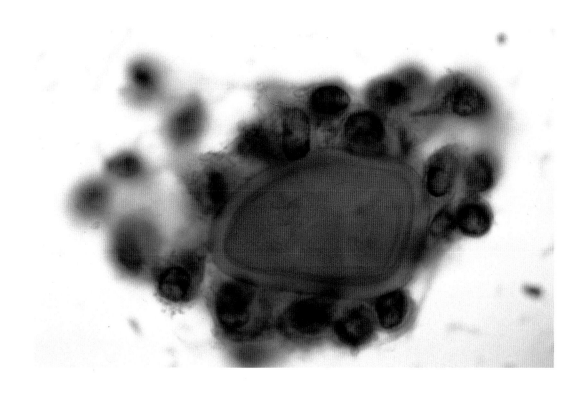

THE KIDNEY, URINE CYTOLOGY

11

THE KIDNEY

The urinary tract comprises two kidneys, two ureters, the urinary bladder, and the urethra (**Fig. 11.1**). The kidney is a bean-shaped organ composed of an outer cortex, an inner medulla, and calyces which drain into the pelvis of the kidney, which in turn drains into the ureter located at the hilum. The cortex of the kidney contains the glomeruli and the convoluted tubules, while the medulla contains the collecting tubules.

Fine needle aspirates of the kidney are now commonplace under image guidance. They should be treated as any other aspirate, the smears being carefully prepared with both wet and dry fixation, and any remaining material sent to the laboratory in the form of needle washings (see Chapter 6). It is extremely useful for a pathologist or cytotechnologist to be present at aspiration to confirm the cellularity of the aspirate.

A fine needle aspirate of a renal lesion may occasionally contain normal kidney structures, such as glomeruli and tubules. **Glomeruli** are composed of a convoluted network of capillaries covered by a capsule of epithelium; they appear in aspirates as tightly clumped, almost lobulated, irregular structures with overlapping small cells (**Figs 11.2, 11.3**). Occasionally, erythrocytes are seen within the glomerulus. The epithelial cells that may be seen in renal aspirates are of two types – from the proximal convoluted tubules and from the collecting tubules. The cells derived from the **convoluted tubules** contain granular cytoplasm and cell borders which are not sharply demarcated (**Figs 11.4, 11.5**). These epithelial cells are uniform with rounded nuclei. **Collecting tubule cells** may also contain granular cytoplasm, but tend to have clear, sharp cytoplasmic borders (**Figs 11.6, 11.7**).

BENIGN LESIONS

Renal cysts are not uncommon, are asymptomatic, and are usually diagnosed on radiological examination. On aspiration they yield a clear, usually colourless fluid which contains varying numbers of foamy macrophages (**Figs 11.8, 11.9**),

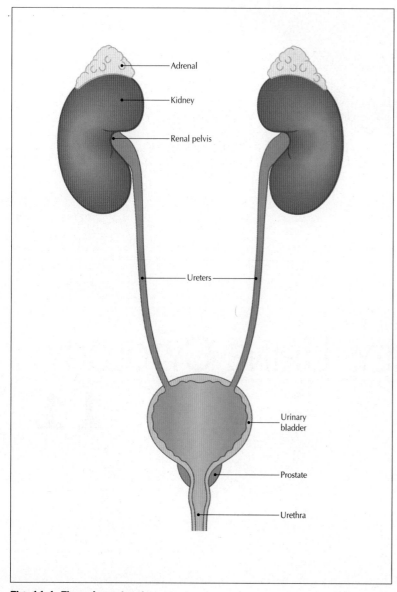

Fig. 11.1 The urinary tract.

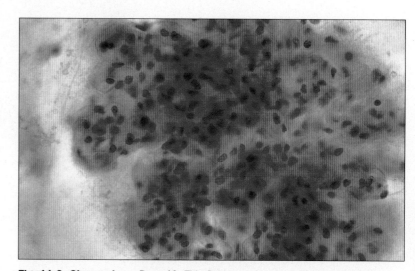

Fig. 11.2 Glomerulus – Pap x40. This field contains an aspirated glomerulus composed of small hyperchromatic cells forming a lobulated structure. The capillaries are not clearly defined in this illustration.

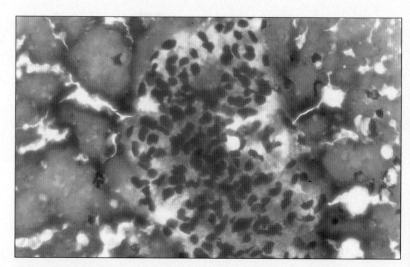

Fig. 11.3 Glomerulus – MGG x40. In air-dried aspirates, glomeruli display the same lobulated appearance and contain small hyperchromatic cells.

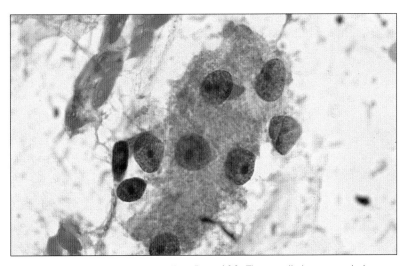

Fig. 11.4 Convoluted tubule cells – Pap x100. These cells have rounded nuclei, clearly visible nucleoli, and granular cytoplasm.

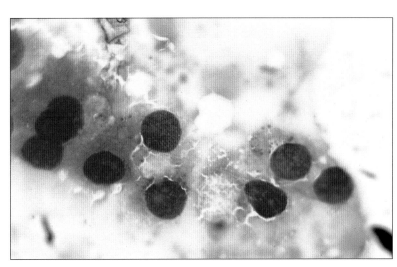

Fig. 11.5 Convoluted tubule cells – MGG x100. The cytoplasm of these cells stains blue with May Grunwald Giemsa. Some granularity is evident and the nuclei are uniform and rounded in outline.

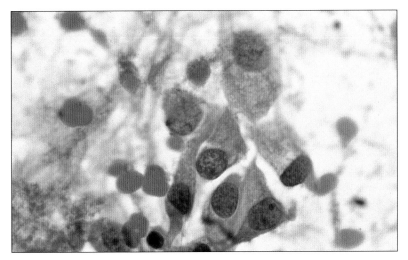

Fig. 11.6 Collecting tubule cells – Pap x100. These cells are smaller than the convoluted tubule cells and have sharper cytoplasmic borders.

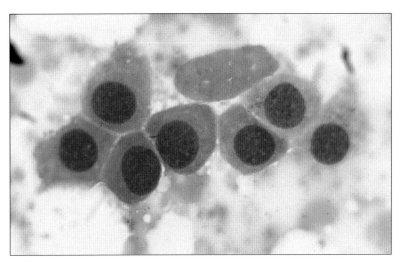

Fig. 11.7 Collecting tubule cells – MGG x100. Note the clearly defined cell borders and granular cytoplasm.

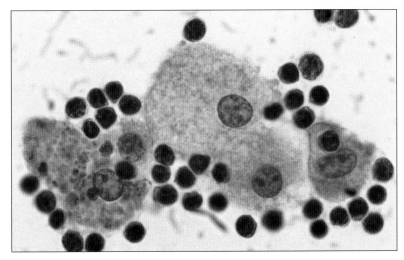

Fig. 11.8 Renal cyst macrophages – Pap x63. This field contains foamy macrophages and small lymphocytes. One of the macrophages contains some yellowish green haemosiderin. Note the clear background.

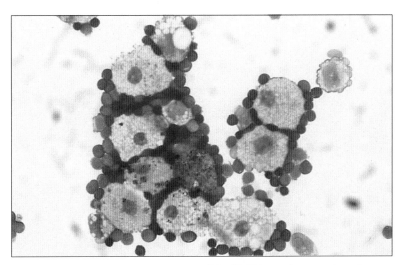

Fig. 11.9 Renal cyst macrophages – MGG x40. This renal cyst aspirate from the same case as shown in **Figure 11.8** displays foamy macrophages with pale foamy cytoplasm and light purple nuclei. One of the macrophages contains fine granules of bluish black haemosiderin. Many small lymphocytes are also present.

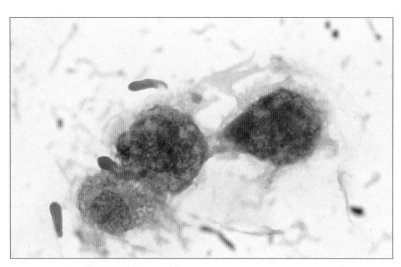

Fig. 11.10 Renal cyst siderophages – Pap x63. These three foamy macrophages contain greenish yellow intracytoplasmic haemosiderin, a common finding when there has been haemorrhage into the cyst.

siderophages [if there has been previous haemorrhage into the cyst (**Figs 11.10, 11.11**)], and a few erythrocytes. Epithelial cells are rarely seen and, when present, may show vacuolar degeneration that simulates macrophages (**Figs 11.12, 11.13**). Macrophages, however, have more delicate, granular cytoplasm and less well-defined cytoplasmic borders. Cyst fluid that is blood-stained or thick and turbid should be examined with great care to exclude necrotic tumour.

Inflammatory processes can be clearly distinguished on cytological preparations, the most problematic being xanthogranulomatous pyelonephritis, which can mimic renal cell carcinoma. Aspirates from a renal abscess show a large number of acute inflammatory cells and histiocytes. Reactive and degenerate epithelial cells may be noted occasionally. The aspirate in xanthogranulomatous

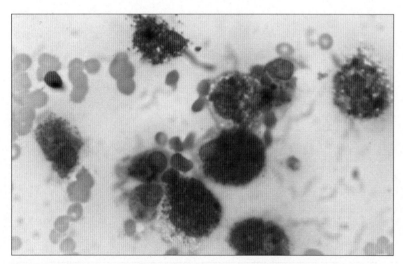

Fig. 11.11 Renal cyst siderophages – MGG x63. The haemosiderin in these foamy macrophages stains bluish black.

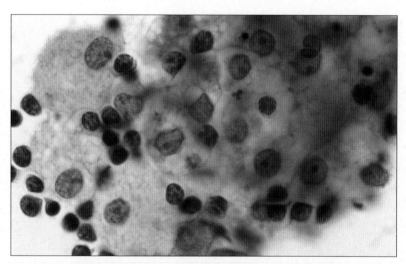

Fig. 11.12 Renal cyst epithelial cells – Pap x100. This cluster consists mostly of benign epithelial cells showing vacuolar degeneration, stimulating the macrophage at the top left. The macrophage has foamy, but not vacuolated, cytoplasm and the nucleus is not central, as in the epithelial cells. Lymphocytes are also visible in this field.

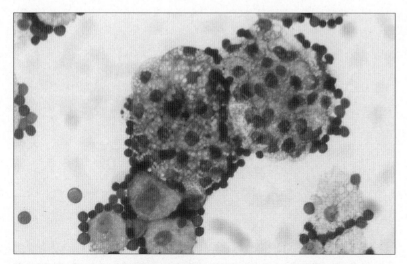

Fig. 11.13 Renal cyst epithelial cells – MGG x40. The air-dried smear better illustrates the difference between degenerate vacuolated epithelial cells and foamy macrophages in renal cyst aspirates. In this field the epithelial cells are smaller with darker nuclei and show honeycomb vacuolation.

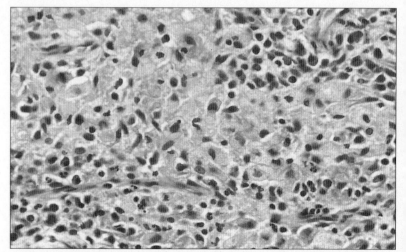

Fig. 11.14 Xanthogranulomatous pyelonephritis – H&E x40. This section illustrates the foamy macrophages and inflammatory cells found in this lesion.

pyelonephritis **(Fig. 11.14)** contains numerous inflammatory cells, foamy macrophages, and debris **(Figs 11.15, 11.16)**. The foamy macrophages may be mistaken for renal carcinoma cells if care is not exercised.

RENAL NEOPLASMS

Angiomyolipoma is a benign neoplasm which can mimic renal cell carcinoma both on radiology and cytology. It contains blood vessels, fat, and smooth muscle **(Fig. 11.17)**. The aspirate is often scanty, heavily blood-stained, and contains a mixture of spindle-shaped cells and round cells accompanied by numerous small fat vacuoles **(Figs 11.18, 11.19)**. When cellular, the aspirate may be

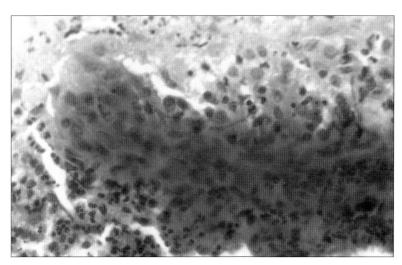

Fig. 11.15 Xanthogranulomatous pyelonephritis – Pap x40. This field contains a group of foamy macrophages mimicking a cluster of epithelial cells, surrounded by lymphocytes and some neutrophils. The foamy macrophages may be mistaken for renal cell carcinoma cells.

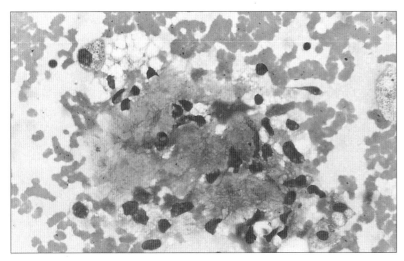

Fig. 11.16 Xanthogranulomatous pyelonephritis – MGG x40. Illustrated here is debris surrounded by foamy macrophages which can mimic renal cell carcinoma cells. Occasional lymphocytes are also noted.

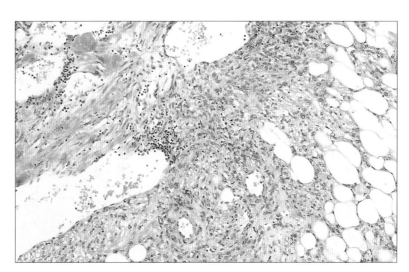

Fig. 11.17 Angiomyolipoma – H&E x10. This benign renal lesion is composed of blood vessels, smooth muscle and fat, as illustrated here.

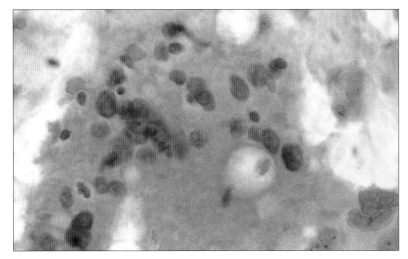

Fig. 11.18 Angiomyolipoma – Pap x100. Illustrated here are the epithelioid cells which may be seen in aspirates from this entity. Fat vacuoles are also present.

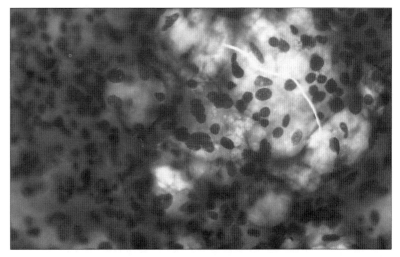

Fig. 11.19 Angiomyolipoma – MGG x40. In this field note the small round cells, occasional spindle cell, and fat cells that constitute an angiomyolipoma.

diagnosed erroneously as suggestive of renal cell carcinoma, since the thick tissue fragments that are often aspirated may appear to be composed of epithelial rather than smooth muscle cells. There are often spindle-shaped bare nuclei in the background and groups of epithelioid cells with abundant cytoplasm.

Renal adenomas are small neoplasms which cannot be distinguished reliably from renal cell carcinomas on cytological material. **Renal oncocytomas (Fig. 11.20)** are composed of cells with abundant eosinophilic cytoplasm and relatively small uniform nuclei **(Figs 11.21, 11.22)**.

Renal cell carcinomas show variable histological appearances, all of which are usually closely matched by the cells in the aspirate. Fine needle aspirates of

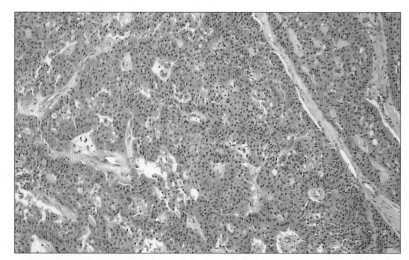

Fig. 11.20 Renal oncocytoma – H&E x10. This section of a renal oncocytoma shows eosinophilic cells with abundant cytoplasm.

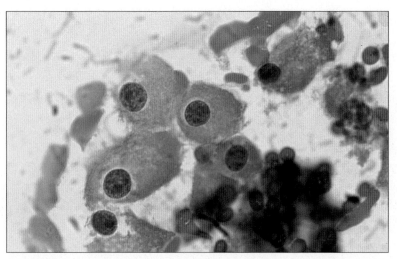

Fig. 11.21 Renal oncocytoma – Pap x100. The oncocytes in this renal aspirate contain abundant granular cytoplasm and round nuclei with nucleoli. There are no features of malignancy in this sample.

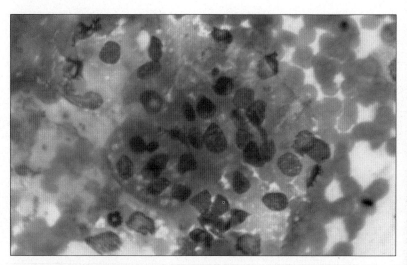

Fig. 11.22 Renal oncocytoma – MGG x40. This aspirate, from the same case as shown in **Figure 11.21**, shows epithelial cells with moderate amounts of cytoplasm, but the oncocytic features are not striking, possibly due to air-drying artefact.

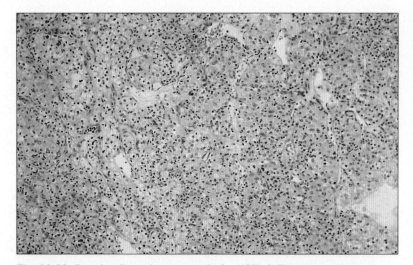

Fig. 11.23 Renal cell carcinoma, grade 1 – H&E x4. This photomicrograph illustrates a low-grade renal cell carcinoma. Even at this low magnification the appearance is fairly uniform.

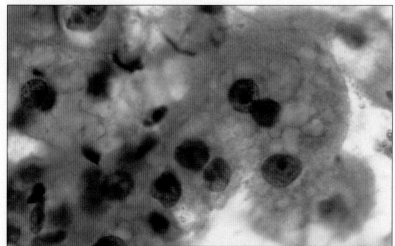

Fig. 11.24 Renal cell carcinoma – Pap x100. The renal carcinoma cells seen here have relatively small nuclei with prominent nucleoli. Note the abundant vacuolated cytoplasm.

these lesions are commonly cellular. **Grade 1** renal cell carcinomas **(Fig. 11.23)** are composed of cells with relatively small nuclei and abundant vacuolated cytoplasm with indistinct borders. The nuclear margins are sharp, with vesicular-to-granular chromatin, and small nucleoli may be clearly visible **(Figs 11.24, 11.25)**. Some cell clusters may exhibit an acinar arrangement **(Fig. 11.26)**. One histological type of renal cell carcinoma is clear cell carcinoma **(Fig. 11.27)**, the cells of which are seen on aspiration to contain very pale, delicately granular cytoplasm **(Fig. 11.28)**. Stromal strands are frequently seen in renal cell carcinomas, but are more obvious on air-dried material **(Fig. 11.29)**. Low-grade renal cell neoplasms can appear cytologically benign with bland round nuclei and small

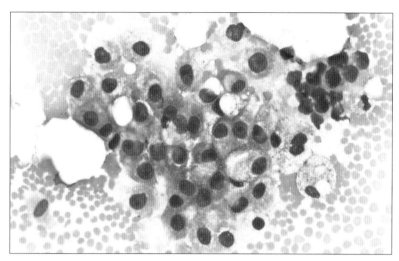

Fig. 11.25 Renal cell carcinoma – MGG x40. These carcinoma cells appear uniform with small nuclei, just visible nucleoli, and abundant foamy cytoplasm.

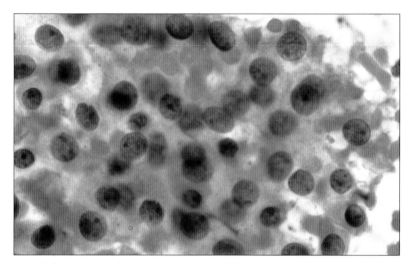

Fig. 11.26 Renal cell carcinoma – Pap x100. This aspirate from a renal cell carcinoma contains well-differentiated malignant cells arranged in acinar clusters. The cytoplasm is granular rather than vacuolated and is ill-defined.

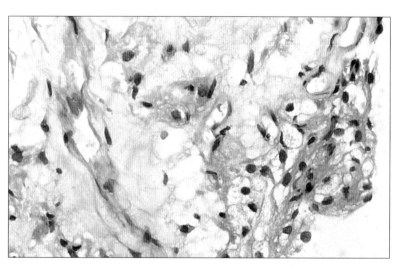

Fig. 11.27 Renal cell carcinoma, clear cell type – H&E x10. This section of a clear cell renal cell carcinoma is composed of cells with small nuclei and abundant, almost colourless cytoplasm. These cells can be mistaken for foamy macrophages, and conversely the foamy macrophages of xanthogranulomatous pyelonephritis may be misinterpreted as clear cell renal cell carcinoma.

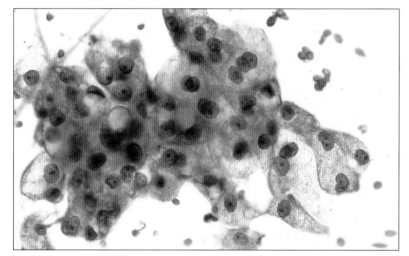

Fig. 11.28 Renal cell carcinoma, clear cell type – Pap x40. In this field cells from a clear cell renal cell carcinoma are visible. They have abundant pale granular cytoplasm, rather than the vacuolated cytoplasm commonly seen in renal cell carcinomas.

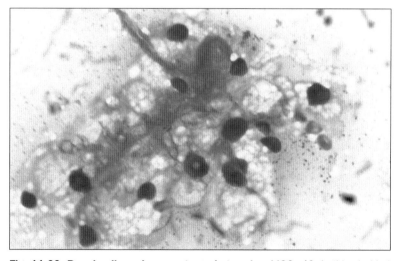

Fig. 11.29 Renal cell carcinoma, stromal strands – MGG x40. In this air-dried sample the cytoplasm of the carcinoma cells appears vacuolated and pink stroma is clearly seen. The nuclei in this field are degenerate.

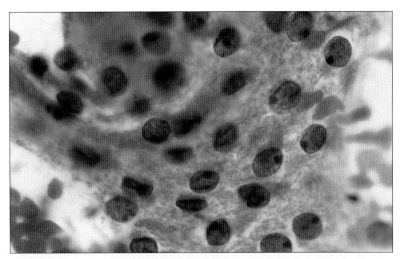

Fig. 11.30 Renal cell carcinoma, low grade – Pap x100. The renal carcinoma illustrated here is low grade, composed of cells with granular cytoplasm and small, round-to-ovoid nuclei with insignificant nucleoli. No cytoplasmic vacuolation is seen. This appearance is deceptive and a careful search must be made for other cells with malignant features.

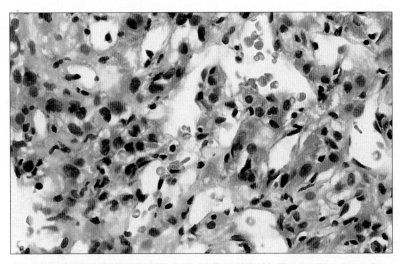

Fig. 11.31 Renal cell carcinoma, grade 2 – H&E x10. This section shows the degree of pleomorphism seen with this grade of tumour.

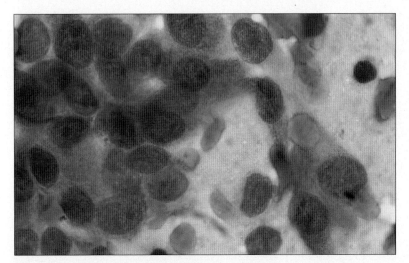

Fig. 11.33 Renal cell carcinoma, grade 2 – MGG x100. The air-dried smear of the same case as shown in **Figure 11.32** shows cells which have a high nuclear–cytoplasmic ratio and prominent nucleoli. The chromatin pattern is granular, but the nuclei do not show much pleomorphism.

nucleoli (**Fig. 11.30**), but there are usually other cells in the aspirate which are more obviously malignant. If there is doubt about the cells being renal in origin, special stains may be performed (such as a PAS and Oil red O stain), both of which will be positive.

Grade 2 renal cell carcinomas (**Fig. 11.31**) produce aspirates with cells which show moderate degrees of pleomorphism. The nuclear–cytoplasmic ratio is increased, the nuclear outlines may be somewhat irregular, the chromatin granular, and red nucleoli can be seen (**Fig. 11.32**). Not all of these features are detectable

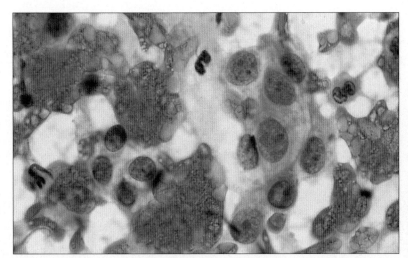

Fig. 11.32 Renal cell carcinoma, grade 2 – Pap x100. These cells have an increased nuclear–cytoplasmic ratio. The cytoplasm is not particularly vacuolated. The nuclei vary in size and some contain conspicuous nucleoli.

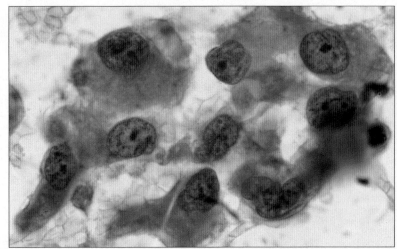

Fig. 11.34 Renal cell carcinoma, grade 3 – Pap x100. These neoplastic cells show marked pleomorphism with irregular nuclear margins, some showing budding. There is clumping of chromatin, with clear areas between the clumps, and the nucleoli are prominent and red. The cytoplasm shows a trace of vacuolation.

on the air-dried smear **(Fig. 11.33)**. Aspirates from **grade 3** renal cell carcinomas contain dissociated pleomorphic epithelial cells with very irregular nuclear margins, nuclear folds, clumping and clearing of chromatin, and red nucleoli **(Fig. 11.34)**. Again, the nuclear features are not as clear on air-dried smears **(Fig. 11.35)**.

Papillary renal cell carcinoma (Fig. 11.36) also yields a cellular aspirate in which papillary fragments are discernible **(Figs 11.37, 11.38)**. Fibrovascular cores are usually seen which stain pale blue with the Papanicolaou stain and bright pink with May Grunwald Giemsa **(Figs 11.39, 11.40)**. The individual cells

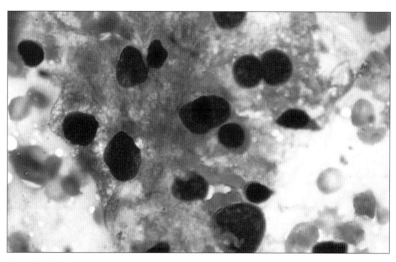

Fig. 11.35 Renal cell carcinoma, grade 3 – MGG x100. The carcinoma cells visible here are pleomorphic with hyperchromatic nuclei. Nucleoli are not seen in this preparation. Note the vacuolated cytoplasm.

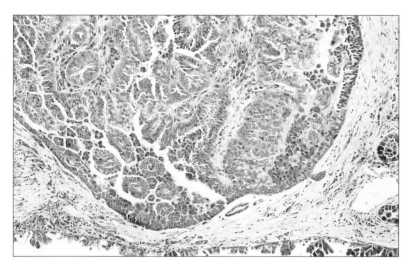

Fig. 11.36 Papillary renal cell carcinoma – H&E x4. This section illustrates beautifully the papillary architecture of these tumours. Note the haemosiderin-laden macrophages, which are stained brown.

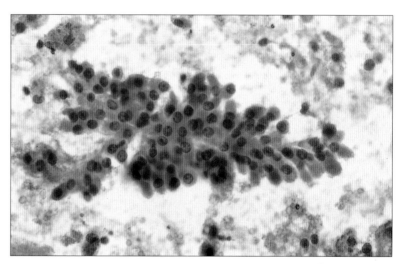

Fig. 11.37 Papillary renal cell carcinoma – Pap x40. In this field there is a papillary cluster of uniform cells with abundant cytoplasm and rounded nuclei. In the background there is altered blood with siderophages.

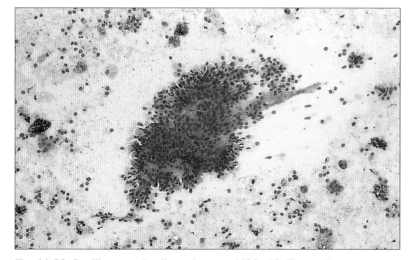

Fig. 11.38 Papillary renal cell carcinoma – MGG x10. The papillary structure of this cluster of cells is illustrated clearly in this field. Note the pink stroma, and the single cells and siderophages in the background.

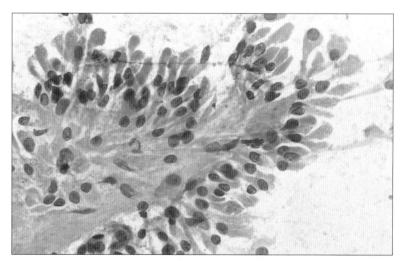

Fig. 11.39 Papillary renal cell carcinoma – Pap x100. With the Papanicolaou stain the fibrovascular cores of this neoplasm stain pale blue, as seen in this example. The epithelial cells look uniform and bland.

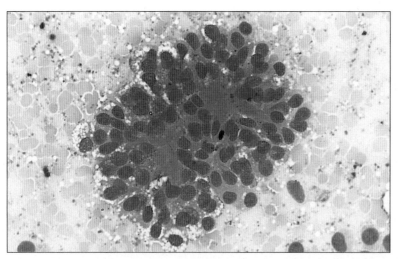

Fig. 11.40 Papillary renal cell carcinoma – MGG x40. In air-dried smears the stromal cores stain bright pink. The tumour cells are small and unremarkable.

may vary considerably, some showing abundant vacuolated cytoplasm and round vesicular nuclei (**Fig. 11.41**), others being more pleomorphic with enlarged irregular nuclei and prominent nucleoli (**Fig. 11.42**). There is often evidence of previous haemorrhage into the tumour, as demonstrated by siderophages (**Fig. 11.43**).

Transitional cell carcinoma (urothelial cell carcinoma) of the kidney is not rare, and usually arises in the renal pelvis. These tumours may be predominantly spindle celled and low grade (**Fig. 11.44**), in which case the aspirate contains similar spindle-shaped cells with somewhat irregular nuclear margins (**Figs 11.45, 11.46**). Grade 2 neoplasms (**Figs 11.47, 11.48**) and grade 3 carcinomas (**Figs 11.49, 11.50**) exhibit increasing degrees of pleomorphism in the aspirated material. Neoplastic cells may be shed into the urine (**Fig. 11.51**), but there are no specific features to differentiate tumours arising in the kidney from those arising in the bladder.

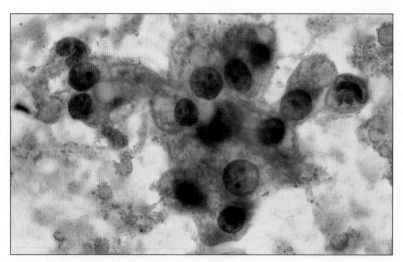

Fig. 11.41 Papillary renal cell carcinoma – Pap x100. The cells in this cluster contain finely vacuolated cytoplasm and round nuclei with small nucleoli.

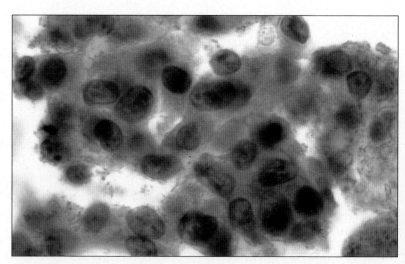

Fig. 11.42 Papillary renal cell carcinoma – Pap x100. This papillary tumour is composed of pleomorphic malignant cells with irregular nuclear outlines and denser cytoplasm.

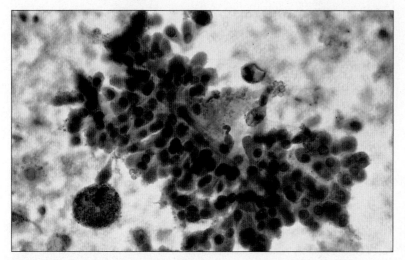

Fig. 11.43 Papillary renal cell carcinoma – Pap x40. Foamy macrophages containing greenish yellow haemosiderin are seen around the papillary cluster of carcinoma cell in this field.

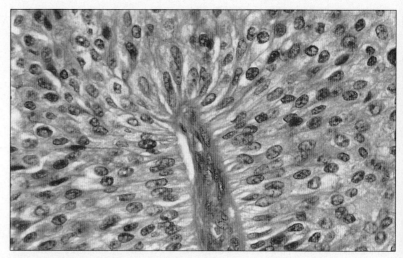

Fig. 11.44 Transitional cell carcinoma – H&E x40. This section of a transitional cell carcinoma of the renal pelvis shows spindle-shaped cells with vesicular, mildly pleomorphic nuclei. Mitoses are not conspicuous.

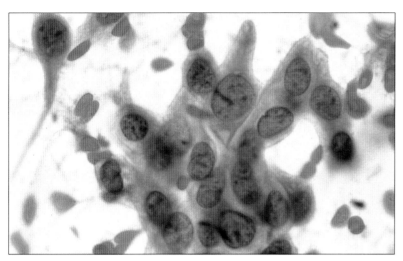

Fig. 11.45 Transitional cell carcinoma – Pap x100. The cells in this field are from the same case as shown in **Figures 11.44** and **11.46**. Some spindle cells are present and the nuclei are vesicular, but the nuclear margins are somewhat irregular. Nucleoli are not prominent and there is no cytoplasmic vacuolation, which is apparent in renal cell carcinomas.

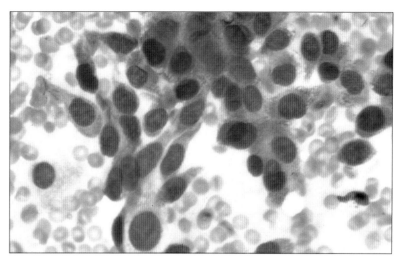

Fig. 11.46 Transitional cell carcinoma – MGG x63. This air-dried smear from the same case as shown in **Figures 11.44** and **11.45** contains spindle-shaped cells with rather bland nuclei. No vacuolation is seen.

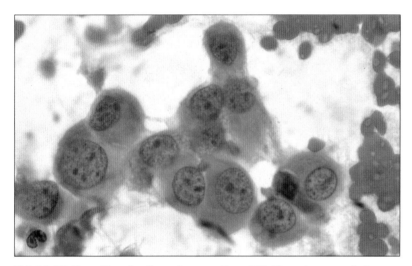

Fig. 11.47 Transitional cell carcinoma – Pap x100. These tumour cells from a grade 2 transitional cell carcinoma of the renal pelvis show moderate pleomorphism with enlarged nuclei, an increased nuclear–cytoplasmic ratio, and chromatin clumping. Nucleoli are noticeable. The cytoplasm is dense and shows no vacuolation.

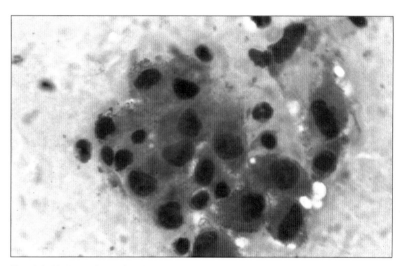

Fig. 11.48 Transitional cell carcinoma – MGG x40. This field of an aspirate from a grade 2 transitional cell carcinoma shows moderately pleomorphic cells with irregular nuclear margins and nucleoli that are just visible.

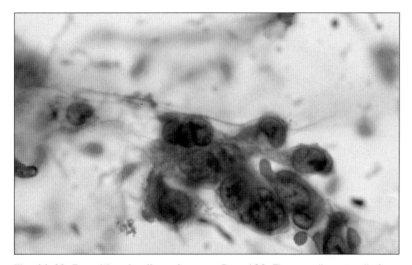

Fig. 11.49 Transitional cell carcinoma – Pap x100. These malignant cells from a grade 3 transitional cell carcinoma of the renal pelvis are small, but pleomorphic with markedly irregular nuclear margins showing budding and clefts. The chromatin pattern is also abnormal.

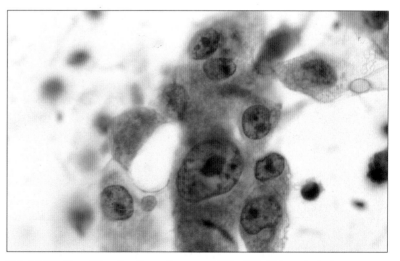

Fig. 11.50 Transitional cell carcinoma – MGG x100. This aspirate from a grade 3 renal cell carcinoma contains pleomorphic cells with huge nucleoli and chromatin clumping.

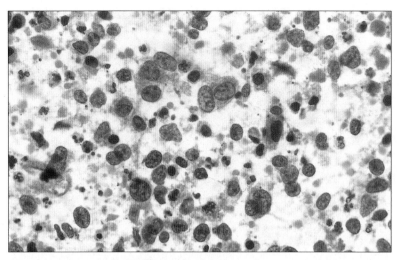

Fig. 11.51 Transitional cell carcinoma, urine – Pap x63. This urine sample contains single pleomorphic transitional carcinoma cells consistent with a grade 3 neoplasm. It is not possible on cytological grounds to establish whether this tumour arose in the bladder, ureter, or renal pelvis.

Primary **squamous cell carcinoma** of the kidney is uncommon. Squamous differentiation may be noted in urothelial cell carcinomas, however. The aspirates are cellular and contain predominantly single cells which are often keratinized (**Figs 11.52, 11.53**). Necrotic cellular debris is a frequent finding.

Wilms' tumour is a neoplasm of childhood which produces a cellular aspirate composed of small hyperchromatic cells; in theory these are supposed to demonstrate two patterns. The aspirates in practice contain cohesive clusters of small cells without demonstrable cytoplasm, as well as a few single cells (**Fig. 11.54**). The chromatin pattern appears granular and the cells mimic other small, round cell types of neoplasm (**Fig. 11.55**).

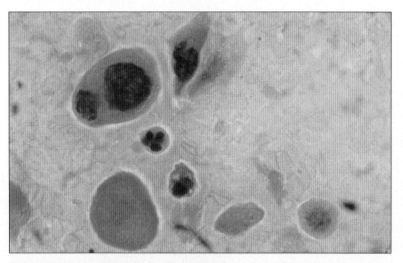

Fig. 11.52 Squamous cell carcinoma, kidney – Pap x40. In this field there are degenerate squamous carcinoma cells with orange–pink dense cytoplasm and sharply demarcated cell borders. There is much necrotic cellular debris in the background.

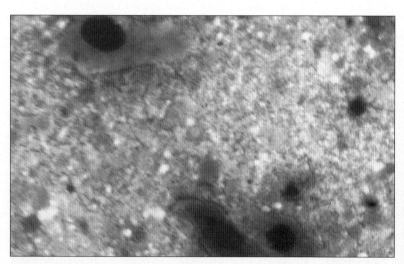

Fig. 11.53 Squamous cell carcinoma, kidney – MGG x100. Some of the malignant cells in the aspirate show keratinization with blue cytoplasm and well-defined cell borders.

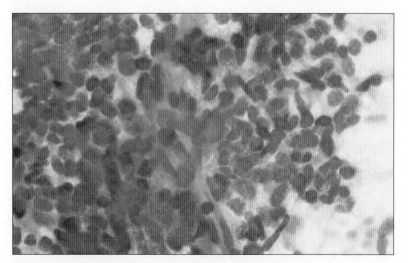

Fig. 11.54 Wilms' tumour – Pap x100. This rather poorly preserved aspirate is composed of small undifferentiated cells with inconspicuous cytoplasm and round-to-ovoid nuclei. It would not be possible to accurately type this tumour without clinical details, including the patient's age.

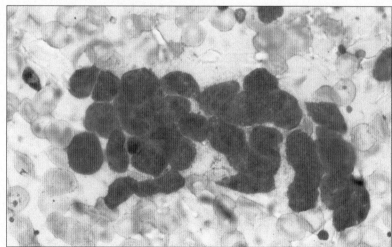

Fig. 11.55 Wilms' tumour – MGG x100. This group of cells shows granular chromatin and nuclei slightly larger than the erythrocytes in the background. No specific features are seen.

URINE CYTOLOGY

The cytological examination of urine reveals changes that may have taken place anywhere in the urinary tract. Urine is produced in the kidneys, and passes through the ureters into the urinary bladder, where it is stored and then voided through the urethra. Cells that are exfoliated into urine may originate from the kidney, ureter, bladder, prostate, or urethra.

Normal urine contains very few cells from the urinary bladder; any found are of squamous or urothelial type. It is essential that urine cytology should be performed on freshly voided urine, preferably **not** an early morning sample as the cells will have been lying in urine for hours, rapidly degenerating. A mid-morning sample is the most useful – three specimens should be taken on three separate days to optimize the likelihood of detecting abnormalities. Samples should be collected in a clean container and sent to the laboratory immediately. If, for any reason, the specimen has to be transported or kept overnight, alcohol should be added to preserve the cells.

The colour and quantity of the sample are recorded in the laboratory before the urine is processed by centrifugation. In some laboratories a membrane filter is used to collect all the cells that are present, but this type of preparation produces a dark background with much debris so the cell features are often difficult to interpret. A cytospin produces good results, with the cells concentrated in a small area and therefore easy to find. The smears are stained using the Papanicolaou method, which maintains the translucency of the cytoplasm while highlighting the chromatin pattern of the nucleus.

To recognize the cells present in urine it is necessary to be familiar with the histology of the urinary bladder, as most of the cells in urine originate from this organ. The ureters and bladder are lined by urothelium, formerly referred to as transitional epithelium. This is a multilayered epithelium with small basal cells in the deeper layers, slightly larger cells in the upper layers, and very large multinucleated cells at the surface (**Fig. 11.56**). These large cells on the surface are also known as umbrella cells, as each one of them overlies several smaller intermediate cells. They can contain up to 55 nuclei each. The trigone of the bladder, which is the base of the bladder, is often lined by squamous epithelium (**Fig. 11.57**) which accounts partly for the squamous cells seen in urine in males, some being of urethral origin. In females the abundance of squamous cells sometimes seen in urine is often due to vaginal contamination. Parts of the urinary bladder may show areas lined by mucin-secreting columnar-type epithelial cells, which explains the columnar cells and mucin which are occasionally seen in urine.

The **deeper layer cells** of the urothelium are small with fairly dense, cyanophilic cytoplasm and a single round-to-ovoid nucleus. The chromatin pattern is vesicular and the nuclear margin is smooth and sharp (**Fig. 11.58**). These cells may appear on the slide singly, or in sheets if the specimen has been collected by catheterization, as this process shears off sheets of urothelial cells. It is important that the laboratory is informed as to the method of urine collection, because catheterized samples can produce cell clusters which mimic papillary structures and lead to a misdiagnosis of neoplasia. Under high magnification the bland nuclear structure is apparent, indicating the benign nature of the cells even though the nuclear–cytoplasmic ratio may appear to be high. The more mature urothelial cells appear larger than those derived from the deeper layers (**Fig. 11.59**). **Superficial urothelial cells** vary greatly in size and number of nuclei present (**Figs 11.60–11.62**). The nuclei are all vesicular and more or less the same size and shape, although the cells may take on bizarre shapes (**Fig. 11.63**).

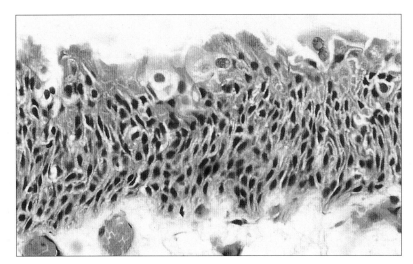

Fig. 11.56 Urinary bladder – H&E x10. This section of a normal urinary bladder shows the various cell layers that comprise the epithelium. The cells at the surface are large and multinucleated, while the deeper layer cells are smaller with less cytoplasm and relatively large nuclei.

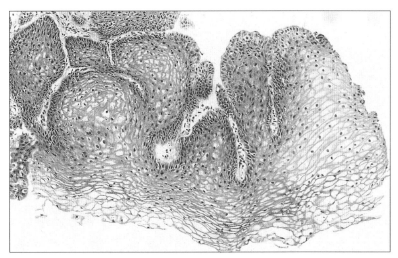

Fig. 11.57 Urinary bladder – H&E x4. This section shows squamous epithelium lining the bladder, a feature not uncommonly seen in the trigone of the bladder.

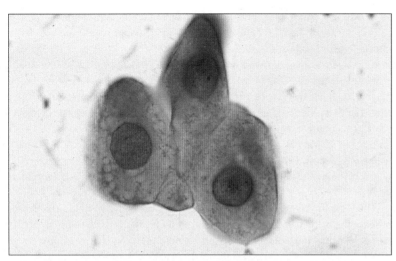

Fig. 11.58 Deeper layer urothelial cells – Pap x100. These cells are from the deeper layer of urothelium and are small with relatively large nuclei. The nuclear outlines are round and sharply defined, and the chromatin is dense. The cytoplasm is usually denser than that of intermediate squamous cells, although in this illustration some degenerative vacuolation is present.

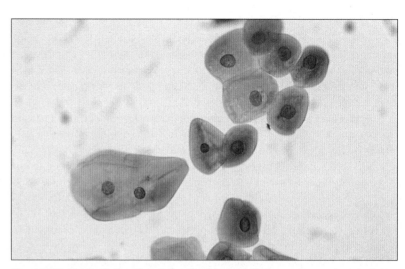

Fig. 11.59 Urothelial cells – Pap x40. This field displays a range of urothelial cells varying in size. The large binucleate cell on the left is from the superficial layer, the other smaller cells are deeper layer cells.

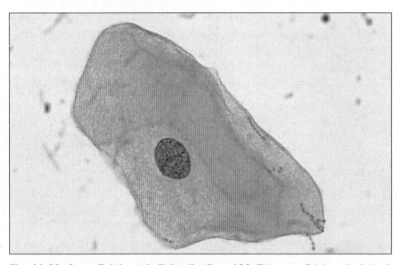

Fig. 11.60 Superficial urothelial cell – Pap x100. This superficial urothelial cell is much larger than deeper layer cells (see **Figure 11.58**), but displays the same sharply defined cell borders, fairly dense cytoplasm, and round nucleus. These cells may be mistaken for intermediate squamous cells.

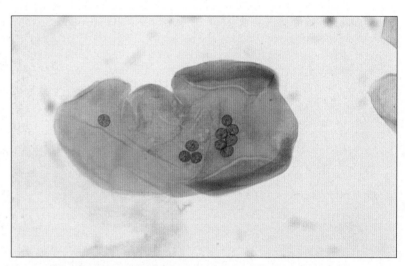

Fig. 11.61 Superficial urothelial cell – Pap x40. This is a very large cell with several nuclei, exfoliated from the superficial layer of urothelium. Note the clearly defined cell margin and the uniform nuclei.

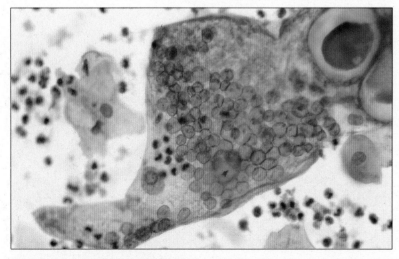

Fig. 11.62 Superficial urothelial cell – Pap x40. This enormous superficial cell contains abundant nuclei, all vesicular and of the same size. It has also phagocytosed some debris.

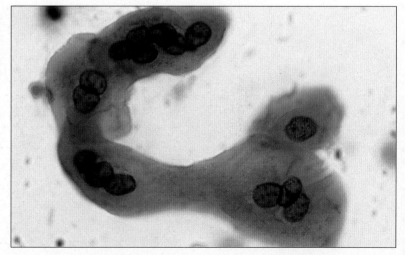

Fig. 11.63 Superficial urothelial cell – Pap x100. This superficial urothelial cell has a bizarre shape and nuclei in little groups scattered along the cytoplasm.

Urothelial cells often contain glycogen, which is bright yellow with the Papanicolaou stain **(Fig. 11.64)**. **Columnar cells**, with their typical wedge shape and basal nuclei, are occasionally seen, sometimes showing cilia if the sample is particularly fresh **(Fig. 11.65)**. **Mucin** is not infrequently seen in urine samples **(Fig. 11.66)**. **Squamous cells** have the same characteristics as those seen in cervical smears; they are usually superficial in type **(Fig. 11.67)**, and may contain keratohyaline granules **(Fig. 11.68)**. Masses of anucleate squames may be visible **(Fig. 11.69)**. Early morning urine specimens or samples that have been stored over a long period contain very degenerate cells which are difficult to interpret. The cytoplasm becomes vacuolated and the nuclei appear pyknotic or structureless,

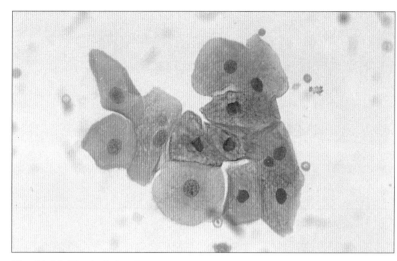

Fig. 11.64 Urothelial cells, glycogen – Pap x40. Some of the urothelial cells in this group contain intracytoplasmic glycogen.

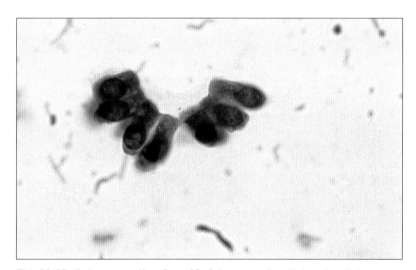

Fig. 11.65 Columnar cells – Pap x40. Columnar cells with basal nuclei are very occasionally noted in normal urine samples. Cilia are not present in this field.

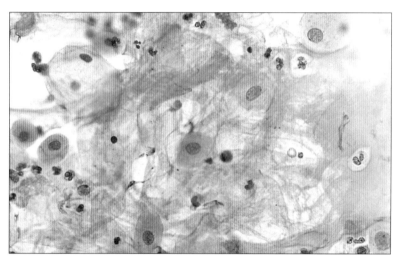

Fig. 11.66 Mucin – Pap x40. Mucin is occasionally seen in urine samples. In this field there are also deeper layer urothelial cells and some inflammatory cells.

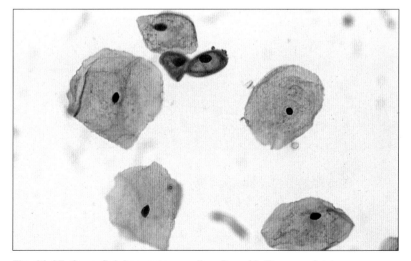

Fig. 11.67 Superficial squamous cells – Pap x40. The superficial squamous cells in this view contain small pyknotic nuclei and are much larger than the small deeper layer urothelial cells also present.

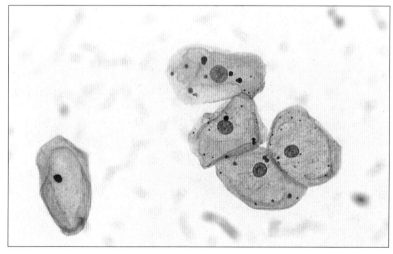

Fig. 11.68 Squamous cells – Pap x40. The intermediate squamous cells in this field contain keratohyaline granules. Note the acidophilic superficial squamous cell.

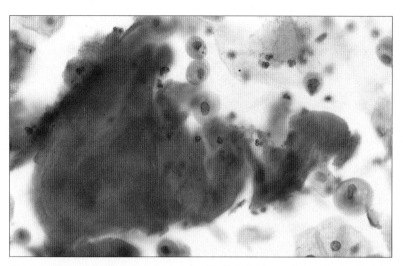

Fig. 11.69 Anucleate squames – Pap x40. This field contains a clump of bright orange keratinized anucleate squames, as well as some urothelial cells and occasional inflammatory cells.

with incomplete nuclear margins (**Fig. 11.70**). A characteristic feature, which is well demonstrated on the Papanicolaou-stained smear, is the presence of well-defined masses of red cytoplasmic inclusions in a variety of shapes and sizes, representing lipofuscin breakdown products (**Fig. 11.71**).

Corpora amylacea derived from the prostate gland are observed not infrequently in urine specimens from males. They vary in size (**Fig. 11.72**), are usually pale blue or pinkish orange, and contain concentric laminations (**Fig. 11.73**).

Spermatozoa are also seen in urine specimens (**Fig. 11.74**), often accompanied by germ cells and seminal vesicle cells. Bacterial chains are commonly observed in urine specimens, either in the background or clearly shown against the pale blue cytoplasm of urothelial or squamous cells (see **Figure 11.74**). These are clearly non-pathogenic if no inflammatory cells are seen.

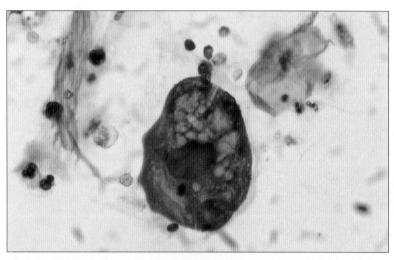

Fig. 11.70 Urothelial cell, degenerative changes – Pap x100. This deeper layer urothelial cell shows cytoplasmic vacuolation as well as loss of continuity of the nuclear margin, due to degeneration.

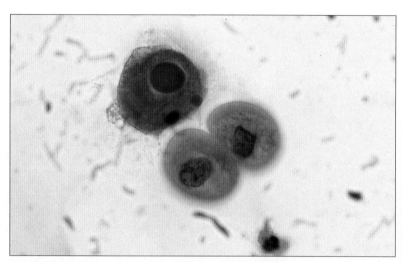

Fig. 11.71 Urothelial cell, cytoplasmic inclusions – Pap x100. Illustrated here is a group of degenerate urothelial cells, two showing degenerative nuclear changes, and the third containing bright red inclusions of varying sizes, believed to be derived from the breakdown of lipofuschin pigments.

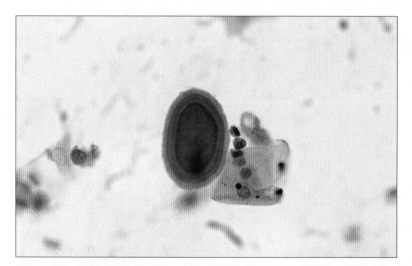

Fig. 11.72 Corpus amylaceum – Pap x40. These bodies, which are frequently seen in urine from males, originate in the prostate gland. Note the clearly defined concentric laminations.

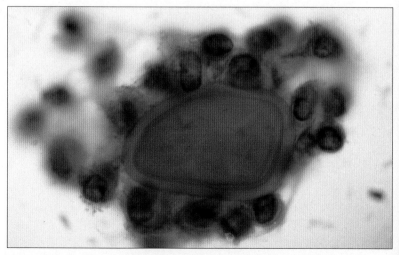

Fig. 11.73 Corpus amylaceum – Pap x100. In this view the red-staining laminated corpus amylaceum is surrounded by inflammatory cells.

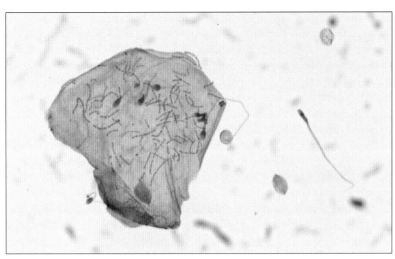

Fig. 11.74 Spermatozoa – Pap x100. A solitary spermatozoon with a tail is seen in this field. Note also the bacteria and a few degenerate spermatozoa on the surface of the squamous cell.

INFLAMMATION

Cystitis produces hazy urine or even haematuria. The sample contains numerous polymorphonuclear leucocytes **(Fig. 11.75)** and histiocytes **(Fig. 11.76)**, accompanied by reactive urothelial cells with enlarged nuclei and a granular chromatin pattern **(Fig. 11.77)**. Other cells show features of degeneration, such as cytoplasmic vacuolation **(Fig. 11.78)**. Bacteria are often present in the background, but these cannot be typed on cytology. Mid-stream urine should be dispatched to the microbiology laboratory for culture and sensitivity tests.

Candida spores and hyphae are sometimes seen in urine samples **(Fig. 11.79)**. The spores may easily be missed on screening if they are unaccompanied by hyphae **(Fig. 11.80)**. **Trichomonads**, either Trichomonas vaginalis or hominis,

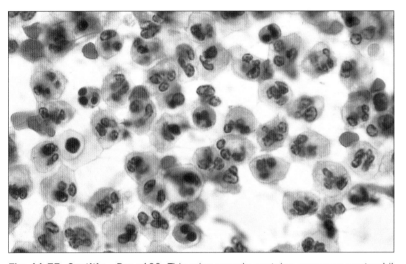

Fig. 11.75 Cystitis – Pap x100. This urine sample contains numerous neutrophil polymorphs, as demonstrated here. Erythrocytes are also present.

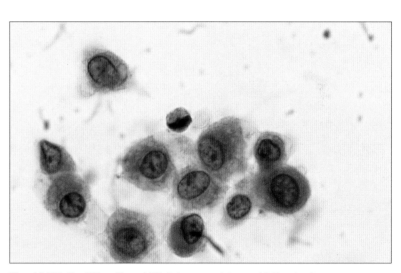

Fig. 11.76 Cystitis – Pap x100. It is unusual to see histiocytes in a group on their own, as illustrated here. Other fields in this smear demonstrated the usual mixture of neutrophils and histiocytes commonly seen in cystitis.

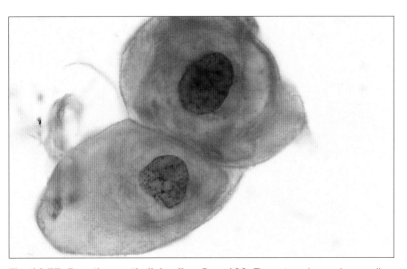

Fig. 11.77 Reactive urothelial cells – Pap x100. These two deeper layer cells exhibit slightly enlarged nuclei with granular chromatin. They should not be mistaken for neoplastic cells.

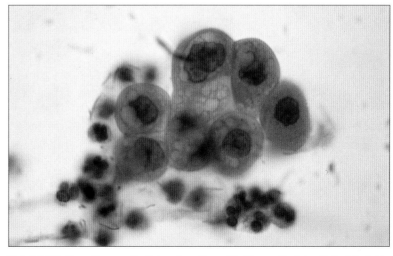

Fig. 11.78 Reactive urothelial cells – Pap x40. The urothelial cells in this field show nuclear enlargement and hyperchromasia that are suggestive of reactive changes, but the cytoplasm is vacuolated, a feature of degeneration. There are neutrophils in the background.

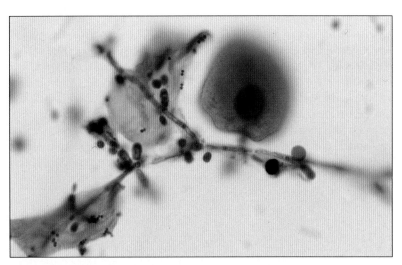

Fig. 11.79 Candida – Pap x100. This field demonstrates Candida spores and hyphae with a deeper layer urothelial cell.

are occasionally noted in urine samples (**Fig. 11.81**). Parasitic ova, for example those of *Enterobius vermicularis* (**pinworm**) (**Fig. 11.82**) and *Schistosoma haematobium* (**Fig. 11.83**), are seldom seen in urine samples in this country. Both of these infestations are accompanied by erythrocytes and masses of acute inflammatory cells in the urine, including haemosiderin-laden macrophages (**Fig. 11.84**). A rare finding in urine samples is the presence of epithelial cells infected by **herpes simplex**, with their typical multinucleated, ground glass, moulded nuclei (**Fig. 11.85**). Background inflammation can obscure these cells.

Casts may be noted in urine samples, reflecting damage to the kidneys. There are various types of casts that may be seen – hyaline, granular, and red cell casts (**Figs 11.86–11.88**). They are often accompanied by erythrocytes and debris, as well as by inflammatory cells.

Crystals of different types are frequently seen in urine preparations. These may be matrix-type crystals, composed of proteins which form an organic matrix. These crystals are transparent, but not birefringent (**Fig. 11.89**). Birefringent uri-

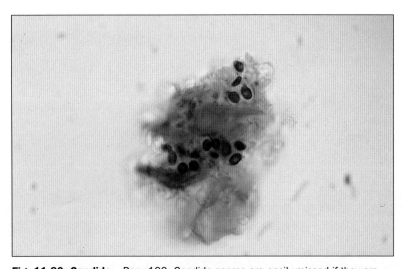

Fig. 11.80 Candida – Pap x100. Candida spores are easily missed if they are unaccompanied by hyphae, as in this view. The spores are overlying some anucleate squames.

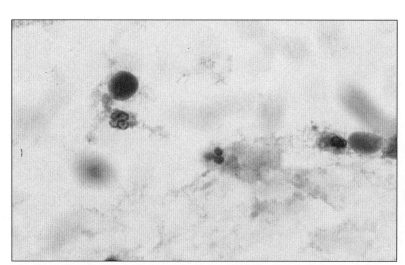

Fig. 11.81 Trichomonas – Pap x100. These pear-shaped organisms are very occasionally seen in urine samples.

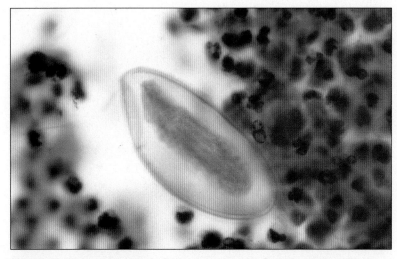

Fig. 11.82 *Enterobius vermicularis* ovum – Pap x100. This urine sample contained numerous neutrophils, histiocytes, and erythrocytes, obscuring much of the cellular detail. This type of pale-staining ovum is liable to be missed in such inflammatory specimens. Note the characteristic convex and flat sides, with one edge folded over.

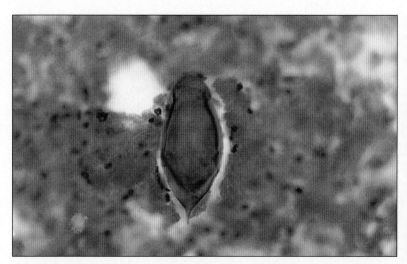

Fig. 11.83 *Schistosoma haematobium* – Pap x40. This heavily blood-stained urine sample contained many schistosome ova, with the terminal spine that characterizes *Schistosoma haematobium*. These ova are much larger than those of *Enterobius vermicularis* and stain mauve as opposed to yellowish orange.

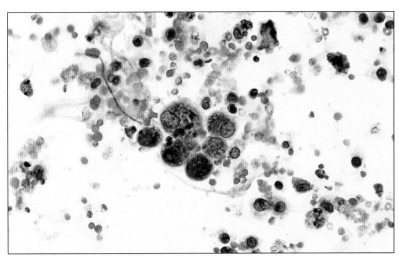

Fig. 11.84 Siderophages – Pap x40. There are several haemosiderin-filled macrophages in this field, accompanied by inflammatory cells and erythrocytes.

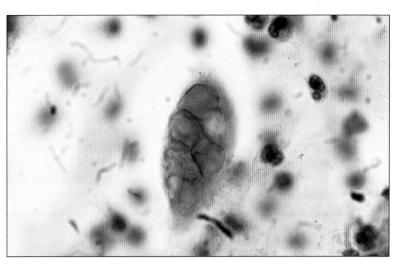

Fig. 11.85 Herpes simplex – Pap x100. This urine specimen contained mostly inflammatory cells with occasional epithelial cells, such as the one illustrated here, exhibiting multinucleation with nuclear moulding and a ground-glass appearance.

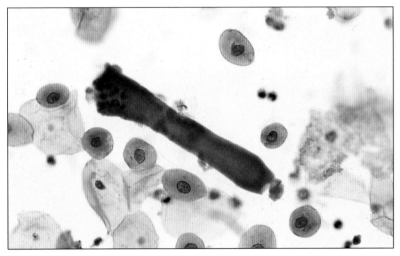

Fig. 11.86 Hyaline cast – Pap x40. This field illustrates a hyaline cast accompanied by deeper layer urothelial cells.

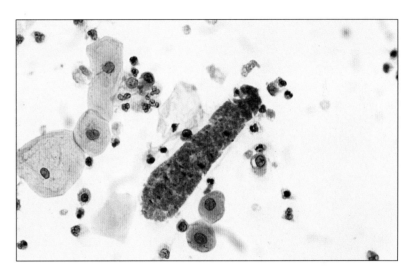

Fig. 11.87 Granular cast – Pap x40. In the centre of this field is a granular cast accompanied by some inflammatory cells and urothelial cells.

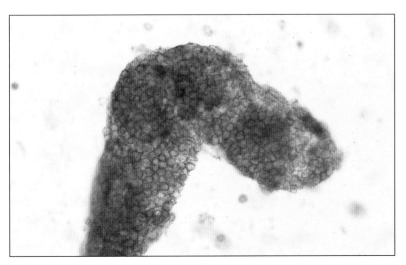

Fig. 11.88 Red cell cast. PAP X40 This large cast is composed of erythrocytes. There are single erythrocytes in the background.

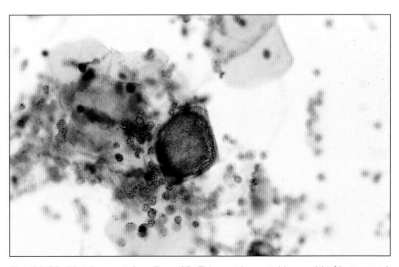

Fig. 11.89 Matrix crystals – Pap x40. This matrix crystal is non-birefringent and is accompanied by erythrocytes and inflammatory cells.

nary crystals that may be seen are cholesterol (**Fig. 11.90**), oxalate, and triple phosphate crystals. Crystals may also be seen in the presence of bladder stones or calculi. Other varieties of unidentifiable crystals are often present and may be related to medication. **Calcium** is very occasionally seen in urine samples (**Figs 11.91, 11.92**).

Calculi are clearly demonstrated on intravenous pyelograms (IVPs) and on cystoscopy. However, cytological changes due to urinary bladder calculi can present problems of interpretation on cytology if the clinical details are not known. The cells in these urine samples may be shed in papillary clusters, mimicking a low-grade urothelial carcinoma (**Fig. 11.93**). They have enlarged, somewhat hyperchromatic nuclei with vacuolar degenerative cytoplasmic changes. The nuclear margins, however, are smooth, the chromatin is clumped evenly (not the irregular clumping and clearing of malignancy), and the borders of the clusters are usually smooth, not ragged (**Fig. 11.94**). It must be remembered, however, that low-grade papillary carcinomas can also have bland, pale nuclei, but they are unlikely to be accompanied by the erythrocytes and inflammatory cells noted with calculi. Single abnormal urothelial cells in the background are seen more frequently with carcinoma than with calculi, but they are reactive or show degeneration only in the latter.

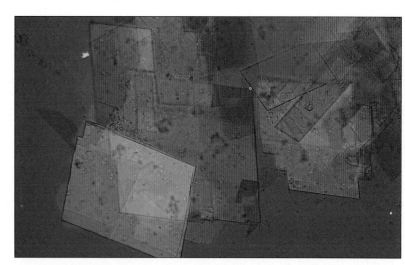

Fig. 11.90 Cholesterol crystals – Polarized light x40. These large envelope-shaped crystals characteristically have a corner chipped off.

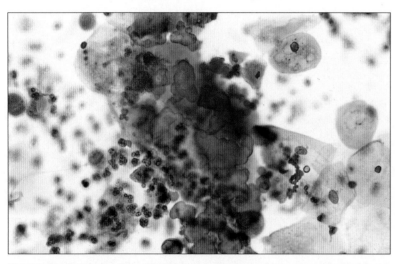

Fig. 11.91 Calcium – Pap x40. This urine sample contains numerous particles of calcium which have stained orange–red. Many inflammatory cells are present.

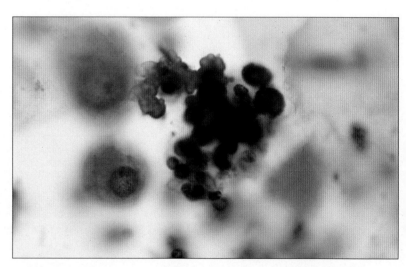

Fig. 11.92 Calcium – Pap x40. In this specimen the calcium stains bluish purple. Both this patient and the one in the case shown in **Figure 11.91** had urinary calculi.

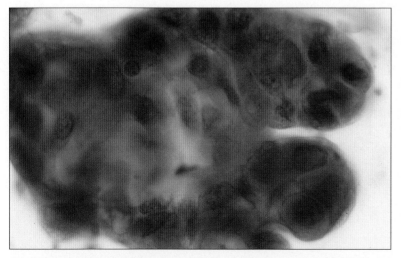

Fig. 11.93 Papillary cluster – Pap x100. This papillary cluster is composed of urothelial cells which show reactive changes, but no malignant features. This should not be interpreted as suspicious of papillary carcinoma, but rather as a result of bladder calculi.

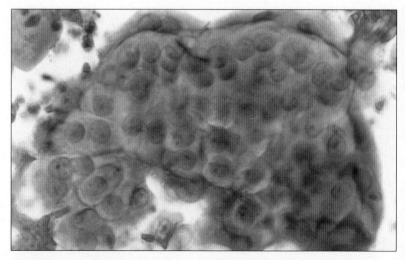

Fig. 11.94 Papillary cluster – Pap x100. This smooth-edged cluster of urothelial cells with bland nuclei and abundant cytoplasm is from the urine of a patient with bladder calculi. Reactive cellular changes may be marked in some cases.

UROTHELIAL CARCINOMA

Cytology is especially useful for detecting malignant cells in the urine; it is part of the work-up of any patient with haematuria. Urothelial neoplasms, formerly referred to as transitional cell carcinomas, can arise at any site within the urothelium – the renal calyces, pelvis, ureters, and bladder. They may be multiple and often recur. These tumours may be papillary, *in situ,* or invasive. *In situ* carcinomas are not always distinguishable on cystoscopy, but the other types are discernible fairly easily. IVPs are another means of identifying tumours other than those *in situ.* Urothelial carcinomas are classified into three grades, grade 1 being the best differentiated and grade 3 the worst.

Grade 1 urothelial carcinoma

Low-grade and papillary carcinomas (also *in situ* neoplasms) tend to show a clean background on cytological examination, unlike the messy background of erythrocytes and inflammatory cells which accompanies high-grade lesions. Papillary carcinomas are usually low-grade. Histological sections of grade 1 carcinoma show urothelium composed of mildly pleomorphic cells, an increase in the number of cell layers being the diagnostic feature **(Fig. 11.95)**. The urine contains numerous bland urothelial cells, many single and others in small clusters **(Figs 11.96,**

11. 97). The clusters usually, but not always, have irregular edges, unlike the smooth-edged clusters of cells seen with bladder calculi. Hyperchromasia is often absent and nucleoli are not prominent **(Figs 11.98–11.100)**, while the background is free from blood and inflammatory cells. The sheer number of cells present should be a warning signal that there may be underlying neoplasia, because normal urine contains very few cells. Yet there may be insufficient criteria for a firm diagnosis of malignancy, in which case the report has to fall into the 'suspicious' category.

Grade 2 urothelial carcinoma

Histologically, these tumours show more atypia than the grade 1 carcinomas do. There is an even greater increase in the number of cell layers in the urothelium, with features of malignancy such as pleomorphism and loss of polarity **(Fig. 11.101)**. The cytological features correspond to the histological appearances, with many moderately pleomorphic urothelial cells exhibiting irregular nuclear outlines and abnormal chromatin, either pale or coarsely clumped **(Figs 11.102, 11.103)**. The cells are usually single **(Fig. 11.104)**, with papillary clusters being relatively uncommon, although small groups of carcinoma cells may be seen **(Figs 11.105, 11.106)**. Blood may be seen in the background, but inflammatory cells are not common.

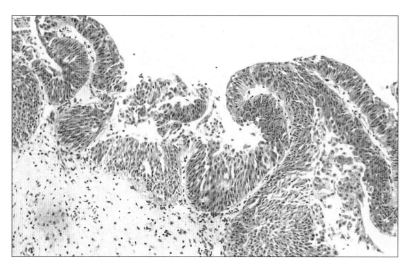

Fig. 11.95 Papillary carcinoma, grade 1 – H&E x10. This section shows a grade 1 papillary urothelial carcinoma with an increased number of cell layers in the epithelium. The cells are mildly pleomorphic and mitoses are not obvious.

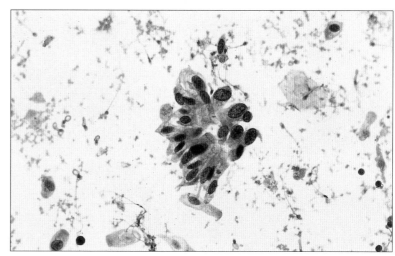

Fig. 11.96 Grade 1 carcinoma – Pap x40. In this field there is a papillary cluster of elongated urothelial cells with mildly pleomorphic, slightly hyperchromatic nuclei. A few single cells are seen in the background. The cells look vaguely columnar and may be mistaken for benign columnar epithelial cells.

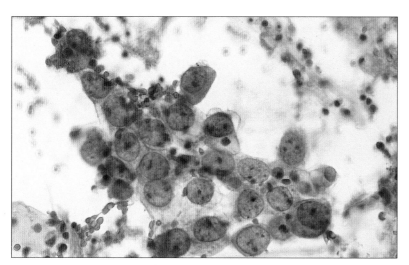

Fig. 11.97 Grade 1 carcinoma – Pap x40. The malignant urothelial cells in this cluster have rounded nuclei (which are uniform in size), small nucleoli, and vesicular chromatin. The edges of the cluster are irregular, not smooth as in clusters of cells seen with calculi.

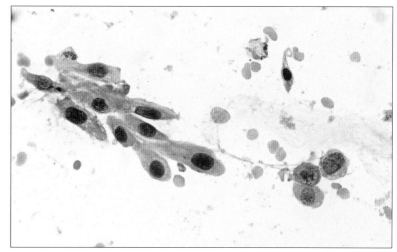

Fig. 11.98 Grade 1 carcinoma – Pap x40. This group of epithelial cells from a grade 1 urothelial carcinoma contains hyperchromatic nuclei, but the cells are mostly uniform in size. They are seen to be quite small when their nuclei are compared with the surrounding erythrocytes. This sort of appearance of elongated cells is common with papillary carcinoma, even when papillary clusters are absent.

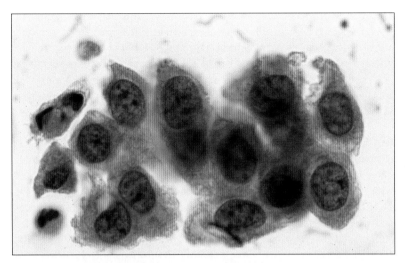

Fig. 11.99 Grade 1 carcinoma – Pap x100. Illustrated is a group of urothelial cells with enlarged, but smooth nuclei and a clumped chromatin pattern. These features are in keeping with a grade 1 carcinoma.

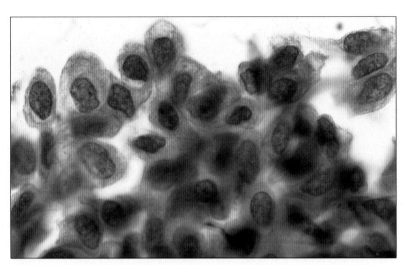

Fig. 11.100 Grade 1 carcinoma – Pap x100. This cellular urine sample is composed of abnormal urothelial cells with enlarged, somewhat irregular nuclear margins and granular chromatin. The appearance is consistent with a grade 1 carcinoma.

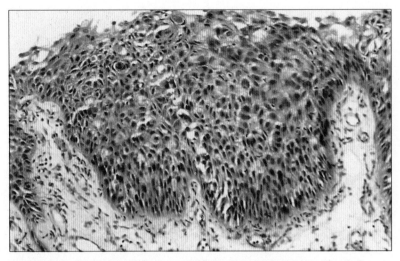

Fig. 11.101 Grade 2 carcinoma – H&E x10. This section shows a grade 2 urothelial carcinoma displaying a marked increase in the number of cell layers and moderate pleomorphism.

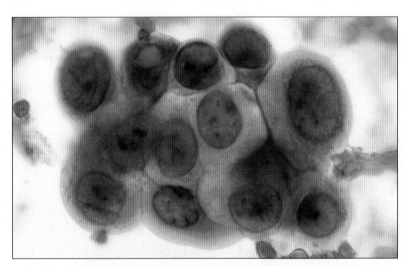

Fig. 11.102 Grade 2 carcinoma – Pap x100. The cells illustrated here have greatly enlarged nuclei with grooves and buds. The chromatin is predominantly pale euchromatin with clumps of heterochromatin.

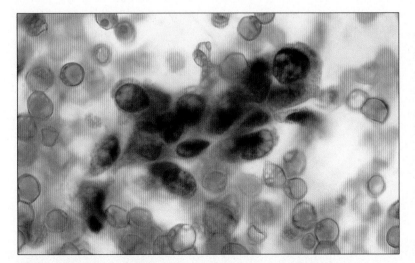

Fig. 11.103 Grade 2 carcinoma – Pap x100. These cells from a grade 2 urothelial carcinoma are small with irregular nuclear margins and clumped chromatin.

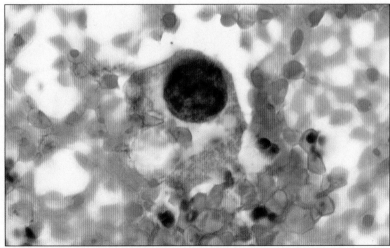

Fig. 11.104 Grade 2 carcinoma – Pap x100. Single cells are often seen in grade 2 carcinomas, as shown here. Note the hyperchromasia and large chromatin clumps.

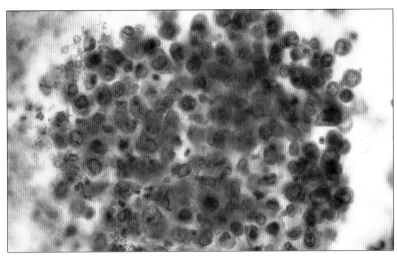

Fig. 11.105 Grade 2 carcinoma – Pap x40. This field shows the pleomorphism that may be seen in grade 2 tumours. Some of the cells have prominent nucleoli.

Grade 3 urothelial carcinoma

These tumours have typical histological features, with many cell layers, loss of polarity, and markedly pleomorphic cells (**Fig. 11.107**). Numerous mitoses may be seen. These tumours are rarely papillary, but are often invasive. Cytological examination of the urine shows much debris, blood, and inflammatory cells admixed with neoplastic cells (**Fig. 11.108**), and sometimes almost obscuring them. The carcinoma cells are often single with bizarre shapes (**Fig. 11.109**), pleomorphism is common, and cell clustering may also occur (**Fig. 11.110**). The cells have irregular nuclear outlines and abnormally clumped chromatin, with areas of parachromatin clearing (**Fig. 11.111**). Mitoses may be present, although not necessarily abnormal in form (**Fig. 11.112**). Spindle-shaped cells and vacuolated cells, almost signet ring in appearance, are often seen (**Figs 11.113, 11.114**).

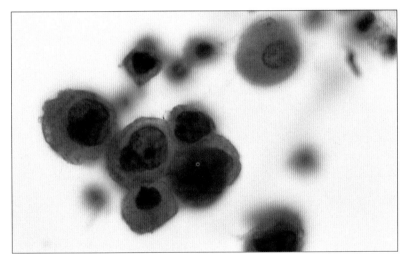

Fig. 11.106 Grade 2 carcinoma – Pap x100. These cells display prominent nucleoli and hyperchromasia. Note the clean background.

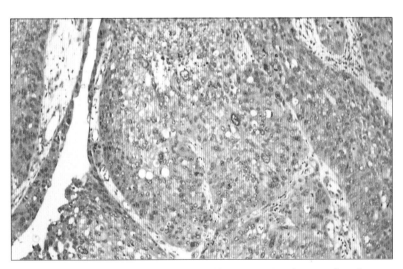

Fig. 11.107 Grade 3 carcinoma – H&E x10. This section shows an invasive grade 3 urothelial carcinoma, with loss of polarity and marked pleomorphism.

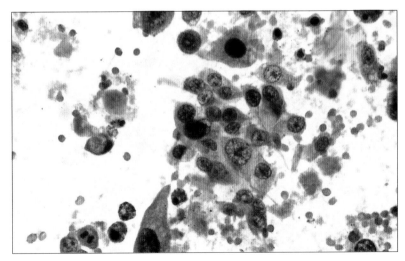

Fig. 11.108 Grade 3 carcinoma – Pap x40. This field is typical of a grade 3 urothelial carcinoma, with extremely pleomorphic malignant cells, and blood and necrotic cellular debris in the background.

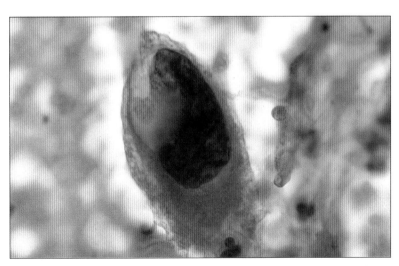

Fig. 11.109 Grade 3 carcinoma – Pap x100. This enormous carcinoma cell contains a huge irregular hyperchromatic nucleus.

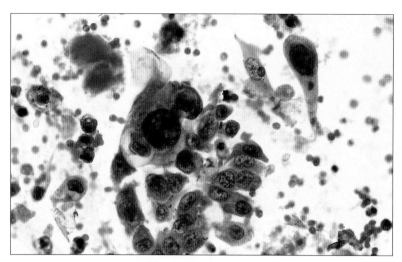

Fig. 11.110 Grade 3 carcinoma – Pap x40. The cells in the group are pleomorphic with prominent nucleoli and clumped chromatin. Degenerate cells and necrotic debris are also seen.

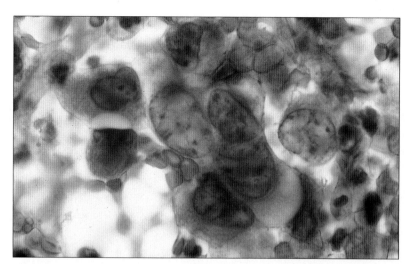

Fig. 11.111 Grade 3 carcinoma – Pap x100. These carcinoma cells have huge nuclei, filling up most of the cell. The chromatin is almost colourless, being composed of active euchromatin. Pleomorphism is obvious and there are inflammatory cells and erythrocytes in the background.

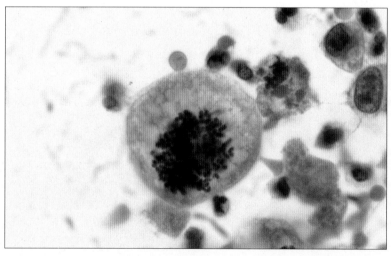

Fig. 11.112 Grade 3 carcinoma – Pap x100. This beautifully preserved mitotic figure is from a case of grade 3 urothelial carcinoma. Some neutrophils and erythrocytes are also visible.

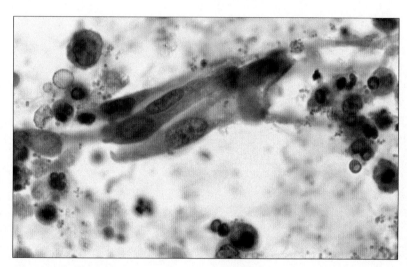

Fig. 11.113 Grade 3 carcinoma – Pap x100. Spindle-shaped neoplastic cells are visible in this field.

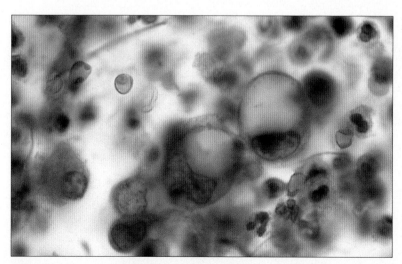

Fig. 11.114 Grade 3 carcinoma – Pap x100. This field shows yet another variation in the morphology of these malignant cells. These cells show vacuolation, with the nucleus being pushed to the periphery to produce a signet-ring appearance.

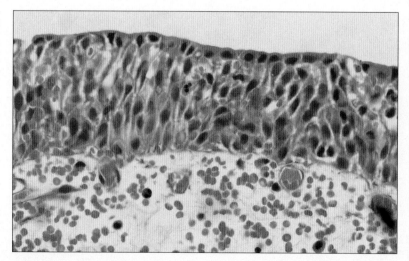

Fig. 11.115 Carcinoma-in-situ – H&E x40. This is a section of carcinoma-in-situ of the bladder. There is loss of polarity, but mitotic figures are not obvious in this field.

Carcinoma-in-situ

This flat lesion varies in thickness on histological sections **(Fig. 11.115)**. It is composed of pleomorphic urothelial cells showing loss of polarity and many mitotic figures. The cytological features in urine include pleomorphic urothelial cells in sheets, with clumped chromatin and irregular nuclei, but the nucleoli may not be prominent **(Fig. 11.116)**. The background is typically clean with none of the blood and debris associated with grade 3 carcinomas, although the cells may look identical **(Fig. 11.117)**. These lesions, as mentioned above, are not always detectable on cystoscopy, so positive cytology should be carefully followed up.

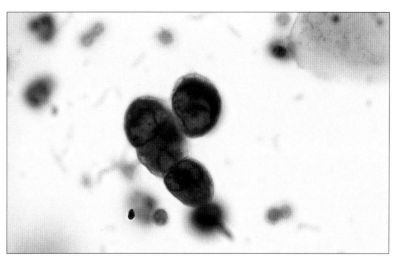

Fig. 11.116 Carcinoma-in-situ – Pap x100. These malignant cells contain large nuclei with abnormal chromatin. The few erythrocytes and neutrophils seen in the background are unusual for this neoplasm.

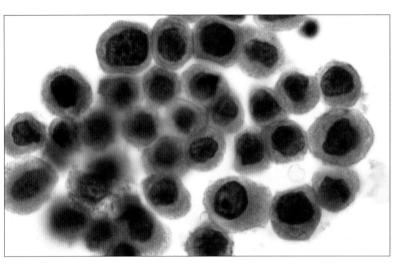

Fig. 11.117 Carcinoma-in-situ – Pap x100. These carcinoma cells contain large, hyperchromatic, irregular nuclei. Note the clean background.

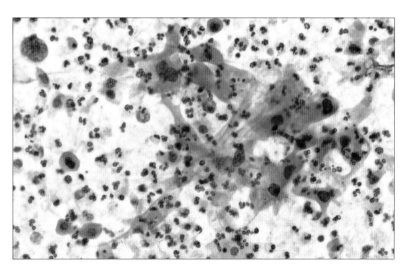

Fig. 11.118 Squamous differentiation – Pap x40. In this field there are keratinized squamous carcinoma cells with an occasional urothelial carcinoma cell. Note the inflammatory background.

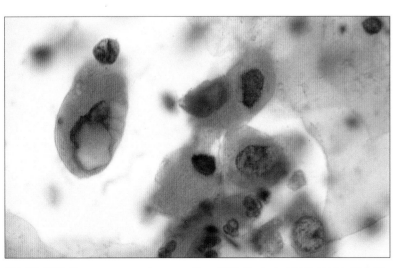

Fig. 11.119 Squamous carcinoma – Pap x100. Illustrated here are keratinized squamous carcinoma cells with bright orange cytoplasm. The appearances are identical in both primary and metastatic squamous carcinoma.

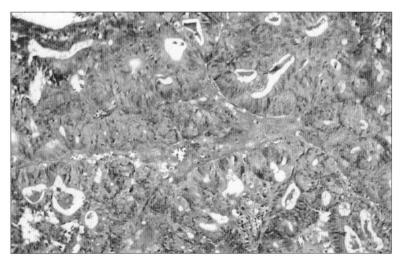

Fig. 11.120 Adenocarcinoma – H&E x10. This section is of a primary adenocarcinoma of the bladder, an uncommon neoplasm at this site.

Urothelial carcinomas may show squamous differentiation and, in such cases, the urine contains a combination of malignant urothelial and squamous cells, the latter with keratinized cytoplasm (**Fig. 11.118**). Pure squamous carcinomas of the bladder are uncommon, but are diagnosed easily from their cytological appearances (**Fig. 11.119**), the only problem being distinguishing them from metastatic squamous carcinoma from the uterine cervix, for example.

Primary **adenocarcinomas** of the bladder (**Fig. 11.120**) are very rare. The cytological features of adenocarcinoma, whether primary or metastatic, include acinar groups and papillary clusters of vacuolated malignant cells with prominent nucle-

oli (**Figs 11.121, 1.122**). Metastatic adenocarcinoma cells from carcinomas of the breast (**Fig. 11.123**), ovary (**Fig. 11.124**), rectum, and prostate have been noted in urine samples. Cells from renal cell carcinomas are seen very rarely in urine.

Cellular changes due to treatment, such as chemotherapy or radiotherapy, are detectable in urine and can mimic malignancy. The cells show bizarre enlargement, both nuclear and cytoplasmic, but the nuclei show degenerative vacuolation, although they may be hyperchromatic (**Fig. 11.125**) or pale and structureless (**Fig. 11.126**). Clinical details should be provided always to eliminate the possibility of false positive reporting.

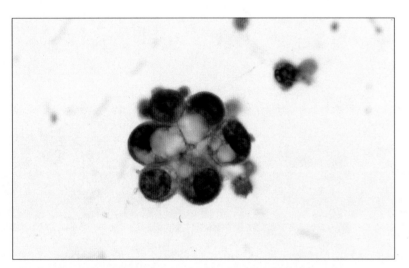

Fig. 11.121 Adenocarcinoma – Pap x100. This is a small cluster of adenocarcinoma cells with vacuoles and peripherally placed nuclei.

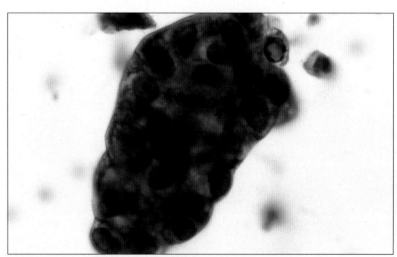

Fig. 11.122 Adenocarcinoma – Pap x100. These cells are from the same case as shown in **Figure 11.121**. The cluster is larger and the cells exhibit honeycomb vacuolation, rather than a single vacuole. They also have prominent nucleoli.

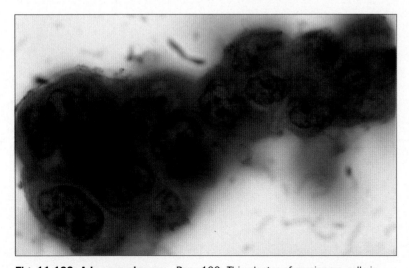

Fig. 11.123 Adenocarcinoma – Pap x100. This cluster of carcinoma cells is from metastatic carcinoma of the breast. There are no distinguishing features which would provide clues as to whether this is primary or metastatic disease.

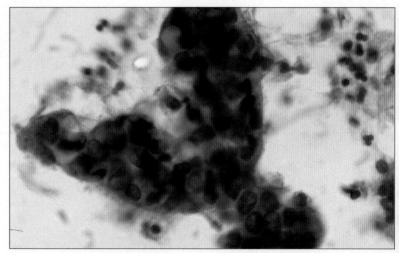

Fig. 11.124 Adenocarcinoma – Pap x63. This papillary cluster of cells shows marked vacuolation, similar to that seen in the primary ovarian carcinoma.

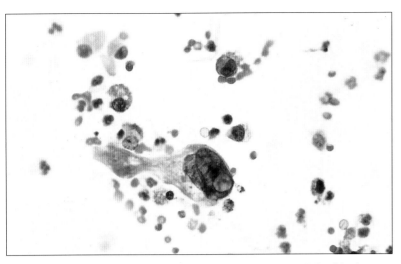

Fig. 11.125 Radiation changes – Pap x100. The large urothelial cell in the centre of the field has an abnormal hyperchromatic, but degenerate nucleus showing vacuolation. This type of change is seen following radiotherapy.

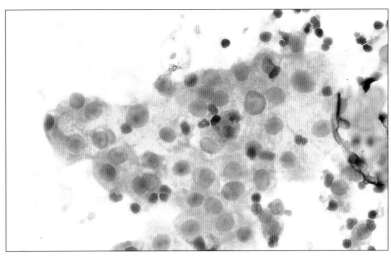

Fig. 11.126 Radiation changes – Pap x40. Illustrated here are the bland, structureless nuclei seen in degenerate cells following radiation treatment.

SUGGESTED READING

Highman W, Wilson E. Urine cytology in patients with calculi. *J Clin Pathol* 1982; **35**: 350–356.

Kannan V, Bose S. Low grade transitional cell carcinoma and instrument artefact: A challenge in urinary cytology. *Acta Cytol* 1993; **37**: 899–902.

McKee G, Trott P. Urinary tract cytology. In: Gray W, ed. *Diagnostic Cytopathology*. Edinburgh: Churchill Livingstone; 1995: 455–478.

Murphy WM. Current status of urinary cytology in the evaluation of bladder neoplasms. *Human Pathol* 1990; **21**: 886–895.

Ro JY, Staerkel GA, Ayala AG. Cytologic and histologic features of superficial bladder camcer. *Urol Clin North America* 1992; **19**: 435–453.

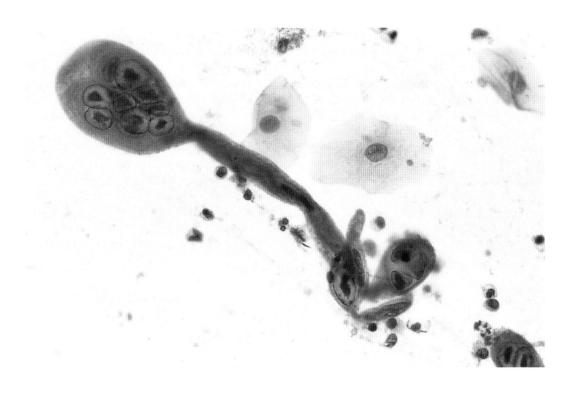

THE RESPIRATORY SYSTEM
AND MEDIASTINUM

12

THE RESPIRATORY SYSTEM AND MEDIASTINUM

Cytology of the respiratory system includes interpretation of cells derived from the trachea, bronchi, bronchioles, and alveoli (**Fig. 12.1**). There are various methods of collecting cytological material – sputum (with its exfoliated cells), bronchial brushings, bronchial washings, and fine needle aspiration of the lung. There are differences in the cytological features of these specimens, which must be taken into account when the material is being screened in the laboratory. Deep cough rather than salivary (which are unsatisfactory) sputum samples should be collected and sent immediately to the laboratory to discourage the overgrowth of fungal and other contaminants. Physiotherapy may be necessary to encourage deep coughing. Bronchial brushings and washings are usually collected before any biopsies are performed to avoid heavy blood-staining.

The brush specimen is spread on one or two glass slides and immediately fixed in alcohol, preferably by immersion to prevent air-drying. Only wet-fixed material is examined routinely, except for fine needle aspirates of the lung of which air-dried smears are also examined. Bronchial washings are processed in the laboratory and wet-fixed smears prepared. If the washings are heavily blood-stained (**Fig. 12.2**), Carnoy's solution may be used to lyse the erythrocytes, usually with excellent results (**Fig. 12.3**).

Fine needle aspiration of the lung is a common diagnostic procedure performed by radiologists for a variety of lesions – cavities or masses within the lung or pleural thickenings. Cytological material is sent to the laboratory in the form of wet-fixed and air-dried smears with needle washings (see Chapter 6).

When it is thought that the aspiration might be difficult, for example, if the lesion is deep-seated or near vital organs, or the patient is too unwell or unwilling for a repeat aspirate to be done later because of inadequate sampling, the cytopathologist or cytotechnologist should be present to assess cellularity.

NORMAL CONSTITUENTS OF RESPIRATORY TRACT SPECIMENS

Mature **squamous cells** from the trachea and larynx are seen frequently in samples from the respiratory tract. The bronchi are lined by respiratory epithelium, which is pseudostratified and contains **columnar epithelial cells** interspersed with **goblet cells** (**Fig. 12.4**), the former often being ciliated. These cells are seen in abundance in bronchial brushings, often in the same pseudostratified arrangement (**Fig. 12.5**), whereas in the other specimens, such as sputum and bronchial washings, a mixture of cell types is present, including macrophages and squamous cells. Fine needle aspirates of the lung usually contain pulmonary macrophages and benign bronchial epithelial often cells, in addition to the lesional cells. Respiratory epithelium often is ciliated (**Fig. 12.6**) and well-preserved ciliated columnar cells are frequently noted in all types of respiratory specimens, especially brushings. These benign cells are usually seen in the form of sheets in brushings (**Fig. 12.7**) and as clusters in bronchial washings. Occasionally, these glandular clusters appear hyperchromatic and therefore suspicious, but under oil immersion cilia are often seen, which confirms their benign nature (**Fig. 12.8**).

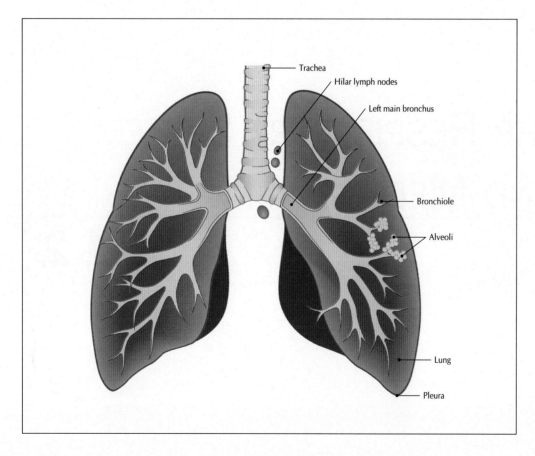

Fig. 12.1 **The respiratory system.**

Trachea
Hilar lymph nodes
Left main bronchus
Bronchiole
Alveoli
Lung
Pleura

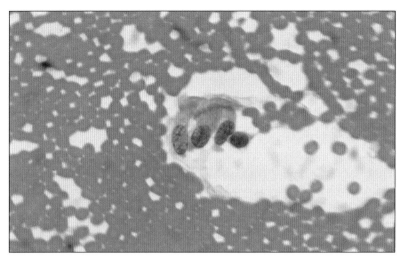

Fig. 12.2 Bronchial wash – Pap x40. This type of heavily blood-stained specimen can be difficult to interpret and is also liable to obscure diagnostic cells. A small group of benign, ciliated, bronchial epithelial cells is shown here.

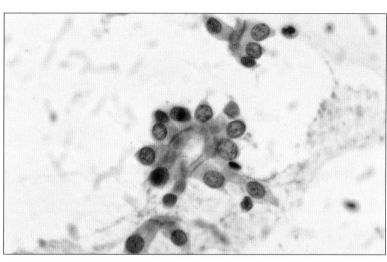

Fig. 12.3 Bronchial wash, Carnoy's solution – Pap x40. This simple procedure ensures that the diagnostic material is visible clearly, as the erythrocytes are lysed and the background becomes clear. The ciliated bronchial epithelial cells in this smear are well-preserved.

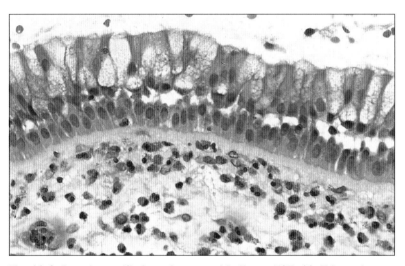

Fig. 12.4 Pseudostratified respiratory epithelium – H&E x10. This section demonstrates the pseudostratifed epithelium that lines the larger bronchi. Note the basal cells just above the stroma, and also the tall columnar and goblet cells, the latter with vacuolated cytoplasm containing mucin. There are large numbers of eosinophils in the submucosa.

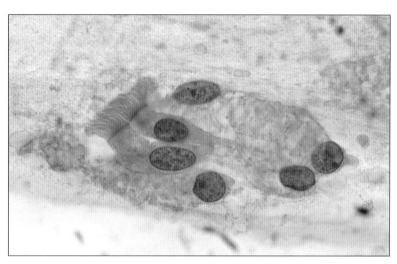

Fig. 12.5 Respiratory epithelial cells – Pap x100. This group of epithelial cells from a bronchial brush specimen exhibits the same arrangement as that seen in the histology (see **Figure 12.2**). The tall columnar cells are ciliated, while the goblet cells contain foamy mucin-filled cytoplasm.

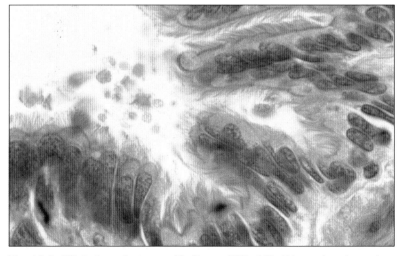

Fig. 12.6 Ciliated respiratory epithelium – H&E x100. This section shows the ciliated, tall columnar epithelial cells lining a bronchiole. No goblet cells are seen.

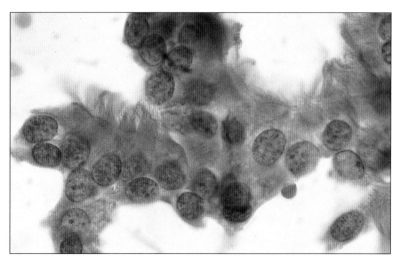

Fig. 12.7 Ciliated bronchial epithelial cells – Pap x100. These tall columnar cells, from a bronchial brush specimen, are wedge-shaped with basal nuclei and long pink cilia.

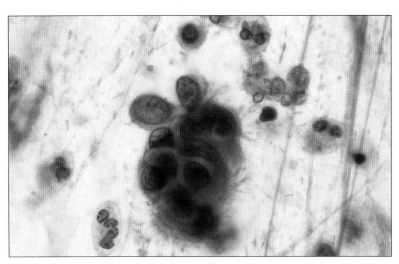

Fig. 12.8 Ciliated bronchial epithelial cells – Pap x100. In bronchial washings the epithelial cells often present as small balls of cells, but the cilia are still evident. The presence of cilia precludes the possibility of malignancy.

Squamous metaplasia is a common occurrence in the respiratory tract, often occurring as a defence mechanism, especially in smokers. Squamous metaplastic cells are exfoliated into sputum and are also seen in bronchial washings. These cells are smaller than mature squamous cells and contain larger nuclei, resulting in an increased nuclear–cytoplasmic ratio. The cytoplasm is fairly dense and may be acidophilic or cyanophilic **(Fig. 12.9)**. These cells should not be considered suspicious or malignant even though they often show some atypia **(Fig. 12.10)**. Benign **squamous pearls** are noted occasionally in bronchial washings **(Fig. 12.11)**.

Mucus is frequently seen in sputum and in bronchial washings and brushings as delicate pale pink or blue wispy material. It may be sometimes be present in bronchial washings in an apparently more solid form, seeming to take on the shape of bronchioles **(Fig. 12.12)**.

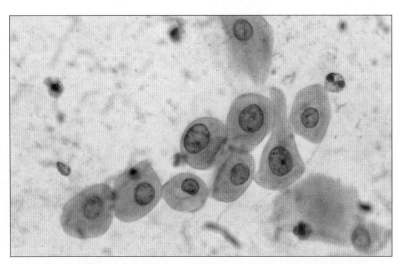

Fig. 12.9 Squamous metaplastic cells – Pap x63. These metaplastic squamous cells are similar to those seen in cervical smears. The nuclear–cytoplasmic ratio is high and the cells may be misinterpreted as being suspicious of malignancy. These cells are frequently seen in bronchial washings and sputum, but are not common in bronchial brushings.

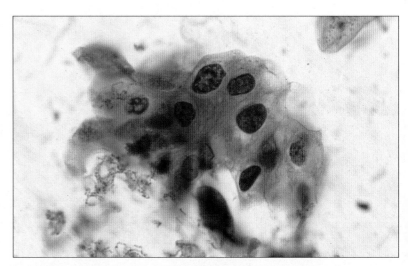

Fig. 12.10 Atypical squamous metaplastic cells – Pap x100. These squamous metaplastic cells in bronchial washings show enlarged, hyperchromatic nuclei, but nevertheless should not be regarded as malignant or even suspicious of malignancy. They are commonly seen in the washings of smokers and in chronic respiratory illnesses.

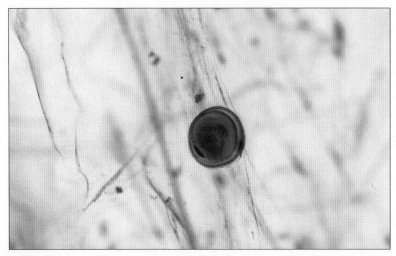

Fig. 12.11 Squamous pearl – Pap x40. These benign whorls of squamous cells are seen frequently in sputum and bronchial washings.

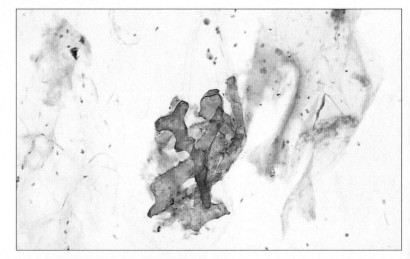

Fig. 12.12 Mucin – Pap x40. The blue mucin seen here in a bronchial wash specimen outlines the shape of tiny bronchioles. Mucin in sputum specimens tends to be more wispy and ill-defined.

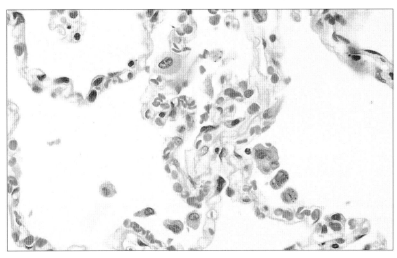

Fig. 12.13 Pulmonary macrophages – H&E x40. This section of normal lung shows alveoli containing free pulmonary alveolar macrophages.

Pulmonary macrophages are present in the alveolar spaces in a normal lung (**Fig. 12.13**) and should be present in a sputum sample for the sample to be deemed satisfactory. These scavenger cells are usually small, with either bean-shaped or round nuclei (**Fig. 12.14**) and delicate foamy cytoplasm, which often contains carbon pigment (**Fig. 12.15**). They are also seen in bronchial washings, but are not common in brushings.

Food debris is unfortunately often seen in sputum samples, sometimes obscuring all other detail. It displays a variety of forms, such as vegetable matter with thickened cellulose membranes (**Fig. 12.16**) and meat showing the typical cross-striations of voluntary muscle (**Fig. 12.17**). Other plant material may also be seen which can be mistaken for hyperchromatic malignant cells (**Fig. 12.18**). The size of the apparent cells and the thick walls are a clue to their foreign nature.

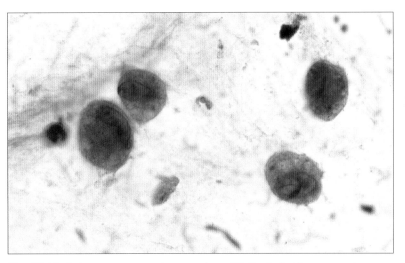

Fig. 12.14 Pulmonary macrophages – Pap x40. Illustrated here are pulmonary macrophages with round to bean-shaped nuclei and abundant vacuolated cytoplasm.

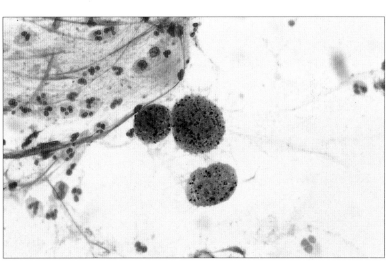

Fig. 12.15 Pulmonary macrophages – Pap x40. The three pulmonary macrophages in the centre of the field contain abundant carbon pigment. These cells are seen frequently in the sputum and bronchial washings of smokers.

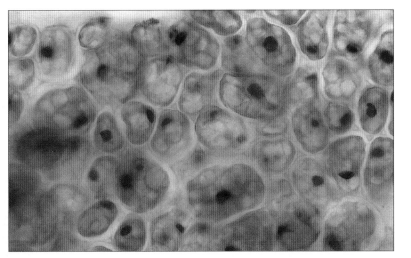

Fig. 12.16 Food debris – Pap x40. This sputum sample contains much vegetable material in the form of large cells with thick cellulose walls.

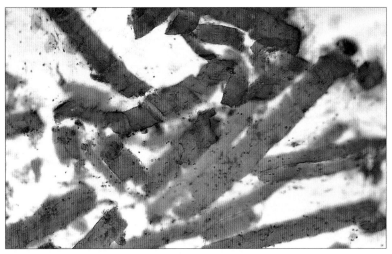

Fig. 12.17 Food debris – Pap x10. These thick fibres are skeletal muscle derived from ingested meat.

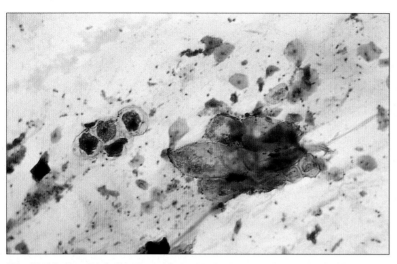

Fig. 12.18 Food debris – Pap x10. In this field there is a cluster of thick-walled, large vegetable cells and a smaller group of structures which appear to be cells with hyperchromatic malignant nuclei. However, these are not human cells as they are much larger than the squamous cells in the background.

INFLAMMATORY PROCESSES

A few **neutrophil polymorphs** are invariably found in normal sputum samples. Large numbers are seen in the sputum of smokers, and they constitute most of the smear in pneumonia and other acute inflammatory conditions. In chronic bronchitis and bronchiectasis, neutrophils and chronic inflammatory cells are seen together with **Curschmann's spirals**, which are mucus casts of bronchioles. These vary considerably in length (**Fig. 12.19**) and consist of a darker inner spiral with a delicate outer layer. Curschmann's spirals are also seen in asthma and may be noted in both bronchial washings and in sputum samples. In inflammatory conditions, reactive bronchial epithelial cells with enlarged nuclei and visible nucleoli are often seen (**Fig. 12.20**). They may be multinucleated (**Fig. 12.21**) and sometimes occur as rounded clusters.

Lung abscess is one of the causes of radiological cavities in the lung which produce a characteristic aspirate that is composed predominantly of neutrophils with some histiocytes and debris. Epithelial cells are found rarely. Material should also be sent for bacteriological examination. A careful search should be made for any evidence of underlying tumour, such as necrotic cellular debris, as inflammatory cells can mask tumour cells.

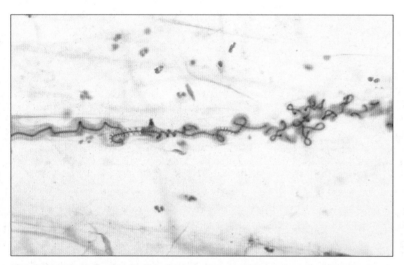

Fig. 12.19 Curschmann's spiral – Pap x10. This Curschmann's spiral is extremely long and coiled, like a length of unravelled knitting yarn. Even at low magnification the darker inner spiral and its pale outer covering are visible.

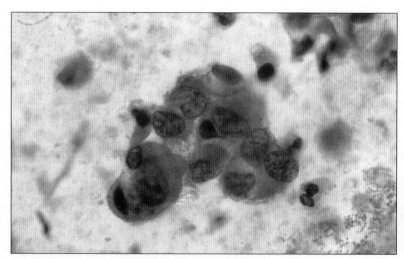

Fig. 12.20 Reactive bronchial epithelial cells– Pap x 100. This is a group of atypical bronchial epithelial cells with varying nuclear size. They are not malignant, however, as cilia are clearly visible.

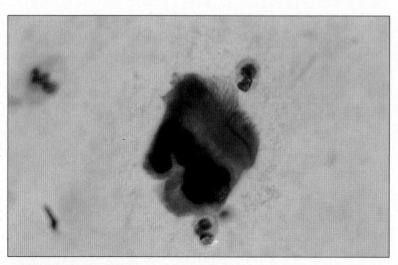

Fig. 12.21 Bronchial epithelial cells – Pap x100. This strip of bronchial epithelial cells shows cilia and multinucleation.

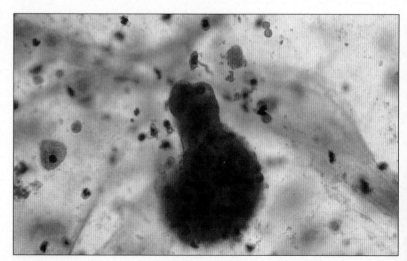

Fig. 12.22 Creola body – Pap x40. This arrangement of bronchial epithelial cells in a ball is seen commonly in bronchial asthma. The cells are all benign.

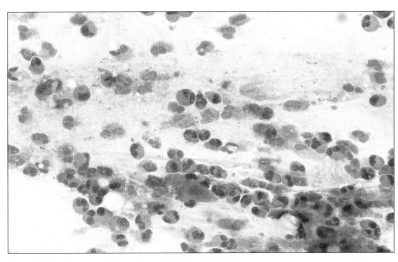

Fig. 12.23 Eosinophils – Pap x40. This field shows a mixture of neutrophil polymorphs and eosinophils. The eosinophils are generally bilobed and show pale, greenish yellow granules.

BRONCHIAL ASTHMA

Bronchial asthma has characteristic features in sputum and bronchial washings. The bronchial epithelial cells are reactive with enlarged nuclei, often in the form of small balls called **Creola bodies (Fig. 12.22)**. Curschmann's spirals may be seen and **eosinophils** often abound **(Fig. 12.23)**. They are difficult to differentiate from neutrophils in Papanicolaou-stained specimens but, if suspected, a smear stained with May Grunwald Giemsa will demonstrate them clearly **(Fig. 12.24)**. **Charcot-Leyden crystals**, which are formed from the granules in eosinophils, are also seen commonly in bright pinkish orange with the Papanicolaou stain **(Figs 12.25, 12.26)**.

ORGANISMS, INFECTIOUS PROCESSES

Candida hyphae and spores are not uncommon in small numbers in sputum samples and may be ignored **(Fig. 12.27)**. If they are present in abundance it usually means the sample has been lying around at room temperature for more than a day before being sent to the laboratory. Candida is seen in large amounts in the bronchial washings of immunocompromised patients.

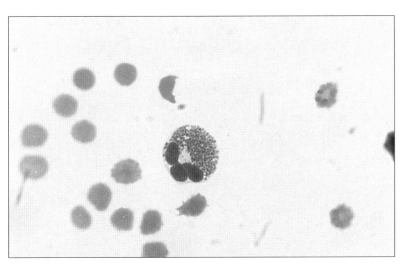

Fig. 12.24 Eosinophil – MGG x100. This eosinophil has a three-lobed nucleus and coarse granules.

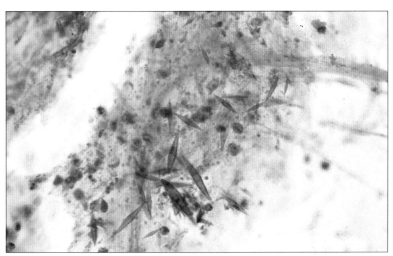

Fig. 12.25 Charcot-Leyden crystals – Pap x40. Illustrated here is a collection of Charcot-Leyden crystals in sputum from a patient with bronchial asthma.

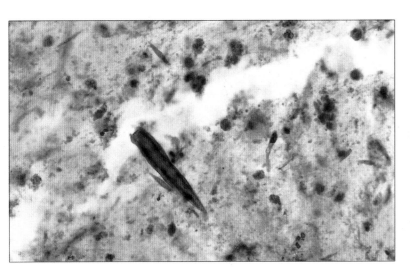

Fig. 12.26 Charcot-Leyden crystals – Pap x40. This field demonstrates the marked variability in size of Charcot-Leyden crystals.

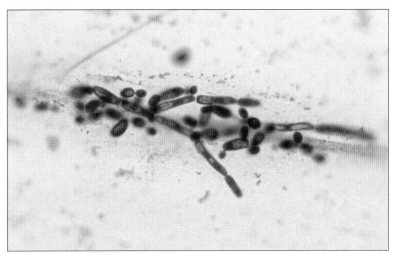

Fig. 12.27 Candida – Pap x100. Candida hyphae and spores are commonly seen in sputum samples.

Viral changes are non-specific. It is suggested that viral infections can produce a cytological feature known as ciliocytophthoria – detachment of the terminal plate with attached cilia from the rest of the bronchial epithelial cell. By itself, this is insufficient evidence of viral infection. **Herpes virus** changes can affect respiratory cells, so ground-glass nuclei with typical inclusions may be seen (**Figs 12.28, 12.29**). Under low magnification these changes may be misinterpreted as malignant.

Tuberculosis is now becoming more common. No characteristic features are seen in sputum, or in bronchial wash or brush specimens, but lung aspirates may be diagnostic. A fine needle aspirate of an involved lung shows epithelioid histiocytes (**Fig. 12.30**), Langhans' giant cells (**Fig. 12.31**), and caseation necrosis. A Ziehl–Neelsen stain usually reveals acid-fast bacilli (**Fig. 12.32**). The differential diagnosis must include sarcoid when only granulomata are seen.

Actinomyces are seen in the form of thick clusters of filamentous organisms (**Fig. 12.33**), which stain bright pink with a PAS stain (**Fig. 12.34**).

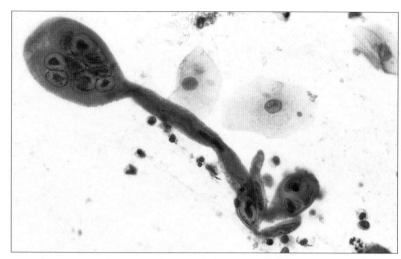

Fig. 12.28 Herpes simplex virus – Pap x40. This huge herpes virus infected cell contains several nuclei with large inclusions.

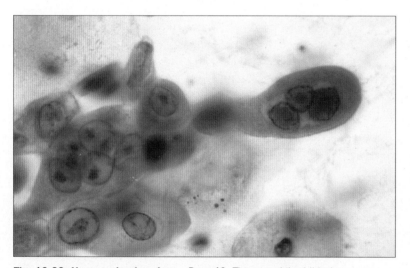

Fig. 12.29 Herpes simplex virus – Pap x40. These nuclei exhibit the characteristic ground-glass appearance seen in such infections.

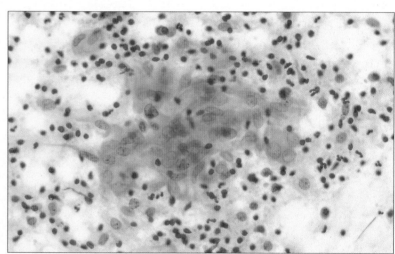

Fig. 12.30 Tuberculosis, epithelioid cells – Ziehl–Neelsen x40. This lung aspirate illustrates a granuloma composed of epithelioid histiocytes in a patient with a cavitating lung mass.

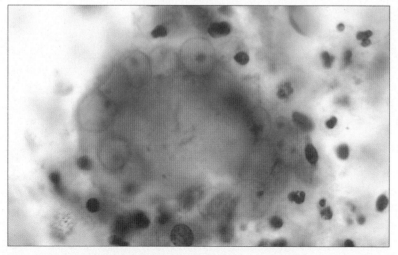

Fig. 12.31 Tuberculosis, Langhans' giant cell – Ziehl–Neelsen x40. This type of giant cell, with peripherally arranged nuclei, is characteristic of tuberculosis.

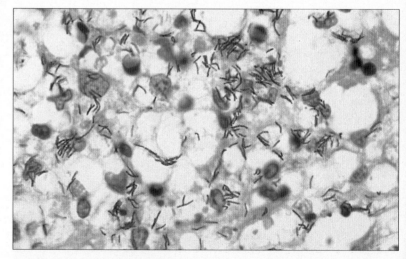

Fig. 12.32 Tuberculosis, acid-fast bacilli – Ziehl–Neelsen x100. This field from the same case as shown in **Figures 12.30** and **12.31** shows numerous, beaded acid-fast bacteria, confirming the diagnosis of tuberculosis.

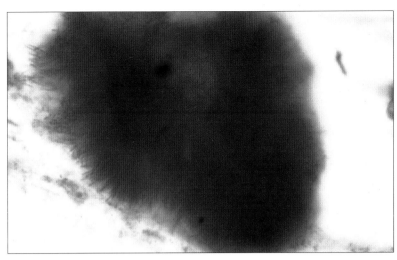

Fig. 12.33 Actinomyces – Pap x100. These organisms may be seen in bronchial washings and show typical colonies with club-shaped filaments at the periphery and small bacillary bodies in the centre.

Aspergillomas are not infrequent in the lung (**Fig. 12.35**). The characteristic wide, flat fungal hyphae with their 45° branches are well-demonstrated in both sputum and bronchial brushings, and also in fine needle aspirates of the lung (**Fig. 12.36**), but the aspergillum is rarely seen as well as it is in histological sections.

Cytomegalovirus infection is another complication seen in immunocompromised patients. The involved cells are large with a single nuclear inclusion surrounded by a halo.

Pneumocystis is an infection which is also rampant in immunocompromised patients. Sputum is not the best material for identifying the cysts, although good results are obtained by using immunofluorescence methods. Bronchial washings are preferable, as the material can be spread thinly on the slide and then stained either with a Grocott or Pap–Grocott stain. The cysts are small, approximately the size of erythrocytes, and are often empty, but may contain a small black speck (**Fig. 12.37**). These cysts are most commonly found in the areas of the smear that contain foamy material.

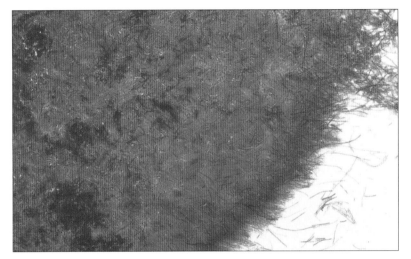

Fig. 12.34 Actinomyces – PAS x100. This stain demonstrates clearly the filamentous structure of these organisms.

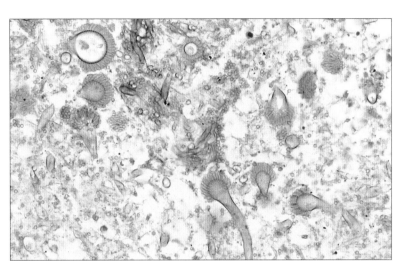

Fig. 12.35 Aspergilloma – H&E x40. This section of lung reveals aspergillus hyphae and several examples of the characteristic aspergillum which gives the fungus its name.

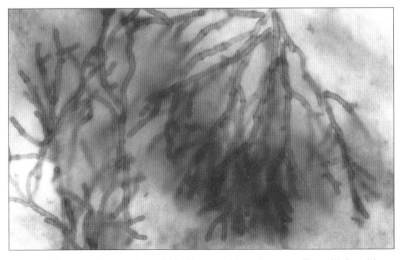

Fig. 12.36 Aspergillus – Pap x100. Illustrated here is aspergillus with its wide hyphae and 45° branching pattern. It is rare to see an aspergillum in cytological samples.

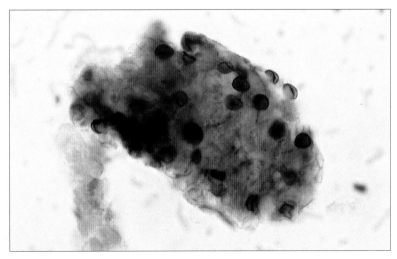

Fig. 12.37 Pneumocystis cysts – Grocott x100. These tiny cysts are approximately the size of erythrocytes and are usually empty. They are difficult to identify on thick smears as there is often much background staining.

NEOPLASMS

Neoplasms of the bronchus and lung may be benign or malignant. They may be diagnosed on sputum, brushings, washings or fine needle aspirate samples. A cellular, well-preserved aspirate is essential for accurate diagnosis. As with other sites it may only be possible to state that an aspirate is malignant without identifying the tumour type, as there is usually insufficient material for special stains.

Hamartomas of the lung usually produce diagnostic material in the form of cartilage or more myxoid material containing spindle cells (**Figs 12.38, 12.39**), fat cells, and benign epithelial cells (**Fig. 12.40**).

Carcinoid tumours (Fig. 12.41) can sometimes present diagnostic difficulties with cytological material. Sputum, bronchial brushings, and bronchial washings often contain no neoplastic cells, even when the tumour is visible on bronchoscopy as the overlying respiratory epithelium may be intact. Fine needle aspirates or washings and brushings taken **after** biopsy produce diagnostic cells.

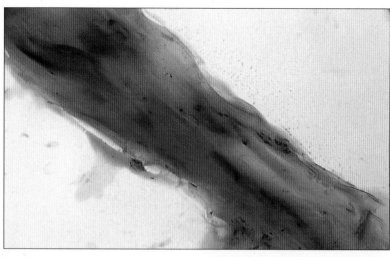

Fig. 12.38 Hamartoma – Pap x10. This lung aspirate contains myxoid material which is pinkish orange with the Papanicolaou stain. No cartilage is seen in this field.

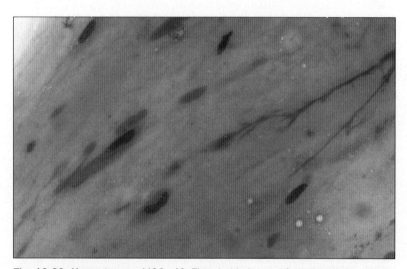

Fig. 12.39 Hamartoma – MGG x40. The air-dried smear from the same case as shown in **Figure 12.38** displays magenta myxoid material within which are spindle cells.

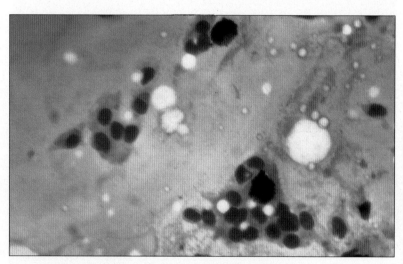

Fig. 12.40 Hamartoma – MGG x63. This field demonstrates benign epithelial cells which form part of the aspirate in a hamartoma.

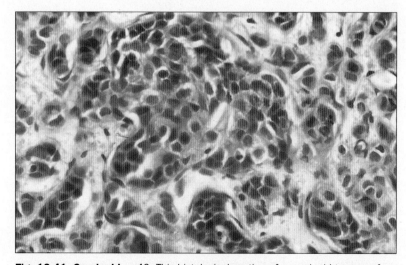

Fig. 12.41 Carcinoid – x40. This histological section of a carcinoid tumour of the lung shows small cells arranged in a trabecular pattern.

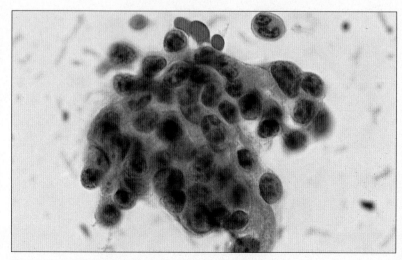

Fig. 12.42 Carcinoid – Pap x100. Illustrated is a cluster of small neoplastic cells with eccentric nuclei and pale blue cytoplasm. The chromatin pattern is speckled and the nuclei are small, just larger than the erythrocytes in the field.

The sample is usually cellular, composed of small cells in clusters (Figs 12.42, 12.43) and acinar groups (Fig. 12.44), but also lying singly. The cells have a plasmacytoid appearance because of their eccentric nuclei, which are round or ovoid. Nucleoli are not prominent and the chromatin pattern is speckled, not unlike that of small cell carcinoma. The cytoplasm is pale and cyanophilic. In air-dried material, the tumour cell clusters are occasionally seen to contain pink-staining material (Fig. 12.45). This neoplasm is characteristically chromogranin and Grimelius positive.

Adenoid cystic carcinoma of the bronchus has similar features to such carcinomas found in the breast and salivary gland (Fig. 12.46). The aspirate is usually cellular, with globules and cylinders of hyaline material surrounded by small neoplastic cells. The hyaline material is best seen in the air-dried smear as it stains bright pink or magenta; on the wet-fixed smear it is pale and may be missed (Figs 12.47, 12.48).

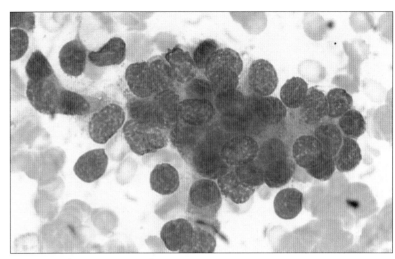

Fig. 12.43 Carcinoid – MGG x100. In air-dried smears, cells from carcinoid tumours show speckled chromatin and very pale cytoplasm, only discernible in the centre of the cluster here. The plasmacytoid appearance of the cells is therefore not visible in these preparations.

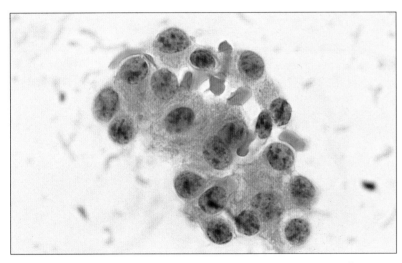

Fig. 12.44 Carcinoid – Pap x100. This field shows small neoplastic cells arranged in a vaguely acinar fashion. The speckled chromatin and eccentric nuclei are well-demonstrated.

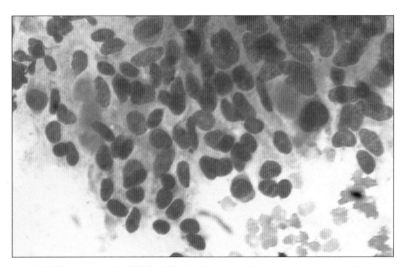

Fig. 12.45 Carcinoid – MGG x100. In this air-dried preparation the nuclei are more spindle-shaped than rounded and small blobs of pink-staining material are evident.

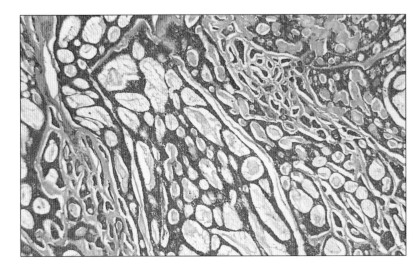

Fig. 12.46 Adenoid cystic carcinoma – H&E x10. This histological section shows the characteristic features of adenoid cystic carcinoma, with cribriform holes filled with hyaline material.

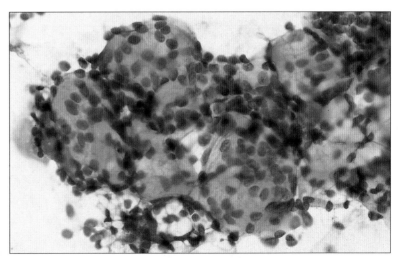

Fig. 12.47 Adenoid cystic carcinoma – Pap x40. This field displays small uniform cells arranged around spheres of pale blue hyaline material. The hyaline material can easily be overlooked on the wet-fixed smear and the diagnosis therefore missed.

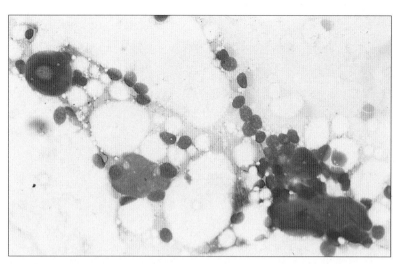

Fig. 12.48 Adenoid cystic carcinoma – MGG x40. The hyaline spheres or globules seen in this tumour stain bright pink or magenta with the May Grunwald Giemsa stain and make the diagnosis obvious.

Muco-epidermoid carcinomas are not common. The aspirate contains two cell types, malignant squamous cells (**Fig. 12.49**) and neoplastic vacuolated glandular cells (**Fig. 12.50**). If the aspirate is composed predominantly of one cell type it is easy to miss the second type and a diagnosis of either squamous or adenocarcinoma may be made.

Squamous cell carcinoma is a common neoplasm of the bronchus (**Fig. 12.51**), which can be diagnosed from sputum, brushing, and washing specimens, as well as on fine needle aspirates. The cellular features are dependent on the differentiation of the tumour. In well-differentiated squamous carcinomas the cells are keratinized with abundant, orange refractile cytoplasm with the Papanicolaou stain (**Fig. 12.52**), which is azure blue on the air-dried smear (**Fig. 12.53**). The nuclei are enlarged, irregular, hyperchromatic, and often pyknotic. The cells are usually single, but may be in sheets or clumps. Much pleomorphism may be seen,

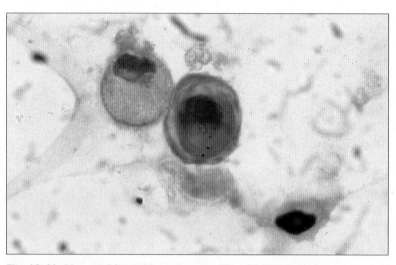

Fig. 12.49 Muco-epidermoid carcinoma – Pap x40. This field shows a keratinized squamous carcinoma cell next to a vacuolated adenocarcinoma cell.

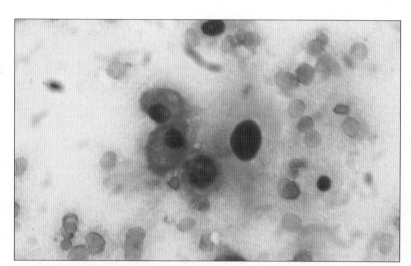

Fig. 12.50 Muco-epidermoid carcinoma – MGG x40. Illustrated here is a small group of vacuolated adenocarcinoma cells adjacent to a squamous cell, which has a hyperchromatic nucleus and pale blue cytoplasm.

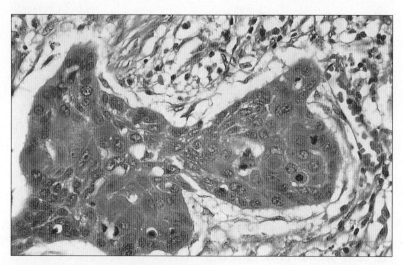

Fig. 12.51 Squamous carcinoma – Pap x25. This section of lung shows a nest of well-differentiated squamous carcinoma cells.

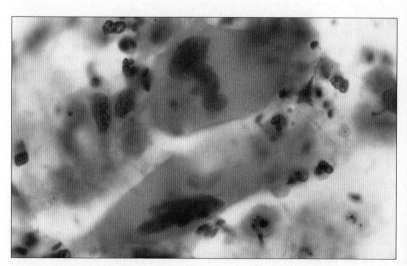

Fig. 12.52 Squamous carcinoma – Pap x100. These are keratinized squamous carcinoma cells with bright orange refractile cytoplasm and irregular hyperchromatic nuclei. This appearance may be seen in any type of cytology specimen – bronchial washings and brushings, sputum, and fine needle aspirates of the lung.

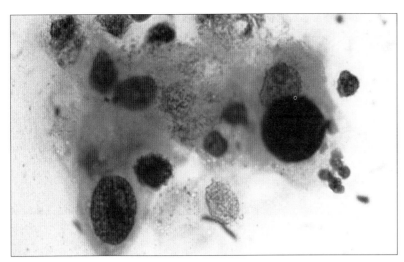

Fig. 12.53 Squamous carcinoma – MGG x100. Keratinized cells exhibit a characteristic shade of blue cytoplasmic staining, as illustrated in these squamous carcinoma cells.

including fibre cells. A clue often noticed when the smear is screened is the presence of ghost cells which are keratinized squames that are either anucleate or show karyolysis **(Fig. 12.54)**. Poorly differentiated tumours contain cells that are often in clusters, with prominent nucleoli and moderate amounts of cytoplasm, which is not keratinized and may be cyanophilic on the wet-fixed preparation **(Figs 12.55, 12.56)**. However, even in poorly differentiated neoplasms, a careful search is often rewarded by finding a few keratinized malignant cells. Fine needle aspirates of squamous cell carcinoma also contain necrotic cellular debris and foamy macrophages which have ingested keratin **(Fig. 12.57)**. The necrotic debris and macrophages may obscure malignant cells and simulate a lung abscess. **Dysplasia** of the bronchial epithelium is difficult to diagnose in cytological material, but can manifest as dyskaryotic squamous cells in sputum and bronchial washings **(Fig. 12.58)**.

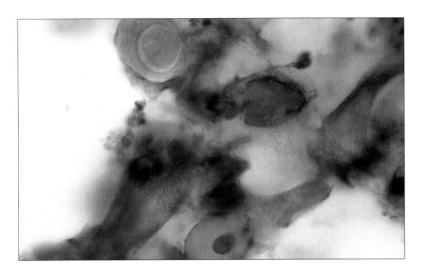

Fig. 12.54 Squamous carcinoma – Pap x100. The orange cell at the top of the field without a nucleus is a 'ghost' cell; it represents a degenerate squamous carcinoma cell.

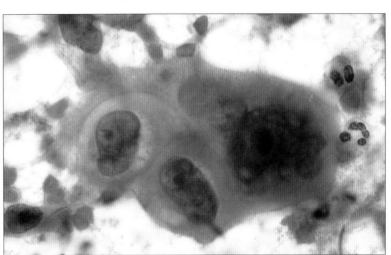

Fig. 12.55 Squamous carcinoma – Pap x100. Non-keratinizing squamous carcinoma cells exhibit dense cyanophilic cytoplasm with sharp cytoplasmic borders. The nuclei of these cells show marked irregularity, hyperchromasia and huge nucleoli.

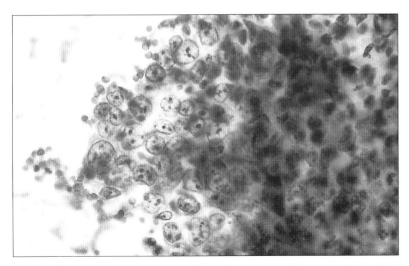

Fig. 12.56 Squamous carcinoma – Pap x40. Another variation in cell type in squamous carcinoma is shown here. The cluster demonstrates pale, almost colourless nuclear chromatin with prominent nucleoli. The cytoplasm is ill-defined. These are features of poorly differentiated squamous carcinoma.

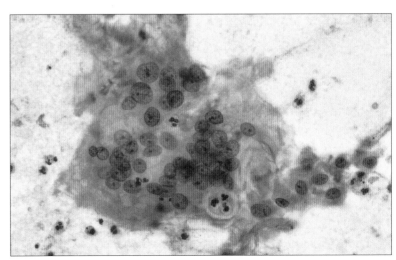

Fig. 12.57 Squamous carcinoma – Pap x40. This field displays a large multinucleated giant histiocyte which has engulfed squamous carcinoma cells, as evidenced by the residual keratin within its cytoplasm. This feature is seen only in fine needle aspirates of squamous carcinoma and lymph nodes with metastatic squamous carcinoma, not in sputum, brushings, or washings.

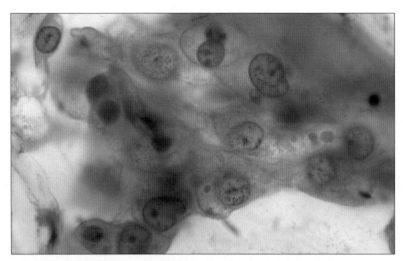

Fig. 12.58 Dysplasia – Pap x100. Dysplastic changes in bronchial epithelium are difficult to diagnose on cytology. The cells seen here are dyskaryotic with abnormal, hypochromatic nuclei, the changes falling short of malignancy.

Adenocarcinoma of the lung (**Fig. 12.59**) may be diagnosed in sputum samples, bronchial brushings and washings, and fine needle aspirates. The tumour cells tend to be in three-dimensional clusters and are usually vacuolated (**Fig. 12.60**). In smaller clusters the nuclei are pushed to the periphery by the large vacuoles (**Fig. 12.61**). The cytoplasm is delicate and the nuclei, which are often rounded but may exhibit varying degrees of irregularity of their margins (depending on the differentiation of the tumour), contain prominent central nucleoli which are often red (**Fig. 12.62**). Single cells (**Fig. 12.63**) are seen infrequently. As in endometrial adenocarcinoma, tumour cells from adenocarcinoma of the lung may exhibit phagocytosis with engulfed neutrophils (see **Figure 12.62**). It is not possible to differentiate between primary and metastatic adenocarcinomas from cytological samples.

Primary **papillary adenocarcinoma** of the lung is not common. The aspirates are cellular with papillary fronds of material, visible even under low power

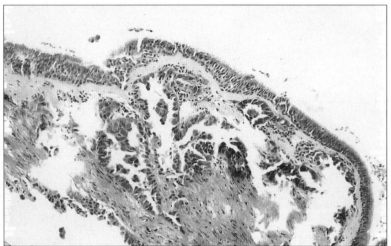

Fig. 12.59 Adenocarcinoma – H&E x10. This bronchial biopsy shows invasive adenocarcinoma beneath an epithelium which is intact in the visible area.

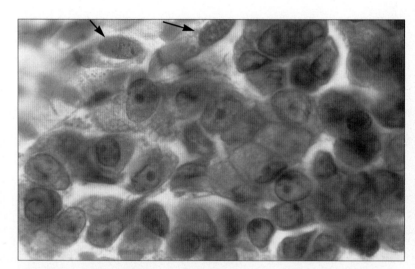

Fig. 12.60 Adenocarcinoma – Pap x100. This smear prepared from bronchial brushings shows a cluster of vacuolated adenocarcinoma cells with large, red central nucleoli and finely vacuolated cytoplasm. Note the two benign bronchial epithelial cells at the top of the neoplastic cluster (arrowed).

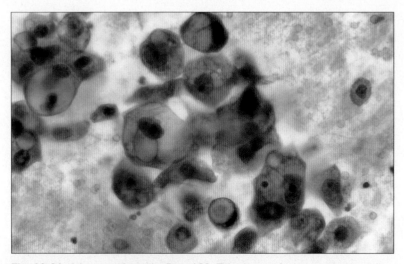

Fig. 12.61 Adenocarcinoma – Pap x100. This cluster of adenocarcinoma cells shows the large vacuoles characteristic of this neoplasm; in many cases these push the nucleus to the edge of the cell. This feature is seen commonly in bronchial washings and sputum samples.

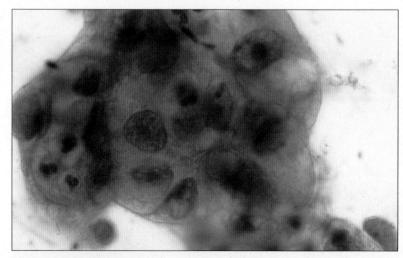

Fig. 12.62 Adenocarcinoma – Pap x100. This bronchial brushing specimen shows large adenocarcinoma cells with vacuoles and huge red central nucleoli. Note the neutrophils that have been phagocytosed by the neoplastic cells.

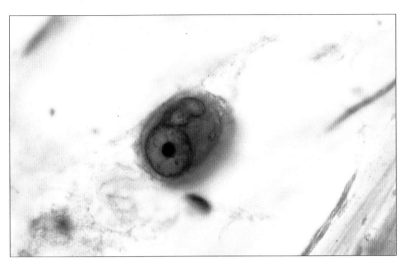

Fig. 12.63 Adenocarcinoma – Pap x100. The adenocarcinoma cell in this field from a bronchial wash sample is unusual in that it is a single cell, rather than in a cluster. The nucleus is abnormal in outline and there is a huge nucleolus.

(Fig. 12.64). The cells in the clusters show features typical of adenocarcinoma, as described above **(Figs 12.65, 12.66)**.

A special type of adenocarcinoma seen in the lung is **bronchiolo-alveolar carcinoma**. The histological section shows a well-differentiated tumours growing along the alveolar walls, composed of either tall columnar or mucin-secreting cells **(Fig. 12.67)**. This tumour has cytological features which are characteristic if they are borne in mind, but otherwise may be missed. The first unusual finding is an abundance of what appear to be foamy or pulmonary macrophages, both single and in loosely associated groups **(Figs 12.68–12.70)**. Clusters of small glandular cells may be noted; these resemble bronchial epithelial cells **(Fig. 12.71)**. On higher magnification these cells are seen to have prominent nucleoli and an abnormal chromatin pattern, as well as cytoplasmic vacuolation **(Fig. 12.72)**. Bronchiolo-alveolar carcinomas may present as clusters of bland, vacuolated cells **(Fig. 12.73)**.

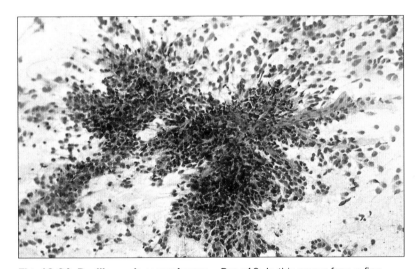

Fig. 12.64 Papillary adenocarcinoma – Pap x10. In this smear from a fine needle aspirate of lung, papillary fronds of cells are clearly visible.

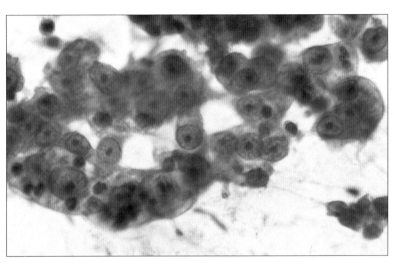

Fig. 12.65 Papillary adenocarcinoma – Pap x63. These cells are from bronchial washings obtained from a patient with papillary adenocarcinoma of the lung. The cells have rounded nuclei with prominent central nucleoli; many phagocytosed neutrophils are also visible.

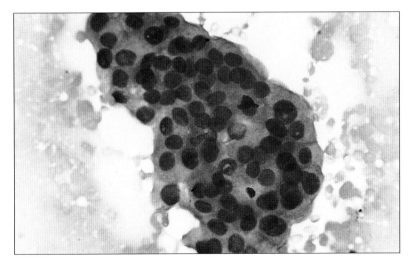

Fig. 12.66 Papillary adenocarcioma – MGG x40. This fine needle aspirate from the same case as shown in **Figure 12.65** contains a cluster of adenocarcinoma cells. Nucleoli are not visible in this preparation.

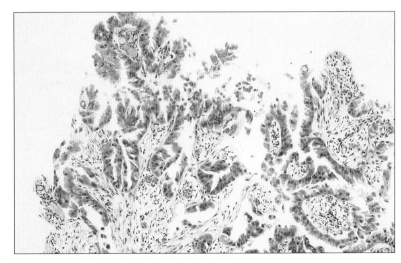

Fig. 12.67 Bronchiolo-alveolar carcinoma – H&E x10. This histological section of lung demonstrates the growth pattern of this tumour, which is composed of tall columnar cells.

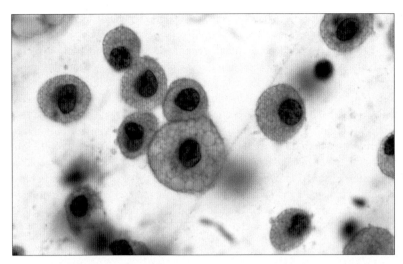

Fig. 12.68 Bronchiolo-alveolar carcinoma – Pap x100. This field, from a bronchial washing smear, demonstrates the cells with relatively small nuclei and abundant foamy cytoplasm which constitute this tumour. They can be mistaken easily for pulmonary macrophages, but do not contain pigment.

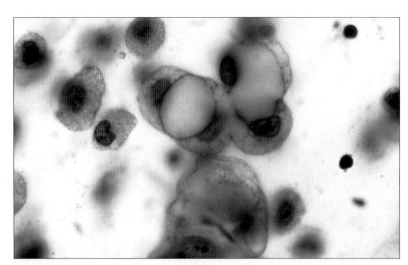

Fig. 12.69 Bronchiolo-alveolar carcinoma – Pap x100. Illustrated are single foamy neoplastic cells, as well as small groups of two to three vacuolated cells (again from a bronchial washing sample).

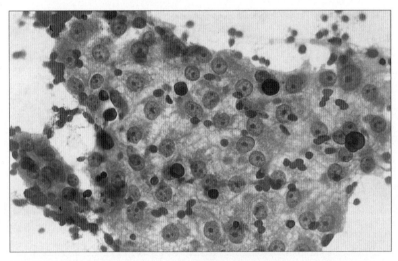

Fig. 12.70 Bronchiolo-alveolar carcinoma – Pap x40. This bronchial brush smear shows a sheet of finely vacuolated cells with abundant cytoplasm, rounded nuclei, and prominent nucleoli. The clustering of cells seen in washings is not apparent here.

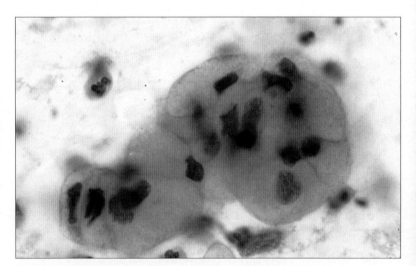

Fig. 12.71 Bronchiolo-alveolar carcinoma – Pap x100. The cells seen here are from a fine needle aspirate of the lung. The neoplastic cells have small nuclei and appear to be distended with mucin, resembling normal bronchial epithelial cells.

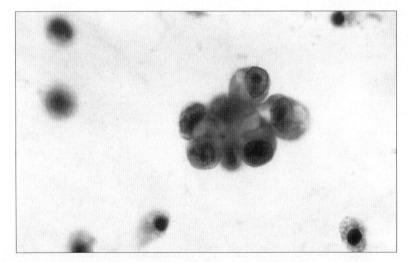

Fig. 12.72 Bronchiolo-alveolar carcinoma – Pap x100. This cluster of tiny cells is characteristic of adenocarcinoma, exhibiting vacuoles and prominent red nucleoli.

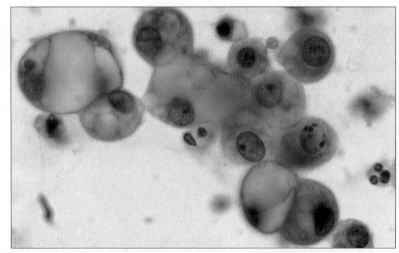

Fig. 12.73 Bronchiolo-alveolar carcinoma – Pap x100. In this variety of bronchiolo-alveolar carcinoma the tumour cells are in clusters with large vacuoles and small, bland nuclei. These cells resemble reactive bronchial epithelial cells, rather than pulmonary macrophages.

Small cell carcinoma (oat cell type) of the lung (**Fig. 12.74**) shows characteristic cytological features. On sputum smears, streaks of small darkly staining tumour cells are seen (**Fig. 12.75**), which (under higher magnification) are approximately the size of lymphocytes, show little or no cytoplasm (**Fig. 12.76**), and exhibit nuclear moulding with a speckled or 'salt and pepper' chromatin pattern (**Fig. 12.77**). Nucleoli are not visible. These cells may be mistaken for lymphocytes unless examined under high power. On bronchial brush specimens, the neoplastic cells are often interspersed with benign bronchial epithelial cells, while in fine needle aspirates, usually only the tumour cells are seen. They may be present in tight or loose clusters (**Fig. 12.78**) and not infrequently show a streak artefact, with the chromatin pulled out of the delicate cells, if the smearing technique is too vigorous. The differential diagnosis includes lymphoma, which does not show nuclear moulding or speckled chromatin and is positive with lymphoid markers, whereas small cell carcinomas are positive with neuroendocrine markers.

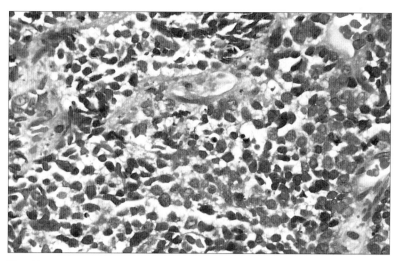

Fig. 12.74 Small cell carcinoma – H&E x10. This section of lung shows the small hyperchromatic cells seen in this neoplasm.

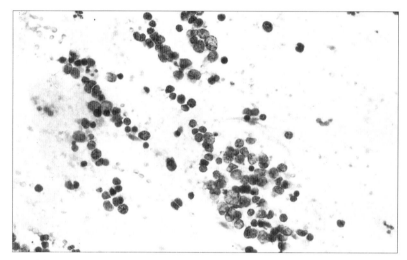

Fig. 12.75 Small cell carcinoma – Pap x10. In this sputum sample the tumour cells are seen in streaks and groups, resembling lymphocytes.

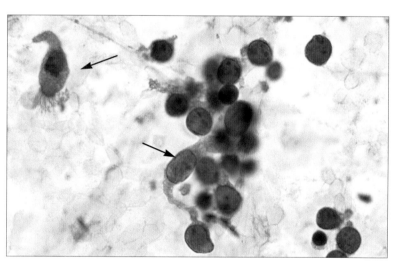

Fig. 12.76 Small cell carcinoma – Pap x100. This field, from a bronchial brush sample, displays small neoplastic cells with nuclei of varying sizes, and two benign, ciliated bronchial epithelial cells (arrowed).

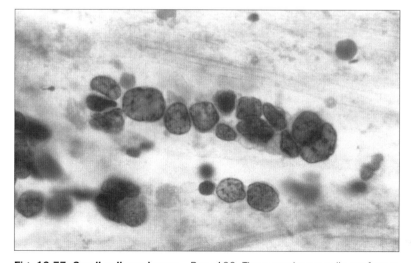

Fig. 12.77 Small cell carcinoma – Pap x100. These carcinoma cells are from a sputum specimen and show moulding of nuclei, as well as speckled, 'salt and pepper' chromatin.

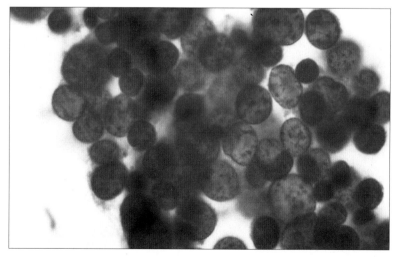

Fig. 12.78 Small cell carcinoma – Pap x100. This cluster of tumour cells does not exhibit moulding, but is composed of neoplastic cells of varying sizes. The speckled chromatin is demonstrated clearly.

The intermediate type of small cell carcinoma has cells which are slightly larger than the oat cell type and contain nucleoli and more cytoplasm (**Figs 12.79, 12.80**). The third variety of small cell carcinoma is the combined type, in which a small cell neoplasm and another tumour, such as squamous or adenocarcinoma, are both present. Following treatment, recurrent small cell carcinomas often show features of the intermediate cell type, namely nucleoli and larger cells.

Large cell undifferentiated carcinoma of the lung yields large carcinoma cells, which are usually in clusters (**Fig. 12.81**), can be pleomorphic with an abnormal

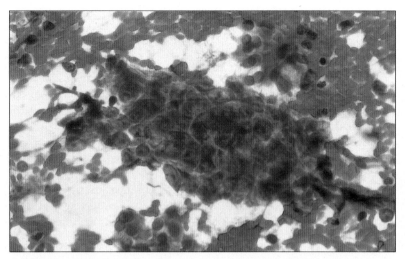

Fig. 12.79 Small cell carcinoma – Pap x40. In this bronchial brush specimen the tumour cells show some evidence of streak artefact due to the vigorous smearing technique. Note the nucleoli in most of the cells, which indicates they are the intermediate type of small cell carcinoma.

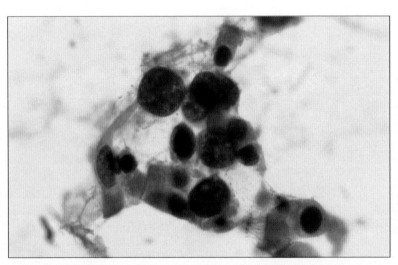

Fig. 12.80 Small cell carcinoma – Pap x100. This smear, prepared from bronchial washings, shows large nuclei in some of the tumour cells. There are a few benign, ciliated bronchial epithelial cells which enable comparison of nuclear size.

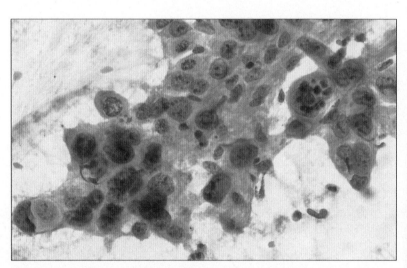

Fig. 12.81 Large cell undifferentiated carcinoma – Pap x40. The cluster of carcinoma cells illustrated here consists of large, pleomorphic cells (compare the nuclear size with the surrounding erythrocytes) with moderate amounts of cytoplasm. The chromatin pattern is abnormal. Neither mucin production nor keratinization are evident.

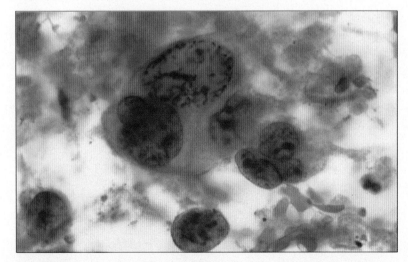

Fig. 12.82 Large cell undifferentiated carcinoma – Pap x100. The cells in this field show marked pleomorphism with irregular nuclear outlines, abnormal clumping and clearing of chromatin, and prominent nucleoli. A mitotic figure is also present.

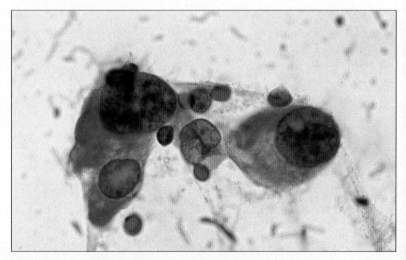

Fig. 12.83 Large cell undifferentiated carcinoma – Pap x100. These cells are from a bronchial brush smear. They have huge nuclei and an abnormal chromatin pattern. The cytoplasmic margins are well-defined, but the cytoplasm is somewhat wispy. Nucleoli are not prominent in these cells.

chromatin pattern (**Figs 12.82, 12.83**), have irregular nuclei with prominent, multiple nucleoli (**Fig. 12.84**), and may contain occasional cytoplasmic vacuoles. The amount of cytoplasm present is variable (**Figs 12.85, 12.86**), but no keratinization or mucin production is seen. Tumour giant cells may be noted occasionally.

Giant cell carcinoma is a variant of large cell undifferentiated carcinoma of the lung (**Fig. 12.87**) and is readily diagnosed on fine needle aspirates. The tumour cells are enormous and pleomorphic, with abundant cytoplasm, irregular, often multiple nuclei, and nucleoli (**Figs 12.87, 12.88**).

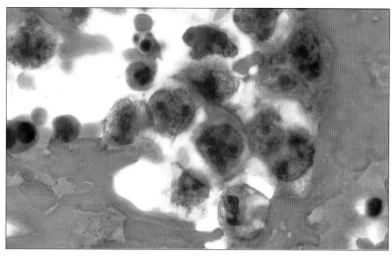

Fig. 12.84 Large cell undifferentiated carcinoma – Pap x100. This sputum sample contains carcinoma cells which have large, multiple nucleoli and abnormally granular chromatin.

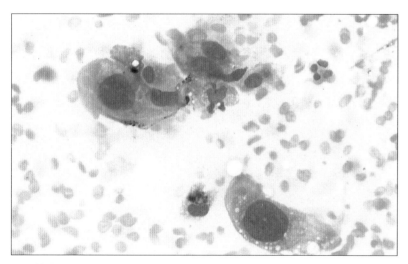

Fig. 12.85 Large cell undifferentiated carcinoma – MGG x100. This fine needle aspirate contains large cells with moderate amounts of cytoplasm. Neither keratinization nor mucin vacuoles are seen.

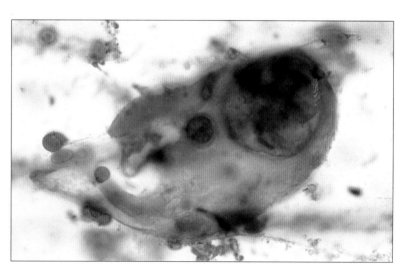

Fig. 12.86 Large cell undifferentiated carcinoma – Pap x100. These neoplastic cells are occasionally single. This cell has abundant cytoplasm and an abnormally pale chromatin pattern.

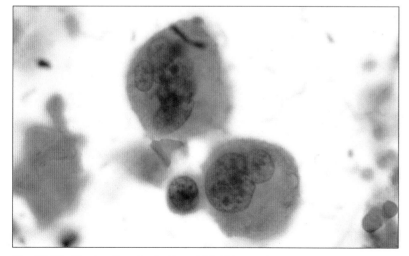

Fig. 12.87 Giant cell variant – Pap x100. This neoplasm, which is a variant of large cell undifferentiated carcinoma of the lung, is composed of huge, often multinucleated, pleomorphic neoplastic cells with abundant cytoplasm, as demonstrated in this fine needle aspirate of the lung.

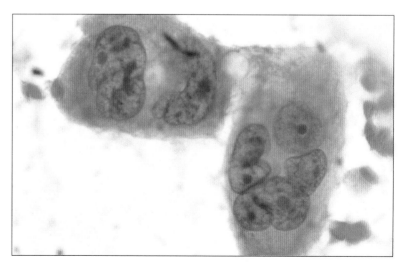

Fig. 12.88 Giant cell variant – Pap x100. The enormous cells shown here are multinucleated, with large red nucleoli and irregular nuclear margins.

Lymphoma of the lung is not uncommon (**Fig. 12.89**). The cytological features depend on the histological type, but in general the cells are fairly uniform with little cytoplasm and are single rather than in clusters (**Figs 12.90, 12.91**). Diagnostic cells may be seen in sputum, as well as in washings, brushings, and aspirates. Hodgkin's disease requires the identification of Reed–Sternberg cells or Hodgkin's cells in the smear (see Chapter 10).

Sarcoma of the lung is a rare entity. The cells in the aspirate are spindle-shaped (**Fig. 12.92**) or pleomorphic, with irregular nuclei showing grooving, budding, and

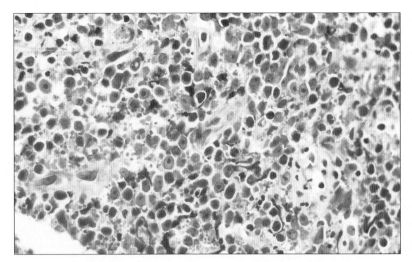

Fig. 12.89 Lymphoma – H&E x40. This bronchial biopsy shows an infiltrate composed of small malignant cells with the features of lymphoma.

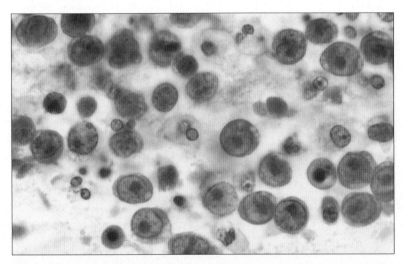

Fig. 12.90 Lymphoma– Pap x100. This sputum sample from the same patient as shown in **Figure 12.89** displays single malignant cells, each of which contains a prominent nucleolus and a small rim of cytoplasm. The cytological features are those of a lymphoma composed of immunoblastic lymphoid cells.

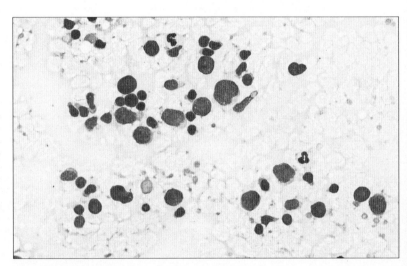

Fig. 12.91 Lymphoma – MGG x40. Illustrated here is a fine needle aspirate of the lung composed of large abnormal lymphoid cells with some scattered small lymphocytes, consistent with the diagnosis of lymphoma.

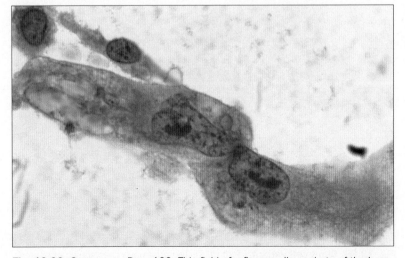

Fig. 12.92 Sarcoma – Pap x100. This field of a fine needle aspirate of the lung shows two enormous, somewhat spindle-shaped cells with delicate cytoplasm and huge irregular nuclei. It is not possible to type sarcomas reliably on cytology.

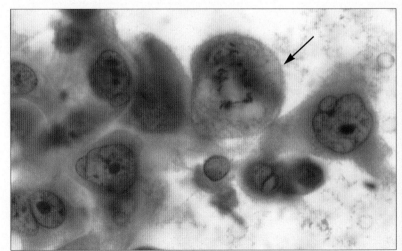

Fig. 12.93 Sarcoma – Pap x100. These cells, which are from the same case as shown in **Figure 12.92**, are more rounded, with very irregular nuclear outlines, pale nuclei with finely granular heterochromatin, and red nucleoli. Note the abnormal mitotic figure (arrowed).

abnormal nucleoli (**Figs 12.93, 12.94**). It is not possible to type sarcomas reliably on cytology. Occasionally, the aspirate produces bland spindle-shaped cells with vesicular chromatin and small nucleoli (**Fig. 12.95**). In such cases a description of the cells with a cytological diagnosis of mesenchymal neoplasm, probably benign, with a recommendation for biopsy, is all that can be expected of the cytopathologist.

Metastatic carcinomas in the lung frequently show typical 'cannon ball' shadowing on radiographs. The more common ones include adenocarcinomas from the breast (**Fig. 12.96**), prostate (**Fig. 12.97**), gastrointestinal tract (**Fig. 12.98**),

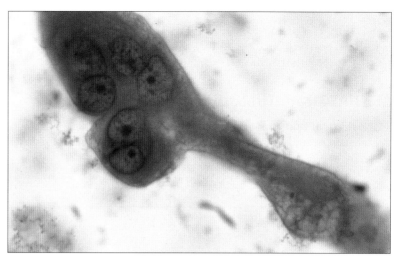

Fig. 12.94 Sarcoma – Pap x100. Sarcoma cells may exhibit bizarre shapes, as illustrated here. The nuclei are clustered at one end of the cell and display the same abnormal chromatin pattern and red nucleoli seen in the rounded cells of **Figure 12.93**.

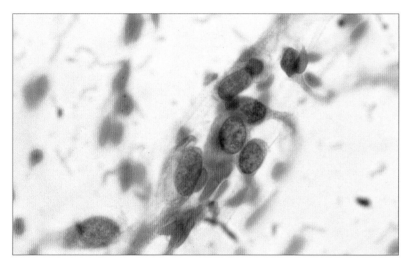

Fig. 12.95 Mesenchymal neoplasm – Pap x40. These spindle-shaped cells contain ovoid, smooth-rimmed nuclei with a bland chromatin pattern. Nucleoli are not prominent. As with sarcomas, histological examination is essential for an accurate diagnosis.

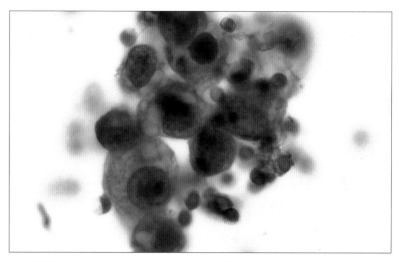

Fig. 12.96 Metastatic breast carcinoma – Pap x100. This bronchial wash specimen contains clusters of adenocarcinoma cells with delicate vacuolated cytoplasm. It is not possible to state the site of the primary tumour from cytological material, but these cells are consistent with spread from adenocarcinoma of the breast. It is always useful to review the primary tumour to establish any cytological similarities.

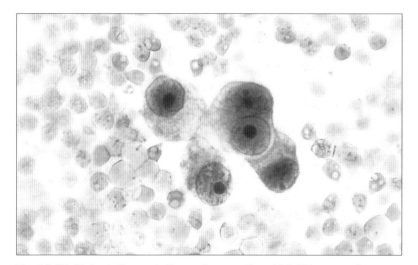

Fig. 12.97 Metastatic prostatic carcinoma – Pap x100. This group of adenocarcinoma cells shows large, red, central nucleoli and granular chromatin. If sufficient material is available, immunocytochemical stains can be performed to confirm the diagnosis of metastatic spread from a prostatic adenocarcinoma.

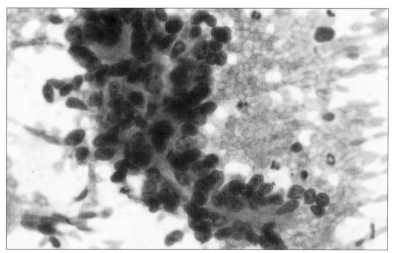

Fig. 12.98 Metastatic colonic carcinoma – Pap x40. This bronchial brush specimen displays a papillary cluster of adenocarcinoma cells. Note the benign columnar epithelial cells in the bottom left corner for comparison of nuclear size. The original colonic carcinoma showed a papillary pattern of growth.

thyroid (**Figs 12.99, 12.100**), melanoma (**Figs 12.101, 12.102**), urothelial carcinoma, renal cell carcinoma (**Fig. 12.103**), and also sarcoma. The features resemble those of the primary tumours (see **Figures 10.48–10.91**).

MEDIASTINAL TUMOURS

Mediastinal tumours include thymomas (epithelial tumours), neuroendocrine neoplasms, germ cell tumours, and thymic lymphomas. Epithelial

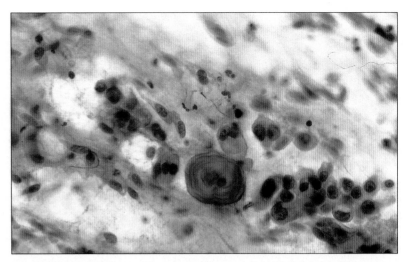

Fig. 12.99 Psammoma body – Pap x40. In the centre of the field in this bronchial brush specimen is a laminated psammoma body surrounded by reactive bronchial epithelial cells.

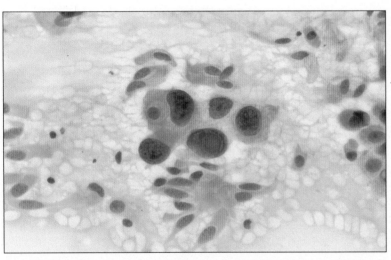

Fig. 12.100 Metastatic adenocarcinoma – Pap x40. Another smear from the same case as shown in **Figure 12.99** contained carcinoma cells, some of which showed intranuclear inclusions. Note the benign bronchial epithelial cells. Distant metastases of papillary carcinoma of the thyroid are rare, but involve the lung when they do occur.

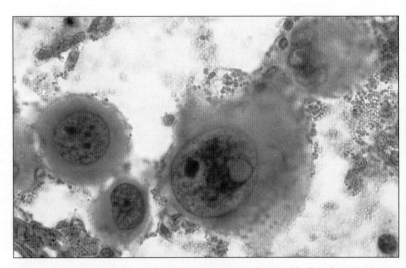

Fig. 12.101 Metastatic malignant melanoma – Pap x100. This fine needle aspirate of a lung mass was composed of large malignant cells with abundant cytoplasm, red nucleoli, and occasional intranuclear inclusions. Even without pigment the features are suggestive of melanoma.

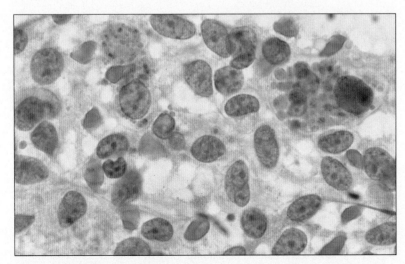

Fig. 12.102 Metastatic malignant melanoma – Pap x100. This is also an aspirate of metastatic melanoma in the lung. These cells contain elongate, ovoid nuclei with visible, but not unduly large, nucleoli and the cytoplasm is indistinct. The clue to the diagnosis here is the melanin pigment.

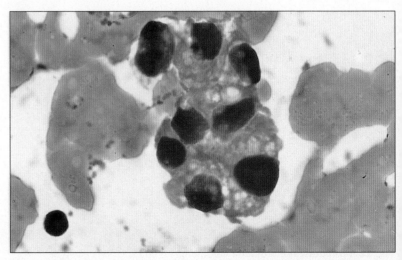

Fig. 12.103 Metastatic renal cell carcinoma – MGG x100. Illustrated here are metastatic renal cell carcinoma cells in a fine needle aspirate of the lung. The cells exhibit the characteristic, finely vacuolated cytoplasm of this neoplasm.

tumours of thymic origin are of various types, one of which is a spindle-cell variety. The neoplasm is composed of spindle cells with fairly bland chromatin and pale cytoplasm (**Figs 12.104, 12.105**). Histological sections confirm the spindle-cell nature of the tumour (**Fig. 12.106**).

The neuroendocrine tumours encountered in the mediastinum include carcinoid (see **Figures 12.42–12.45**) and small cell carcinoma (see **Figures 12.75–12.80**). Germ cell tumours that arise in the mediastinum are seminoma, teratoma (see Chapter 16), embryonal carcinoma and choriocarcinoma. Lymphomas show similar features to those occuring at other sites (see Chapter 10).

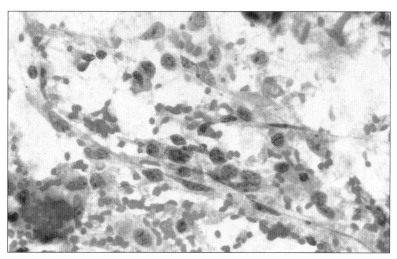

Fig. 12.104 Thymoma – Pap x40. This spindle-cell, thymic epithelial tumour is composed of spindle-shaped cells with delicate cytoplasm and nuclei with vesicular chromatin. A few lymphocytes are seen in the background.

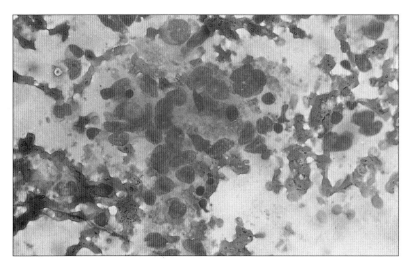

Fig. 12.105 Thymoma – MGG x40. The air-dried preparation of the same case as shown in **Figures 12.104** and **12.106** also shows the spindle-to-ovoid nuclei of this neoplasm, which are much larger in size than the adjacent lymphocytes.

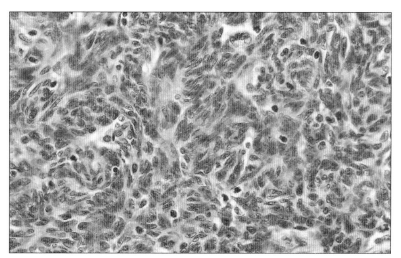

Fig. 12.106 Thymoma – H&E x10. The histological section of the case illustrated in **Figures 12.104** and **12.105** demonstrates the spindle cells comprising this neoplasm.

SUGGESTED READING

Anderson C, Ludwid ME, O'Donnell M, Garcia N. Fine needle aspiration cytology of pulmonary carcinoid tumours. *Acta Cytol* 1990; **34**: 505–510.

Gray W. Normal respiratory tract and inflammatory conditions. In: Gray W, ed. *Diagnostic Cytopathology*. Edinburgh: Churchill Livingstone; 1995: 13–68.

Hirsch FR, Matthews MJ, Aisner S, *et al*. Histopathologic classification of small cell lung cancer: Changing concepts and terminology. *Cancer* 1988; **26**: 973–977.

Johnston WW, Frable WJ, eds. *Diagnostic Respiratory Cytopathology*. New York: Masson; 1979.

Sterrett G, Frost F, Whittaker D. Tumours of lung and mediastinum. In: Gray W, ed. *Diagnostic Cytopathology*. Edinburgh: Churchill Livingstone; 1995: 69–127.

Tao LC, Griffith–Pearson P, Coper JD, *et al*. Cytopathology of thymoma. *Acta Cytol* 1984; **28**: 165–170.

Tao LC, Sanders DE, Weisbrod GL. Value and limitations of transthoracic and transabdominal fine needle aspiration cytology in clinical practice. *Diagn Cytopathol* 1986; **2**: 271–276.

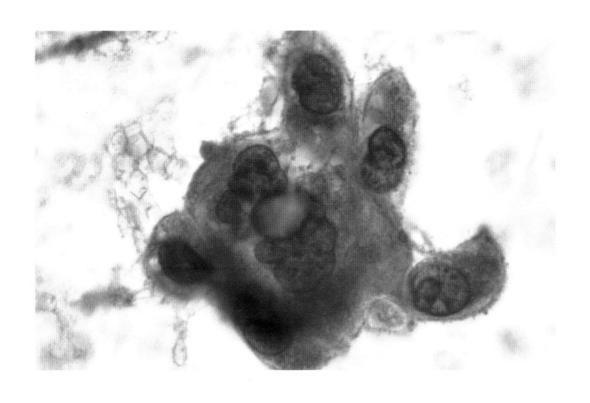

LIVER, PANCREAS, SPLEEN AND ADRENAL GLANDS

13

LIVER

Fine needle aspirates of the liver are now commonplace, performed by radiologists using image-guided techniques. The presence of a pathologist or a cytotechnologist to prepare the smears to check cellularity (see Chapter 6) is extremely useful, as the procedure can be complicated. As with fine needle aspirates from other sites, both wet-fixed and air-dried smears, together with the needle washings, are sent to the cytology laboratory.

Normal liver cells (hepatocytes) are often seen, even in aspirates from abnormal areas in the liver. The cells show the same features on cytology as they do on histology (**Fig. 13.1**) and are often seen in small sheets, but also as single cells. They are large and polygonal with abundant granular cytoplasm, which usually stains pale blue with the Papanicolaou stain and pale purple with May Grunwald Giemsa. Hepatocytes contain a single central nucleus or, not infrequently, two nuclei. The nucleus has a sharp, well-defined margin and a prominent nucleolus, which is often red on the wet-fixed smear. The cells have clearly defined cytoplasmic borders (**Figs 13.2, 13.3**). Normal hepatocytes can appear pleomorphic with fairly marked variation in the size of the nuclei. Intracytoplasmic bile pigment is often seen, which is greenish yellow with the Papanicolaou stain (**Fig. 13.4**) and dark bluish green with May Grunwald Giemsa (**Fig. 13.5**). Extracellular bile may also be present (**Fig. 13.6**). Kupffer cells are noted occasionally among groups of hepatocytes. They are cells of macrophage–monocyte derivation which line the sinusoids in the liver (**Fig. 13.7**). Normal liver aspirates also contain small, flat sheets of benign ductal cells, which are much smaller than hepatocytes, and are uniform with round nuclei and vesicular chromatin (**Figs 13.8, 13.9**). They do not contain bile pigment.

Reactive liver cells may be seen in the aspirate when the needle is inserted into the periphery of a lesion rather than within it. The hepatocytes appear more pleomorphic than do normal liver cells and are often binucleate, with enlarged nuclei, very prominent nuclear margins, and large red nucleoli (**Fig. 13.10**). Intranuclear inclusions (intranuclear cytoplasmic invaginations) are frequently seen. The cytoplasm is abundant and granular, and the cells can appear more worrying than those of a well-differentiated hepatocellular carcinoma (see **Figure 13.15**).

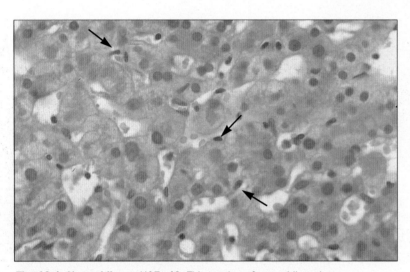

Fig. 13.1 Normal liver – H&E x40. This section of normal liver shows hepatocytes arranged in cords. Note the variability in nuclear size and the occasional Kupffer cell in the sinusoids (arrowed).

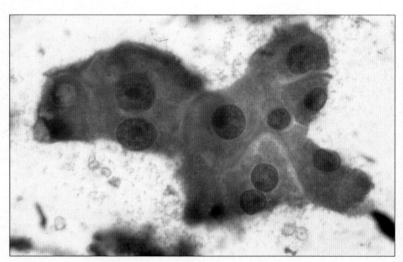

Fig. 13.2 Hepatocytes – Pap x100. This group of benign hepatocytes displays variation in nuclear size, abundant granular cytoplasm, and prominent nucleoli, all of which are normal features for these cells. Note the sharp cytoplasmic borders between adjacent cells.

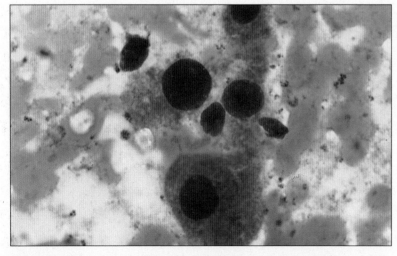

Fig. 13.3 Hepatocytes – MGG x100. This field shows benign hepatocytes with granular cytoplasm, nuclei of variable size, and intracytoplasmic pigment.

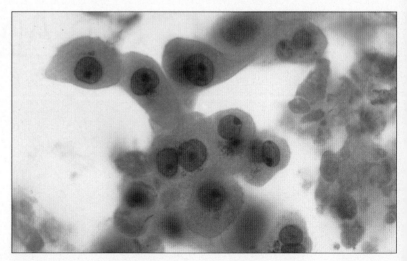

Fig. 13.4 Hepatocytes – Pap x100. The hepatocytes illustrated here have pale blue cytoplasm containing yellowish green bile pigment. Note the clearly defined nuclear and cytoplasmic margins and the prominent nucleoli in these benign cells.

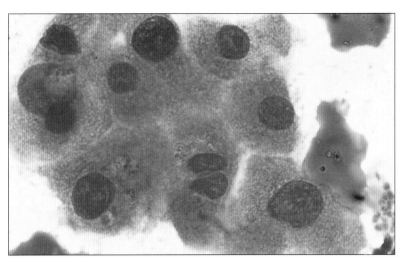

Fig. 13.5 Hepatocytes – MGG x100. This air-dried preparation shows benign hepatocytes with abundant granular cytoplasm and intracytoplasmic bluish black bile pigment. The nucleoli are not as clearly defined in air-dried smears.

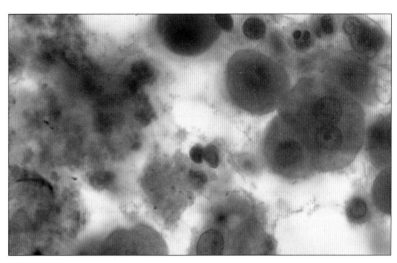

Fig. 13.6 Bile pigment – Pap x100. In this field there are single hepatocytes, some containing intracytoplasmic bile pigment, also masses of extracellular greenish yellow pigment.

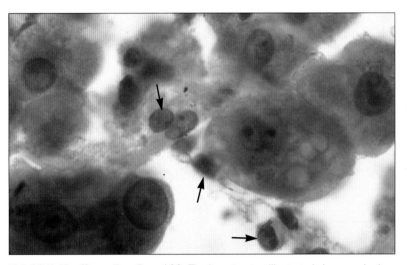

Fig. 13.7 Kupffer cells – Pap x100. The hepatocytes illustrated show marked variation in nuclear size and some have vacuolated cytoplasm. Kupffer cells are the small cells (arrowed) between the hepatocytes.

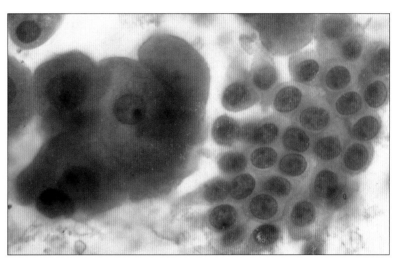

Fig. 13.8 Bile duct cells – Pap x100. Bile duct cells are small cells with uniform rounded nuclei, usually arranged in flat sheets. Their nuclear margins are sharply defined and they may exhibit honeycombing on changing focus in a well-fixed preparation (as do endocervical cells). Note how much smaller the bile duct cells are than hepatocytes.

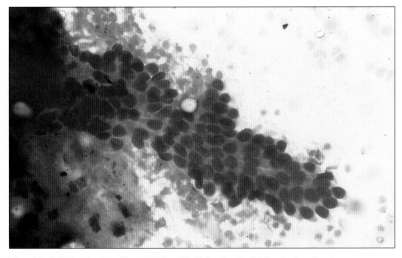

Fig. 13.9 Bile duct cells – MGG x40. This sheet of bile duct cells shows uniformity of nuclear size and shape, but the nuclear details are not clear in this air-dried preparation. The nuclei are slightly larger than the surrounding erythrocytes.

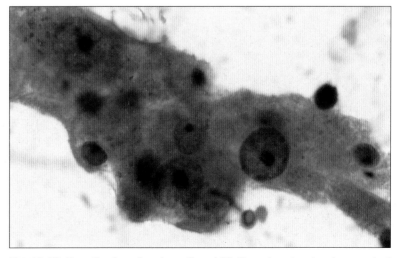

Fig. 13.10 Reactive hepatocytes – Pap x100. These hepatocytes show marked variation in nuclear size, with huge red nucleoli but no evidence of malignancy.

Aspirates from liver that shows **fatty change** contain hepatocytes with vacuoles, which may be large or small (**Fig. 13.11**), but which otherwise resemble normal hepatocytes with clearly defined nuclear margins and prominent nucleoli.

The radiological appearances of a **liver abscess** are characteristic, aspirates being taken for confirmation of the diagnosis. The aspirate consists of thick pus, some of which should be sent for microbiological examination. The smears are composed of large numbers of polymorphs and small histiocytes, with debris and erythrocytes in the background. Few hepatocytes are seen. If a hydatid cyst is mistaken for an abscess and aspirated, typical scolices and hooklets may be seen (**Figs 13.12, 13.13**). Amoebic abscesses, which are rarely aspirated, contain abundant inflammatory cells and blood, with amoebae.

Hepatocellular carcinomas (hepatomas) are primary liver neoplasms (**Fig. 13.14**) which vary in their differentiation; well-differentiated tumours may be very difficult to diagnose on cytology. The cells are often seen in three-dimensional clusters (**Fig. 13.15**), as well as singly (**Figs 13.16. 13.17**). They may be

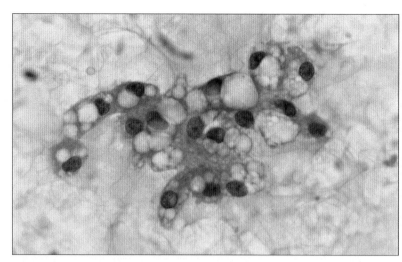

Fig. 13.11 Fatty change – Pap x40. This cluster of hepatocytes shows vacuolated cytoplasm with much variation in the size of the vacuoles. The nuclei show the characteristics of benign hepatocyte nuclei with visible nucleoli.

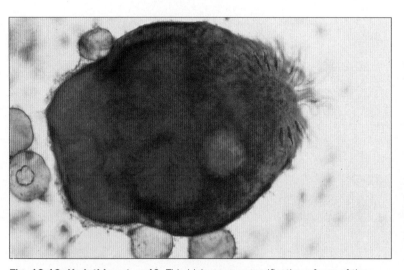

Fig. 13.12 Hydatid cyst – x40. This high-power magnification of one of the scolices seen in a smear of 'hydatid sand' from a hydatid cyst of the liver illustrates clearly the hooklets used for attachment to tissues.

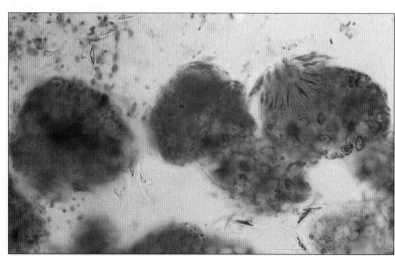

Fig. 13.13 Hydatid cyst – x40. In this field there are several scolices with attached hooklets, and also free hooklets in the background.

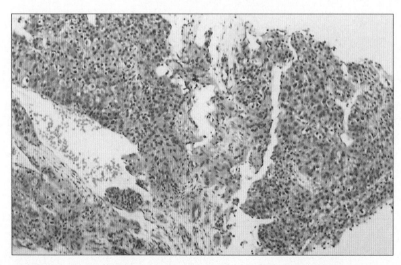

Fig. 13.14 Hepatocellular carcinoma – H&E x10. This section of liver shows a hepatocellular carcinoma displaying the usual trabecular pattern of growth.

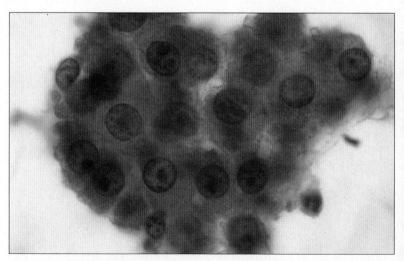

Fig. 13.15 Hepatocellular carcinoma – Pap x100. Illustrated here is a cluster of hepatocytes which show an increased nuclear–cytoplasmic ratio. The nuclei are rounded, but some of them are huge and irregular, some cells have multiple nucleoli, and the chromatin pattern is abnormally clear with granules of heterochromatin.

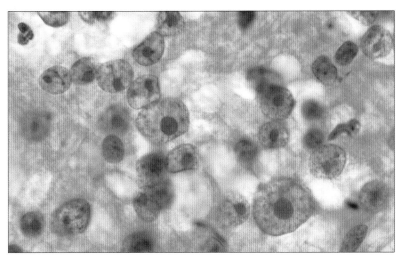

slightly enlarged, with prominent nuclei and nucleoli, or pleomorphic, the pleomorphism being more obvious with the less differentiated neoplasms. Intranuclear inclusions are usually present **(Fig. 13.18)**. The neoplastic cells often contain bile pigment, which differentiates them from cholangiocarcinoma cells; careful examination may reveal endothelial cells at the periphery of some of the cell clusters **(Fig. 13.19)**. The sharp intercellular borders seen in benign groups of hepatocytes may be absent in clusters of hepatoma cells. Biliary ductal cells are rarely seen. Hepatomas composed of signet ring cells rarely occur and, while these are readily diagnosed on histology **(Fig. 13.20)**, the aspirate may be mistaken for a metastatic deposit of signet ring cell adenocarcinoma **(Fig. 13.21)**. **Fibrolamellar hepatocellular carcinoma** occurs in young males **(Fig. 13.22)**; the cytological appearances can be diagnostic, with tumour cells in clusters **(Fig. 13.23)** and showing features such as intranuclear inclusions **(Fig. 13.24)** and the characteristic stromal fragments **(Fig. 13.25)**.

Fig. 13.16 Hepatocellular carcinoma – Pap x100. The cells in this fine needle aspirate are pleomorphic with indefinite cellular borders, almost forming a syncytial group. The nucleoli are very variable in size and the chromatin pattern is granular.

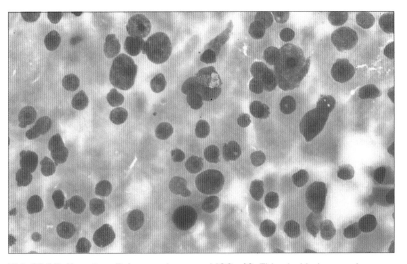

Fig. 13.17 Hepatocellular carcinoma – MGG x40. This air-dried smear is composed of cells showing great variability in nuclear size, but they are still recognizable as hepatocytes. Their cytoplasmic margins are indistinct.

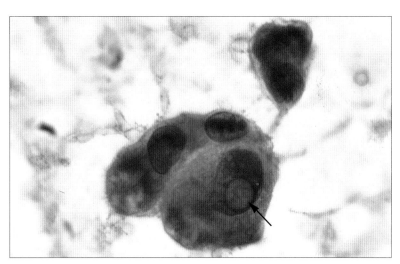

Fig. 13.18 Hepatocellular carcinoma – Pap x100. These pleomorphic cells have irregular nuclei, unlike the usually round nuclei of hepatocytes, and show hyperchromasia. The cytoplasm retains a granular appearance and a large intranuclear inclusion is present (arrowed).

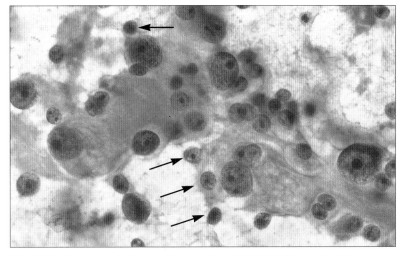

Fig. 13.19 Hepatocellular carcinoma – Pap x100. This liver aspirate is composed of bizarre hepatocytes in a syncytial type of arrangement. The nuclei are extremely variable in size and the cytoplasm is foamy, rather than granular. The small nuclei at the edge of the group may represent endothelial cells (arrowed).

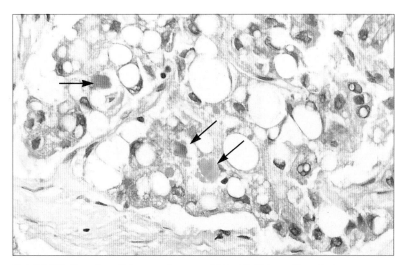

Fig. 13.20 Hepatocellular carcinoma – PAS x10. This section shows an unusual variant of hepatocellular carcinoma composed of signet ring cells. The clear spaces in the cells are not due to glycogen. Note the PAS-positive alpha-1-antitrypsin globules in some of the cells (arrowed).

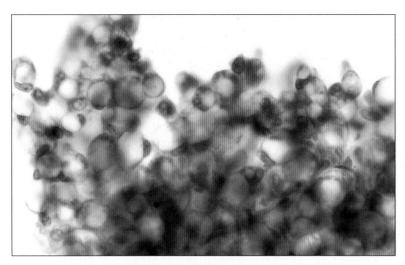

Fig. 13.21 Hepatocellular carcinoma – Pap x40. This aspirate is from the same case as shown in **Figure 13.20**. The cells display a signet ring pattern without features of hepatocytes, mimicking metastatic signet ring cell adenocarcinoma.

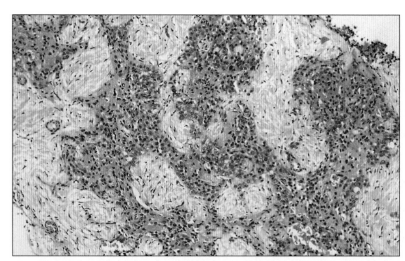

Fig. 13.22 Fibrolamellar hepatocellular carcinoma – H&E x10. This section exhibits the mixture of neoplastic cells and lamellar fibrous stroma which typify this tumour.

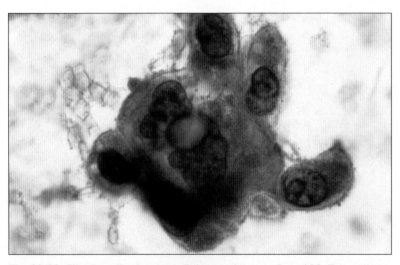

Fig. 13.23 Fibrolamellar hepatocellular carcinoma – Pap x100. This aspirate from the same case as shown in **Figures 13.22** and **13.24** contains pleomorphic cells with irregular budding of the nuclear margins and hyperchromasia. The cytoplasm retains some of the granularity of hepatocytes.

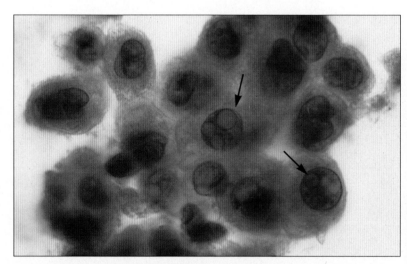

Fig. 13.24 Fibrolamellar hepatocellular carcinoma – Pap x100. These cells, from the same case as shown in **Figures 13.22** and **13.23**, demonstrate the sometimes multiple intranuclear inclusions (cytoplasmic invaginations) seen in neoplasms of the liver (arrowed). Most of the nuclei have irregular margins.

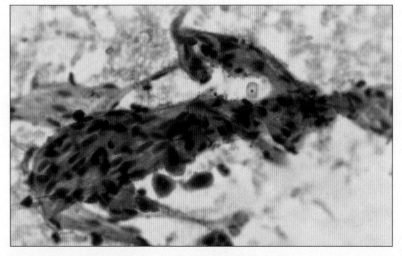

Fig. 13.25 Fibrolamellar hepatocellular carcinoma – Pap x40. Illustrated in this field is a stromal fragment, characteristic of this tumour.

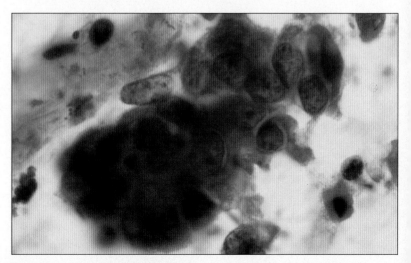

Fig. 13.26 Cholangiocarcinoma – Pap x100. This cytological sample was obtained by fine needle aspiration and shows a cluster of adenocarcinoma cells with foamy cytoplasm, granular chromatin, and small nucleoli. Neither intracytoplasmic bile pigment nor the typical central red nucleoli of hepatocytes is evident.

Cholangiocarcinomas are composed of malignant ductal cells which are much smaller than hepatocytes. Aspirates show clusters of adenocarcinoma cells which display mild to moderate pleomorphism, and also single malignant cells (**Figs 13.26, 13.27**). No bile pigment is seen within the cells, the cytoplasm is not abundant or granular, and intranuclear inclusions are not a feature (**Fig. 13.28**). Reactive hepatocytes may also be present in these aspirates. It is not possible to distinguish cholangiocarcinoma from metastatic adenocarcinoma in the liver.

Other biliary tract lesions may be sampled by brushings or aspiration for cytological diagnosis. Bile is occasionally sent to the cytology laboratry, to be examined for malignant cells. Normal bile duct cells are columnar (**Fig. 13.29**) and may show honeycombing when seen in sheets (**Figs 13.30, 13.31**). These samples may also contain abundant bile pigment (**Fig. 13.32**) and cuboidal glandular cells from bowel mucosa with palisading edges may be noted (**Fig. 13.33**).

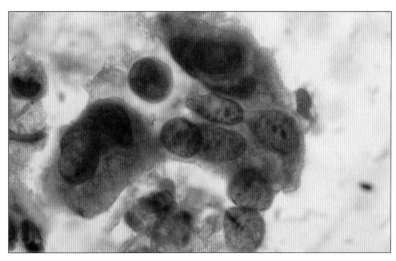

Fig. 13.27 Cholangiocarcinoma – Pap x100. The neoplastic cells in this field exhibit delicate cytoplasm without any pigment, and the nuclei display an abnormal chromatin pattern. There are no features that resemble hepatocytes in these cells.

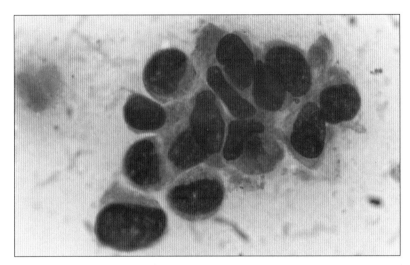

Fig. 13.28 Cholangiocarcinoma – MGG x100. This cluster of cells contains hyperchromatic nuclei which are somewhat irregular in outline. The cytoplasm is delicate and has ill-defined borders. No intracytoplasmic pigment is seen.

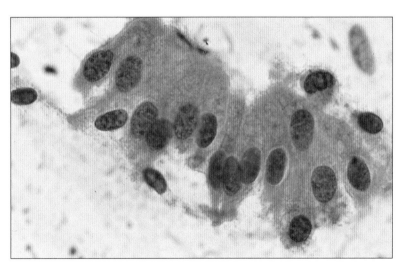

Fig. 13.29 Normal bile duct – Pap x100. The epithelial cells lining the bile ducts are tall columnar in type, as demonstrated here.

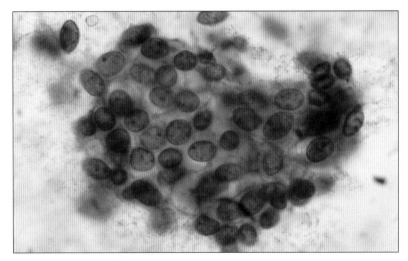

Fig. 13.30 Normal bile duct – Pap x100. The bile duct cells seen here are small with round or ovoid nuclei, which are uniform in size. Cytoplasm is minimal in amount. Honeycombing may be seen on careful focusing.

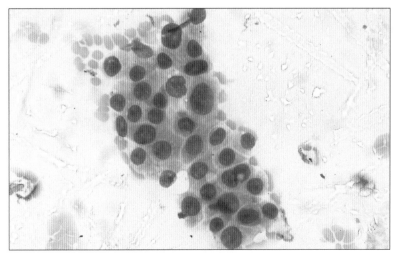

Fig. 13.31 Normal bile duct – MGG x40. These bile ducts cells are in the form of a flat sheet, which does not show honeycombing because it was air-died.

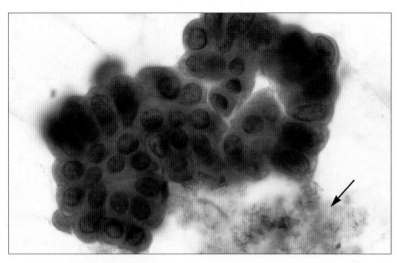

Fig. 13.32 Bile pigment – Pap x100. The benign bile duct cells seen in this field are accompanied by bright, yellowish green bile pigment (arrowed).

The liver is a common site for **metastatic tumours** of various types – adenocarcinomas of the breast and gastrointestinal tract, melanomas, and bronchial neoplasms. The cellular features are usually similar to those of the primary lesion, but it is impossible to be dogmatic about the primary site of a metastatic adenocarcinoma. Metastatic adenocarcinomas do not have the granular cytoplasm and rounded nuclei of hepatocellular carcinomas, but tend instead to have irregular nuclear margins and speckled chromatin (**Fig. 13.34**). They may, however, also show intranuclear inclusions similar to those found in hepatomas (**Fig. 13.35**). Metastatic breast carcinomas are seen as clusters of adenocarcinoma cells with large irregular nuclei and prominent nucleoli (**Fig. 13.36**). Melanoma metastases may or may not be pigmented, but the cells have

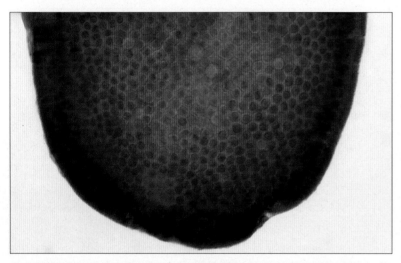

Fig. 13.33 Bowel mucosa – Pap x40. This flat sheet of benign glandular epithelial cells seen in brushings of the ampulla of Vater. Note the palisading around the edge of the sheet.

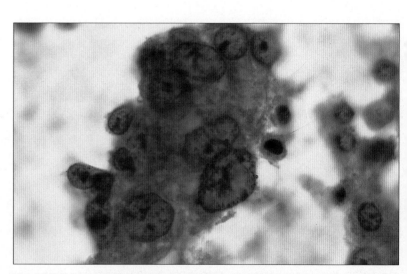

Fig. 13.34 Metastatic breast carcinoma – Pap x100. This liver aspirate from a patient with carcinoma of the breast contains clusters of pleomorphic adenocarcinoma cells with abnormal chromatin and large red nucleoli.

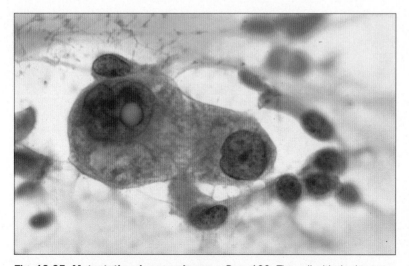

Fig. 13.35 Metastatic adenocarcinoma – Pap x100. The cell with the largest nucleus visible here contains a sharply defined intranuclear inclusion. This is a bile sample hence the columnar cells in the background. The primary was unknown.

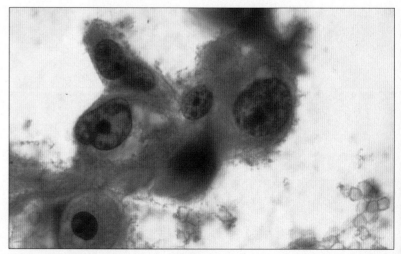

Fig. 13.36 Metastatic adenocarcinoma – Pap x100. The cluster of malignant cells seen in this field displays foamy cytoplasm and pleomorphism. The nuclei show abnormal clumping and clearing of chromatin.

abundant cytoplasm (**Fig. 13.37**) and large nuclei, and are sometimes binucle-ate, occasionally with intranuclear inclusions (see **Figures 10.69–10.81**). Metastatic small cell (oat cell) carcinomas retain their usual characteristics of small cells without apparent cytoplasm, showing nuclear moulding and 'salt and pepper' chromatin (**Fig. 13.38**). Aspirates of carcinoid tumours contain small cells with eccentric nuclei, delicate cytoplasm, and speckled chromatin (**Fig. 13.39**). The neoplastic cells are much smaller than hepatocytes, which contain cytoplasmic pigment (**Figs 13.40, 13.41**). Neoplastic cells from metastatic carcinoma of the colon are typically arranged in large clusters, sometimes in papillary arrangement, composed of glandular cells which occasionally show palisading of the edges (**Fig. 13.42**).

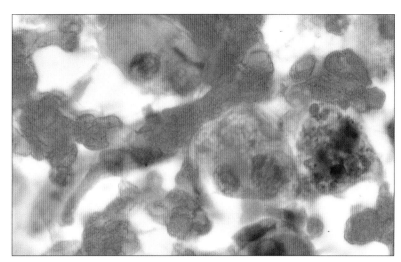

Fig. 13.37 Metastatic melanoma – Pap x100. This liver aspirate is composed of large malignant cells with abundant cytoplasm. Occasional cells contain greenish yellow melanin pigment.

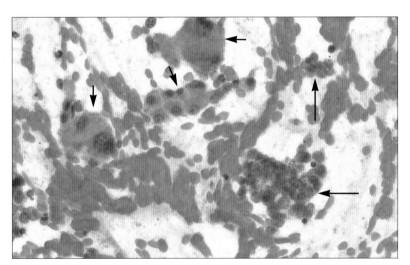

Fig. 13.38 Metastatic small cell carcinoma – Pap x40. This field displays a mixture of large benign hepatocytes containing pigment (short arrows) and clusters of small neoplastic cells with speckled chromatin and no visible cytoplasm (long arrows). These small cells should not be mistaken for bile duct cells or lymphocytes.

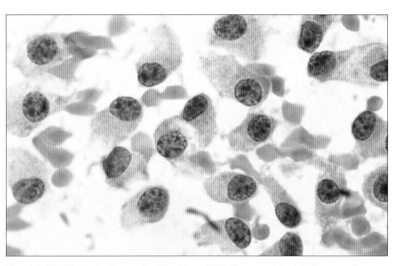

Fig. 13.39 Metastatic carcinoid – Pap x100. Illustrated in this fine needle aspirate of the liver is metastatic carcinoid, with the cells arranged singly, displaying eccentric nuclei and speckled chromatin. They closely resemble plasma cells, but are somewhat larger.

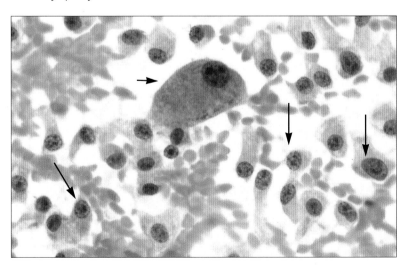

Fig. 13.40 Metastatic carcinoid – Pap x40. In this field the disparity in size between a normal hepatocyte (short arrow) and metastatic carcinoid cells (long arrows) is obvious. Note the variation in nuclear size in the neoplastic cells.

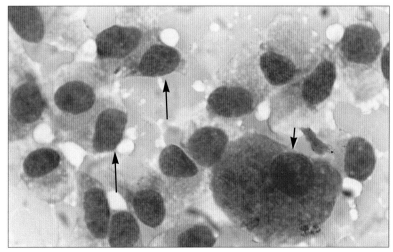

Fig. 13.41 Metastatic carcinoid – MGG x40. The air-dried smear also highlights the difference in size between a hepatocyte (short arrow) and metastatic carcinoid cells (long arrows), but it does not display the subtler features of the latter, such as speckled chromatin and the plasmacytoid appearance.

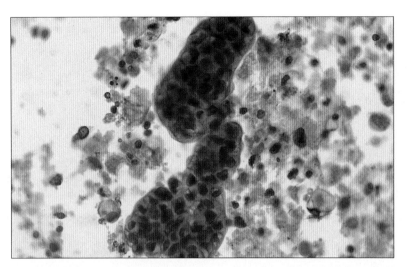

Fig. 13.42 Metastatic adenocarcinoma of the colon – Pap x40. This field shows a papillary type cluster of adenocarcinoma cells with sharply demarcated edges and cytoplasmic vacuolation. There is much necrotic cellular debris in the background.

PANCREAS

Normal pancreas (Fig. 13.43), which is composed of acinar cells and occasional islets of Langerhans, is sometimes sampled during fine needle aspiration of pancreatic and other lesions. Pancreatic epithelial cells are seen in aspirates in the form of small acinar clusters. The cells are wedge-shaped and display delicate granular cytoplasm and small nuclei with vesicular chromatin (Figs 13.44, 13.45). Pancreatic ductal cells are seen in the form of small cohesive sheets (Fig. 13.46). Benign islet cells of the pancreas are rarely seen in aspirates.

Pancreatitis is not usually aspirated. A **pancreatic pseudocyst** aspirate contains inflammatory cells, including polymorphs and histiocytes, mucin, some debris, and degenerate or reactive pancreatic epithelial cells (Fig. 13.47).

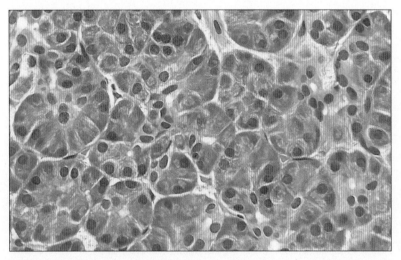

Fig. 13.43 Pancreas – H&E x40. This histological section of a normal pancreas demonstrates rounded clusters of wedge-shaped acinar cells with granular cytoplasm and small round nuclei. No islet cells are seen.

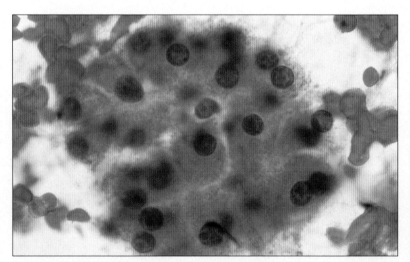

Fig. 13.44 Pancreatic acinar cells – Pap x100. This beautifully preserved pancreatic aspirate shows two clusters of wedge-shaped acinar cells with delicate granular cytoplasm, ill-defined margins, and sharply defined round nuclei. The nuclei are approximately the size of erythrocytes.

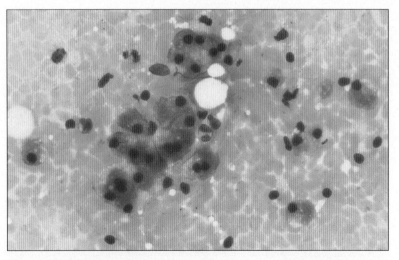

Fig. 13.45 Pancreatic acinar cells – MGG x40. An air-dried preparation also demonstrates the triangular shape of normal acinar cells. The nuclei are small and there are single epithelial cells and bare nuclei in the background.

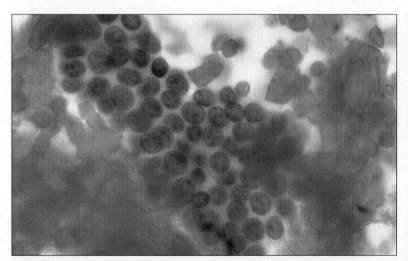

Fig. 13.46 Pancreatic ductal cells – Pap x100. This benign ductal sheet is composed of small uniform cells with rounded nuclei and a vesicular chromatin pattern.

On occasion, the atypia in the epithelial cells may be so marked as to mimic malignancy.

Adenocarcinoma of the pancreas (**Fig. 13.48**) is easily diagnosed on fine needle aspirates when poorly differentiated. Neoplastic cells are usually seen in clusters with scattered single cells and debris (**Figs 13.49, 13.50**). They may be multinucleated with enlarged hyperchromatic nuclei and prominent nucleoli (**Fig. 13.51**). Cytoplasmic vacuolation is sometimes a feature and the cells may appear to be in papillary clusters. Some carcinomas produce mucin, which is seen in the background of the aspirate staining pale pink or blue on the wet-fixed smear and bright pink on the air-dried slide (**Figs 13.52, 13.53**). It is important to screen pancreatic aspirates very carefully, especially when they appear to be composed of inflammatory cells only, suggesting a pancreatic pseudocyst, because some

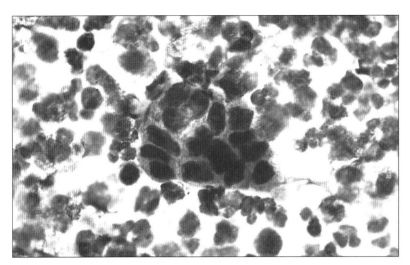

Fig. 13.47 Pancreatic pseudocyst – MGG x40. In this field there are numerous neutrophil polymorphs as well as a cluster of rather degenerate pancreatic epithelial cells.

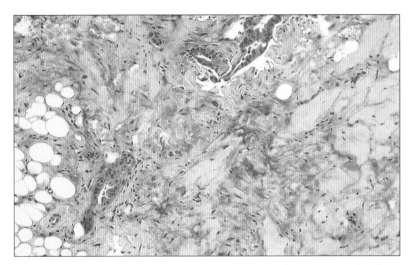

Fig. 13.48 Adenocarcinoma of the pancreas – H&E x10. This section is of a pancreatic adenocarcinoma with infiltrating tubules of malignant cells.

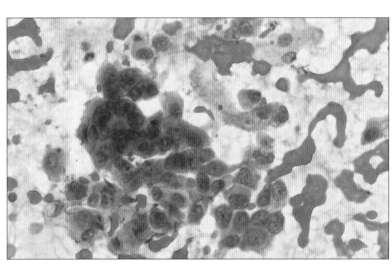

Fig. 13.49 Adenocarcinoma of the pancreas – Pap x40. Illustrated are clusters of small adenocarcinoma cells with irregular nuclear outlines and granular chromatin. There are some single cells, as well as necrotic cellular debris in the background.

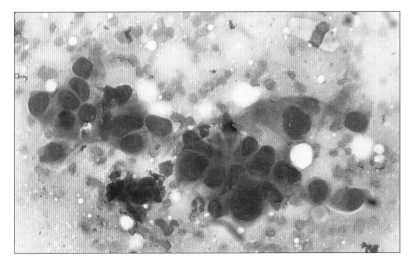

Fig. 13.50 Adenocarcinoma of the pancreas – MGG x40. In this air-dried smear the pleomorphism of the neoplastic cells is highlighted – one of the few advantages of this method of smear preparation. The cells appear to be greatly enlarged, but this is the same case as shown in **Figure 13.49**, in which alcohol fixation demonstrates the true size of the cells compared with erythrocytes.

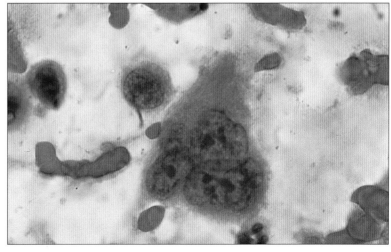

Fig. 13.51 Adenocarcinoma of the pancreas – Pap x100. This aspirate is from a poorly differentiated tumour. The cell in the centre of the field is multinucleated with irregular nuclear margins and multiple red nucleoli.

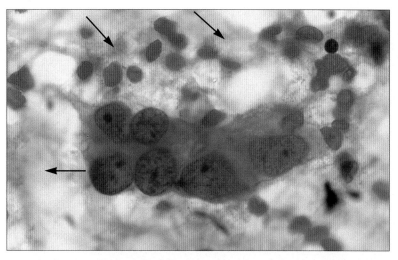

Fig. 13.52 Adenocarcinoma of the pancreas – Pap x100. This cluster of adenocarcinoma cells contains enlarged nuclei with granular chromatin. The pale blue mucin in the background is not obvious (arrowed).

carcinomas exhibit a similar picture with inflammatory cells obscuring the small groups of malignant cells (**Figs 13.54, 13.55**). Anaplastic carcinoma of the pancreas is composed of enormous, bizarre malignant cells (**Fig. 13.56**).

Solid–cystic–papillary tumour of the pancreas is a rare low-grade neoplasm which occurs in young women (**Fig. 13.57**). The aspirate consists of cystic fluid containing papillary clusters of bland cells which can appear benign on low power (**Figs 13.58, 13.59**). Under higher magnification the cells are seen to show mild pleomorphism (**Figs 13.60, 13.61**) and may exhibit nuclear grooves. Foamy macrophages and siderophages may also be present (**Fig. 13.62**). It is important to examine the cells carefully so that the lesion is not mistaken for a benign cyst.

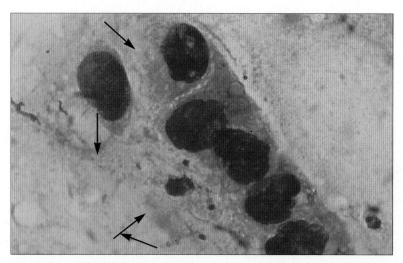

Fig. 13.53 Adenocarcinoma of the pancreas – MGG x100. The carcinoma cells seen here are from the same case shown in **Figure 13.52** and have hyperchromatic irregular nuclei. Note the stringy pink mucin in the background (arrowed).

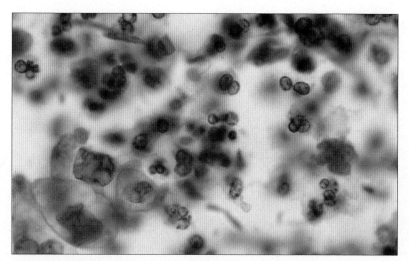

Fig. 13.54 Adenocarcinoma of the pancreas – Pap x100. The first impression made by this aspirate is that it represents an inflammatory process because of the excessive number of neutrophils and histiocytes. However, in the bottom left corner there are some pale carcinoma cells with irregular nuclear margins(arrowed).

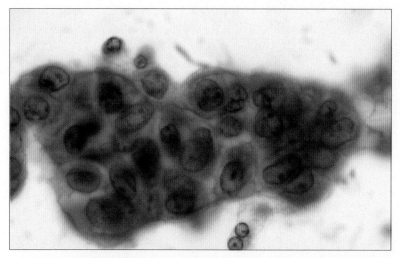

Fig. 13.55 Adenocarcinoma of the pancreas – Pap x100. This cluster of well-preserved carcinoma cells is from the same aspirate as shown in **Figure 13.54** and shows pleomorphism with an abnormal chromatin pattern.

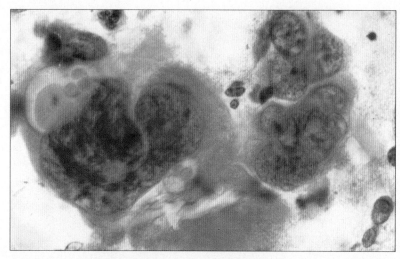

Fig. 13.56 Anaplastic carcinoma of the pancreas – Pap x100. The huge pleomorphic malignant cells visible here are from an anaplastic carcinoma of the pancreas. The amount of cytoplasm present is variable.

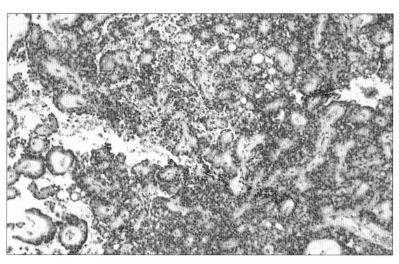

Fig. 13.57 Solid–cystic–papillary tumour – H&E x10. This histological section demonstrates the solid and papillary components of this neoplasm.

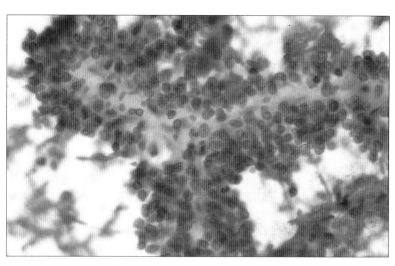

Fig. 13.58 Solid–cystic–papillary tumour – Pap x40. This field displays the papillary fronds of tissue seen in aspirates from this lesion. At this magnification, they appear as connective tissue cores covered with small, deceptively bland epithelial cells.

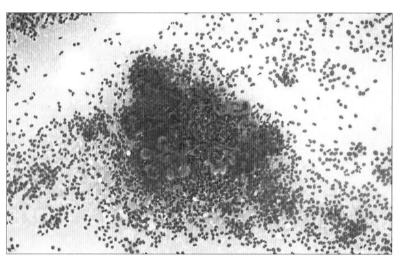

Fig. 13.59 Solid–cystic–papillary tumour – MGG x10. Air-dried smears also show clearly the connective tissue cores within the papillary structures that are common in this tumour. Note also the numerous single cells in the background.

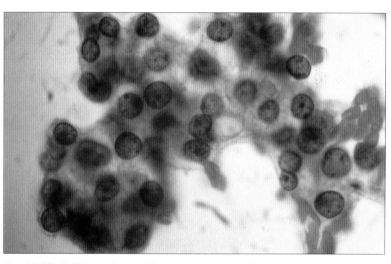

Fig. 13.60 Solid–cystic–papillary tumour – Pap x100. The clusters of tumour cells seen here exhibit mild nuclear pleomorphism with delicate vacuolated cytoplasm, rounded nuclei, and granular chromatin. Nucleoli are visible. Nuclear grooves, which are believed to be characteristic of this tumour, are not visible here.

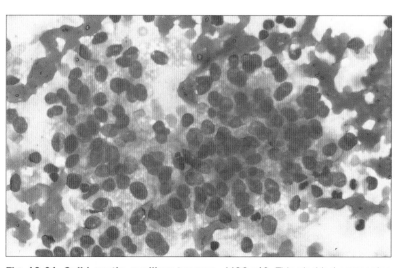

Fig. 13.61 Solid–cystic–papillary tumour – MGG x40. This air-dried smear also shows the small, mildly pleomorphic cells that comprise this tumour. The cytoplasm is indistinct in this preparation.

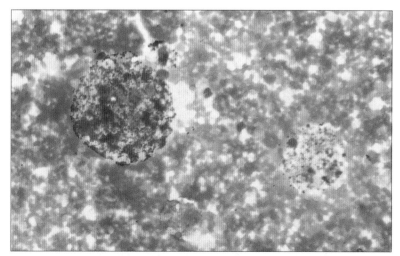

Fig. 13.62 Solid–cystic–papillary tumour – MGG x40. Foamy macrophages and siderophages are seen. These may be abundant, and so obscure the neoplastic cells in the aspirate.

Pancreatic endocrine tumours are not uncommon; some produce insulin or glucagon, which can be identified by immunocytochemical staining of the histological section. The cells in the aspirate have the characteristics of small, well-differentiated carcinoma cells with some of the features of neuroendocrine cells, such as speckled chromatin and ill-defined cytoplasm (**Fig. 13.63**). Attempts at acinus formation may be seen (**Figs 13.64, 13.65**).

SPLEEN

The spleen is rarely aspirated, except when tumour deposits are suspected. Aspirates from normal spleen show only mixed populations of lymphoid cells. Neoplasms which metastasize to the spleen are lymphoma, oat cell carcinoma, and melanoma. These tumours show features similar to those of the primary site. Sarcoid can affect the spleen (**Fig. 13.66**) and must be considered when epithelioid histiocytes are found in the aspirate (**Figs 13.67, 13.68**).

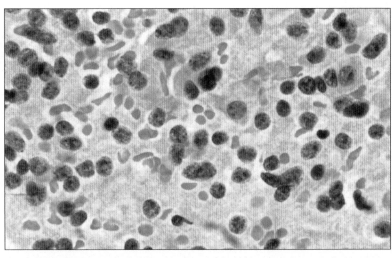

Fig. 13.63 Pancreatic endocrine tumour – Pap x100. This pancreatic aspirate is composed of small cells with ill-defined cytoplasm, round-to-ovoid nuclei, and speckled chromatin.

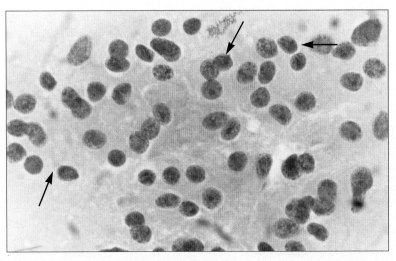

Fig. 13.64 Pancreatic endocrine tumour – Pap x100. In this field the tumour cells are arranged in ill-defined acinar structures (arrowed). Small nucleoli are evident.

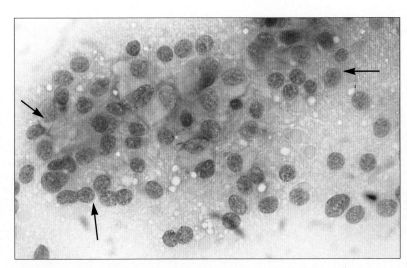

Fig. 13.65 Pancreatic endocrine tumour – MGG x100. The air-dried smear from this tumour displays the mild pleomorphism, delicate cytoplasm, and acinar pattern (arrowed) sometimes seen.

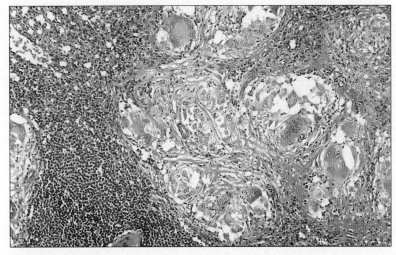

Fig. 13.66 Sarcoid, spleen – H&E x10. This histological section of spleen shows a granulomatous process which, in this case, was due to sarcoidosis.

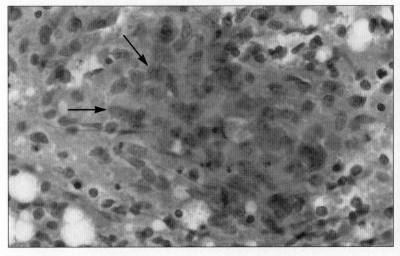

Fig. 13.67 Sarcoid, spleen – Pap x40. The granuloma seen here is composed of a loose collection of epithelioid histiocytes with elongated nuclei and abundant cytoplasm (arrowed). This aspirate is from the same case as shown in **Figures 13.66** and **13.68**.

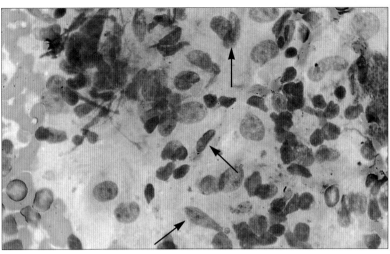

Fig. 13.68 Sarcoid, spleen – MGG x40. This air-dried smear, also from the case illustrated in **Figures 13.66** and **13.67**, shows a granuloma composed of epithelioid histiocytes with pale, indistinct cytoplasm (arrowed).

ADRENAL GLANDS

The histology of the normal adrenal gland **(Fig. 13.69)** may not be fully represented on a fine needle aspirate, depending on the site the tip of the needle samples. Normal cortical cells have small round nuclei and speckled chromatin, with fragile granular cytoplasm and indefinite cell borders **(Fig. 13.70)**.

Adrenal adenomas are composed of uniform cells, similar to normal adrenal cortical cells, arranged in a vaguely acinar pattern **(Figs 13.71, 13.72)**. The cytoplasm is often vacuolated, sometimes showing honeycomb vacuolation which resembles that seen in renal cell carcinoma **(Figs 13.73, 13.74)**. **Adrenal cortical carcinomas (Fig. 13.75)** are much more pleomorphic than adrenal adenomas and the aspirates contain similar, large pleomorphic cells, which may be multinucleated and contain large nucleoli and abundant cytoplasm **(Fig. 13.76)**.

Neuroblastomas are composed of small endocrine cells with round-to-ovoid nuclei and indistinct cytoplasm. The cells are often in tight clusters and are sometimes arranged in acini which may contain fibrillary material **(Figs 13.77, 13.78)**. Many bare nuclei are also seen.

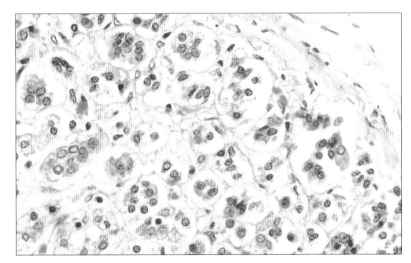

Fig. 13.69 Adrenal cortex – H&E x40. This section shows the zona glomerulosa – the outermost layer of the adrenal cortex. The cells are small with abundant cytoplasm, which contains lipid droplets. The zona fasciculata contains similar cells with vacuolated, lipid-containing cytoplasm. The zona reticulata is composed of cells with eosinophilic cytoplasm and contains brown lipofuscin pigment.

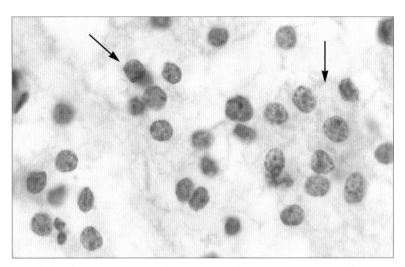

Fig. 13.70 Adrenal cortical cells – Pap x100. These cells are small with round nuclei and speckled chromatin. Although the cytoplasm is faint vacuolation is still evident (arrowed).

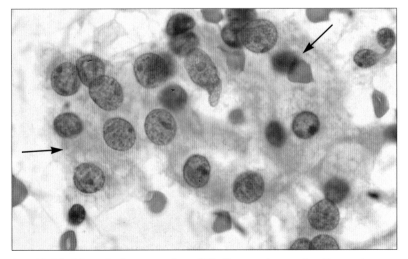

Fig. 13.71 Adrenal adenoma – Pap x100. Illustrated are cells with round nuclei, granular chromatin and delicate vacuolated cytoplasm arranged in an acinar pattern (arrowed) .

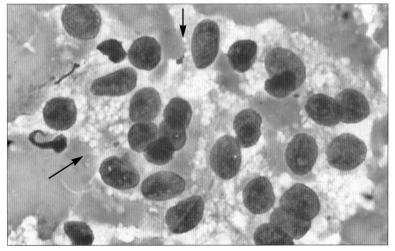

Fig. 13.72 Adrenal adenoma – MGG x100. The cells in this air-dried smear show uniform nuclei and vacuolated cytoplasm. The speckled chromatin is not distinct. Incomplete acini are present (arrowed).

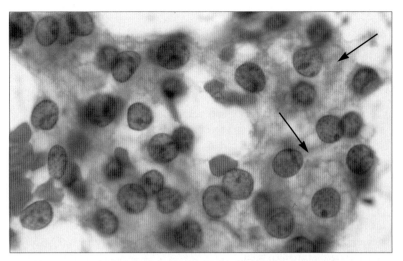

Fig. 13.73 Adrenal adenoma – Pap x100. In this adrenal aspirate the cytoplasmic vacuolation is so marked (arrows) that the cells may be mistaken for a renal cell carcinoma.

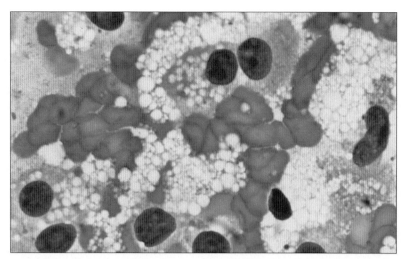

Fig. 13.74 Adrenal adenoma – MGG x100. The abundant, vacuolated cytoplasm of epithelial cells in this aspirate is reminiscent of renal cell carcinoma.

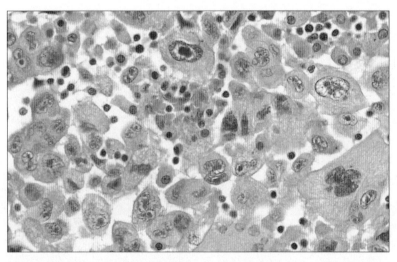

Fig. 13.75 Adrenal cortical carcinoma – H&E x40. This section of an adrenal cortical carcinoma illustrates the marked pleomorphism that may be seen. The cells are very variable in nuclear and cytoplasmic size and shape, and prominent nucleoli are apparent.

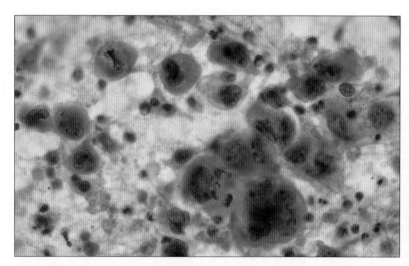

Fig. 13.76 Adrenal cortical carcinoma – Pap x40. This aspirate from the same tumour as shown in **Figure 13.75** contains very large pleomorphic malignant cells, similar to those in the histological section. Note the necrotic debris in the background.

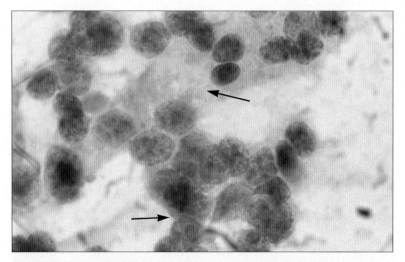

Fig. 13.77 Neuroblastoma – Pap x100. These cells display small nuclei with speckled chromatin, forming incomplete rosettes (arrowed). No fibrillary material is seen.

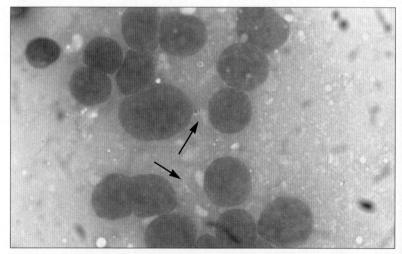

Fig. 13.78 Neuroblastoma – MGG x100. This air-dried aspirate is composed of cells with round nuclei and indistinct cytoplasm, in a vaguely acinar arrangement (arrowed). Fibrillary material is not visible, and neither is the speckled chromatin noticeable.

RETROPERITONEAL ASPIRATES

The retroperitoneum may be involved by retroperitoneal fibrosis and by neoplasms, either primary or secondary. Aspirates of retroperitoneal fibrosis are usually insufficient, composed of fragments of fibrous tissue with no specific features. Primary tumours, such as lymphomas, resemble those arising elsewhere. Aspirates from sarcomas are usually cellular with a mixture of spindle-shaped cells and large pleomorphic cells with abundant cytoplasm. The nuclei may be spindle-shaped or ovoid, with vesicular chromatin and large red nucleoli on the Papanicolaou stain, purple with the May Grunwald Giemsa stain. The cells may be in small groups or aggregates, as well as lying singly.

Metastatic tumours have similar features to the primary neoplasms and are described in Chapter 10.

SUGGESTED READING

Greenberg ML. Pancreas. In: Gray W, ed. *Diagnostic Cytopathology*. Edinburgh: Churchill Livingstone; 1995: 415–434.

Greenberg ML, Rennie Y, Grierson J, *et al*. Solid and papillary epithelial pancreatic tumour. *Diagn Cytopathol* 1993; 9: 541–546.

Katz RL, Patel S, Mackay B, Zornoza J. Fine needle aspiration cytology of the adrenal gland. *Acta Cytol* 1984; 28: 269–282.

Orell SR, Sterrett G, Walters M, Whittaker D. *Manual and Atlas of Fine Needle Aspiration Cytology*. Edinburgh: Churchill Livingstone; 1992: 224–230.

Tao LC. Liver and pancreas. In: Bibbo M, ed. *Comprehensive Cytopathology*. Philadelphia: WB Saunders; 1991: 882–859.

Waters E, Armstrong J. Disorders of the liver. In: Gray W, ed. *Diagnostic Cytopathology*. Edinburgh: Churchill Livingstone; 1995: 353–401.

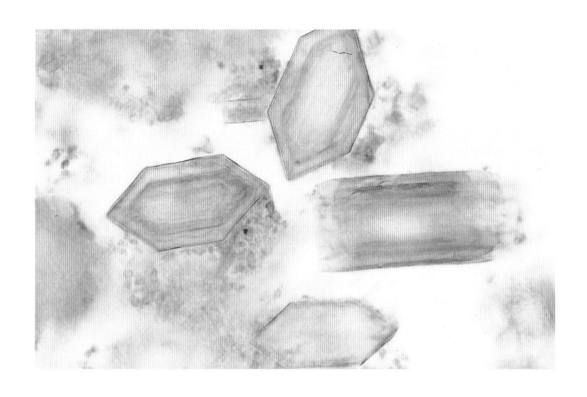

THE SALIVARY GLANDS, OESOPHAGEAL AND GASTRIC CYTOLOGY

14

THE SALIVARY GLANDS

The salivary glands are broadly classified into two categories: the major salivary glands, including the parotid, submandibular, and sublingual glands which are paired, and the numerous minor salivary glands. Histologically, they are composed of acini and ducts (**Fig. 14.1**), the acini containing either serous cells, mucous cells, or a mixture of both. A fine needle aspirate of a normal salivary gland usually contains grape-like clusters of serous acinar cells (**Fig. 14.2**), with small nuclei and abundant, finely vacuolated cytoplasm (**Fig. 14.3**), and also small sheets of uniform ductal cells with very little cytoplasm. Bare nuclei derived from acinar cells may be seen in the background (**Fig. 14.4**).

Retention **cysts** of the salivary gland are not uncommon, the fluid containing macrophages, debris, and some reactive ductal cells. Crystalloids are occasionally seen (**Fig. 14.5**). Atypia and squamous metaplasia have been reported in such cysts, raising the possibility of muco-epidermoid carcinoma if mucin is also present.

Inflammatory processes (sialadenitis) may be acute or chronic. In acute sialadenitis the lesion is usually diagnosed clinically, but if obtained the aspirate contains numerous neutrophil polymorphs and some histiocytes. In chronic sialadenitis lymphocytes are also seen.

Benign lympho-epithelial lesions are characterized by an abundance of small lymphoid cells with a few benign epithelial cells. It is almost impossible from cytological features alone to differentiate between a benign lympho-epithelial lesion and a low-grade lymphoma.

Sarcoidosis involving the salivary glands is not unknown; the cytological features include epithelioid histiocytes and multinucleated histiocytes without the necrosis associated with tuberculosis (**Fig. 14.6**).

Pleomorphic adenoma is the most common benign neoplasm of the salivary gland (**Fig. 14.7**). Aspirates from this lesion tend to be characteristic, with abundant fibrillary myxoid material representing that seen in the histological section, staining pale blue or pink with Papanicolaou (**Fig. 14.8**), and bright magenta with the May Grunwald Giemsa stain (**Fig. 14.9**). The material does not have the sharp, clearly defined margins of the basement membrane mater-ial seen in adenoid cystic carcinoma (see **Figures 14.27–14.29**). Some tumours exhibit chondroid material, as this is a not uncommon change in pleomorphic adenoma. Interspersed with the fibrillary material are epithelial cells, with relatively large nuclei and clearly defined cytoplasm which stains pale blue in the wet-fixed smear (**Fig. 14.10**) and a bright blue in the air-dried preparation. The nuclei may be ovoid or rounded, with clearly defined margins, vesicular chromatin, and small

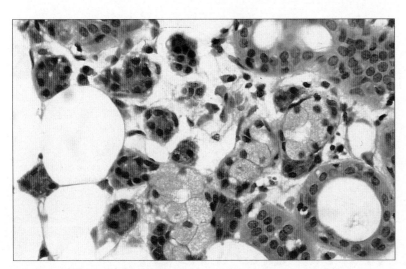

Fig. 14.1 Salivary gland – H&E x10. This section of normal salivary gland illustrates acini and ducts, and also some fat cells.

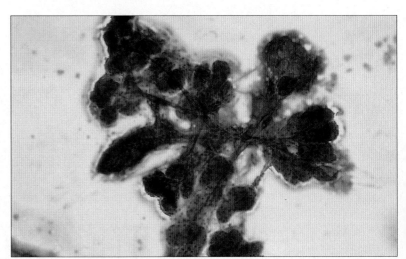

Fig. 14.2 Salivary gland – Pap x10. This fine needle aspirate of normal parotid gland demonstrates the grape-like clusters of serous acinar cells.

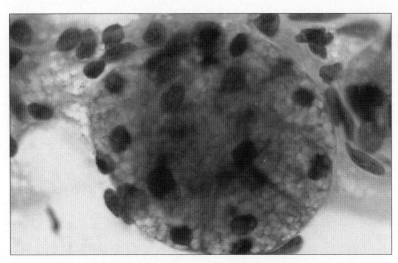

Fig. 14.3 Salivary gland – Pap x100. This cluster of serous acinar salivary gland cells contains relatively small nuclei and abundant, finely vacuolated cytoplasm.

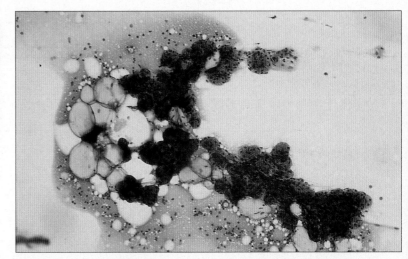

Fig. 14.4 Salivary gland – Pap x10. This low-power view of an aspirate from a normal salivary gland shows, in addition to the clusters of acinar cells, numerous bare nuclei in the background.

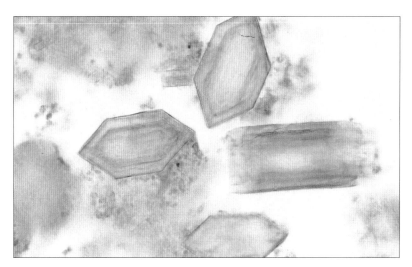

Fig. 14.5 Crystalloids – Pap x40. Retention cysts of the salivary gland often contain crystalloids, as illustrated in this photomicrograph.

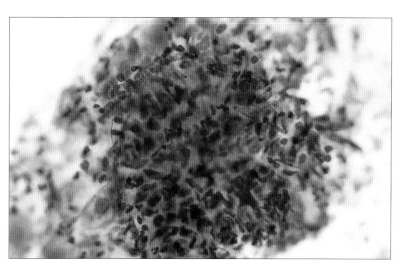

Fig. 14.6 Sarcoid granuloma – Pap x40. This group of epithelioid histiocytes with elongated nuclei is from an aspirate of a parotid gland, which showed sarcoidosis on biopsy.

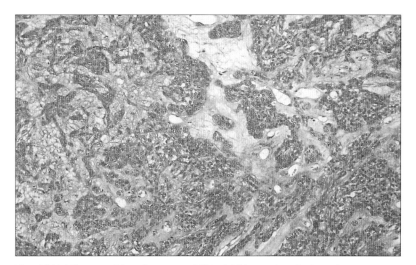

Fig. 14.7 Pleomorphic adenoma – H&E x4. This section displays the characteristic histological features of a pleomorphic adenoma.

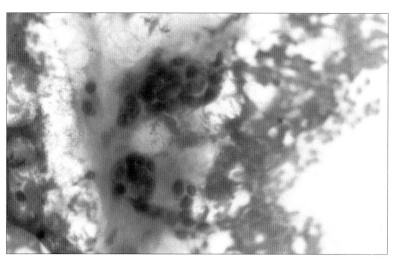

Fig. 14.8 Pleomorphic adenoma – Pap x40. Illustrated is the pale blue fibrillary material commonly seen in aspirates of this neoplasm. A few small groups of epithelial cells are also visible.

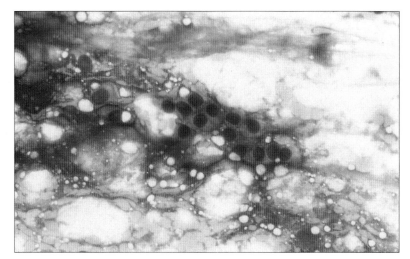

Fig. 14.9 Pleomorphic adenoma – MGG x40. The fibrillary material stains a bright magenta with the May Grunwald Giemsa stain. It has ill-defined margins, unlike the sharp borders of the material in adenoid cystic carcinoma.

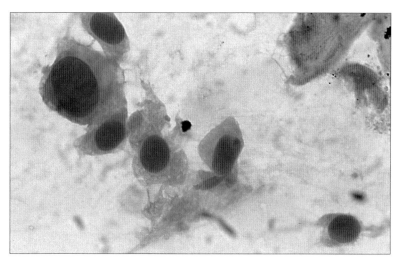

Fig. 14.10 Pleomorphic adenoma – Pap x40. This field contains epithelial cells which are variable in size, but contain bland nuclei and clearly demarcated cytoplasmic borders.

nucleoli (**Figs 14.11, 14.12**). The cellularity is variable depending on the type of area sampled and may be rather scanty or profuse (**Fig. 14.13**). Spindle-shaped mesenchymal cells are also commonly seen (**Fig. 14.14**). Although tyrosine crystals are frequently seen in histological sections (**Fig. 14.15**), they are not visualized in cytological smears. Squamous metaplasia can occur in pleomorphic adenoma, resulting in squamous cells in the aspirate. Carcinoma may arise in pleomorphic adenoma, in which case the smears are seen to contain malignant cells as well as the usual features of the benign neoplasm (see below).

Myoepithelioma (Fig. 14.16) is believed by some authorities to be part of the spectrum of pleomorphic adenomas. The aspirate is cellular, composed of single cells with cigar-shaped, spindle-shaped, or even ovoid nuclei and deli-

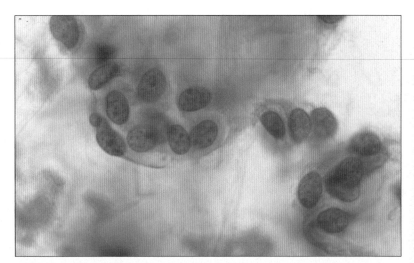

Fig. 14.11 Pleomorphic adenoma – Pap x100. The epithelial cells in this neoplasm are fairly uniform, with ovoid nuclei, vesicular chromatin, and small nucleoli.

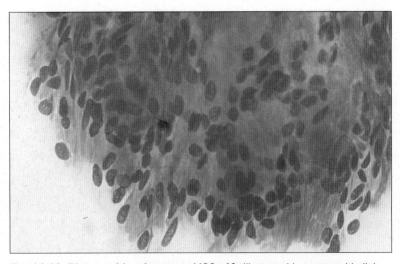

Fig. 14.12 Pleomorphic adenoma – MGG x40. Illustrated here are epithelial cells with ovoid nuclei and blue cytoplasm, overlying bright pink fibrillary material.

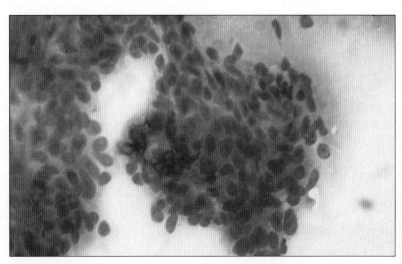

Fig. 14.13 Pleomorphic adenoma – MGG x40. This field illustrates the marked cellularity sometimes seen in aspirates from this neoplasm.

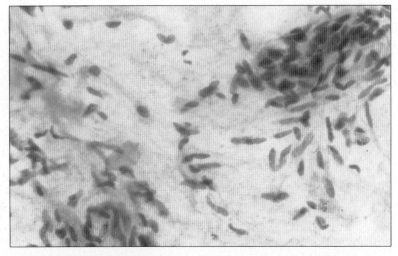

Fig. 14.14 Pleomorphic adenoma – Pap x40. These spindle-shaped cells are most likely to be mesenchymal in origin.

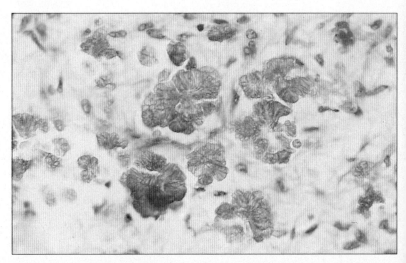

Fig. 14.15 Pleomorphic adenoma – H&E x10. This section of a pleomorphic adenoma demonstrates tyrosine crystals. These are not found in cytological material.

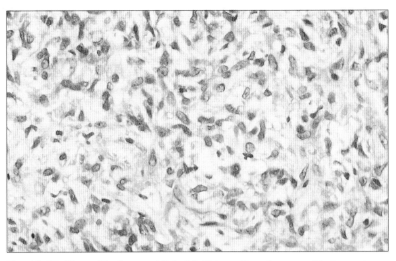

Fig. 14.16 Myoepithelioma – H&E x10. This section of a myoepithelioma shows the spindle-shaped cells that comprise this neoplasm.

cate cytoplasm. The chromatin is vesicular and nucleoli are not prominent (**Figs 14.17, 14.18**). Acinar and ductal epithelial cells are not seen.

Monomorphic adenomas of the salivary gland are uncommon tumours of various types and are not easy to diagnose cytologically. The cells are uniform, with small bland nuclei, and are often plentiful.

Warthin's tumour (adenolymphoma) is not uncommon in the parotid gland. The tumour often appears to be cystic and aspiration produces a murky fluid. Histologically, the lesion is composed of oncocytic cells overlying stroma containing numerous lymphocytes and lymphoid follicles (**Fig. 14.19**). The aspirate typically contains debris (**Figs 14.20, 14.21**) and lymphocytes (**Fig. 14.22**), and also sheets of oncocytes with cytoplasm that stains pink-to-orange

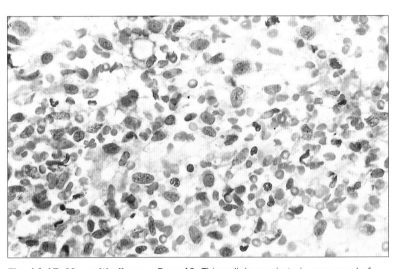

Fig. 14.17 Myoepithelioma – Pap x40. This cellular aspirate is composed of small cells with ovoid to spindle-shaped nuclei, vesicular chromatin, and small nucleoli. The cytoplasm is indistinct. No acinar epithelial cells are found.

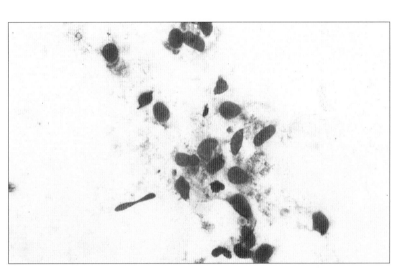

Fig. 14.18 Myoepithelioma – MGG x40. The air-dried smear shows similar features to the wet-fixed preparation, namely cells with ovoid to spindle-shaped nuclei and scanty cytoplasm.

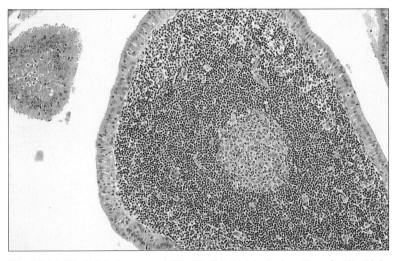

Fig. 14.19 Warthin's tumour – H&E x10. This histological section of a Warthin's tumour clearly demonstrates the oncocytic epithelium overlying stroma infiltrated by lymphocytes and containing a well-defined lymphoid follicle.

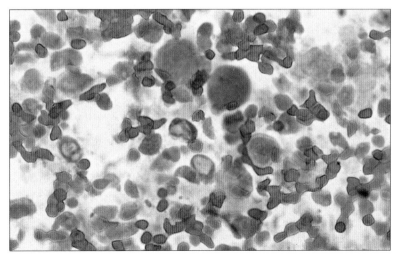

Fig. 14.20 Warthin's tumour – Pap x40. This field shows the 'dirty' background seen in these tumours, with much debris.

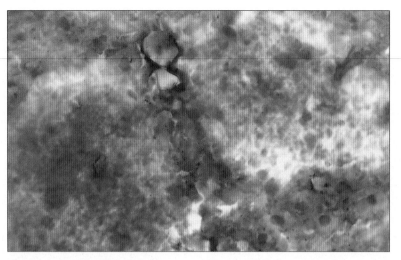

Fig. 14.21 Warthins's tumour – MGG x40. Granular and amorphous debris is also identifiable in the air-dried smear.

on the wet-fixed smear (**Figs 14.23, 14.24**) and blue on the air-dried smear (**Fig. 14.25**). Oncocytes may not be seen in poorly cellular aspirates.

Adenoid cystic carcinoma of the salivary gland has typical histological features (**Fig. 14.26**). Aspirates tend to be cellular with abundant hyaline material in the form of spheres (**Figs 14.27, 14.28**) and cylinders (**Fig. 14.29**). This material stains a pale blue with the Papanicolaou stain and bright pink or magenta with May Grunwald Giemsa, and has sharply demarcated outlines, unlike the fibrillary structure of the myxoid substance in pleomorphic adenoma (see **Figures 14.8, 14.9**) The epithelial cells are small and unremarkable, with little cytoplasm and hyperchromatic nuclei. Nucleoli are not prominent. Often the cells are arranged around the globules of hyaline material, with single cells in the background (**Fig. 14.30**).

Muco-epidermoid carcinoma can be quite difficult to recognize on cytology, although the histological appearances are characteristic (**Fig. 14.31**).

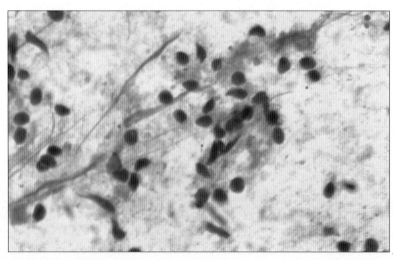

Fig. 14.22 Warthin's tumour – Pap x40. Illustrated here are the lymphocytes which are essential for the diagnosis of this lesion.

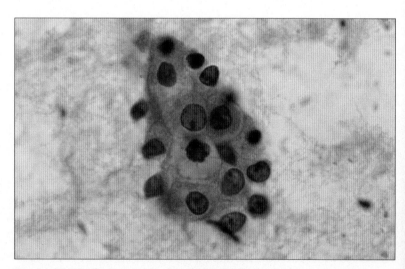

Fig. 14.23 Warthin's tumour – Pap x100. This cluster of oncocytic cells contains abundant, pink granular cytoplasm and rounded, well-defined nuclear margins.

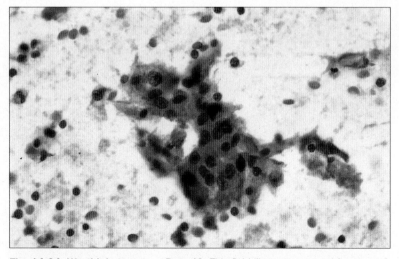

Fig. 14.24 Warthin's tumour – Pap x40. This field illustrates several features of this neoplasm – oncocytes with pinkish–orange cytoplasm, lymphocytes, and background debris.

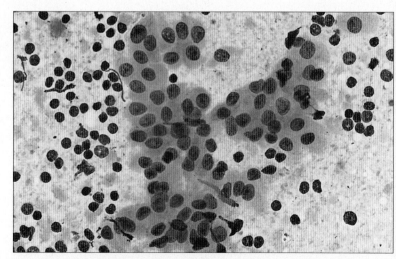

Fig. 14.25 Warthin's tumour – MGG x40. This air-dried smear exhibits a flat sheet of oncocytes, with abundant blue cytoplasm, rounded nuclei and visible nucleoli. In the background are lymphocytes and a small amount of debris.

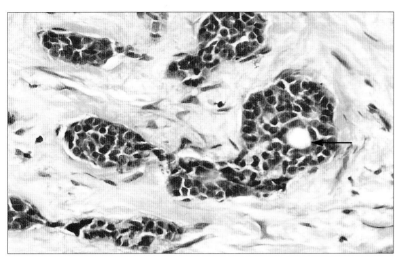

Fig. 14.26 Adenoid cystic carcinoma – H&E x10. This histological section demonstrates the usual features of this neoplasm, which consists of small hyperchromatic cells arranged in small nests around spaces (arrowed).

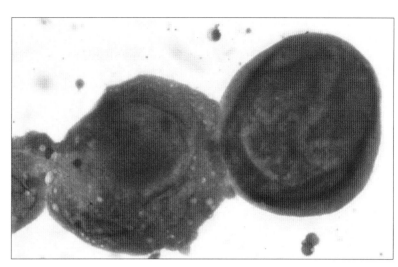

Fig. 14.27 Adenoid cystic carcinoma – MGG x40. These spheres of hyaline material stain bright magenta on air-dried material. They are sharply defined, unlike the fibrillary material of pleomorphic adenoma.

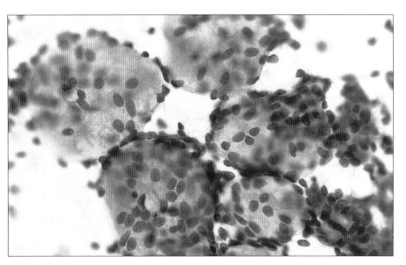

Fig. 14.28 Adenoid cystic carcinoma – Pap x40. The hyaline globules are not seen clearly in wet-fixed preparations, as they stain pale blue. Note, however, the small cells surrounding the globules.

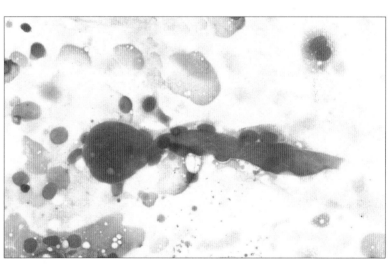

Fig. 14.29 Adenoid cystic carcinoma – MGG x40. In this field are a globule and a cylinder of hyaline material surrounded by small blue-staining nuclei.

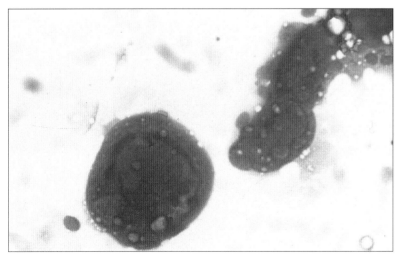

Fig. 14.30 Adenoid cystic carcinoma – MGG x40. The epithelial cells seen here are small and uniform and arranged around the hyaline material, with a few single cells in the background.

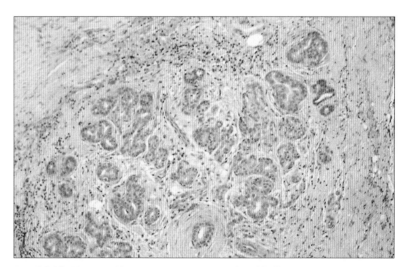

Fig. 14.31 Muco-epidermoid carcinoma – H&E x10. This section shows an area of tumour that is predominantly composed of glands.

The aspirate often contains debris and mucus, with epithelial cells that appear trapped within the mucus. Both glandular, mucin-containing cells (**Figs 14.32, 14.33**), and squamoid cells (**Fig. 14.34**) are present, as well as cells that appear to be intermediate between the two types (**Figs 14.35, 14.36**). Cells that resemble foamy macrophages may predominate, leading to difficulty in making the diagnosis (**Figs 14.37, 14.38**).

Acinic cell carcinoma is uncommon. This tumour is composed of cells that resemble the serous acinar cells of a normal salivary gland (**Fig. 14.39**). Cytologically, the tumour is seen to consist of clusters and sheets of cohesive, fairly uniform cells with finely vacuolated delicate cytoplasm (**Figs 14.40, 14.41**), and occasionally with cytoplasm that appears to be oncocytic.

Adenocarcinoma of the salivary gland may be primary or may develop in a pleomorphic adenoma (carcinoma-ex-pleomorphic adenoma). In the latter case (**Fig. 14.42**) features of pleomorphic adenoma, such as myxoid material, may be seen along with carcinoma cells (**Figs 14.43, 14.44**). The aspirate may be

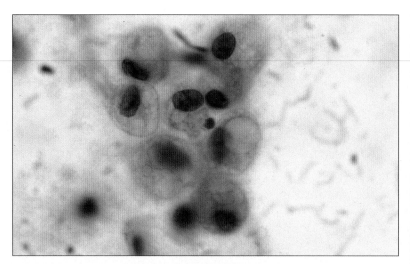

Fig. 14.32 Muco-epidermoid carcinoma – Pap x63. This group of vacuolated glandular cells shows small, but regular, nuclei.

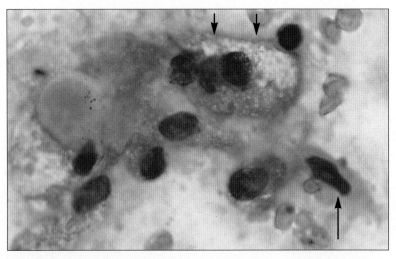

Fig. 14.33 Muco-epidermoid carcinoma – MGG x63. The cells illustrated here are of two types – vacuolated glandular cells (short arrows) and squamoid cells with dense blue cytoplasm (long arrow).

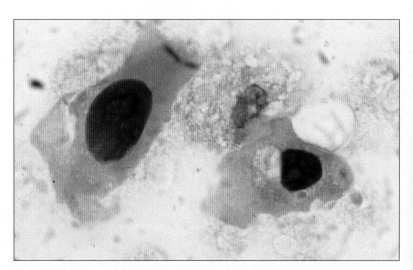

Fig. 14.34 Muco-epidermoid carcinoma – Pap x100. Illustrated here are two squamous carcinoma cells with keratinized cytoplasm and hyperchromatic nuclei.

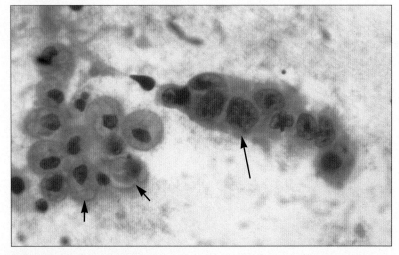

Fig. 14.35 Muco-epidermoid carcinoma – Pap x63. This field contains a group of vacuolated glandular cells (short arrows) and an adjacent cluster of pleomorphic cells with irregular nuclei, representing intermediate cells (long arrow).

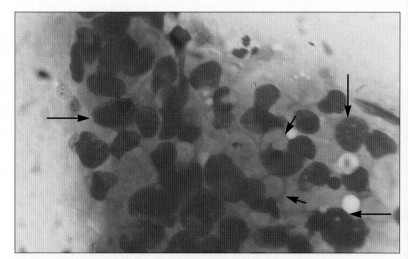

Fig. 14.36 Muco-epidermoid carcinoma – MGG x63. This cluster of hyperchromatic cells contains a few vacuoles (short arrows), with some cells that would be classifiable as intermediate (long arrows).

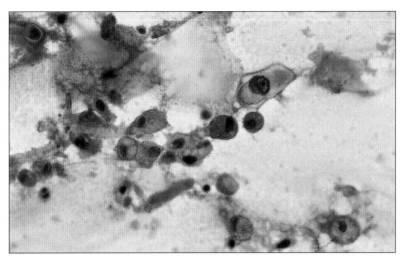

Fig. 14.37 Muco-epidermoid carcinoma – Pap x40. The epithelial cells in this field mimic foamy macrophages. Note the debris in the background.

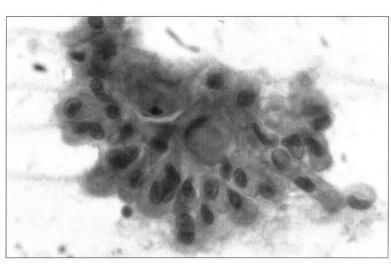

Fig. 14.38 Muco-epidermoid carcinoma – Pap x63. These vacuolated epithelial cells, which resemble foamy macrophages, are surrounding two degenerate keratinized cells.

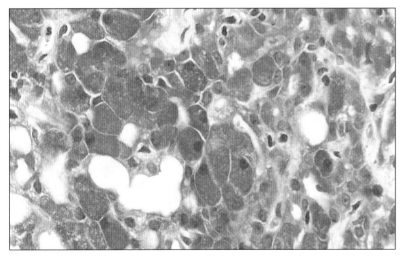

Fig. 14.39 Acinic cell carcinoma – H&E x40. This section shows the acinar cells that comprise this neoplasm. Note the small nuclei and abundant cytoplasm.

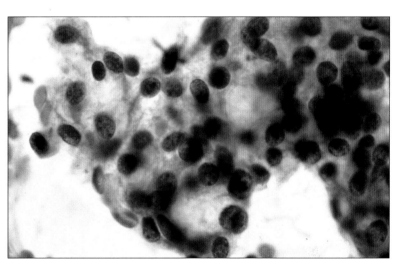

Fig. 14.40 Acinic cell carcinoma – Pap x63. These neoplastic cells contain abundant cytoplasm, which has a foamy appearance. The nuclei are small, but hyperchromatic.

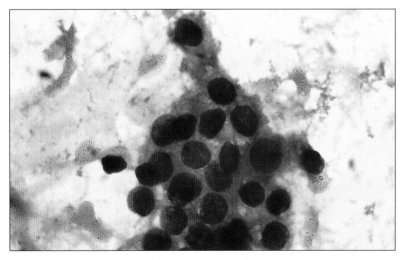

Fig. 14.41 Acinic cell carcinoma – MGG x63. This aspirate contains cells with fairly uniform hyperchromatic nuclei and indistinct cytoplasm. These cells do not closely resemble acinar cells.

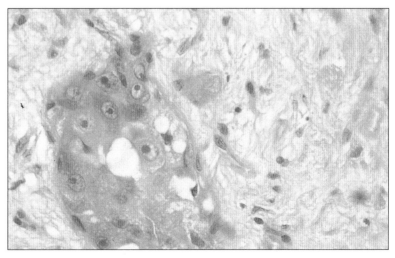

Fig. 14.42 Carcinoma in pleomorphic adenoma. – H&E x40. This histological section shows large malignant cells with prominent red nucleoli.

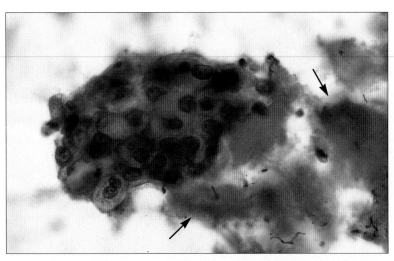

Fig. 14.43 Carcinoma in pleomorphic adenoma – Pap x40. In this field there is a cluster of adenocarcinoma cells adjacent to fibrillary material similar to that seen in pleomorphic adenoma (arrowed).

cellular with clusters of mildly pleomorphic cells. The cells in some carcinomas may appear quite bland and can be mistaken for a benign tumour, such as an adenoma. Other tumours are composed of cells with large nuclei and nucleoli and abnormal chromatin (**Figs 14.45, 14.46**). The aspirate may contain mucin (**Fig. 14.47**).

Other neoplasms of the salivary glands include squamous carcinoma, lymphomas, and metastatic tumours. The features of these are described elsewhere (see Chapter 10).

Amyloid deposits at any site, including the parotid gland, can be diagnosed on fine needle aspirates. The smears show clumps of pale orange amorphous material (**Fig. 14.48**), which exhibits apple-green birefringence with the Congo red stain (**Fig. 14.49**).

OESOPHAGEAL AND GASTRIC CYTOLOGY

Oesophageal brush cytology

Brushings of the oesophagus are performed in cases of oesophagitis to confirm

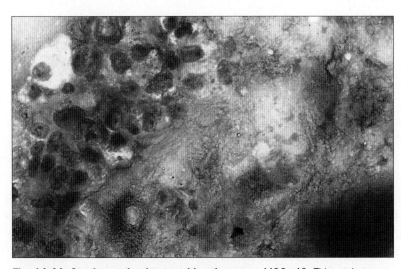

Fig. 14.44 Carcinoma in pleomorphic adenoma – MGG x40. This aspirate from the case illustrated in **Figures 14.42** and **14.43** also shows the magenta fibrillary material associated with pleomorphic adenoma.

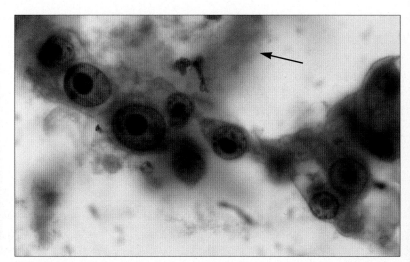

Fig. 14.45 Carcinoma in pleomorphic adenoma – Pap x100. This aspirate contains malignant cells with enormous red nucleoli and clumped chromatin. Some fibrillary material is also seen (arrow).

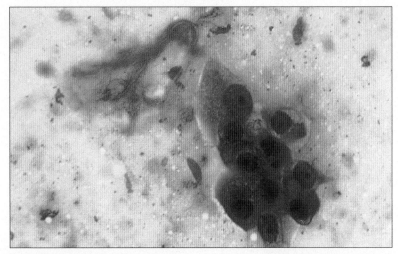

Fig. 14.46 Carcinoma in pleomorphic adenoma – MGG x63. In the air-dried slide from the same case as in **Figure 14.47**, similar neoplastic cells are seen, with large central nucleoli and abundant cytoplasm. Some magenta fibrillary material is also present.

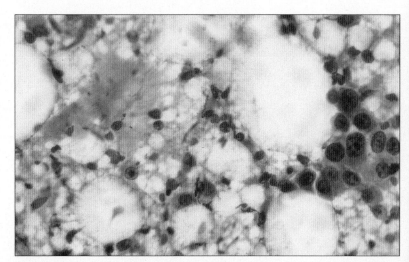

Fig. 14.47 Carcinoma in pleomorphic adenoma – Pap x40. This small group of cohesive neoplastic cells shows mild pleomorphism, with some mucin in the background.

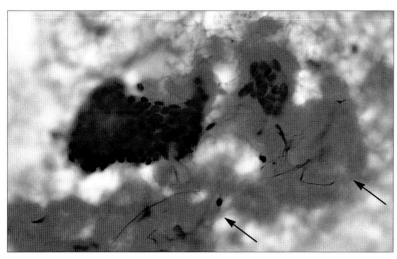

Fig. 14.48 Amyloid – Pap x40. This field shows dense amyloid, with ill-defined edges (arrowed), which appears different from the fibrillary material seen in pleomorphic adenoma. Normal ductal cells are also visible.

Candida infection, in cases of Barrett's oesophagus, and for the diagnosis of carcinoma. The brush specimen is taken at endoscopy and smeared on to glass slides, immediately fixed in alcohol, and then sent to the laboratory.

A brush smear of normal oesophagus shows a mixture of benign squamous and glandular cells. The squamous cells are usually single, while the glandular cells are often in sheets.

Oesophagitis is commonly due to infection with Candida. The inflammatory changes in smears include enlargement of the epithelial cell nuclei, sometimes with binucleation **(Fig. 14.50)** and perinuclear vacuolation **(Fig. 14.51)**, an inflammatory exudate composed of neutrophils and histiocytes, and Candida hyphae and spores **(Fig. 14.52)**. It can be difficult to detect Candida, especially if the fixation and staining of the specimen are not optimal.

Barrett's oesophagus is a clinical diagnosis which can be confirmed by cytology. The brush samples show sheets of glandular cells containing goblet cells produced by intestinal metaplasia (see **Figure 14.57**).

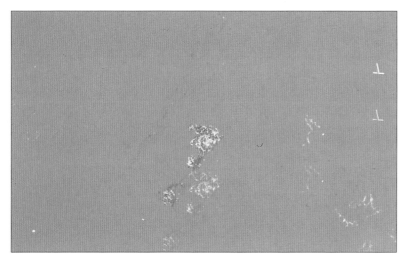

Fig. 14.49 Amyloid – Congo red x40. The amyloid in this aspirate displays apple-green fluorescence.

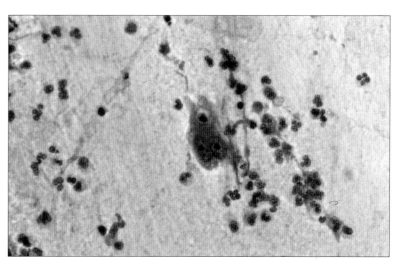

Fig. 14.50 Oesophagitis – Pap x40. This oesophageal brush smear shows acute inflammatory cells and an inflamed binucleate glandular cell in the centre of the field.

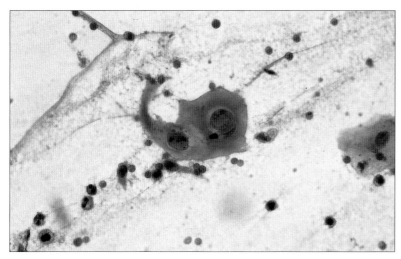

Fig. 14.51 Oesophagitis Pap x40. The squamous cells illustrated in this field show inflammatory changes, including nuclear enlargement and perinuclear haloes. Some inflammatory cells are also present.

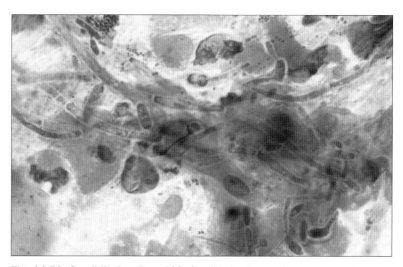

Fig. 14.52 Candidiasis – Pap x100. Candida hyphae and spores are well-illustrated in this oesophageal brush smear.

Squamous carcinoma of the oesophagus is easily diagnosed on cytological material. Well-differentiated tumours are composed of keratinized carcinoma cells with abundant refractile orange cytoplasm (azure blue on air-dried material), which vary in shape (**Fig. 14.53**). Cells derived from poorly differentiated squamous cell carcinomas are often in clusters, contain ovoid nuclei with prominent nucleoli, and lack keratin. The cell margins are sharp, unlike those in adenocarcinoma.

Adenocarcinoma of the oesophagus is also recognized easily on brush samples. Clusters of enlarged pleomorphic carcinoma cells are seen, some showing vacuolation (**Fig. 14.54**). Many of the nuclei contain huge red nucleoli (**Fig. 14.55**) and single cells are not infrequent. Inflammatory cells, sheets of benign glandular cells, and squamous cells may also be present.

Other neoplasms of the oesophagus include **melanoma**, **small cell anaplastic carcinoma**, and lymphoma. Their features have been described elsewhere (see Chapter 10).

Gastric brushings and washings

These methods of sampling gastric lesions are used in conjunction with gastric biopsies; where there is an area of stenosis they are sometimes are more effective than the latter. Wet-fixed smears are prepared by the clinician from the brushings, and the washings are despatched to the cytology laboratory where they are spun down and further wet-fixed smears prepared.

Gastric ulcer is a common reason for sending brush samples to the laboratory. The smears contain abundant inflammatory exudate composed of necrotic cellular

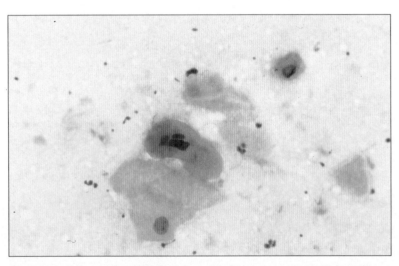

Fig. 14.53 Squamous carcinoma – Pap x40. Squamous cells are illustrated in this field, one showing keratinization and multinucleation suggestive of malignancy, the others displaying degenerative changes.

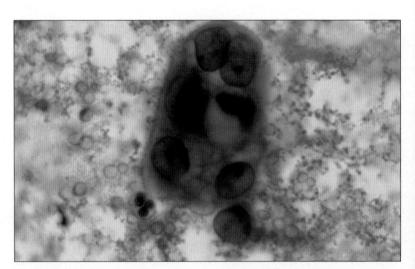

Fig. 14.54 Adenocarcinoma – Pap x100. This cluster of adenocarcinoma cells in an oesophageal brush sample shows vacuolated cytoplasm and prominent nucleoli.

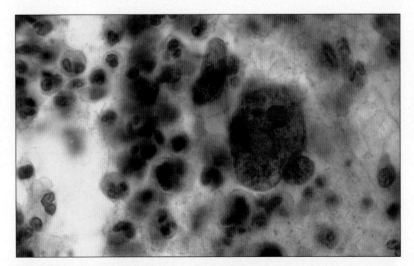

Fig. 14.55 Adenocarcinoma – Pap x100. The large nucleus, containing a huge red nucleolus, in the centre of the field is from an oesophageal adenocarcinoma; it is almost obscured by the inflammatory cells around it.

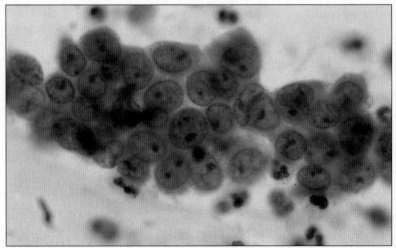

Fig. 14.56 Gastric ulcer – Pap x100. Illustrated here, in a gastric brush sample, is a cluster of reactive glandular cells with enlarged nuclei and well-defined nuclear margins, accompanied by neutrophils.

material, neutrophil polymorphs, and histiocytes. Clusters of reactive glandular cells with enlarged, but regular, nuclei and noticeable nucleoli are seen frequently (**Fig. 14.56**), in addition to sheets of benign columnar or cuboidal epithelial cells. The sheets of benign cells may contain goblet cells (**Fig. 14.57**) suggesting intestinal metaplasia. Food debris is often noted, as are bacteria.

Adenocarcinoma of the stomach shows the same features that are seen in adenocarcinomas elsewhere, with clusters of pleomorphic glandular cells containing vacuoles and prominent red nucleoli (**Fig. 14.58**). There are often Candida hyphae and spores in the background and benign glandular cells may also be seen.

Linitis plastica, being a neoplasm that grows and infiltrates beneath the mucosal surface, is not detectable from brushings or washings, but can be diagnosed by fine needle aspiration cytology. The aspirate contains clusters of pleomorphic adenocarcinoma cells, with typical vacuolation and prominent nucleoli (**Fig. 14.59**).

Lymphoma can be diagnosed from brushings and washings. The features are similar to lymphomas elsewhere, with a monomorphic population of abnormal lymphoid cells (**Fig. 14.60**).

Rare neoplasms, such as **sarcomas**, produce cytological material that contains both spindle cells and others with rounded nuclei (**Figs 14.61, 14.62**). The cytoplasm is delicate and wispy, and large red nucleoli may be present. It is not possible to type sarcomas on cytology and so a biopsy should always be recommended.

Leiomyoblastoma of the stomach is a stromal neoplasm which is possibly of smooth muscle derivation but may be neural in origin. Fine needle aspirates are difficult to interpret, but features that may be seen include epithelioid cells which are usually round (**Figs 14.63, 14.64**) or spindle shaped (**Fig. 14.65**) occasionally accompanied by myxoid material (**Fig. 14.66**).

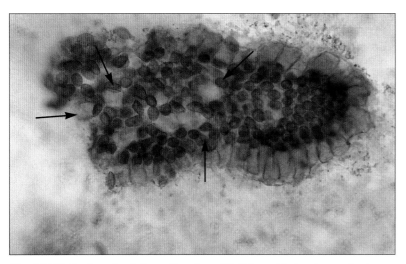

Fig. 14.57 Benign glandular cells – Pap x40. This gastric brush sample shows a sheet of uniform glandular cells with a palisaded edge and some goblet cells in the centre, (arrowed) suggestive of intestinal metaplasia.

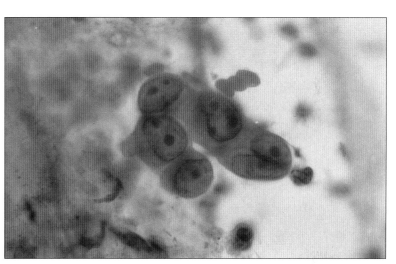

Fig. 14.58 Adenocarcinoma – Pap x100. The adenocarcinoma cells in this brush sample contain nuclei which are irregular in shape, with pale chromatin and large, red, central nucleoli.

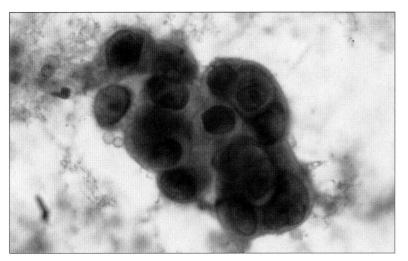

Fig. 14.59 Linitis plastica – Pap x100. Fine needle aspiration of this carcinoma produces a cellular sample with clusters of adenocarcinoma cells. Note the vacuolated cytoplasm and prominent nucleoli.

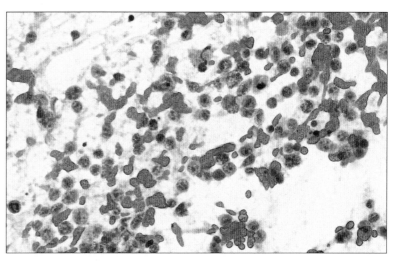

Fig. 14.60 Lymphoma – Pap x40. These gastric brushings show a monomorphic population of small cells with no discernible cytoplasm, suggestive of lymphoma. There were benign glandular cells elsewhere in the sample.

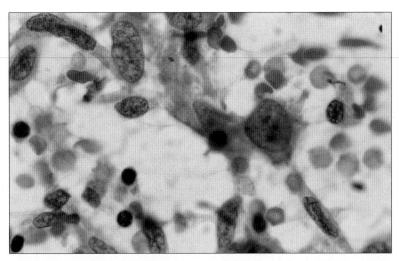

Fig. 14.61 Sarcoma – Pap x100. This fine needle aspirate of an epigastric mass contains spindle cells and other cells with more rounded nuclei. The chromatin pattern is abnormal, but the nuclei are not unduly large. The features are consistent with a sarcoma. The surgical specimen was reported as an epithelioid leiomyosarcoma of the stomach.

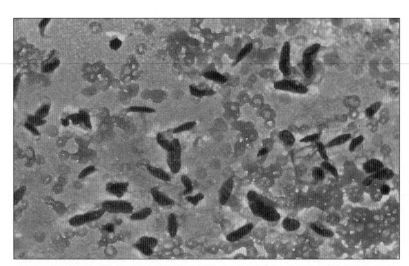

Fig. 14.62 Sarcoma – MGG x40. This field from the air-dried smear of the same aspirate as shown in **Figure 14.61** displays spindle-shaped cells in a myxoid type of stroma.

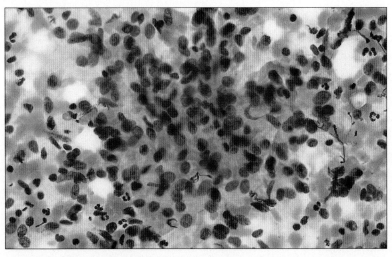

Fig. 14.63 Leiomyoblastoma – Pap x40. This cellular aspirate is composed of small rounded cells with pink cytoplasm. Pleomorphism is not a feature. (Case courtesy of Dr A Salerno, Bolzano, Italy.)

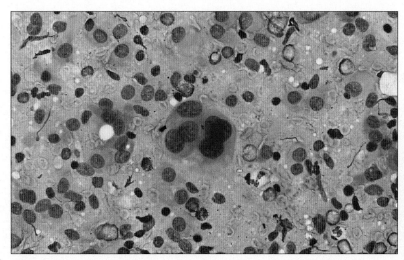

Fig. 14.64 Leiomyoblastoma – MGG x40. The air-dried smear shows pleomorphism with some larger cells i the centre of the field surrounded by small cells. (Case courtesy of Dr A Salerno, Bolzano, Italy.)

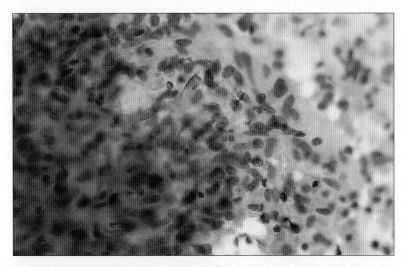

Fig. 14.65 Leiomyoblastoma – Pap x40. This field shows closely packed small spindle cells with little cytoplasm. This feature is believed to suggest neural differentation, (Case courtesy of Dr A Salerno, Bolzano, Italy.)

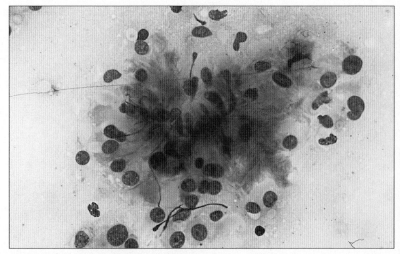

Fig. 14.66 Leiomyoblastoma – MGG x40. The small round cells seen in this field have pale blue cytoplasm and interspersed myoxoid material. (Case courtesy of Dr A Salerno, Bolzano, Italy.)

SUGGESTED READING

Chan MKM, McGuire LJ. Cytodiagnosis of lesions presenting as salivary gland swellings. *Diagn Cytopathol* 1992; **8**: 439–443.

Chan MKM, McGuire LJ, King W, *et al*. Cytodiagnosis of 112 salivary gland lesions: Correlation with histologic and frozen section diagnosis. *Acta Cytol* 1992; **36**: 353–363.

Lowhagen T, Tani EM, Skoog L. Salivary glands and rare head and neck lesions. In: Bibbo M, ed. *Comprehensive Cytopathology*. Philadelphia: WB Saunders; 1991: 621–648.

Palmo O, Reei AM, De Cristofaro JA, Fiaccavanto S. Fine needle aspiration cytology in two cases of acinic-cell carcinoma of the parotid gland: Discussion of diagnostic criteria. *Acta Cytol* 1985; **29**: 516–521.

Singh S, Macleod G, Walker T, *et al*. Endoscopic fine-needle aspiration cytology in the diagnosis of linitis plastica. *Brit J Surg* 1994; **81** : 1010.

Young JA. The salivary glands. In: Young JA, ed. *Fine Needle Aspiration Cytopathology*. Oxford: Blackwell; 1993: 48–67.

Young J. The salivary glands. In: Gray W, ed. *Diagnostic Cytopathology*. Edinburgh: Churchill Livingstone; 1995: 301–304.

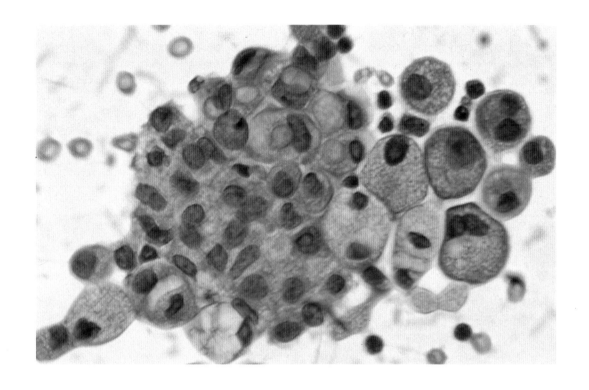

SEROUS CAVITY EFFUSIONS

15

SEROUS CAVITY EFFUSIONS

The intrathoracic and intraperitoneal organs are covered by a single layer of mesothelial cells, which is continuous with the lining of the thoracic and peritoneal cavities. Similar cells line the scrotal sac and the joints (where they are referred to as synovial cells). The potential space between the two layers of epithelium contains a small amount of lubricating fluid. Trauma, infections, or neoplasms result in an increase in the amount of fluid present and the cause of the effusion may be elucidated by examining the fluid. The effusion is aspirated and sent to the cytology laboratory in a clean, dry container. If it is to be kept overnight, it is stored in the refrigerator. The is measured, the colour, clarity, and amount noted, it is then centrifuged, and, if necessary, cytospin smears made, both wet-fixed and air-dried stained with Papanicolaou and May Grunwald Giemsa stains, respectively. Extra smears are reserved for special stains. Any clots present are treated as histological specimens and subjected to sectioning and staining with haematoxylin and eosin. Cell blocks may be prepared from the fluid, but these take a longer time to process than do routine smears, and are therefore mainly used for research purposes. If much blood is present in the effusion Carnoy's fluid should be used to lyse the erythrocytes and unmask any malignant cells present (**Figs 15.1, 15.2**).

Benign effusions contain single **mesothelial cells**, as well as some in small clusters. Mesothelial cells vary in size but, in general, are fairly large, with abundant translucent cytoplasm and a central nucleus with a prominent nuclear margin and nucleolus. In wet-fixed smears the cytoplasm stains blue, in air-dried smears a pale mauve, and the cytoplasmic membrane is surrounded by a frilly or lacy border (**Figs 15.3, 15.4**), which represents the microvilli seen on electron microscopy. Very rarely, mesothelial cells exhibit long processes resembling

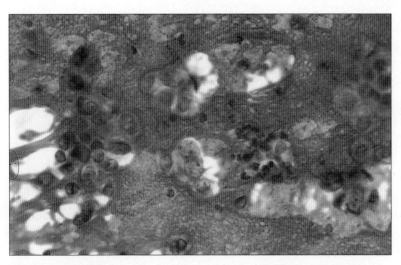

Fig. 15.1 Ascitic fluid – Pap x40. This sample of ascitic fluid is heavily blood-stained and therefore difficult to interpret. The background cells may be epithelial or mesothelial.

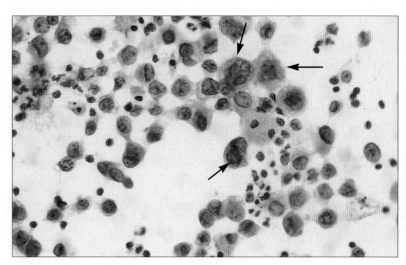

Fig. 15.2 Ascitic fluid (after Carnoy's) – Pap x40. This fluid is from the same case as shown in **Figure 15.1,** but has been treated with Carnoy's solution to lyse the blood cells. Note the clean background and the well-preserved malignant cells now visible (arrowed).

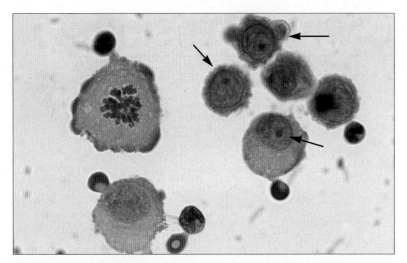

Fig. 15.3 Mesothelial cells – Pap x40. This benign pleural effusion contains mesothelial cells of varying sizes, with rounded nuclei and abundant blue cytoplasm with frilly or lacy borders. Note the visible nucleoli in the nucleii of the smaller cells (arrows) and also the normal mitotic figure.

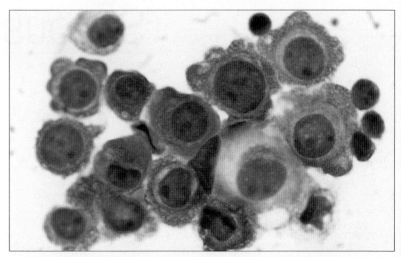

Fig. 15.4 Mesothelial cells – MGG x40. This air-dried preparation contains benign mesothelial cells with prominent frilly borders. The nuclear–cytoplasmic ratio is high and there are conspicuous nucleoli.

cilia, which are elongated microvilli (**Fig. 15.5**). Within the cell groups there are clear spaces or gaps between adjacent cells, known as cell windows – an important method of differentiating between mesothelial cells and metastatic adenocarcinoma cells (**Figs 15.6, 15.7**). In serous cavity samples, such as peritoneal or Pouch of Douglas washings, mesothelial cells may be seen in large flat or folded sheets with uniform nuclei (**Figs 15.8, 15.9**). Mesothelial cells occasionally contain vacuoles and can exhibit marked variation in size, as well as in the number of nuclei present (**Fig. 15.10**), especially when reactive. Papillary clusters of benign mesothelial cells showing atypia, such as nuclear enlargement, and prominent nucleoli may be seen in reactive conditions. A typical feature of mesothelial cell clusters is the presence of hyaline material in the centre, which represents collagen and stains blue in wet-fixed smears and mauve in air-dried smears (**Figs 15.11, 15.12**). Benign mesothelial cells often show mitoses (**Figs 15.13, 15.14**).

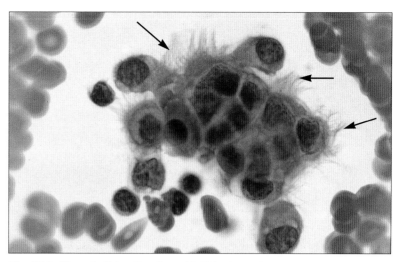

Fig. 15.5 Mesothelial cells – Pap x40. This sheet of benign mesothelial cells exhibits long cytoplasmic processes resembling cilia, but which are probably long microvilli (arrowed).

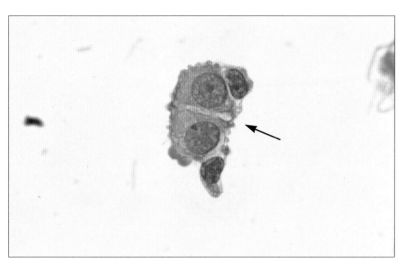

Fig. 15.6 Mesothelial cells – Pap x40. The two benign mesothelial cells illustrated here show a clear gap between their borders, commonly termed a window (arrow).

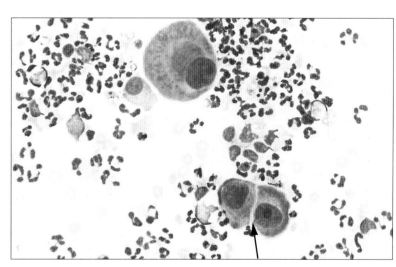

Fig. 15.7 Mesothelial cells – MGG x40. This field contains three mesothelial cells, two of which are closely apposed with a window or gap between them (arrow). Note the variation in cell size.

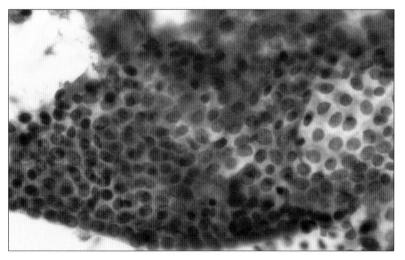

Fig. 15.8 Mesothelial cells – Pap x40. Illustrated here is a sheet of mesothelial cells which are uniform in size and shape. Note the palisaded edge – a sign that it is benign.

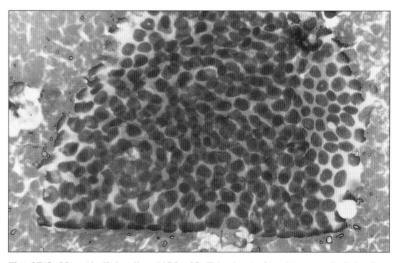

Fig. 15.9 Mesothelial cells – MGG x40. This sheet of benign mesothelial cells is flat, composed of regular cells. These sheets are more commonly seen in peritoneal washings than in ascitic or pleural effusions.

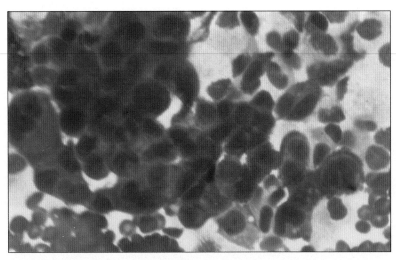

Fig. 15.10 Mesothelial cells – MGG x40. This three-dimensional cluster of mesothelial cells shows reactive changes, with some variation in nuclear size.

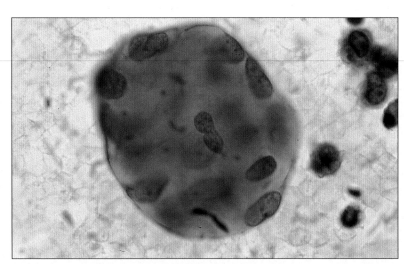

Fig. 15.11 Mesothelial cells – Pap x40. This ascitic fluid specimen contains a cluster of mesothelial cells arranged around a core of collagen, a feature which is extremely useful in differentiating benign mesothelial cells from adenocarcinoma.

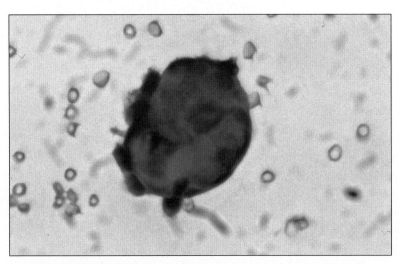

Fig. 15.12 Mesothelial cells – MGG x40. This field shows a collagen core in an air-dried preparation of a pleural effusion.

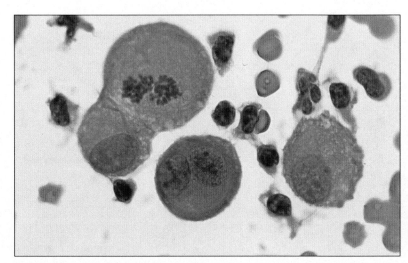

Fig. 15.13 Mesothelial cells – Pap x40. The four mesothelial cells seen here demonstrate a variety of appearances: the one in the centre is binucleate with amphophilic staining, probably due to degeneration. The cell on the right has a lacy border and the larger cell in the group of two is undergoing mitosis.

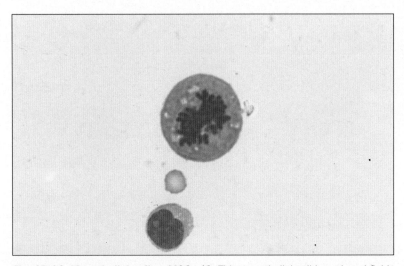

Fig. 15.14 Mesothelial cells – MGG x40. This mesothelial cell in a pleural fluid sample shows mitosis.

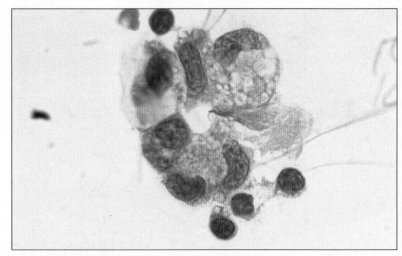

Fig. 15.15 Histiocytes – Pap x40. Illustrated here is a group of histiocytes with elongated and bean-shaped nuclei. Note the delicate foamy cytoplasm.

PLEURAL AND PERITONEAL CAVITY EFFUSIONS

It used to be fashionable to subdivide these effusions into transudates and exudates but the features usually overlap, making clear distinction between the two impossible.

Histiocytes are commonly noted in effusions. They vary in size, but are usually smaller than mesothelial cells, with either bean-shaped or ovoid nuclei, visible nucleoli, and abundant delicate or foamy cytoplasm (**Figs 15.15, 15.16**). Occasionally, histiocytes appear to be in cohesive sheets, probably a result of centrifugation rather than a cellular process. **Multinucleated histiocytes** may be seen, usually as part of reactive changes.

Small **lymphocytes** are very common in reactive effusions (**Fig. 15.17**), but when present in large numbers necessitate careful examination to differentiate between a lymphocytic effusion and a lymphoma. Proteinaceous background material is also seen in effusions.

In acute inflammatory conditions the fluid may be turbid and purulent – known clinically as **empyema** when it involves pleural fluid and **peritonitis** when the abdominal cavity is affected. The smears contain large numbers of neutrophil polymorphs and small histiocytes, obscuring all other cellular detail (**Figs 15.18, 15.19**). Organisms may be seen, but cannot be identified on cytology. Care should be taken to search for necrotic cellular debris which may rep-

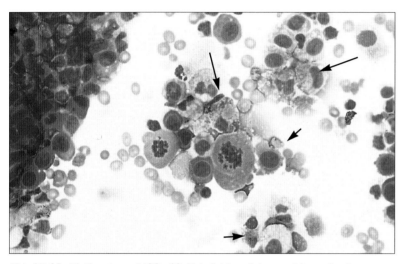

Fig. 15.16 Histiocytes – MGG x40. This field contains a mixture of cells – mesothelial cells with frilly borders (short arrows), mesothelial cells in mitosis, histiocytes (long arrows), and some erythrocytes.

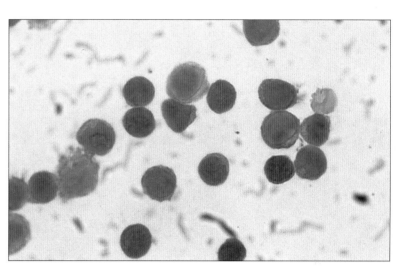

Fig. 15.17 Lymphocytes – MGG x100. This pleural effusion contains many benign lymphocytes which are variable in size and have a thin rim of cytoplasm.

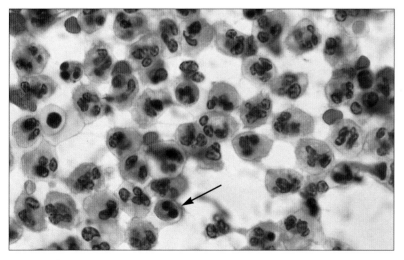

Fig. 15.18 Empyema – Pap x100. In this acute inflammatory process involving the pleural cavity, the cell population consists of neutrophils with an occasional eosinophil (arrow).

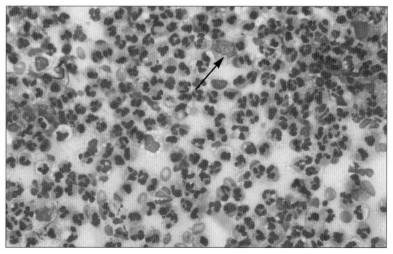

Fig. 15.19 Empyema – MGG x40. In this air-dried smear the neutrophil nuclei stain purple. The pale smudged cells in the background are probably histiocytes (arrow).

resent an underlying malignancy, but it must be remembered that mesothelial cells in such conditions may look very atypical and simulate malignancy. Similar cytological features are seen in ascitic fluid in **acute pancreatitis (Figs 15.20, 15.21)**.

Eosinophilic effusions are not uncommon. They may represent an allergic process, but are also associated with pneumothorax. The wet-fixed smear under low power appears to contain many neutrophils **(Fig. 15.22)**, but at higher magnification these are seen to be bilobed eosinophils with pale granules **(Fig. 15.23)**.

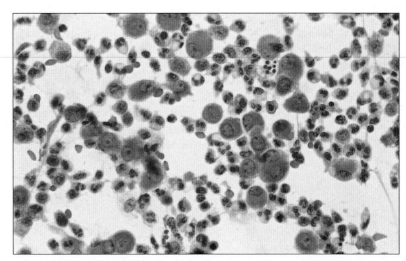

Fig. 15.20 Acute pancreatitis – Pap x40. This ascitic fluid preparation contains reactive mesothelial cells, some of which are binucleate, and numerous neutrophils. The features are non-specific.

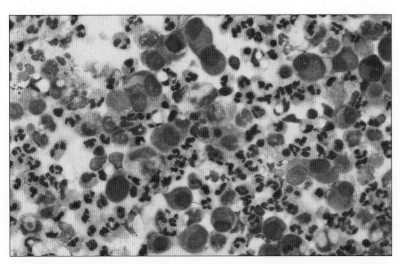

Fig. 15.21 Acute pancreatitis – MGG x40. This air-dried preparation of ascitic fluid from the case illustrated in **Figure 15.19** also shows mesothelial cells and numerous acute inflammatory cells.

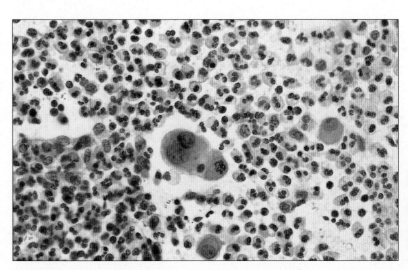

Fig. 15.22 Eosinophilic effusion – Pap x40. At this magnification, this pleural effusion appears to contain many neutrophil polymorphs and some reactive mesothelial cells.

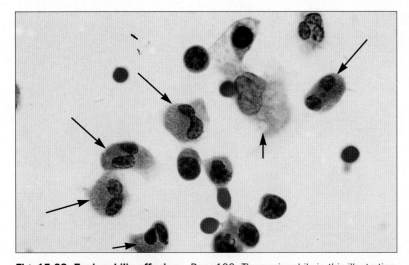

Fig. 15.23 Eosinophilic effusion – Pap x100. The eosinophils in this illustration are bilobed with greenish yellow granules (long arrows). There are also a few lymphocytes, a histiocyte (short arrows), and a neutrophil polymorph in this field.

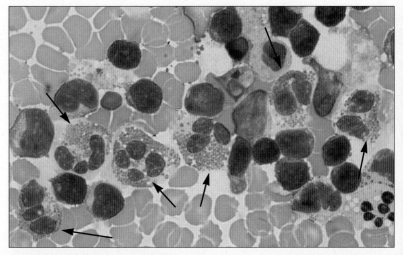

Fig. 15.24 Eosinophilic effusion – MGG x100. Illustrated here are several eosinophils with nuclear lobes that vary in number from two to four (arrows). The granules are coarse and stain pink. There are also a few histiocytes and lymphocytes in this field.

The granules are orange-to-pink are usually much more easily detectable in the DiffQuik and May Grunwald Giemsa smears (**Fig. 15.24**). Where there are eosinophils there are usually **Charcot-Leyden crystals**, which are needle-shaped, variable in size and number, and stain a pale pink to orange with the Papanicolaou stain and blue with May Grunwald Giemsa (**Figs 15.25–15.27**). Distorted erythrocytes should not be mistaken for Charcot-Leyden crystals (**Fig. 15.28**).

Rheumatoid arthritis has characteristic features. The smears show amorphous granular debris in the background (**Fig. 15.29**) and contain, in addition,

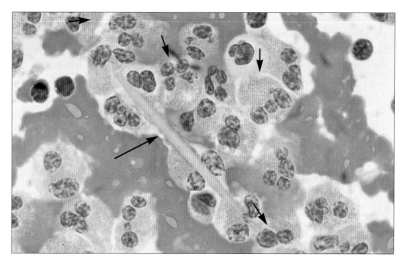

Fig. 15.25 Charcot-Leyden crystals – Pap x100. The Charcot-Leyden crystal in this field is rather pale (long arrow) and might easily be missed. Note the surrounding eosinophils with their refractile greenish yellow granules (short arrows).

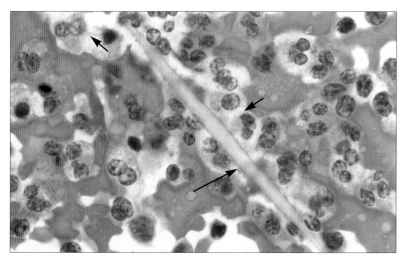

Fig. 15.26 Charcot-Leyden crystals – Pap x100. The crystal illustrated here is very large and clearly defined (long arrow), but the granules of the eosinophils are not particularly prominent (short arrows).

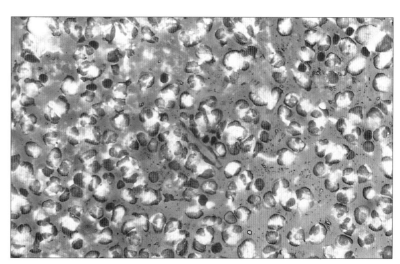

Fig. 15.27 Charcot-Leyden crystals – MGG x40. In air-dried smears Charcot-Leyden crystals are not easily found. They are pale blue and may be obscured by the surrounding cells, some of which are eosinophils.

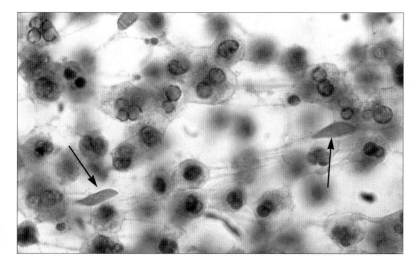

Fig. 15.28 Erythrocytes – Pap x100. The erythrocytes pictured here are distorted with pointed edges (arrows), mimicking Charcot-Leyden crystals.

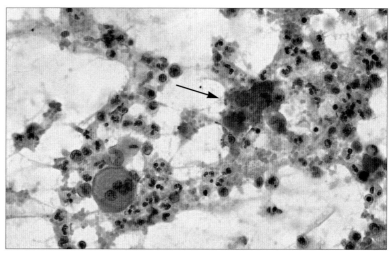

Fig. 15.29 Rheumatoid arthritis – Pap x40. This pleural effusion shows background debris, (arrow) multinucleated histiocytes, neutrophils, and some lymphocytes.

many inflammatory cells and enlarged multinucleated histiocytes and spindle cells (Figs 15.30–15.32), as well as epithelioid histiocytes. Reactive mesothelial cells are seen frequently.

Conditions in which there has been previous haemorrhage into the serous cavity, such as **haemothorax** or **endometriosis**, produce effusions which contain numerous haemosiderin-filled macrophages – siderophages (Figs 15.33, 15.34). Reactive mesothelial cells are also present and can be mistaken for malignancy. Endometrial cells may be seen in the peritoneal fluid in endometriosis (Figs 15.35, 15.36).

Benign conditions, such as **endosalpingiosis**, can result in atypical appearances in peritoneal effusions. The mesothelial cells appear very reactive, occur-

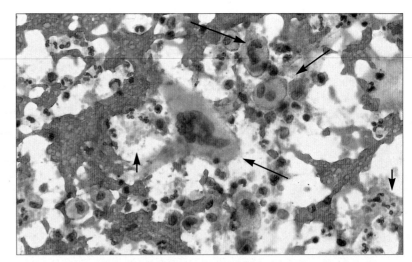

Fig. 15.30 Rheumatoid arthritis – Pap x40. Multinucleated cells with varying numbers of nuclei are seen in this field (long arrows). Some necrotic debris is also present (short arrows).

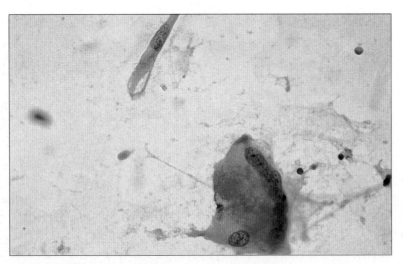

Fig. 15.31 Rheumatoid arthritis – Pap x40. In this field there is a large, bizarre, multinucleated histiocyte with most of its nuclei lining one side of the cell, as well as a spindle-shaped cell (possibly also histiocytic in origin).

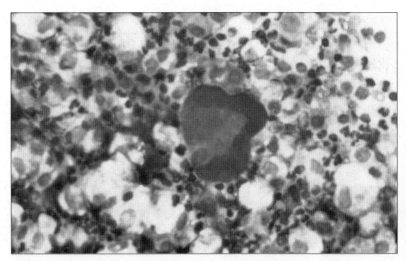

Fig. 15.32 Rheumatoid arthritis – MGG x40. The large multinucleated histiocyte in the centre of the field displays an unusual arrangement of its nuclei at the periphery of the cell. Note also the inflammatory cells in the background.

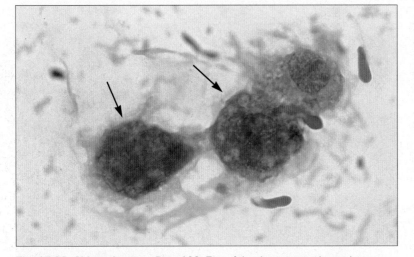

Fig. 15.33 Siderophages – Pap x100. Two of the three macrophages have foamy cytoplasm containing greenish yellow haemosiderin pigment (arrows), suggestive of previous haemorrhage into the peritoneal cavity.

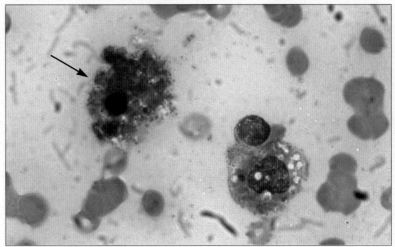

Fig. 15.34 Siderophages – MGG x100. In air-dried smears haemosiderin takes on a bluish black colour, obscuring the nucleus of the macrophage (arrow).

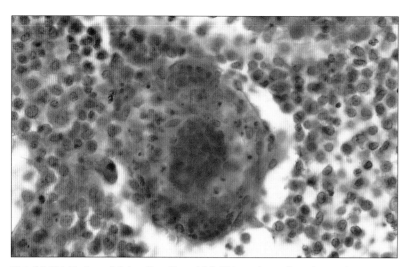

Fig. 15.35 Endometrial cells – Pap x100. This peritoneal wash sample contains much blood, histiocytes, and a cluster of endometrial cells with darker stromal cells and outer glandular cells, similar to their appearance in cervical smears.

ring in papillary clusters with enlarged nuclei, and psammoma bodies may be present (**Figs 15.37, 15.38**). Clusters of small glandular epithelial cells may also be seen, believed to be tubal in origin (**Fig 15.39**).

One of the most taxing cytological problems is the differentiation between adenocarcinoma and mesothelial cell proliferation, either benign or malignant (**Fig. 15.40**). Detailed descriptions, with illustrations, of the differences between the two tumours, are provided below (see **Figures 15.89–15.99**). These are useful, but may not always distinguish between the two.

Adenocarcinomas from various sites frequently metastasize to the pleural and peritoneal cavities. **Metastatic adenocarcinomas** vary in their appearance. **Carcinoma of the breast** typically presents as spherical balls of small, mildly

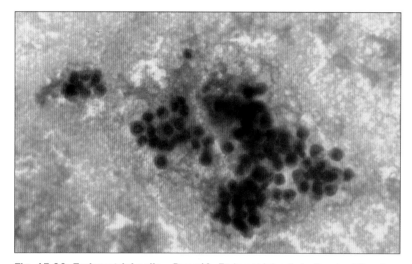

Fig. 15.36 Endometrial cells – Pap x40. Endometrial cells in Pouch of Douglas fluid are often small and degenerate, as illustrated here.

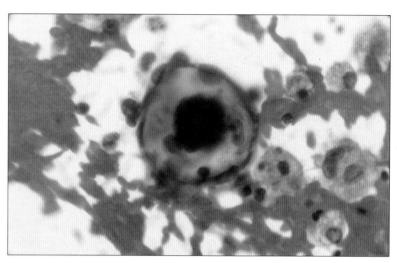

Fig. 15.37 Endosalpingiosis – Pap x63. This field contains a rounded cluster of glandular cells surrounding a psammoma body. In the background are histiocytes, some containing haemosiderin. No definite evidence of malignancy is apparent.

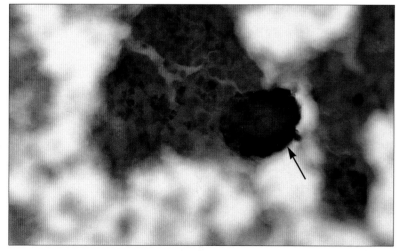

Fig. 15.38 Endosalpingiosis – Pap x40. Illustrated here are groups of small glandular cells with a superimposed psammoma body (arrow). These appearances closely resemble those of metastatic serous cystadenoma of the ovary.

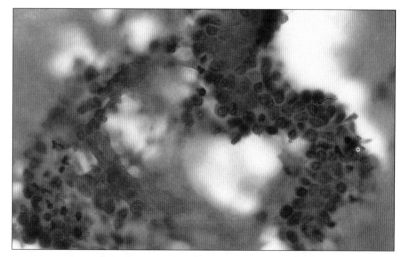

Fig. 15.39 Endosalpingiosis – Pap x40. The clusters of cells seen in peritoneal fluid in endosalpingiosis appear glandular, but ciliated cells may be seen occasionally as this condition is believed to be composed of tubal-type epithelial cells.

pleomorphic carcinoma cells without vacuolation or prominent nucleoli (**Figs 15.41, 15.42**). High-grade metastatic breast neoplasms may display clusters of pleomorphic vacuolated adenocarcinoma cells with enlarged nucleoli (**Fig. 15.43**). Single malignant cells may be seen (**Fig. 15.44**), accompanied by mesothelial cells and histiocytes. Ovarian adenocarcinomas are characteristically pleomorphic with huge vacuolated cells, either single or in small clusters, often with very few mesothelial or other cells in the background (**Figs 15.45, 15.46**). Sometimes little pleomorphism and lack of vacuolation are noted, especially in tumours such as serous cystadenocarcinomas (**Figs 15.47, 15.48**). Mitoses are frequent in the pleomorphic forms (**Fig. 15.49**). Metastases from clear cell adenocarcinoma of the ovary are composed of clusters of malignant cells, with clear cytoplasm surrounding collections of mucin (**Figs 15.50, 15.51**). **Psammoma bodies** may be seen, usually laminated, surrounded by pleomorphic carcinoma cells (**Figs 15.52, 15.53**), or by small bland epithelial cells (**Figs 15.54**), in which case the diagnosis could be either borderline serous cystadenocarcinoma or endosalpingiosis. A dogmatic report cannot be issued in such cases.

Some metastatic adenocarcinomas are composed of cells with cytoplasm showing honeycomb vacuolation and relatively small nuclei, resembling histiocytes (**Figs 15.55, 15.56**). Higher magnification usually reveals at least a few cells with pleomorphic nuclei. If not, immunocytochemical stains are necessary to prove that the cells are glandular (**Fig. 15.57**). Cells derived from **carcinoma of the colon** often fall into this category (**Fig. 15.58**). **Signet ring cell adenocarcinoma of the stomach**, which metastasizes to the peritoneum, sheds signet ring cells into ascitic fluid (**Figs 15.59, 15.60**).

ADENOCARCINOMA	MESOTHELIOMA
Two cell populations	One cell population
Cells usually in clusters	Cells usually in clusters
Scalloping of cluster edges common	Scalloping of cell clusters may be present
No 'windows' between cells	'Windows' between cells
No central core of collagen in clusters	Central core of collagen may be present
Large vacuoles indenting the nucleus	Vacuolation may be seen
Smooth cell margins	Frilly cell borders
Nuclei usually peripheral	Nuclei usually central
Cytoplasm is delicate and pale	Cytoplasm is more dense
HMFG2 usually positive	HMFG2 usually negative
BerEP4 usually positive	BerEP4 usually negative

Fig. 15.40 Metastatic adenocarcinoma versus mesothelioma.

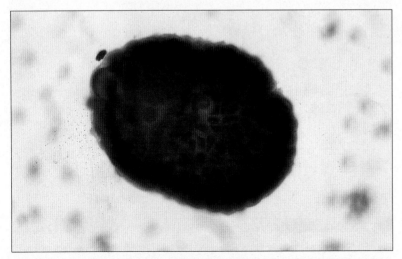

Fig. 15.41 Metastatic breast carcinoma – Pap x40. This illustrates the typical appearance of metastatic breast carcinoma in serous fluids with balls of small, apparently uniform cells. They are difficult to distinguish from mesothelial cell proliferation, unless a second population of mesothelial cells is found in the sample.

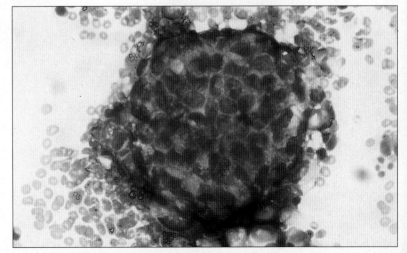

Fig. 15.42 Metastatic breast carcinoma – MGG x40. This pleural fluid contains a ball of adenocarcinoma cells which has metastasized from carcinoma of the breast. A search must be made for mesothelial cells to differentiate this from proliferating mesothelial cells.

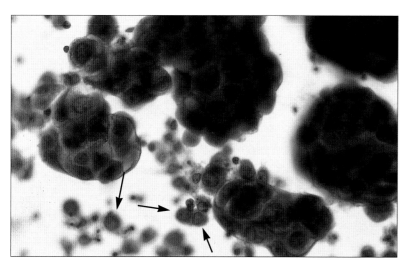

Fig. 15.43 Metastatic breast carcinoma – Pap x40. In this sample the carcinoma cells show more pleomorphism with some vacuolation. The windows between cells may cause problems in distinguishing this from mesothelioma, but there are benign mesothelial cells in the background (arrows).

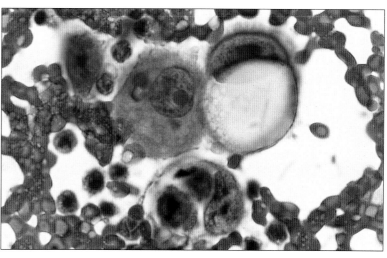

Fig. 15.44 Metastatic breast carcinoma – Pap x100. Illustrated are metastatic adenocarcinoma cells derived from a high-grade breast carcinoma. The cells have huge nuclei (compared with the lymphocytes in the background) and large nucleoli, and some are vacuolated.

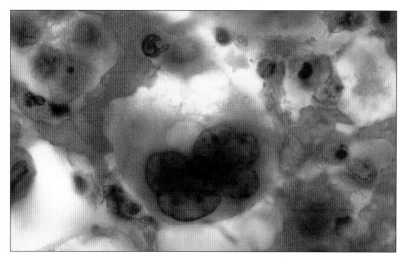

Fig. 15.45 Metastatic ovarian carcinoma – Pap x100. This field shows a large binucleate malignant cell with vacuoles. The nuclei are irregular in shape and the chromatin pattern is abnormally clear.

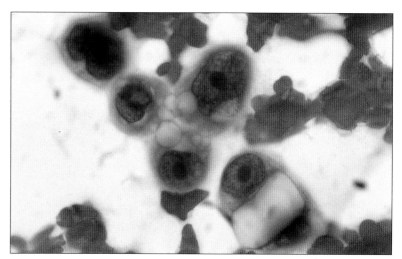

Fig. 15.46 Metastatic ovarian carcinoma – Pap x100. These cells are vacuolated and contain large red nucleoli.

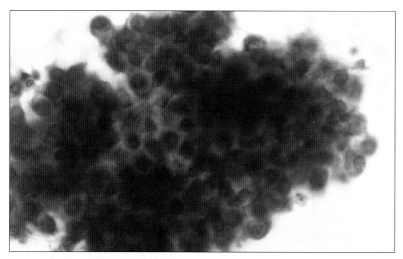

Fig. 15.47 Metastatic ovarian serous cystadenocarcinoma – Pap x40. This field contains a large cluster of small, mildly pleomorphic adenocarcinoma cells. No vacuolation is present.

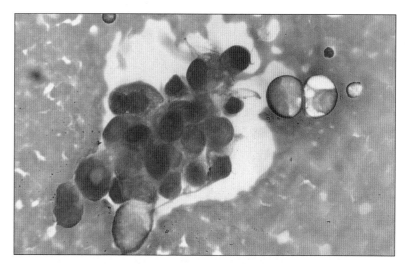

Fig. 15.48 Metastatic ovarian serous cystadenocarcinoma – MGG x40. This air-dried preparation of ascitic fluid displays a cluster of mildly pleomorphic adenocarcinoma cells and a few single malignant cells.

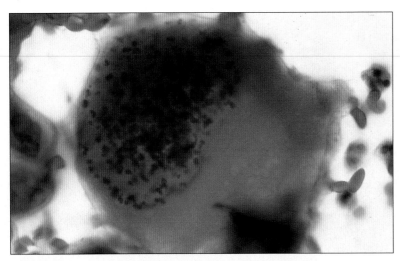

Fig. 15.49 Metastatic ovarian carcinoma – Pap x100. This enormous cell undergoing mitosis is from an ovarian carcinoma metastasizing to the peritoneal cavity.

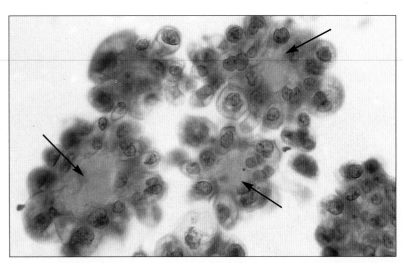

Fig. 15.50 Metastatic clear cell carcinoma of the ovary – Pap x40. This aspirate contains clusters of small adenocarcinoma cells with irregular nuclei and vacuolated cytoplasm. They are surrounding collections of mucinous material (arrows).

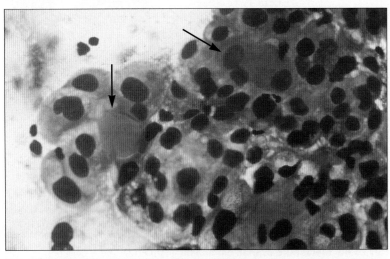

Fig. 15.51 Metastatic clear cell carcinoma of the ovary – MGG x40. In this field there are clusters of mildly pleomorphic adenocarcinoma cells with vacuolated cytoplasm, some surrounding mucin globules (arrows).

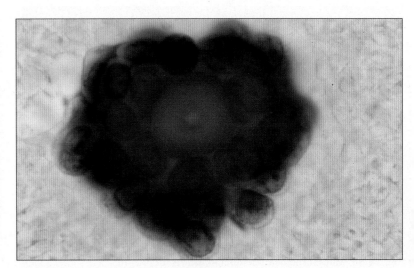

Fig. 15.52 Psammoma body – Pap x100. Illustrated here is a psammoma body composed of concentric rings of calcium, surrounded by adenocarcinoma cells with irregular nuclei and large red nucleoli.

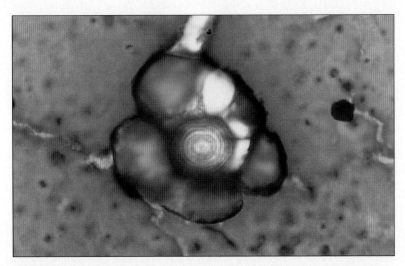

Fig. 15.53 Psammoma body – MGG x40. Psammoma bodies are detectable on air-dried material, as well as on wet-fixed smears. The laminations are clearly visible. Adenocarcinoma cells surround the calcospherite (psammoma body).

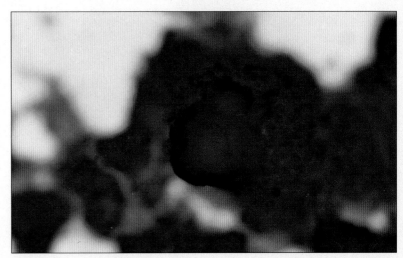

Fig. 15.54 Psammoma body – Pap x40. This cellular ascitic fluid contains large clusters of small, bland glandular cells and a laminated psammoma body (arrow). It is not possible to state definitely whether these cells are benign, from a lesion such as endosalpingiosis, or whether they are from a low-grade adenocarcinoma.

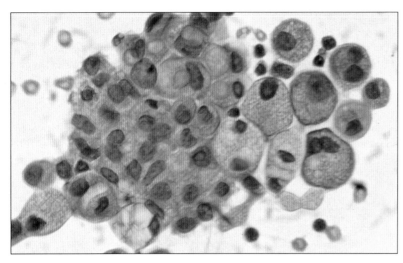

Fig. 15.55 Adenocarcinoma – Pap x100. The cells in this fluid have a low nuclear–cytoplasmic ratio with abundant honeycomb-type cytoplasmic vacuolation. Some of the nuclei appear to be bean-shaped, resembling histiocytes.

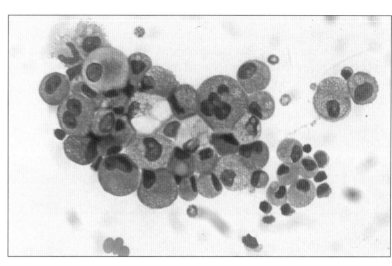

Fig. 15.56 Adenocarcinoma – MGG x40. This air-dried smear is prepared from the same ascitic fluid as that seen in **Figures 15.55** and **15.57**. The cells demonstrated here show abundant vacuolated cytoplasm and bland nuclei, similar to that of histiocytes.

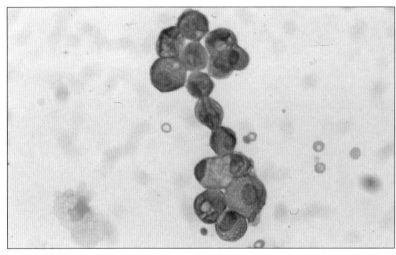

Fig. 15.57 Adenocarcinoma – BerEP4 x40. This cluster of cells from the same fluid as in **Figures 15.55** and **15.56** shows positive staining with this marker, confirming that these are adenocarcinoma cells, not histiocytes.

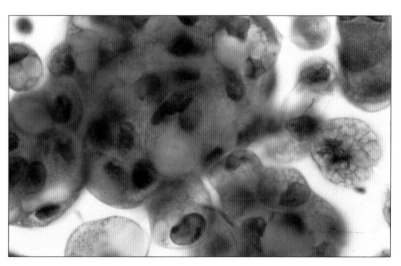

Fig. 15.58 Adenocarcinoma – Pap x100. This ascitic fluid contains adenocarcinoma cells which have spread from carcinoma of the colon. Note the abundant vacuolated cytoplasm.

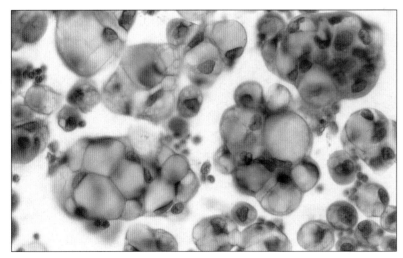

Fig. 15.59 Signet ring cell adenocarcinoma of the stomach – Pap x40. The clusters of malignant cells illustrated here are composed of signet ring type cells with large vacuoles distending the cytoplasm.

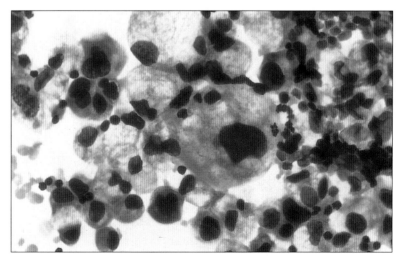

Fig. 15.60 Signet ring cell adenocarcinoma of the stomach – MGG x40. The signet ring cell shape is not as obvious in air-dried preparations (this case is the same as that illustrated in **Figure 15.59**).

Peritoneal washings are a useful method of detecting whether borderline or malignant ovarian carcinomas have spread outside the surface; they are also useful in following-up patients after treatment. Sometimes, peritoneal washings can produce papillary clusters of reactive mesothelial cells, which may appear suspicious of malignancy; immunocytochemical stains will help to identify those that are malignant.

In **pseudomyxoma peritonei** the peritoneal fluid is composed of thick, gelatinous material which can be very difficult to aspirate. Smears are composed of abundant mucin, which varies in colour from pale pink to pale blue on the Papanicolaou-stained smear and is bright pink with May Grunwald Giemsa (**Fig. 15.61**). The epithelial cells may be few and far between and appear quite bland, with delicate foamy cytoplasm and small vesicular nuclei. These cells are occasionally seen trapped in pools of mucin. Mucin may also be seen in peritoneal fluid in **mucinous cystadenocarcinomas of the ovary (Figs 15.62, 15.63)**, but in smaller amounts than in pseudomyxoma peritonei. **Endometrial adenocarcinoma** cells are usually smaller than cells from ovarian carcinoma (**Figs 15.64, 15.65**). **Renal cell carcinoma** metastases have cells with foamy cytoplasm and comparatively small nuclei (**Figs 15.66, 15.67**), which are PAS positive (**Fig. 15.68**) and diastase–PAS negative. Metastatic **malignant melanoma** cells have large nucleoli and often contain pigment (**Figs 15.69–15.71**). Metastatic adenocarcinomas from unknown primary neoplasms occasionally present as single cells without vacuoles in serous fluids and may

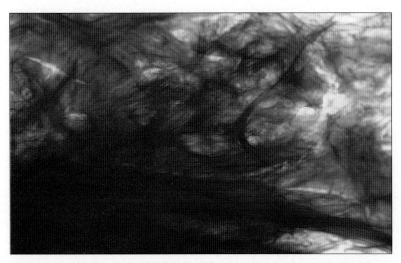

Fig. 15.61 Pseudomyxoma peritonei – MGG x40. This smear shows the abundant mucin seen in these aspirates. Often no cells are seen, but when they are present they are bland and may be columnar in type.

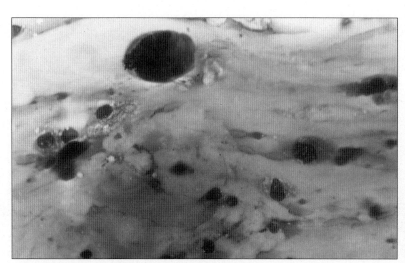

Fig. 15.62 Mucinous cystadenocarcinoma of the ovary – MGG x40. Small amounts of mucin may be seen in the ascitic fluid from these tumours. The malignant cells, however, are usually pleomorphic and not bland.

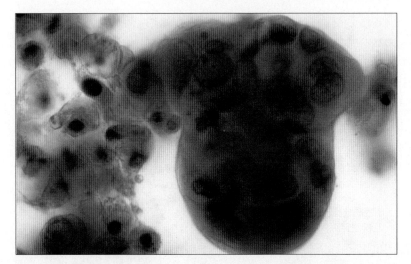

Fig. 15.63 Mucinous cystadenocarcinoma of the ovary – Pap x100. The cells illustrated here are pleomorphic glandular cells with vacuolated cytoplasm and prominent nucleoli. Background mucin is not identified easily in wet-fixed smears.

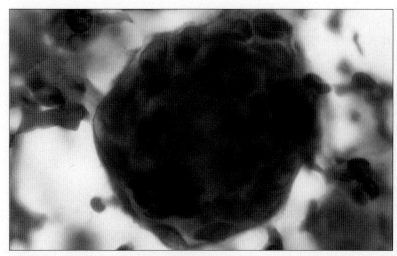

Fig. 15.64 Endometrial carcinoma – Pap x100. This field shows a three-dimensional ball-like cluster of small mildly pleomorphic adenocarcinoma cells.

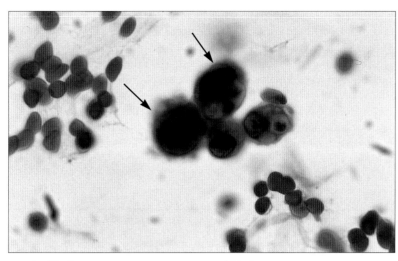

Fig. 15.65 Endometrial carcinoma – Pap x100. The small cells seen here exhibit cytoplasmic vacuoles, some containing phagocytosed erythrocytes (arrows). The cells are much smaller than ovarian carcinoma cells.

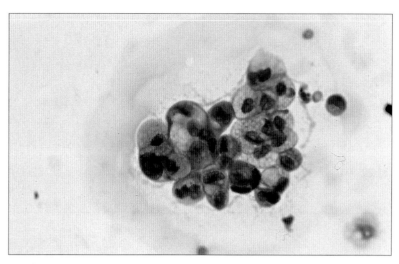

Fig. 15.66 Renal cell carcinoma – Pap x40. The neoplastic cells shown here have abundant, vacuolated cytoplasm and relatively small nuclei, closely resembling those of renal cell carcinoma.

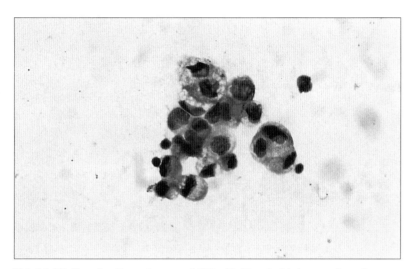

Fig. 15.67 Renal cell carcinoma – MGG x40. The air-dried smear from the same case as shown in **Figure 15.66** shows similar features with vacuolated cytoplasm, but the nuclei appear to be more pleomorphic.

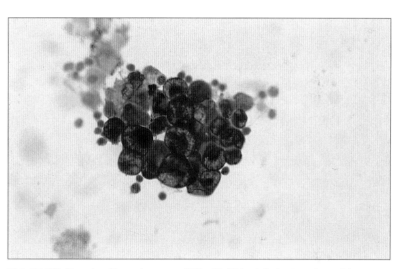

Fig. 15.68 Renal cell carcinoma – PAS x40. This stain is strongly positive because of the glycogen within the tumour cells, the diastase–PAS was negative. An Oil red O stain would also be positive because of the lipid content of the cells.

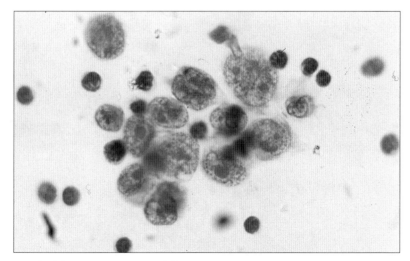

Fig. 15.69 Melanoma – Pap x100. This loosely cohesive group of pale-staining cells exhibits large nucleoli with an abnormal granular chromatin pattern. Very little cytoplasm is visible. There are no specific features to indicate that this is a metastatic malignant melanoma and without a history this specimen would have to be reported as containing undifferentiated malignant cells.

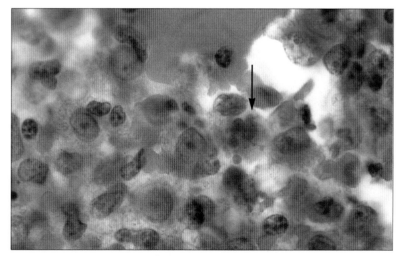

Fig. 15.70 Melanoma – Pap x100. In this case the pleural fluid contains malignant cells with abundant cytoplasm and coarse, brownish yellow melanin pigment granules (arrow).

be difficult to distinguish from mesothelioma (**Figs 15.72, 15.73**). In such cases, a positive BerEP4 or HMFG2 immunocytochemical stain identifies these cells as adenocarcinoma (**Fig. 15.74**).

Other tumours that metastasize to the serous cavities include lung carcinomas. **Squamous carcinoma** cells in effusions show the usual features of keratinization and a single-cell population when they are well-differentiated (**Figs 15.75, 15.76**). **Small cell anaplastic carcinoma** cells of the oat cell type may be missed on the wet-fixed smear, as they are small and may be single or in small groups, resembling lymphocytes (**Fig. 15.77**). These cells are easier to detect on the air-dried smear stained with May Grunwald Giemsa, in which

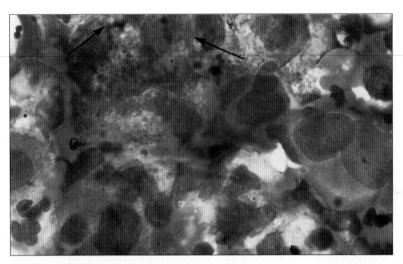

Fig. 15.71 Melanoma – MGG x100. This air-dried smear from the same case as shown in **Figure 15.70** displays similar large malignant cells and coarse, bluish black melanin pigment (arrows).

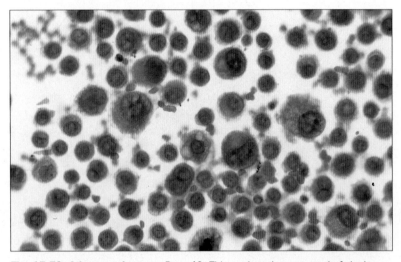

Fig. 15.72 Adenocarcinoma – Pap x40. This aspirate is composed of single malignant cells with pleomorphic nuclei, some vacuolation, and apparent microvilli around some of the cells. The differential diagnosis includes mesothelioma and adenocarcinoma.

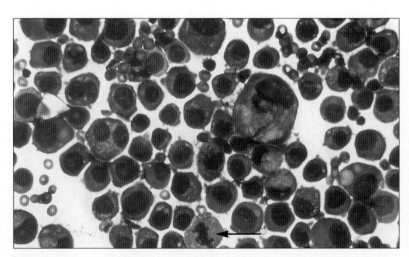

Fig. 15.73 Adenocarcinoma – MGG x40. The air-dried smear of the same case as shown in **Figure 15.72** shows identical features to the wet-fixed preparation, with single cells. Note the mitotic figure at the bottom of the field (arrowed).

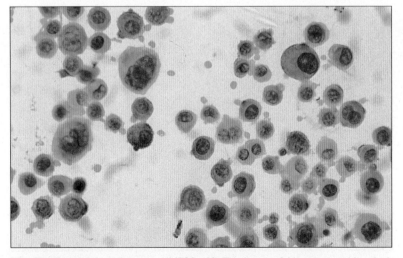

Fig. 15.74 Adenocarcinoma – HMFG2 x40. This is a useful immunocytochemical stain to differentiate between adenocarcinoma, in which it is usually positive (as demonstrated here), and mesothelioma, in which it is usually negative.

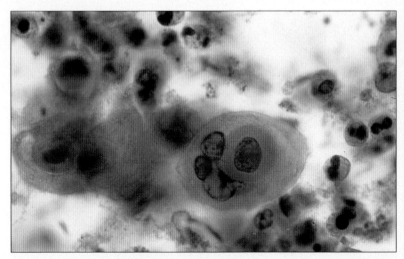

Fig. 15.75 Squamous carcinoma – Pap x100. These malignant cells exhibit keratinization, a feature diagnostic of well-differentiated squamous carcinoma.

they are larger than lymphocytes and stain a paler shade of mauve (**Fig. 15.78**). The malignant cells show the nuclear moulding, 'salt and pepper' chromatin, and paucity of cytoplasm associated with oat cell carcinomas (**Fig. 15.79**). An interesting feature is the change seen in the morphology of the cells when the tumour recurs after treatment – they are larger, with more cytoplasm and visible nucleoli , similar to the intermediate-type cell of small cell anaplastic carcinoma (**Fig. 15.80**). **Hepatoma** cells cannot be distinguished reliably from other adenocarcinomas in effusions (**Fig. 15.81**).

Leukaemic infiltrates may be seen in effusions in the form of blast cells containing prominent nucleoli. **Lymphoma** not infrequently metastasizes to

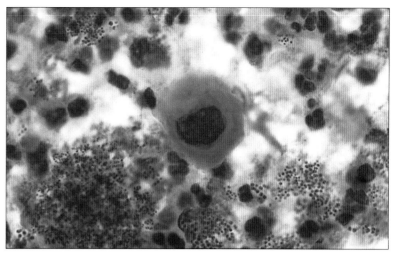

Fig. 15.76 Squamous carcinoma – MGG x100. The carcinoma cell in the centre of the field displays blue keratinized cytoplasm. There are neutrophils and bacteria in the background.

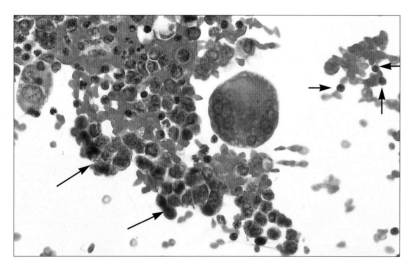

Fig. 15.77 Small cell carcinoma – Pap x40. In the centre of the smear, prepared from a pleural effusion, is a large multinucleated histiocyte, adjacent to which are small cells which appear hyperchromatic and clumped. These are carcinoma cells which have metastasized from a small cell carcinoma of lung (long arrows). They may be mistaken for lymphocytes, although there are a few lymphocytes at the top of the field (short arrows).

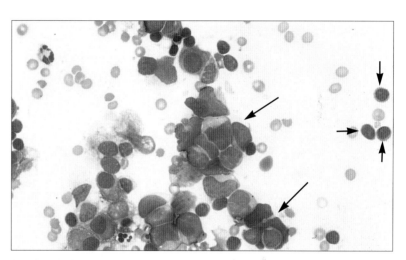

Fig. 15.78 Small cell carcinoma – MGG x40. This air-dried preparation is from the same case as shown in **Figure 15.77**. The neoplastic cells are disproportionately enlarged compared with the lymphocytes due to air-drying, which is one of the few advantages of this preparation. The carcinoma cells show moulding and irregular outlines, with very little cytoplasm (long arrows). By comparison, the lymphocytes are small and round (short arrows).

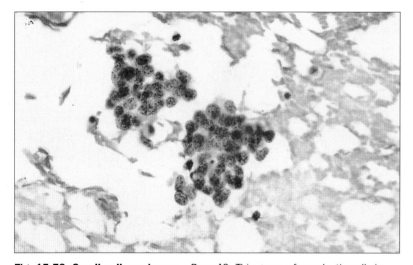

Fig. 15.79 Small cell carcinoma – Pap x40. This group of neoplastic cells in pleural fluid from a small cell carcinoma exhibits the characteristic 'salt and pepper' chromatin and moulding of this neoplasm. Note the nucleus size – slightly larger than that of a lymphocyte.

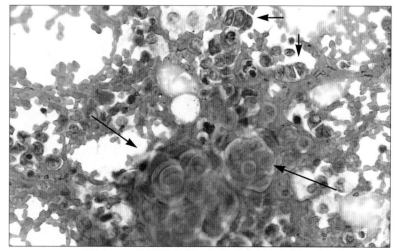

Fig. 15.80 Small cell carcinoma – Pap x40. This sample of pleural fluid is from a patient with recurrent small cell carcinoma (oat cell type) after treatment. Some of the neoplastic cells appear larger with increased amounts of cytoplasm, (large arrows) simulating the intermediate type of small cell carcinoma. There are small tumour cells of the usual small-cell type in the background (short arrows).

the serous cavities. The smears contain an almost exclusive population of abnormal lymphoid cells – mesothelial and other cells types may be obscured. The cells are single with large nuclei, prominent nucleoli, and a thin rim of cytoplasm (**Figs 15.82–15.84**). The diagnosis can be confirmed using immunocytochemical markers for lymphoid cells (**Fig. 15.85**). **Hodgkin's disease** can involve serous cavities with the characteristic Reed–Sternberg cells seen in the aspirate. **Sarcomas** may also spread to serous cavities; the smears contain spin-

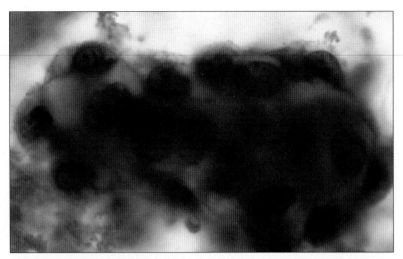

Fig. 15.81 Hepatocellular carcinoma – Pap x40. These tumour cells cannot be distinguished confidently from other adenocarcinoma cells in peritoneal fluid. They are vacuolated, with nuclei pushed to the periphery of the cluster, and may contain large nucleoli. Intracytoplasmic bile pigment, if present, may provide a clue to the diagnosis.

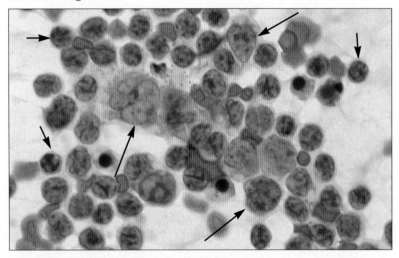

Fig. 15.82 Lymphoma – Pap x100. Illustrated here are abnormal, enlarged lymphoid cells with irregular nuclear outlines (long arrows). Occasional small lymphocytes are also present (short arrows).

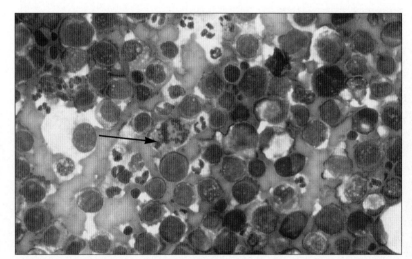

Fig. 15.83 Lymphoma – MGG x100. This field shows single abnormal lymphoid cells, which are much larger than the neutrophils also present. Note the abnormal mitotic figure in the centre of the field (arrow).

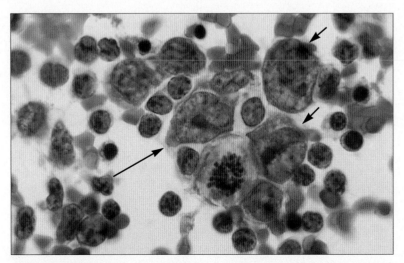

Fig. 15.84 Lymphoma – Pap x100. In this sample some of the neoplastic cells are huge with large nucleoli, resembling centroblasts (short arrows); there is an immunoblast in the centre of the field (long arrow) and numerous centrocytes. A few normal lymphocytes are also present. Note the mitotic figure.

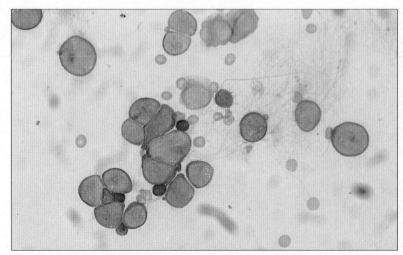

Fig. 15.85 Lymphoma – LCA (leucocyte common antigen) x40. This is the same effusion as that shown in **Fig. 15.84**. The neoplastic cells and small lymphocytes show positive staining, confirming their lymphoid origin.

dle cells and pleomorphic sarcoma cells with ovoid-to-round nuclei and large nucleoli **(Figs 15.86, 15.87)**.

Mesotheliomas are neoplasms which develop following exposure to asbestos. The causative fibres, coated with iron and protein, known as asbestos bodies or ferruginous bodies, may be detected in pleural fluid, sputum, or lung aspirates **(Fig. 15.88)**. As already stated, one of the most difficult cytological problems is to differentiate between adenocarcinoma and mesothelial cell pro-

liferations, either benign or malignant, in serous effusions. Adenocarcinomas tend to have two cell populations – carcinoma cells and mesothelial cells – while mesotheliomas are composed of mesothelial cells, malignant and reactive.

Reactive mesothelial cells may form papillary clusters, but the individual cells show no features of malignancy. Mesotheliomas may be composed predominantly of single cells **(Fig. 15.89)**, as may adenocarcinomas **(Fig. 15.90)**, or may form large or small clusters of cells. The cells within the clusters are

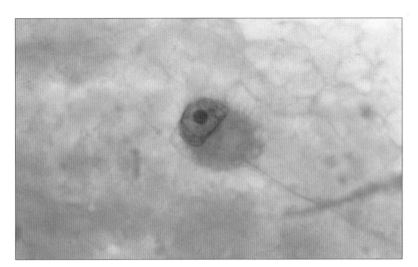

Fig. 15.86 Sarcoma – Pap x40. This single cell with a large red nucleolus and rounded nucleus was seen in ascitic fluid which contained metastases from an endometrial sarcoma NOS (not otherwise specified).

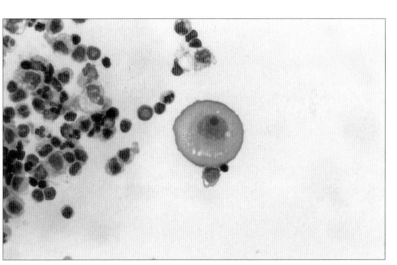

Fig. 15.87 Sarcoma – MGG x40. The air-dried smear from the same case as shown in **Figure 15.86** also demonstrates the rounded nucleus that may be seen in sarcoma cells. Often, however, the cells and nuclei are spindle-shaped. This cell may be mistaken for a mesothelial cell, but it lacks the frilly border and the nucleolus is too large for a mesothelial cell.

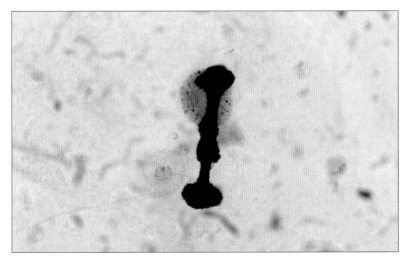

Fig. 15.88 Asbestos (ferruginous) body – Perl's stain x63. The asbestos body seen here was found in a sputum sample from a patient who had been exposed to asbestos 15 years previously.

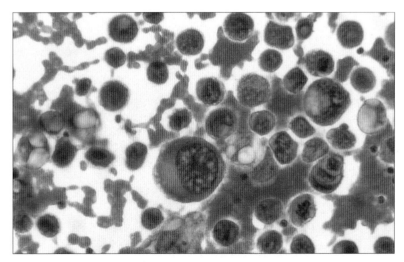

Fig. 15.89 Mesothelioma – Pap x40. This is a wet-fixed smear of pleural fluid from a patient with mesothelioma. In the centre of the field is a large malignant mesothelial cell with a greatly enlarged nucleus and chromatin clumps. Note the frilly border around the cell. In the background are smaller mesothelial cells, some reactive and others showing features of malignancy, including an abnormal chromatin pattern. The vacuolated cells are also mesothelial in origin.

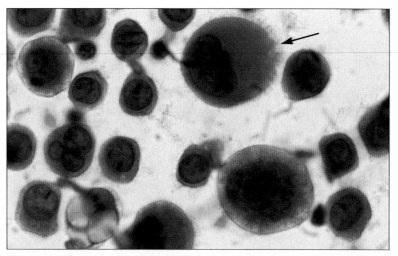

Fig. 15.90 Metastatic adenocarcinoma – Pap x100. This pleural fluid is from a patient with metastatic breast carcinoma. The pattern is single celled with much pleomorphism, but the cells do not display the characteristic microvilli around their borders, except for one of the large cells which appears to have a tuft of microvilli (arrow).

delineated clearly, with windows between individual cells, central nuclei, and frilly or lacy cytoplasmic borders **(Figs 15.91, 15.92)**. In adenocarcinomas, the cell clusters form a syncytial arrangement without clear cytoplasmic borders, the nuclei are pushed to the periphery by vacuoles, and there are no frilly margins **(Fig. 15.93)**. Vacuolation, which is a characteristic feature of adenocarcinomas, may be noted in mesotheliomas, but is usually accompanied by the frilly borders characteristic of mesothelial cells **(Fig. 15.94)**. Multinucleation may be seen **(Fig. 15.95)** and intranuclear inclusions are very occasionally noted **(Fig. 15.96)**. Special stains, such as PAS and diastase–PAS, are useful, but may not always help to distinguish between the two. The presence of collagen balls (see **Figures 15.11, 15.12**) is more common with mesothelial cells. Immuno-cytochemical stains are useful in distinguishing between the two types of malignancy, as mesotheliomas are negative with CEA and BerEP4 markers. Cell blocks may

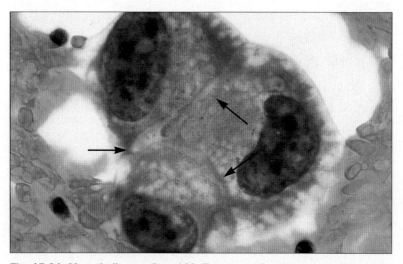

Fig. 15.91 Mesothelioma – Pap x100. This group of malignant mesothelial cells displays the clearly defined cell borders (windows) (arrows) and lacy margins characteristic of their origin. The nuclei are large, irregular in shape, and contain clumped chromatin with several large red nucleoli.

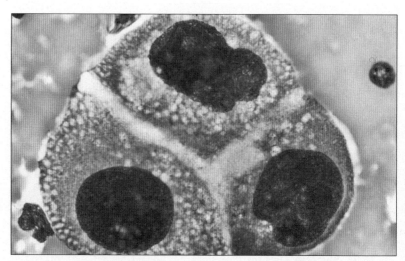

Fig. 15.92 Mesothelioma – MGG x100. The air-dried smear from the same case as shown in **Figure 15.91** shows the same characteristics – well-defined gaps between cells, irregular nuclear borders, huge, multiple nucleoli, and lacy cell margins.

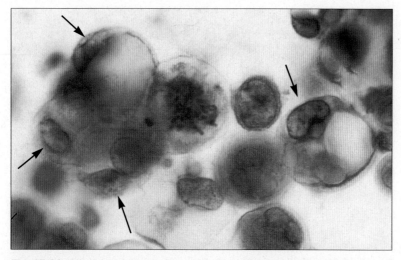

Fig. 15.93 Adenocarcinoma – Pap x100. This smear was prepared from pleural fluid in a patient with metastatic ovarian carcinoma and shows vacuolated carcinoma cells, both single and in clusters. The nuclei are pushed to the periphery of the clusters by the vacuoles (arrows). Note the mitotic figure and the pale chromatin.

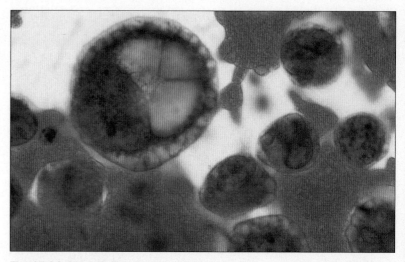

Fig. 15.94 Mesothelioma – Pap x100. The largest mesothelioma cell visible here is vacuolated, but it has a very obvious lacy border. The smaller cells also display the same cytoplasmic border.

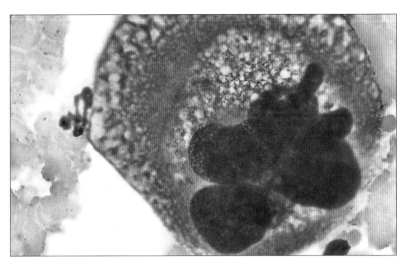

Fig. 15.95 Mesothelioma – MGG x100. This enormous mesothelioma cell is multinucleated and has vacuolated cytoplasm, which makes the lacy border difficult to distinguish.

be prepared, but this procedure takes time and removes the diagnosis from the field of cytology. However, there are many instances where cytology can provide only an indication of the type of neoplasm present, so histological confirmation should then be requested. Solid pleural plaques of mesothelioma may be aspirated with a fine needle, but this procedure may not sample both the areas in a biphasic tumour (**Fig. 15.97**). If only spindle cells are seen in the aspirate, an accurate diagnosis may not be possible until a biopsy has been performed (**Figs 15.98, 15.99**).

Peritoneal washings are a useful diagnostic tool to detect the spread of ovarian carcinomas, and also for following-up patients after surgery. Sometimes the washings contain papillary clusters of reactive mesothelial cells which may appear suspicious, especially if degenerate. Unequivocal features of carcinoma should be seen to make a diagnosis of metastatic tumour.

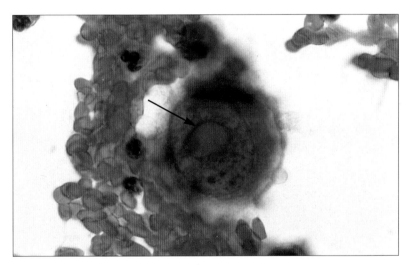

Fig. 15.96 Mesothelioma – Pap x100. This field from a sample of pleural fluid in a patient with mesothelioma shows a cell with a large intranuclear inclusion (intranuclear cytoplasmic invagination) (arrow) and the dense cytoplasm and lacy border characteristic of mesothelial cells.

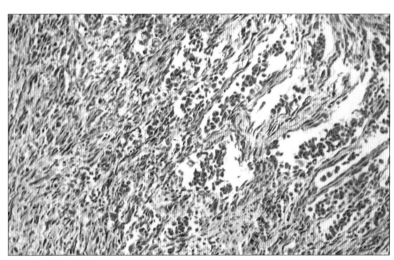

Fig. 15.97 Mesothelioma – H&E x10. This section of a pleural mass shows the features of a biphasic mesothelioma, confirmed by immunocytochemical stains.

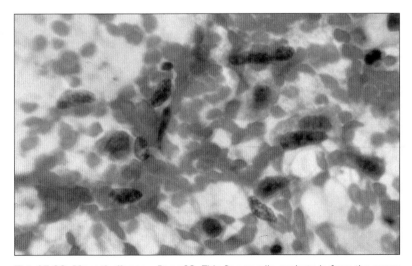

Fig. 15.98 Mesothelioma – Pap x63. This fine needle aspirate is from the same mass as that shown in **Figures 15.97** and **15.99**. The cells seen here are single and spindle-shaped, with ovoid to spindle-shaped nuclei. No cytological features of mesothelioma are visible in this sample.

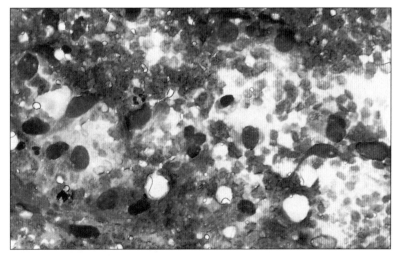

Fig. 15.99 Mesothelioma – MGG x40. The air-dried smear from the same sample as shown in **Figures 15.97** and **15.98** also contains single cells with ovoid to spindle-shaped nuclei.

JOINT EFFUSIONS

Hydrocoele and spermatocoele are discussed in Chapter 16.

Synovial fluid aspirated from joints is sent frequently to the cytology laboratory for identification of crystals under polarized light. Smears prepared from synovial fluid are rich in proteinaceous material (**Figs 15.100, 15.101**); they contain synovial cells (**Fig. 15.102**) and, sometimes, cartilage cells (**Figs 15.103, 15.104**). In **gout** the smear contains some polymorphs, as well as synovial cells; polarized light microscopy shows the typical needle-shaped urate crystals associated with this condition (**Fig. 15.105**). In pseudogout the fluid contains the same cells, but the calcium pyrophosphate crystals seen under polarized light are smaller, often intracellular, and rod shaped (**Figs 15.106, 15.107**). In rheumatoid arthritis the smears show numerous polymorphs, known as ragocytes, which contain debris. No crystals are seen, but hyperplastic synovial cells may be present, as well as lymphocytes. Septic arthritis effusions contain very large numbers of polymorphs and histiocytes. Fluid from joints which have been subjected to long-standing haemorrhage display cholesterol crystals (**Fig. 15.108**).

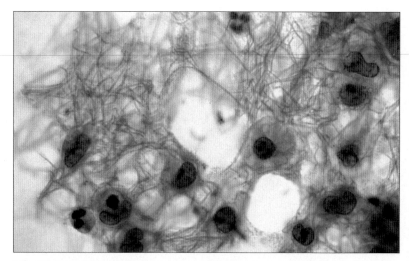

Fig. 15.100 Synovial fluid – Pap x100. This wet-fixed smear of synovial fluid contains neutrophils, histiocytes, and strands of proteinaceous material.

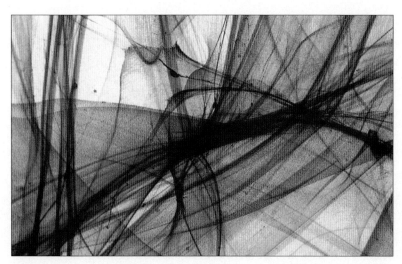

Fig. 15.101 Synovial fluid – Toluidine blue x40. The proteinaceous material in synovial fluid is magenta-coloured with this stain.

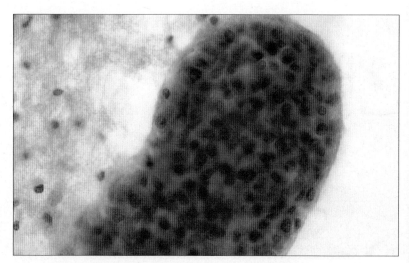

Fig. 15.102 Synovial cells – Pap x40. This cluster of benign synovial cells shows uniform nuclei and moderate amounts of cytoplasm.

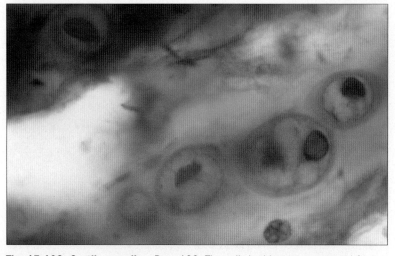

Fig. 15.103 Cartilage cells – Pap x100. The cells in this smear prepared from synovial fluid display a prominent clear area (lacuna) around the nucleus.

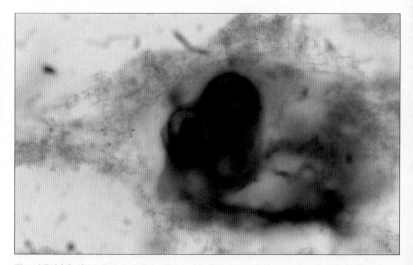

Fig. 15.104 Cartilage cells – Pap x40. There are three cartilage cells in this field, each of which exhibits the typical lacuna around the nucleus.

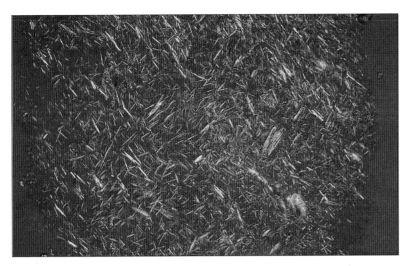

Fig. 15.105 Urate crystals – Polarized light x40. Illustrated here are the characteristic needle-shaped urate crystals seen in gout.

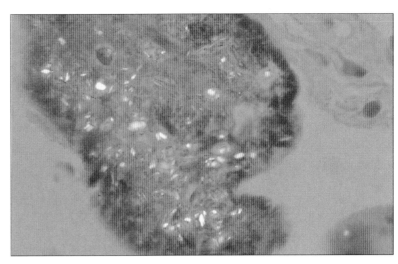

Fig. 15.106 Calcium pyrophosphate arthropathy – H&E x40. This stained section of synovial tissue shows birefringent calcium pyrophosphate crystals under polarized light.

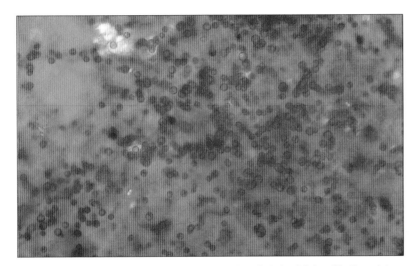

Fig. 15.107 Calcium pyrophosphate crystals – Polarized light x40. Synovial fluid from the same case as shown in **Figure 15.106** also contains calcium pyrophosphate crystals, which are small, usually rod-shaped, and often intracellular.

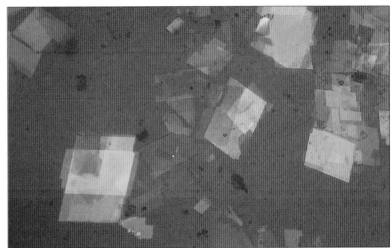

Fig. 15.108 Cholesterol crystals – Polarized light x40. The cholesterol crystals illustrated here are from an aspirate from a knee joint into which there had been previous haemorrhage. The crystals are typically square in shape with a corner missing.

SUGGESTED READING

DiBonito L, Falconieri G, Colautti I, *et al*. Cytopathology of malignant mesothelioma: A study of its patterns and histological basis. *Diagn Cytopathol* 1993; **9**: 25–31.

Krausz T, Barker F. Reactive effusions. In: Gray W, ed.: *Diagnostic Cytopathology*. Edinburgh: Churchill Livingstone; 1995: 131–148.

Naylor B. Pleural, peritoneal and pericardial fluids. In: Bibbo M, ed.: *Comprehensive Cytopathology*. Philadelphia: WB Saunders; 1991: 590–610.

Schofield J, Krausz T. Metastatic disease and lymphomas. In: Gray W, ed.: *Diagnostic Cytopathology*. Edinburgh: Churchill Livingstone; 1991: 149–194.

Spriggs AI, Boddington MM. Atlas of serous fluid cytopathology. Dordrecht: Kluwer Academic Publishers; 1989.

Soosay GN, Griffiths M, Padaki L, *et. al.* The differential diagnosis of epithelial type mesothelioma form adenocarcinoma and mesothelial proliferation *J. Pathol* 1991; **163**: 299–305.

Whitaker D, Sterret GF, Shilkin KB. Cytological appearances of malignant mesothelioma. In: Henderson DW, Shilkin KB, Langlois SLeP, Whitaker D eds. *Malignant mesothelioma*. New York: Hemisphere; 1992: 167–182.

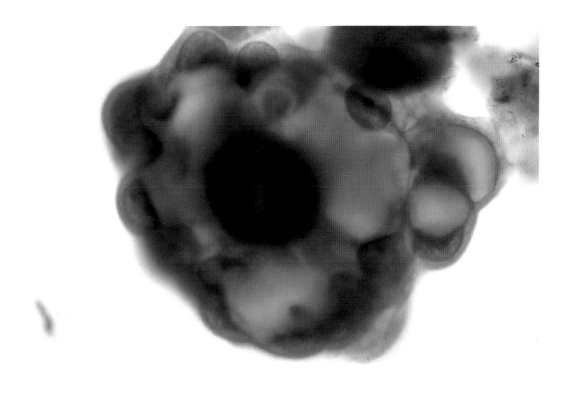

CYTOLOGY OF THE OVARY, TESTIS AND PROSTATE GLAND

16

OVARY

The normal structure of the ovary is quite simple, being composed of fibrous stroma arranged in a storiform pattern with scattered oocytes (**Fig. 16.1**) and follicles in various stages of developement. An aspirate from a normal ovary would be acellular.

Ovarian cysts are fairly common and benign cysts are usually aspirated either transabdominally or transvaginally. It is important that the cytopathologist is informed about the method of aspiration used, as squamous cells are seen commonly in transvaginal aspirates and may suggest a benign teratoma. Cysts that are suspected clinically of being malignant are not aspirated, because of the risk of tumour seeding during the procedure. If care is taken when a malignant cyst is removed surgically, it can be aspirated postoperatively, either in the theatre or in the laboratory, for a rapid cytology result. Cyst fluid is sent to the laboratory in a clean container without any additives. It is spun down, both wet-fixed and air-dried smears are prepared, and the extra material is reserved for special stains and immunocytochemistry.

Ovarian cysts may be neoplastic or non-neoplastic. Non-neoplastic cysts are of various types. **Simple cysts** may contain only small amounts of fluid, which is usually clear. In this category are included fimbrial and parovarian cysts, as they show the same cytological features. The smears contain a few foamy macrophages (**Figs 16.2, 16.3**), proteinaceous material or debris, and a few erythrocytes. The background is usually very clean. Rarely, a few small sheets of degenerate cuboidal epithelial cells are found (**Fig. 16.4**). Evidence of previous haemorrhage is seen in the form of siderophages (**Fig. 16.5**). Mesothelial cell sheets are sometimes seen in aspirates of fimbrial cysts (**Fig. 16.6**).

Functional cysts, such as follicular cysts, are often cellular with clusters of granulosa cells derived from the lining of the follicle and single cells (**Figs 16.7, 16.8**). Granulosa cells are small with delicate cytoplasm and irregular nuclei, and small nucleoli may be present also. Mitoses are frequent and are not a cause for alarm. When luteinized, granulosa cells have abundant vacuolated cytoplasm (**Figs 16.9, 16.10**).

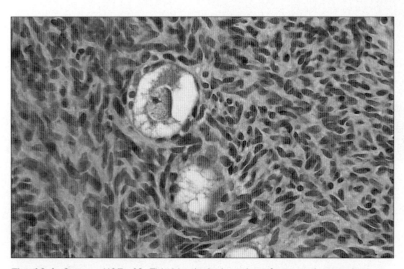

Fig. 16.1 Ovary – H&E x40. This histological section of a normal ovary shows two oocytes, each surrounded by a single layer of granulosa cells which comprise primordial follicles. They are within a cellular stroma that displays a storiform pattern of spindle cells.

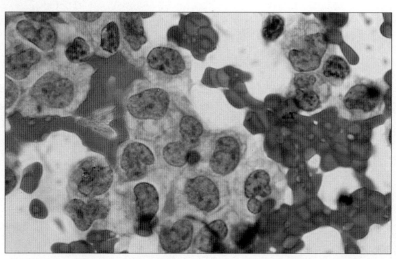

Fig. 16.2 Simple cyst – Pap x100. These ovarian (and fimbrial) cysts contain clear fluid, which is seen on cytological preparations to have varying numbers of histiocytes with foamy cytoplasm. Note the nuclear outlines, which are bean-shaped in some cells and irregular in others.

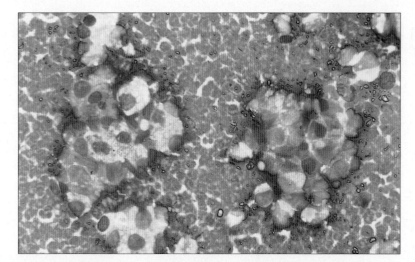

Fig. 16.3 Simple cyst – MGG x40. In this air-dried preparation the delicate vacuolated cytoplasm of foamy macrophages is well-illustrated. These cells appear to be clustering, but this is a result of centrifugation.

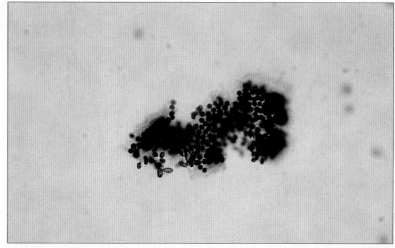

Fig. 16.4 Simple cyst – Pap x40. This aspirate from a simple cyst of the ovary contains a cluster of small, degenerate epithelial cells.

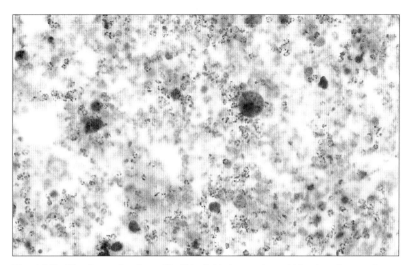

Fig. 16.5 Simple cyst – Pap x40. This field shows altered blood and several foamy macrophages that contain greenish yellow haemosiderin, indicative of previous haemorrhage into the cyst.

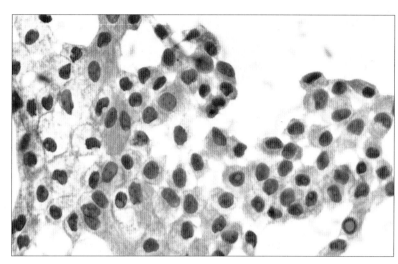

Fig. 16.6 Simple cyst – Pap x63. This is a sheet of benign epithelial cells which was found in an aspirate from a fimbrial cyst.

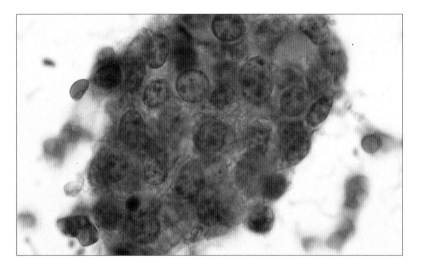

Fig. 16.7 Follicular cyst, granulosa cells – Pap x100. Granulosa cells contain apparently active nuclei, with clumped chromatin and visible nucleoli, but the nuclear margins are usually round-to-oval. The blue blob within the cluster is probably secretory material and may be related to the Call–Exner bodies seen in granulosa cell tumours.

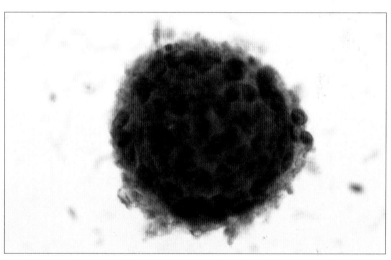

Fig. 16.8 Follicular cyst, granulosa cells – Pap x63. Follicular cysts contain tight clusters of small, hyperchromatic granulosa cells, as illustrated here.

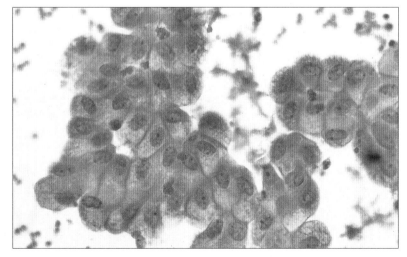

Fig. 16.9 Luteinized granulosa cells – Pap x40. These cells have abundant cytoplasm, uniform nuclei, and small nucleoli.

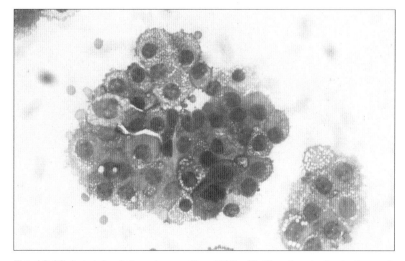

Fig. 16.10 Luteinized granulosa cells – MGG x40. The abundant cytoplasm of these cells is evident on the air-dried smears, but appears to be vacuolated, possibly due to degenerative changes.

Endometriotic cysts (chocolate cysts) produce a thick brown fluid aspirate which contains much altered blood, some erythrocytes, and foamy macrophages, including haemosiderin-filled macrophages **(Figs 16.11, 16.12)**. Endometrial cells are not always seen and are often degenerate when present. If the aspirate is performed after a recent haemorrhage, macrophages with ingested erythrocytes are usually seen, with intact erythrocytes in the background **(Figs 16.13, 16.14)**.

Dermoid cysts (benign teratomas) (Fig. 16.15) yield a characteristic thick, greasy, often unpleasant smelling aspirate, which can be very difficult to retain on the slide during staining. The smears show anucleate squames, thick back-

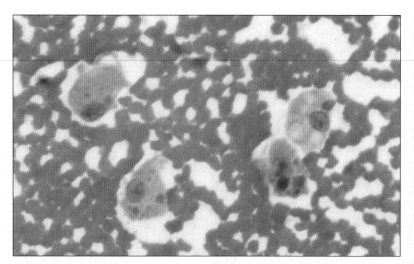

Fig. 16.11 Endometriotic cyst, siderophages – Pap x63. Three of the four foamy macrophages in this field contain greenish yellow haemosiderin.

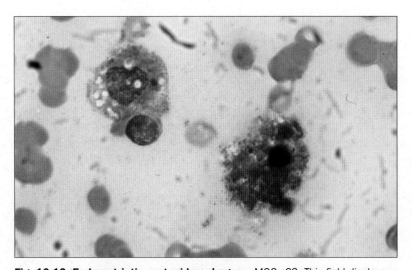

Fig. 16.12 Endometriotic cyst, siderophages – MGG x63. This field displays a lymphocyte and two foamy macrophages, one of which contains abundant bluish black haemosiderin.

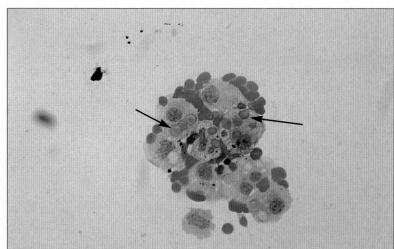

Fig. 16.13 Endometriotic cyst – Pap x40. The macrophages in this aspirate of an endometriotic cyst have phagocytosed erythrocytes (arrows) and some debris. There is fresh blood in this aspirate, in the form of intact erythrocytes, rather than altered blood.

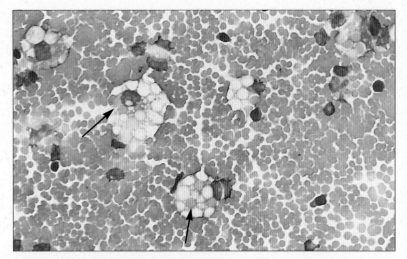

Fig. 16.14 Endometriotic cyst – MGG x40. The foamy macrophages in this field show ingested erythrocytes (arrows). Note the numerous background erythrocytes, indicative of fresh haemorrhage.

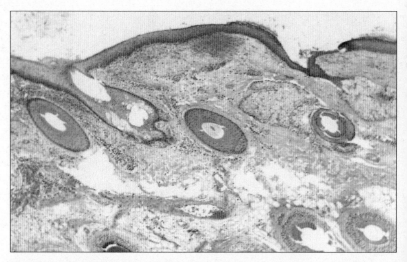

Fig. 16.15 Dermoid cyst – H&E x10. This section of a dermoid cyst of the ovary displays epithelium with sebaceous glands and hair follicles.

ground material (**Fig. 16.16**) and inflammatory cells, and may include columnar and respiratory epithelial cells.

Serous cystadenoma is a benign neoplastic process (**Fig. 16.17**) which is disappointingly poor in cellularity. The smears contain a few clusters of cuboidal epithelial cells with uniform nuclei. The cells often look less sinister than those in a follicular cyst and no mitoses are seen. Occasionally, the cells are noted in papillary clusters and may show mild nuclear atypia (**Figs 16.18, 16.19**). Psammoma bodies may be present, either within cell clusters (**Figs 16.20, 16.21**) or lying free (**Figs 16.22, 16.23**). Aspirates with atypical features should be reported as suspicious of a borderline lesion, although the final diagnosis can be made only on histology.

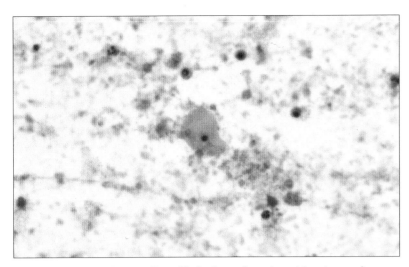

Fig. 16.16 Dermoid cyst – Pap x40. Aspirates from dermoid cysts are often disappointing, as in this case in which only occasional squamous cells and much debris are seen.

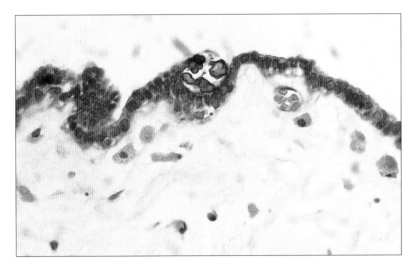

Fig. 16.17 Serous cystadenoma – H&E x10. This section of the wall of a serous cystadenoma demonstrates the mildly atypical cells that constitute the cyst lining. Note the psammoma bodies.

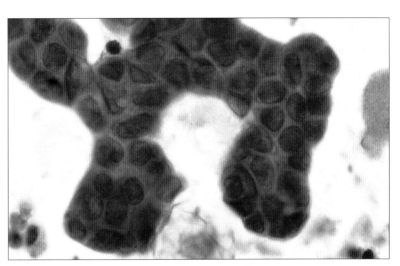

Fig. 16.18 Serous cystadenoma – Pap x100. This papillary group of mildly pleomorphic epithelial cells is cohesive and displays vesicular chromatin without prominent nucleoli.

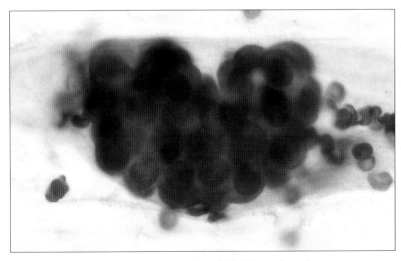

Fig. 16.19 Serous cystadenoma – Pap x100. This aspirate from a serous cystadenoma contains clusters of hyperchromatic cells showing some variation in nuclear size and chromatin pattern.

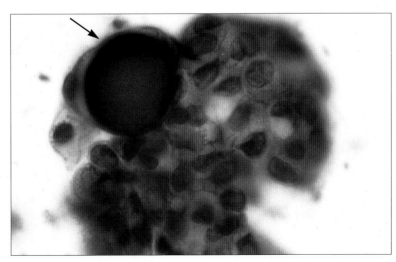

Fig. 16.20 Serous cystadenoma – Pap x100. This cluster of mildly pleomorphic glandular cells encloses a round, laminated, red-staining psammoma body (arrow).

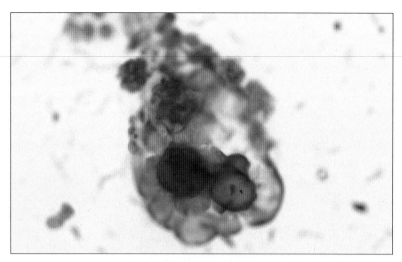

Fig. 16.21 Serous cystadenoma – MGG x63. In the air-dried smear from the same case as shown in **Figure 16.20**, the rounded psammoma bodies stain blue. The glandular cells are poorly preserved here.

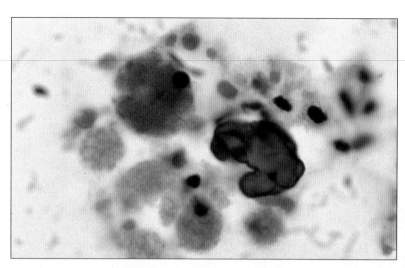

Fig. 16.22 Serous cystadenoma – Pap x100. Psammoma bodies are often found lying loose in the cyst fluid, as illustrated here. Note the irregular outlines of this psammoma body (arrow), in contrast to the laminated appearance in **Figure 16.20**.

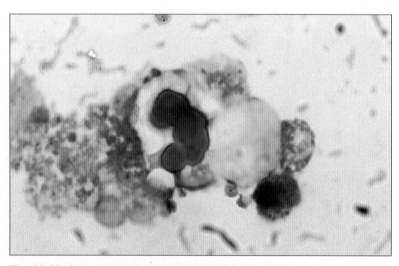

Fig. 16.23 Serous cystadenoma – MGG x100. This aspirate shows laminated psammoma bodies which appear to be interconnected. The epithelial cells in the background are degenerate and some debris is also visible.

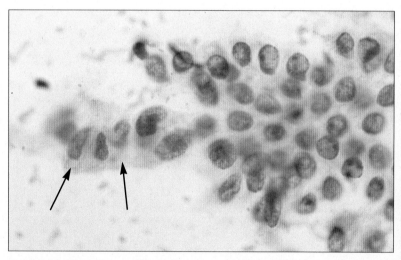

Fig. 16.24 Mucinous cystadenoma – Pap x100. This illustrates, at the edge of the cluster, the tall columnar cells that comprise this lesion (arrows). The cluster contains cells with vesicular nuclei and pale cytoplasm.

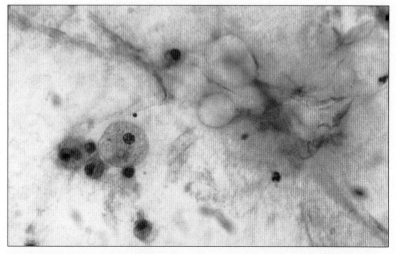

Fig. 16.25 Mucinous cystadenoma – Pap x63. The mucin in this field is pale pink and ill-defined, so can be missed easily on screening the slide. There are some cells with foamy cytoplasm in the background, which may be either histiocytic in origin or neoplastic.

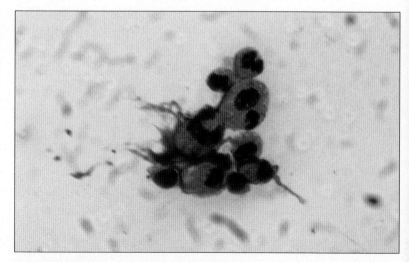

Fig. 16.26 Mucinous cystadenoma – MGG x63. This air-dried smear displays a group of cells with foamy cytoplasm, probably epithelial, and some bright pink strands of mucin.

Mucinous cystadenoma is also benign, but the fluid is often thick and gelatinous and the cells in the smear are tall and columnar in type **(Fig. 16.24)**. The mucin is pale blue or pink on the wet-fixed smear **(Fig. 16.25)** and bright pink or purple on the smear stained with May Grunwald Giemsa **(Fig. 16.26)**. A PAS stain highlights the mucin within the cytoplasm **(Fig. 16.27)**. Any tumours that show cellular pleomorphism should, as above, be regarded as borderline.

Serous cystadenocarcinoma of the ovary **(Fig. 16.28)** is not usually aspirated pre-operatively, but a rapid diagnosis can be made on fluid aspirated from the intact cyst once it is sent to the laboratory. The smears are cellular, containing groups or papillary clusters of pleomorphic epithelial cells with prominent nucleoli and irregular nuclei **(Fig. 16.29)**. The cells may contain vacuoles **(Fig. 16.30)**, acinar structures may be seen **(Fig. 16.31)**, and mitoses may be present. Psammoma bodies are often present **(Figs 16.32–16.34)**.

Mucinous cystadenocarcinoma aspirates contain abundant mucin **(Figs 16.35, 16.36)** and columnar cells, both single and in clusters. Tumour cells that may be present in ascitic fluid are impossible to differentiate from other mucin-secreting carcinomas **(Fig. 16.37)**.

Other malignant, solid neoplasms of the ovary are not usually aspirated.

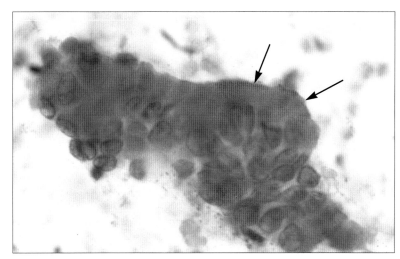

Fig. 16.27 Mucinous cystadenoma – PAS x100. This stain highlights the mucin content of the tall columnar cells that comprise this tumour (arrows).

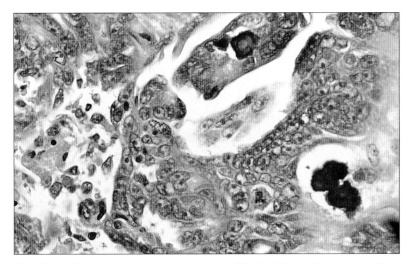

Fig. 16.28 Serous cystadenocarcinoma – H&E x40. This section of a papillary serous cystadenocarcinoma of the ovary illustrates pleomorphism of the epithelial cells, with irregular, hyperchromatic nuclei.

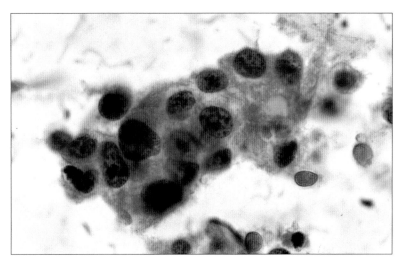

Fig. 16.29 Serous cystadenocarcinoma – Pap x100. This cluster of cells shows marked pleomorphism, with irregular nuclear margins and clumped chromatin.

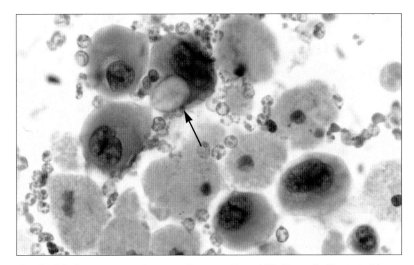

Fig. 16.30 Serous cystadenocarcinoma – Pap x100. The cells illustrated here are a mixture of single carcinoma cells with markedly irregular nuclei and abnormal chromatin and foamy macrophages. Note the vacuole in the cytoplasm of one of the carcinoma cells (arrow).

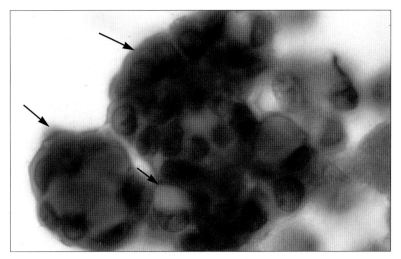

Fig. 16.31 Serous cystadenocarcinoma – Pap x100. The cells seen here are forming acinar clusters (long arrows). Some vacuolation is visible (short arrow).

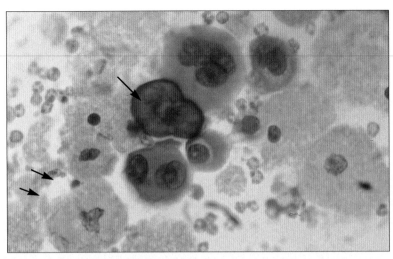

Fig. 16.32 Serous cystadenocarcinoma – Pap x100. This field shows multinucleated carcinoma cells and a psammoma body (long arrow). There are some foamy macrophages in the background (short arrows).

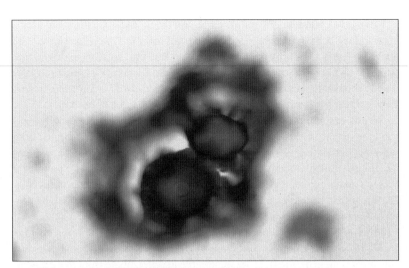

Fig. 16.33 Serous cystadenocarcinoma – MGG x40. The psammoma bodies seen here are surrounded by glandular cells, which are poorly preserved and show no definite features of malignancy. It is sometimes difficult on air-dried smears to distinguish benign from malignant neoplasms (see **Figure 16.21**).

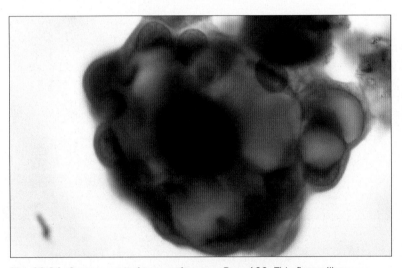

Fig. 16.34 Serous cystadenocarcinoma – Pap x100. This flower-like arrangement of adenocarcinoma cells around a psammoma body is frequently seen in papillary serous cystadenocarcinomas. The cells in this aspirate are vacuolated.

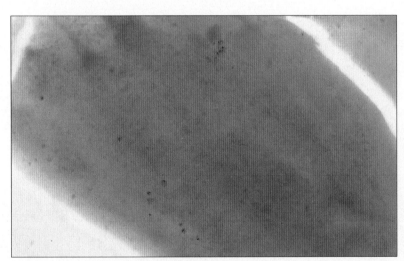

Fig. 16.35 Mucinous cystadenocarcinoma – Pap x10. This imprint smear from a mucinous cystadenocarcinoma of the ovary shows abundant mucinous material, which stains pink in the wet-fixed smear.

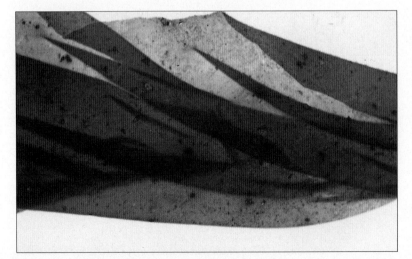

Fig. 16.36 Mucinous cystadenocarcinoma – MGG x10. Mucin in air-dried smears stains a magenta or purple shade.

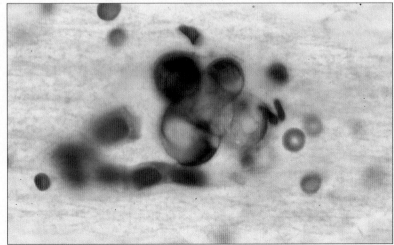

Fig. 16.37 Mucinous cystadenocarcinoma – Pap x100. These adenocarcinoma cells are greatly distended with mucin and do not display the usual columnar appearance seen in this neoplasm.

TESTIS

Fine needle aspiration of the testis is not widely practised but is performed in a few centres. It is not advocated for testicular neoplasms, but may be used in the evaluation of spermatogenesis.

The normal testis is composed mainly of seminiferous tubules lined by many layers of cells, including spermatogonia, spermatocytes, and spermatids, with intervening support cells known as Sertoli cells (**Fig. 16.38**). Spermatozoa may also be seen. Leydig cells may be identified between the tubules.

Inflammatory lesions of the testis are not usually aspirated. Granulomatous inflammation is represented by thickened blood vessels accompanied by inflammatory cells and epithelioid histiocytes (**Figs 16.39, 16.40**).

Hydrocoele of the testis is a not uncommon problem. The fluid that is aspirated is usually clear, and often straw-coloured. Smears prepared from hydrocoele fluid show scanty cellularity; they contain mesothelial cells in small clusters and histiocytes (**Fig. 16.41**). Spermatozoa are often seen, as the epididymis or testis is not infrequently punctured (**Fig. 16.42**). If there has been haemorrhage into the hydrocoele, an interesting finding is the outline of cholesterol crystals in an air-dried smear of the aspirate (**Fig. 16.43**).

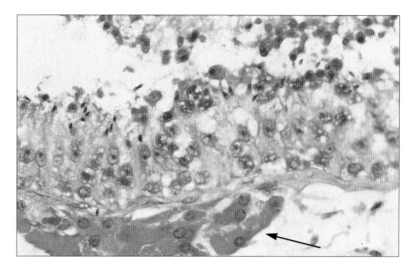

Fig. 16.38 Normal testis – H&E x40. This section of testis shows part of a seminiferous tubule with germ cells of varying maturity, including spermatogonia, spermatocytes, and spermatids. Some spermatozoa are also visible. Note the eosinophilic cytoplasm of the Leydig cells (arrow) adjacent to the seminiferous tubule.

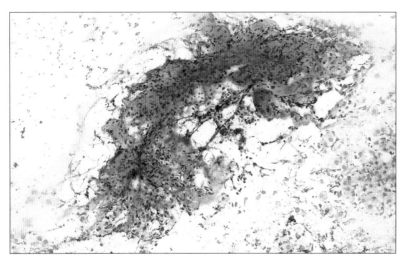

Fig. 16.39 Testis, granulomatous inflammation – Pap x10. This low-power view of a testicular aspirate shows thickened blood vessels and an inflammatory infiltrate.

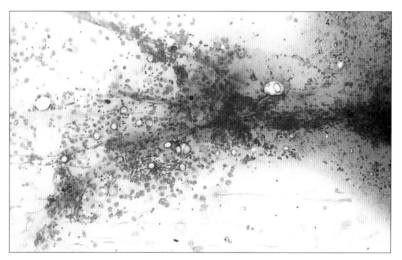

Fig. 16.40 Testis, granulomatous inflammation – MGG x10. Thickened blood vessels are clearly visualized in this air-dried smear. Note the numerous inflammatory cells in the background.

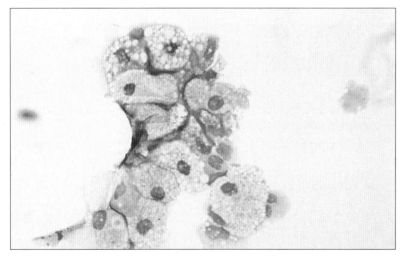

Fig. 16.41 Hydrocoele – Pap x63. This field shows a group of histiocytes with foamy cytoplasm.

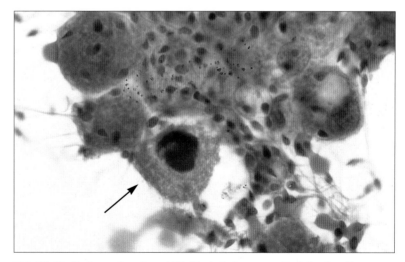

Fig. 16.42 Hydrocoele – Pap x100. Illustrated are mesothelial cells with numerous spermatozoa, the latter indicating puncture of the testis or epididymis. The cell with a large hyperchromatic nucleus is a seminal vesicle cell (arrow).

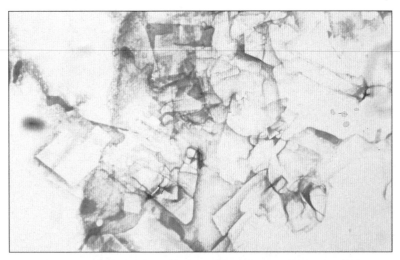

Fig. 16.43 Hydrocoele – MGG x40. Although cholesterol crystals are much prettier under polarized light, they can be detected in air-dried smears as negative images.

Spermatocoele smears contain abundant spermatozoa.

Testicular neoplasms are not common, but are seen more frequently in young males. The two main types that may be seen in cytological specimens are seminomas and teratomas. These are not aspirated, but imprint smears are sometimes made at operation for a rapid diagnosis. **Seminoma (Fig. 16.44)** imprints are very cellular, composed of large single cells with huge, sometimes multiple, red nucleoli. The chromatin pattern is vesicular or finely granular and the cytoplasm is very delicate and ill-defined (**Figs 16.45, 16.46**). Lymphocytes are seen scattered in the background. The cells are fragile and easily disrupted

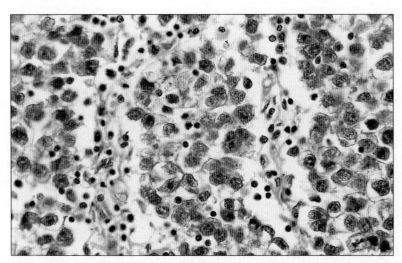

Fig. 16.44 Seminoma – H&E x40. This histological section of testis shows the features of a seminoma, consisting of large cells with prominent nucleoli, and a lymphocytic infiltrate.

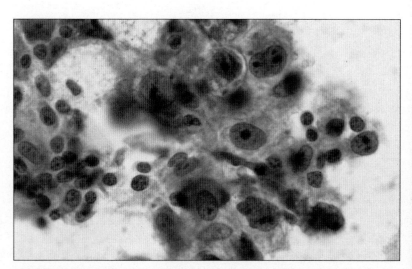

Fig. 16.45 Seminoma – Pap x63. This aspirate is composed of large cells with delicate, ill-defined cytoplasm and huge red nucleoli. There are also many lymphocytes in this field.

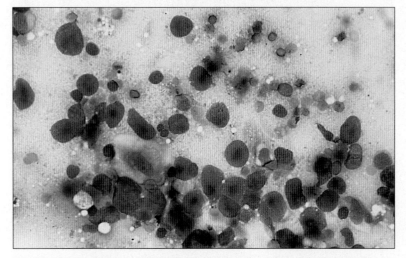

Fig. 16.46 Seminoma – MGG x40. An air-dried smear shows the single-cell pattern of this neoplasm, with prominent nucleoli, no visible cytoplasm, and scattered lymphocytes.

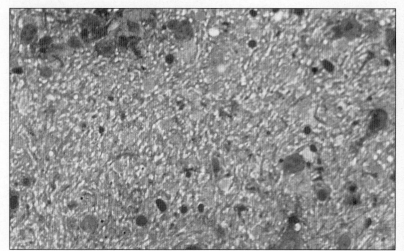

Fig. 16.47 Seminoma – MGG x40. The so-called 'tigroid' pattern of the background of this tumour is well-illustrated here.

by vigorous smearing techniques. Under low magnification the air-dried smear shows a pattern described as 'tigroid' (**Fig. 16.47**), which is typical of seminoma aspirates.

Teratomas of the testis (**Fig. 16.48**) yield cells which are pleomorphic, with enormous red nucleoli and irregular nuclear margins (**Figs 16.49, 16.50**). The cells may be in clusters and may contain abundant cytoplasm (**Fig. 16.51**).

Lymphoma is occasionally seen in the testis. The cells are usually single with minimal cytoplasm and resemble cytological preparations of lymphomas from other sites (**Fig. 16.52**).

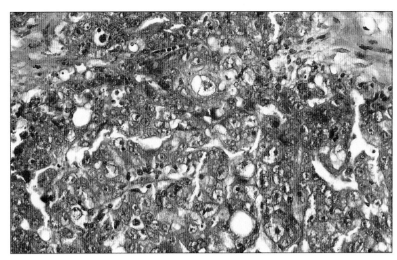

Fig. 16.48 Teratoma – H&E x10. This section of a malignant teratoma, undifferentiated, is composed of large, pleomorphic, malignant cells.

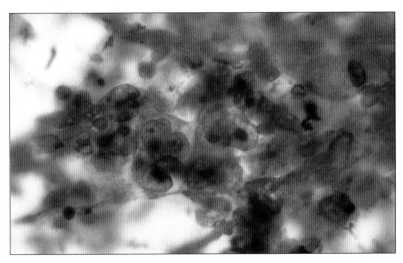

Fig. 16.49 Teratoma – Pap x100. These testicular imprint smears display large malignant cells, with huge red nucleoli, irregular nuclear outlines, and pale chromatin.

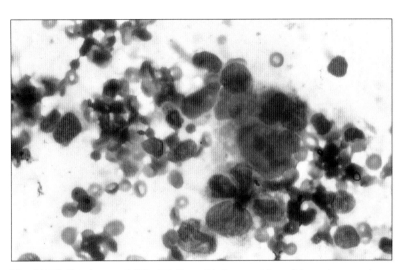

Fig. 16.50 Teratoma – MGG x63. The wild pleomorphism of these tumours is well-represented in this air-dried imprint smear. Multiple nucleoli are seen in some of the cells.

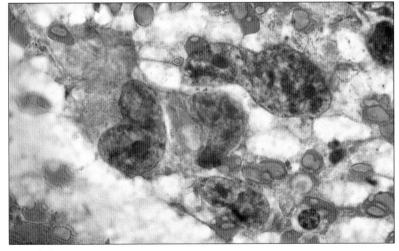

Fig. 16.51 Teratoma – Pap x100. In this field large cells with irregular nuclear margins, huge red multiple nucleoli, and moderate amounts of cytoplasm are visible.

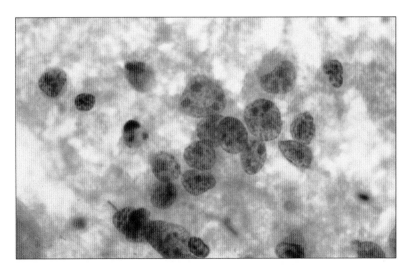

Fig. 16.52 Lymphoma – Pap x63. In this imprint smear of a testicular lymphoma the cells retain a lymphoid appearance, with no visible cytoplasm, and multiple nucleoli. This should not be mistaken for a seminoma.

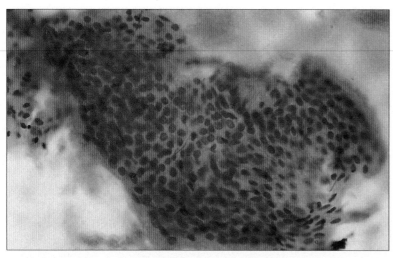

Fig. 16.53 Normal prostate – Pap x40. This is a benign sheet of ductal cells showing uniform nuclei with palisading around the edges.

PROSTATE GLAND

Fine needle aspirates of the prostate are no longer performed in most centres, as they have been replaced by gun biopsies. Prostatic aspirates are fairly straightforward to interpret, the benign ones containing sheets of uniform ductal cells, which often display palisaded edges (**Fig. 16.53**). Honeycombing may be seen (**Fig. 16.54**) and the cells look obviously benign (**Fig. 16.55**).

Adenocarcinoma of the prostate displays the usual features of this neoplasm: nuclear enlargement, irregularity of nuclear outline, loss of cohesion, large nucleoli; the severity of features is related to the grade (**Figs 16.56–16.58**).

Tumours from other sites may metastasize to the prostate, for example small cell carcinoma of the bronchus (**Fig. 16.59**).

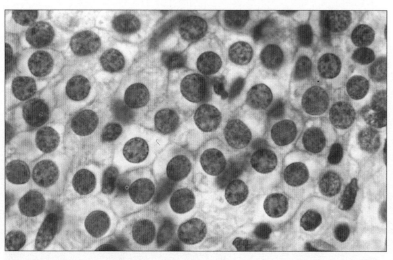

Fig. 16.54 Normal prostate – Pap x100. This high magnification view of normal prostatic ductal cells demonstrates round uniform nuclei and a honeycomb-type appearance to the cytoplasm.

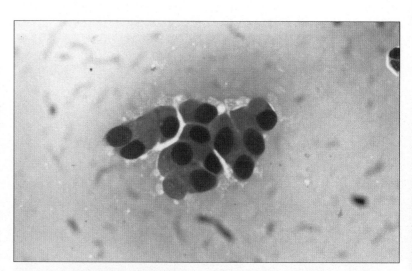

Fig. 16.55 Normal prostate – MGG x63. This air-dried smear of an aspirate from a normal prostate displays cells with moderate amounts of cytoplasm and uniform nuclei.

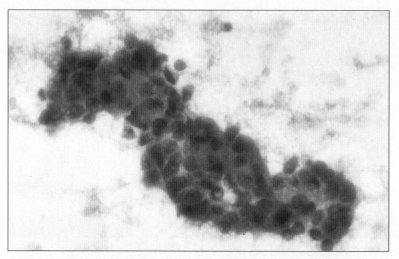

Fig. 16.56 Adenocarcinoma – Pap x40. Illustrated is a three-dimensional cluster of small adenocarcinoma cells with some nuclear pleomorphism. There is hyperchromasia, but nucleoli are not prominent.

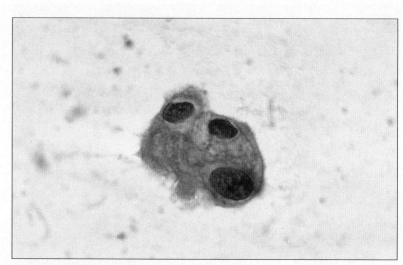

Fig. 16.57 Adenocarcinoma – Pap x100. These cells are from a high-grade adenocarcinoma, and display marked pleomorphism with clumped chromatin.

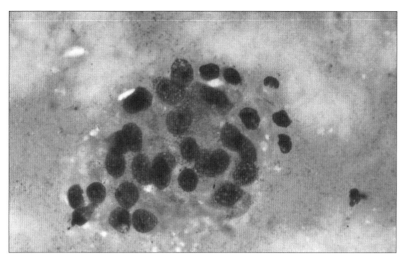

Semen analysis is rapidly becoming a part of the service provided by cytology laboratories. Elaboration of the various techniques employed to analyze semen samples is not appropriate in an atlas of cytopathology, but illustrations of sperm morphology are relevant. Papanicolaou-stained semen smears are used to examine sperm morphology. A normal spermatozoon consists of a head and a tailpiece, the latter being responsible for motility (**Fig. 16.60**). The head of the sperm contains the acrosomal cap and the postacrosomal region, which lies in the nucleus.

Abnormal sperm morphology includes head and tailpiece abnormalities, such as absence of the acrosome (**Figs 16.61, 16.62**), an abnormal postacrosomal region (**Fig. 16.63**), a cytoplasmic extrusion mass (**Figs 16.64, 16.65**), and a coiled tailpiece (**Fig. 16.66**).

Fig. 16.58 Adenocarcinoma – MGG x63. In this aspirate the cells are less cohesive and contain nucleoli.

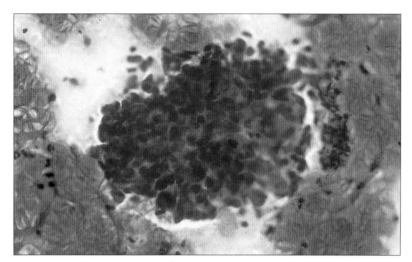

Fig. 16.59 Metastatic small cell carcinoma – Pap x40. This field demonstrates a cluster of cells from a small cell carcinoma (oat cell type), which has metastasized from the bronchus.

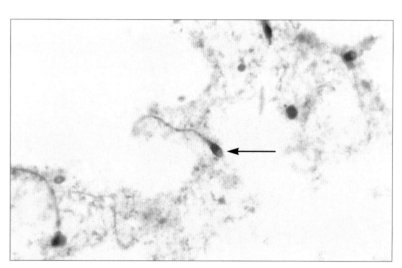

Fig. 16.60 Normal sperm – Pap x100. The spermatozoon in the centre of the field has an ovoid head with a clear acrosome. (arrow)

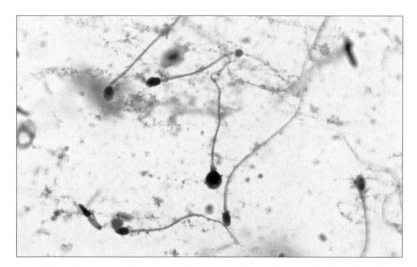

Fig. 16.61 Sperm with acrosomal deficiency – Pap x100. At least three of the sperm illustrated here have acrosomal deficiencies, including pointed headpieces and one with a large and flattened headpiece.

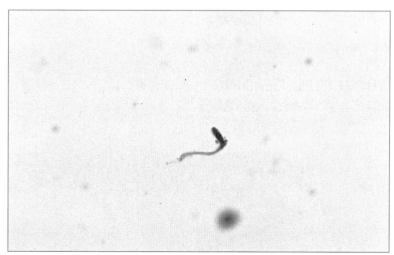

Fig. 16.62 Sperm with acrosomal deficiency – Pap x100. This sperm has a tapered head and very short tailpiece.

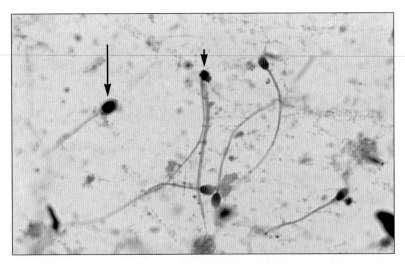

Fig. 16.63 Sperm with abnormal postacrosomal region – Pap x100. In this field there is a sperm on the left with a large head and no acrosome (long arrow), and also another one to its right with a small head and no acrosome (short arrow).

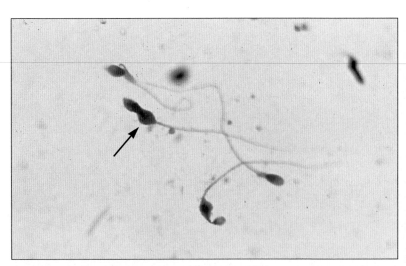

Fig. 16.64 Sperm with cytoplasmic extrusion mass – Pap x100. The sperm lying horizontally across the field has excessive cytoplasm around the midpiece region (arrow). This usually is due to a problem with epididymal function.

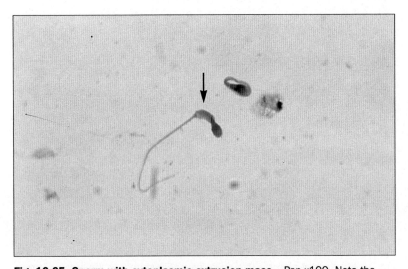

Fig. 16.65 Sperm with cytoplasmic extrusion mass – Pap x100. Note the excess cytoplasm in the midpiece region of the lower sperm (arrow).

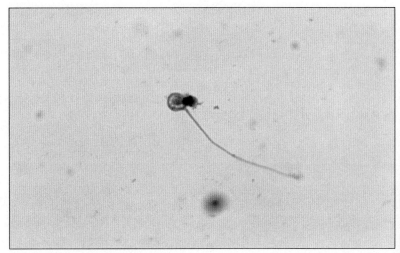

Fig. 16.66 Sperm with coiled tailpiece – Pap x100. This sperm displays, in addition to its coiled tailpiece, an acrosomal abnormality.

SUGGESTED READING

Abdul-Karim FW, Ng ABP. Ovaries and fallopian tubes. In: Gray W, ed. *Diagnostic Cytopathology*. Edinburgh: Churchill Livingstone; 1995: 811–819.

Adelman MM, Cahill EM. *Atlas of Sperm Morphology*. Chicago: American Society of Clinical Pathologists; 1989.

Greenbaum E, Mayer JR, Stangel JJ, Hughes P. Aspiration cytology of ovarian cysts in *in vitro* fertilization patients. *Acta Cytol* 1992; 36: 11–18.

Nunez C, Diaz J. Ovarian follicular cysts: A potential source of false positive diagnoses in ovarian cytology. *Diagn Cytopathol*, 1992; 8: 532–537.

Selvaggi SM. Cytology of non-neoplastic cysts of the ovary. *Diagn Cytopathol* 1990; 6: 77–85.

Smith R, Melcher D. Cytology of testis and scrotum. in Diagnostic Cytology, n: Gray W, ed. *Diagnostic Cytopathology*. Edinburgh: Churchill Livingstone; 1995: 609–628.

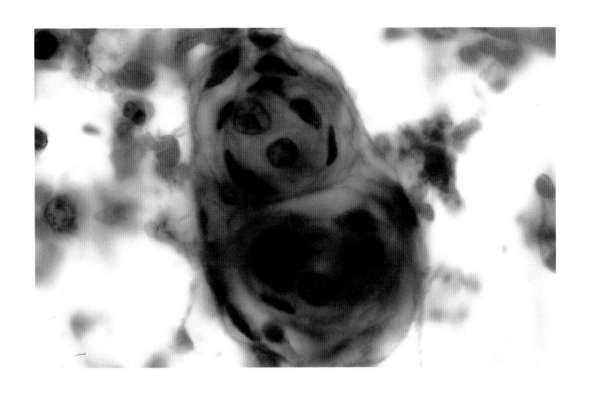

SKIN, BONE AND SOFT TISSUE LESIONS

17

SKIN AND SUBCUTANEOUS LESIONS

Skin lesions are easily sampled, either by scraping or by fine needle aspiration for a rapid diagnosis, with the understanding that in many cases the cytology report can only provide a differential diagnosis rather than a definite one. There are often instances when the clinician needs to know whether a mass is inflammatory or neoplastic, which can usually be done reliably by cytological examination.

Eczema of the nipple is sometimes difficult to differentiate clinically from Paget's disease of the breast; however, a firm nipple scrape of the affected area to give wet-fixed and air-dried smears is usually diagnostic. In eczema, the smear contains anucleate squames, inflamed squamous cells, and inflammatory cells, including neutrophils and histiocytes (see **Figure 8.146**). With Paget's disease of the nipple, the smears show large carcinoma cells with abundant clear cytoplasm (see **Figures 9.164, 9.165**), as well as anucleate squames. Occasionally, inflammatory cells are also present.

Herpetic vesicles can be punctured and the material smeared on to glass slides for cytological examination. The smears contain many inflammatory cells and also both multinucleated giant cells with moulded, ground-glass nuclei (**Fig. 17.1**) and cells that exhibit intranuclear eosinophilic inclusions (**Fig. 17.2**).

Molluscum contagiosum is another viral infection which is sometimes aspirated. The smears contain cells with large intranuclear inclusions (**Fig. 17.3**). These inclusions stain pink with the Papanicolaou stain.

There are several types of benign cysts that are superficial and easily aspirated: epidermoid, pilar, branchial and thyroglossal duct cysts. It is helpful to know the site of cysts in the neck, whether lateral or midline. Cyst fluids should be examined under polarized light for cholesterol crystals, as well as being centrifuged for wet-fixed and air-dried smears.

Epidermoid cysts (see **Figure 8.49**) contain abundant anucleate squames, debris, and keratinized squamous cells. Inflammatory cells, including neutrophils, histiocytes, and multinucleated giant histiocytes, are also often in evidence (**Figs 17.4, 17.5**). These aspirates should not be mistaken for metastatic squamous carcinoma with necrosis. **Pilar cysts** contain pink debris, but not keratinized squamous cells. Inflammatory cells may be present.

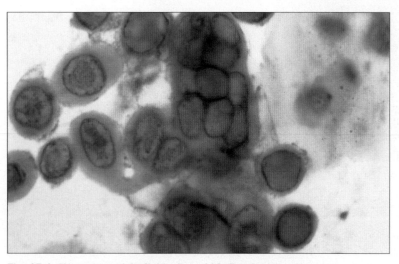

Fig. 17.1 Herpetic vesicle fluid – Pap x100. This field illustrates the characteristic multinucleated cells seen in material obtained from herpetic vesicles before secondary bacterial infection sets in. The cells contain moulded nuclei with crisp nuclear outlines and a homogeneous, ground-glass appearance, without chromatin detail.

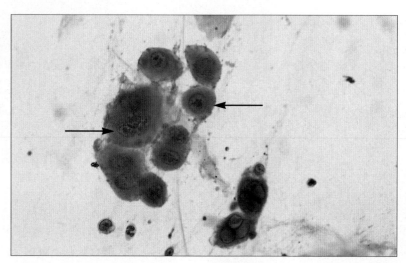

Fig. 17.2 Herpetic vesicle fluid – Pap x40. All the cells in this field are infected with herpes simplex virus. Some are multinucleated and contain red intranuclear inclusions (arrows), while others show only a ground-glass nuclear appearance. Some of the cells with single nuclei also contain inclusions.

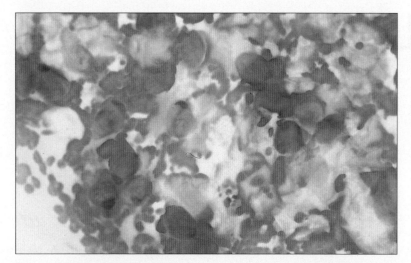

Fig. 17.3 Molluscum contagiosum – Pap x40. This poorly fixed skin scrape of a lesion of molluscum contagiosum shows a mixture of erythrocytes, keratinized squamous cells, and large, pale pink bodies which represent the intracellular inclusions of this infection.

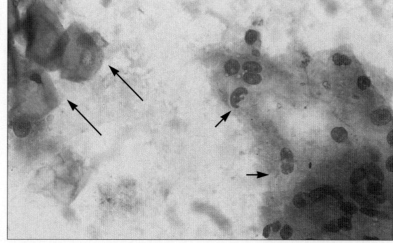

Fig. 17.4 Epidermoid cyst – MGG x40. Illustrated here are anucleate squames with sharp cytoplasmic margins and translucent cytoplasm (long arrows), macrophages with foamy cytoplasm and indistinct cell borders are also visible (short arrows).

Branchial cysts are lined by squamous (**Fig. 17.6**) or respiratory (**Fig. 17.7**) epithelium, or both, and have an underlying lymphoid infiltrate. Aspirates from these cysts usually contain debris, squamous cells (**Figs 17.8, 17.9**), rarely columnar epithelial cells (**Fig. 17.10**), and lymphocytes (see **Figures 17.15, 17.16**). Squamous pearls may also be found (**Fig. 17.11**).

Acquired cysts are infrequent, but when aspirated are seen to contain debris and crystalline material (**Fig. 17.12**).

Lymphocoeles may develop post-operatively, simulating recurrent tumour; cytology in these cases can provide rapid reassurance. The fluid is usually clear and the smear contains abundant lymphocytes (**Fig. 17.13**).

Chyle is a milky fluid which also contains large numbers of lymphocytes (**Fig. 17.14**) and shows strong positivity with an Oil-red-O stain (**Fig. 17.15**).

Following surgery for malignant disease, nodules may develop beneath the scar. These may be due to fibrosis but should be aspirated to rule out recurrent tumour. Following radiotherapy for carcinoma of the breast, areas of thickening may develop, which may be difficult to distinguish from recurrent tumours. A fine neddle aspirate of such a lesion is often acellular but may contain stromal fragments with foamy macrophages. In reactive and/or inflammatory conditions the aspirate shows proliferating blood vessels with acute inflammatory cells (**Fig. 17.16**). Eosinophils may be prominent (**Fig. 17.17**). Cells that may cause concern are regenerating striated muscle cells, with their multiple hyperchromatic nuclei (**Figs 17.18, 17.19**). However, cross-striations are often visible.

Aspirates of superficial lesions often produce non-diagnostic normal tissues, such as mature fat cells (**Fig. 17.20**), striated muscle (**Figs 17.21, 17.22**), and fibroblasts (**Fig. 17.23**). Fat cells and striated muscle are often sampled when aspirates are taken from lesions in the axilla. Fat cells may also be seen when the central portion of a lymph node is sampled.

Panniculitis can produce subcutaneous nodules, which are occasionally aspirated; the smears contain degenerate fat cells (**Figs 17.24, 17.25**), sometimes with deposits of calcium (**Figs 17.26, 17.27**). Panniculitis is often associated with pancreatic disease. Fat necrosis is not uncommon in the breast (see Chapter 8) and is usually related to trauma. Rarely, fat necrosis is accompanied by the deposition of osteoid as well as of calcium.

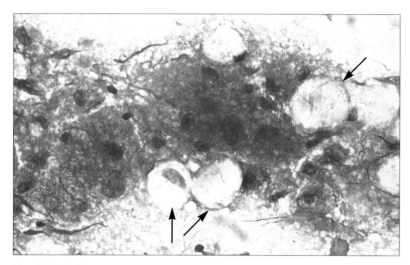

Fig. 17.5 Epidermoid cyst – MGG x40. Here the anucleate squames appear colourless and can be mistaken for fat cells (arrows). Numerous macrophages are also present.

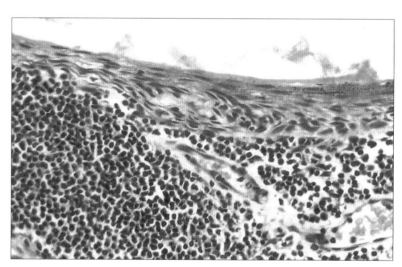

Fig. 17.6 Branchial cyst – H&E x10. This histological section of the wall of a branchial cyst displays a stratified squamous epithelial lining with an underlying infiltrate of lymphocytes.

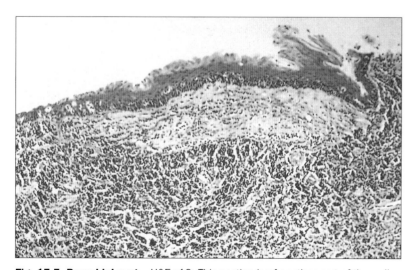

Fig. 17.7 Branchial cyst – H&E x10. This section is of another part of the wall of the cyst illustrated in **Figure 17.6**, showing respiratory epithelium and squamous metaplasia, again with underlying lymphocytes.

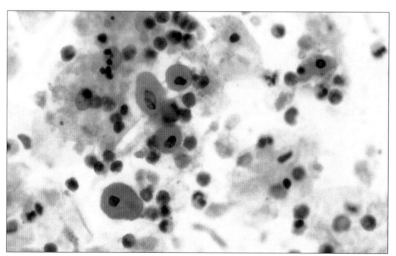

Fig. 17.8 Branchial cyst – Pap x40. This aspirate shows keratinized squamous cells with pyknotic nuclei, lymphocytes, and debris. Although the nuclei of the squamous cells appear somewhat enlarged, this is just a degenerative feature and should not be mistaken for metastatic squamous cell carcinoma in a lymph node.

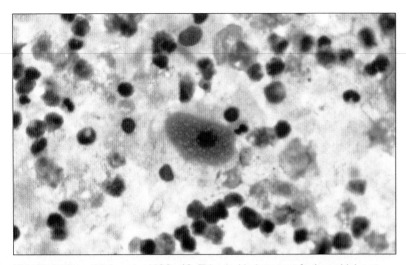

Fig. 17.9 Branchial cyst – MGG x40. This air-dried smear of a branchial cyst aspirate shows numerous lymphocytes and a single keratinized benign squamous cell.

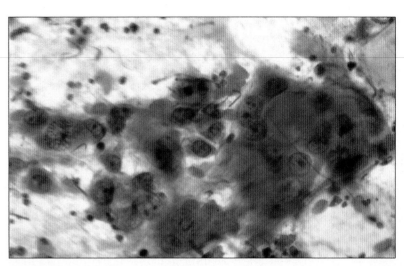

Fig. 17.10 Branchial cyst – Pap x63. Illustrated here are benign glandular cells surrounding some anucleate squames. A few inflammatory cells are seen in the background.

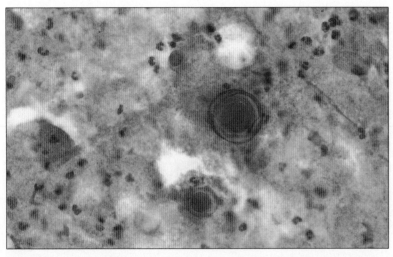

Fig. 17.11 Branchial cyst – Pap x40. This field from an aspirate of an inflamed branchial cyst shows two perfectly formed squamous epithelial pearls surrounded by debris and some inflammatory cells.

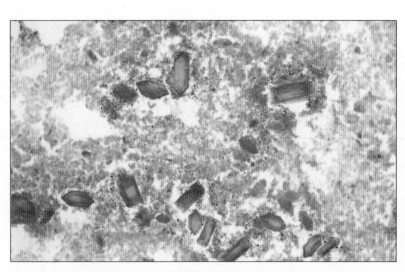

Fig. 17.12 Acquired cyst – Pap x40. The aspirate illustrated here is from a cyst in the neck, acquired post-operatively. This field shows debris and crystalline material, which is non-birefringent, and there is no evidence of an inflammatory or reactive process.

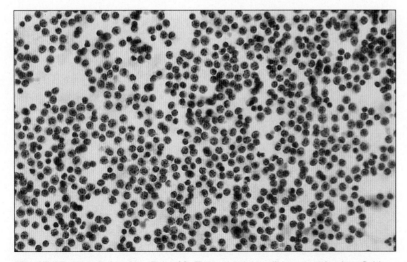

Fig. 17.13 Lymphocoele – Pap x40. These cystic swellings contain clear fluid which is composed of numerous small lymphocytes in a clean background, as illustrated here.

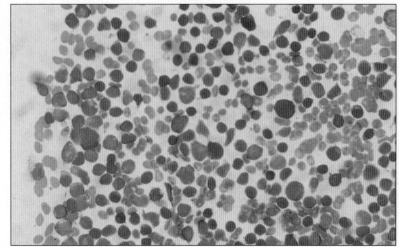

Fig. 17.14 Chyle – MGG x40. The air-dried smear contains a mixture of lymphoid cells and erythrocytes, with no evidence of malignancy. The gross appearance of the fluid provides a clue to the diagnosis.

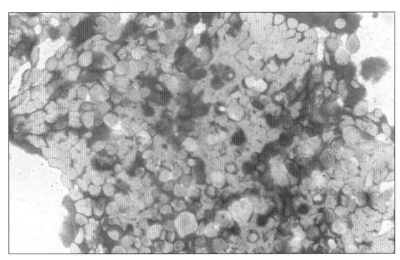

Fig. 17.15 Chyle – Oil-red-O x40. This smear from the same case as shown in **Figure 17.14** shows strongly positive red globules of fat interspersed with lymphocytes and erythrocytes.

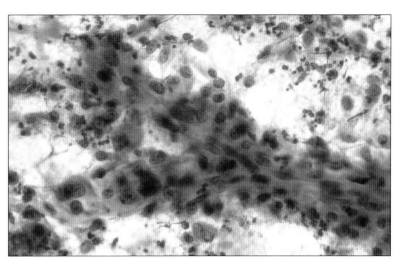

Fig. 17.16 Post-operative inflammation – Pap x40. Illustrated here is an aspirate from a tender mass which had developed adjacent to a surgical scar. There is a large, proliferating blood vessel in the centre of the field, surrounded by degenerate neutrophils and histiocytes. No malignant cells are seen.

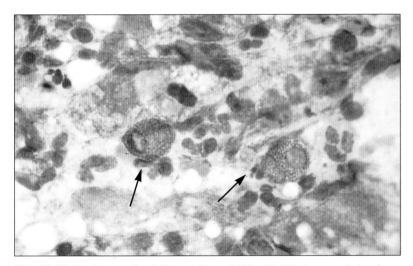

Fig. 17.17 Post-operative inflammation – MGG x63. This is an aspirate of a thickened area adjacent to a surgical scar. In the centre of the field, there are two eosinophils with coarse granules (arrows), surrounded by neutrophils and proteinaceous background material.

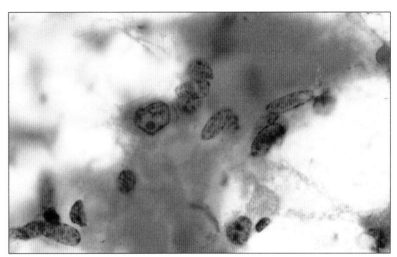

Fig. 17.18 Regenerating striated muscle cells – Pap x63. A consequence of surgical procedures is that subsequent aspirates may contain cells, such as those seen here, which could be mistaken for neoplastic cells surrounding mucin. These are regenerating striated muscle cells; cross-striations may be visible with careful focusing.

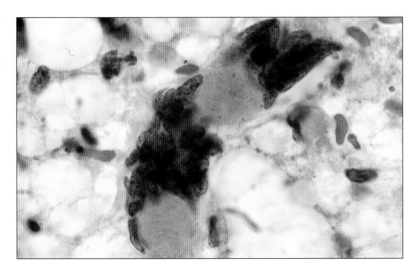

Fig. 17.19 Regenerating striated muscle cells – Pap x63. This field, from the same aspirate as shown in **Figure 17.18**, shows the hyperchromatic clusters of elongated nuclei that are sometimes seen; these may be misinterpreted as abnormal.

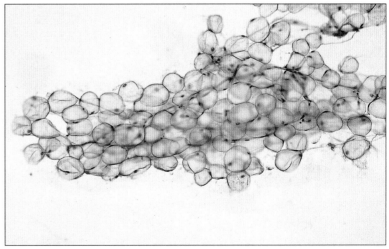

Fig. 17.20 Fat cells – Pap x40. This is an aspirate of a superficial mass which shows only mature fat cells, resembling soap suds, and no diagnostic material. Note the capillaries traversing the fat. The lesion was not a lipoma, normal fat had been aspirated.

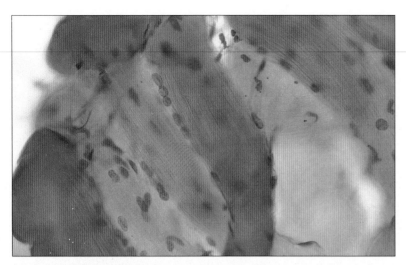

Fig. 17.21 Striated muscle – Pap x63. Illustrated here are several striated muscle fibres with peripheral nuclei and clearly visible cross-striations.

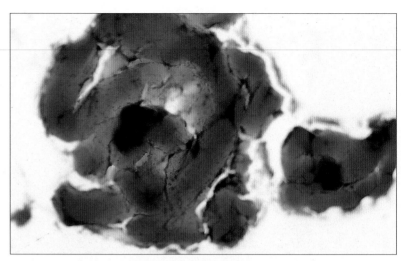

Fig. 17.22 Striated muscle – MGG x40. Striated muscle fibres stain rather deeply with May Grunwald Giemsa, so cross-striations are not distinct.

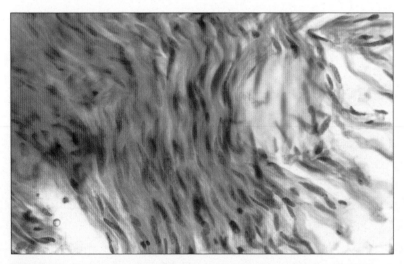

Fig. 17.23 Fibroblasts – Pap x40. Fibroblasts are seen as bundles of spindle-shaped cells with elongated, thin nuclei.

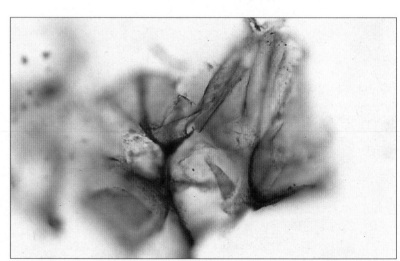

Fig. 17.24 Degenerate fat cells – MGG x40. In panniculitis, especially that related to pancreatic disease, aspirates may yield degenerate fat cells, as seen here.

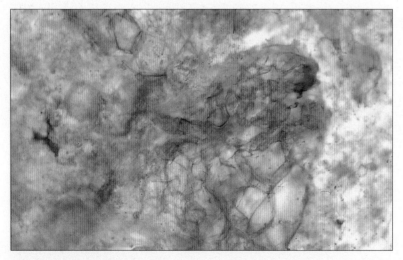

Fig. 17.25 Degenerate fat cells – Pap x40. This field demonstrates degenerate fat cells and debris. The smear may be thought to contain only debris if the fat cells are not recognized.

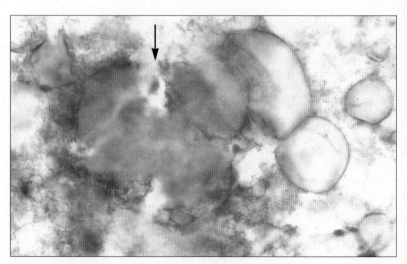

Fig. 17.26 Calcium – Pap x40. In the centre of the field (arrow) is a fragmented calcium particle. These are fragile and easily crushed by the slightest pressure on the coverslip. The fat cells in this field are not degenerate.

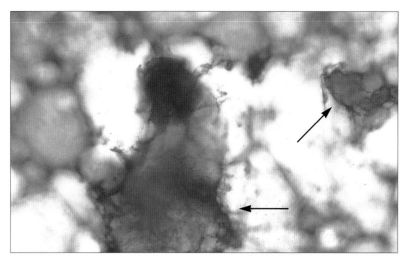

Fig. 17.27 Calcium – MGG x40. The calcium in air-dried smears is more difficult to recognize. (arrows) It is blue in colour and is here surrounded by degenerate fat cells, which are also blue.

An aspirate from a **ganglion** is composed of thick, glairy fluid which, when spun down, is composed of mucinous material (**Figs 17.28, 17.29**). Cells are rarely seen.

Gouty tophi produce chalky aspirates which, under polarized light, are seen to contain large numbers of urate crystals (**Fig. 17.30**).

Primary neoplasms of the skin that are commonly sampled for cytological evaluation are squamous and basal cell carcinomas. The usual problem with skin scrape specimens is that they are often too rigorously spread, causing streak artefact, and are not infrequently poorly fixed. **Basal cell carcinoma** has characteristic histological appearances (**Fig. 17.31**), which are usually well represented and should be searched for in skin-scrape specimens. The tumour cells are small and hyperchromatic, usually in three-dimensional clusters (**Figs 17.32, 17.33**).

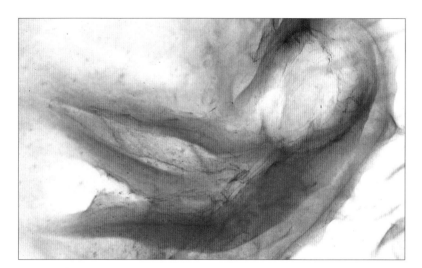

Fig. 17.28 Ganglion – Pap x10. This field shows the pinkish orange staining of the mucinous contents of a ganglion.

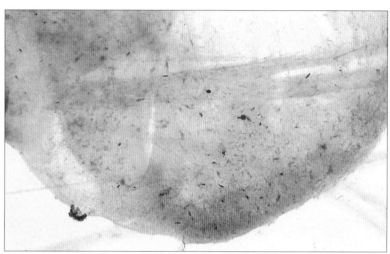

Fig. 17.29 Ganglion – MGG x10. In an air-dried smear mucinous material stains a pale magenta shade.

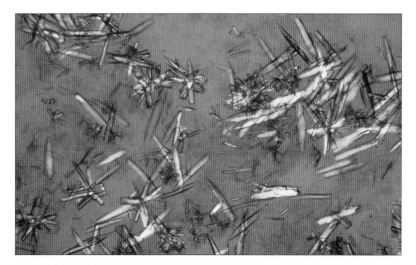

Fig. 17.30 Gouty tophus – Polarized light x40. These needle-shaped urate crystals are typical of gout.

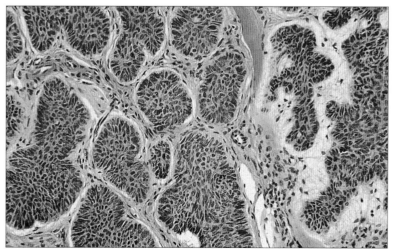

Fig. 17.31 Basal cell carcinoma – H&E x25. This histological section demonstrates the islands of small tumour cells and peripheral palisading characteristic of this neoplasm. (Courtesy of Dr PH McKee, St. Thomas' Hospital, London, UK.)

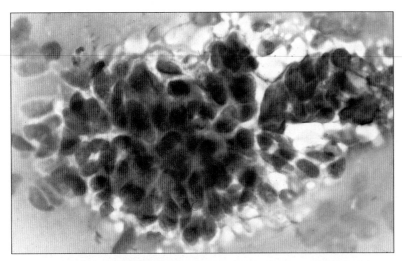

Fig. 17.32 Basal cell carcinoma – Pap x63. This is a skin scrape from a basal cell carcinoma showing the small hyperchromatic nuclei that comprise this tumour. The chromatin pattern is granular and nucleoli are not prominent. The nuclei are about the same size as the erythrocytes in the field.

A vague hint may be seen of the palisading usually present in histological sections (**Fig. 17.34**). Anucleate squames may be present.

Squamous cell carcinoma scrape smears often contain abundant anucleate squames (**Figs 17.35, 17.36**), which may be accompanied by inflammatory cells. The neoplastic cells are often in thick clumps, but have abundant keratinized cytoplasm and abnormal, although often degenerate, nuclei (**Fig. 17.37**). There are usually single keratinized malignant cells (**Figs 17.38, 17.39**), but these may be difficult to classify in poorly differentiated tumours (**Fig. 17.40**). An unusual presentation of squamous cell carcinoma is in the form of a blister, the aspirate containing proteinaceous material, inflammatory cells, and single squamous carcinoma cells. Scrapes from **keratoacanthoma** show identical features to those squamous carcinoma, namely anucleate squamous and keratinised carcinoma cells (**Figs 17.41, 17.42**). The clinical impresion and duration of the lesion are more useful than cytology for distinguishing between the two.

Merkel cell tumour (primary neuroendocrine carcinoma) of the skin produces aspirates composed of small cells resembling lymphocytes (**Figs 17.43, 17.44**)

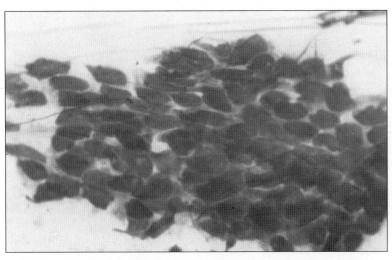

Fig. 17.33 Basal cell carcinoma – MGG x63. The neoplastic cells in this preparation are somewhat dispersed and variable in size. There is distortion of some of the nuclei due to vigorous smearing. These cells are unlike squamous carcinoma cells, as they have very little cytoplasm.

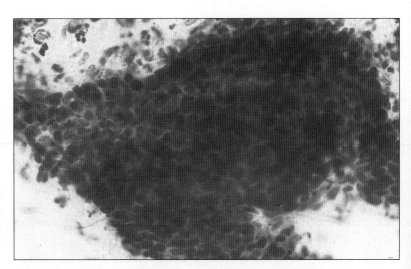

Fig. 17.34 Basal cell carcinoma – MGG x40. The tight cluster, rather darkly stained, of neoplastic cells seen in this field shows peripheral palisading, identical to that seen in tissue sections.

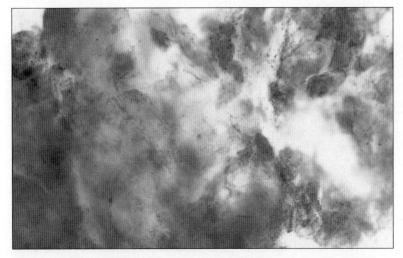

Fig. 17.35 Squamous cell carcinoma – Pap x40. Illustrated here is a thick clump of anucleate squames in a scrape taken from the surface of the lesion. The features are non-diagnostic.

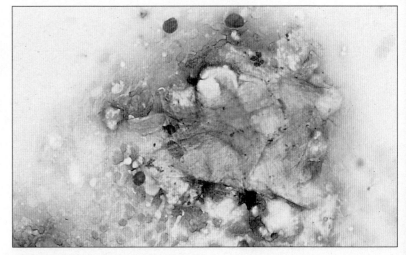

Fig. 17.36 Squamous cell carcinoma – MGG x40. Anucleate squamous cells in air-dried material stain pale blue and may appear translucent.

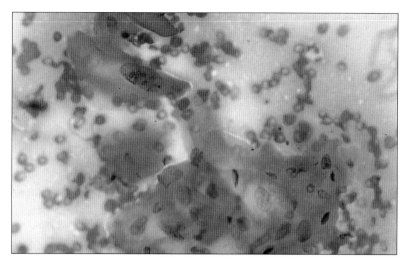

Fig. 17.37 Squamous cell carcinoma – Pap x43. These malignant cells have abundant keratinized cytoplasm and abnormal nuclei, but are very degenerate, so should be reported as suspicious rather than diagnostic of squamous cell carcinoma. Atypical squamous cells are occasionally seen in skin scrapes from a basal cell carcinoma.

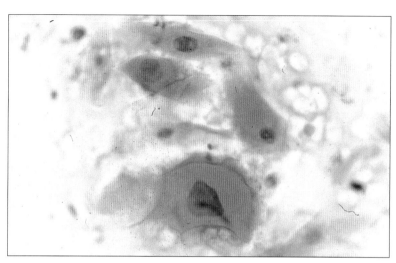

Fig. 17.38 Squamous cell carcinoma – Pap x40. Illustrated here are keratinized squamous carcinoma cells in a skin scrape.

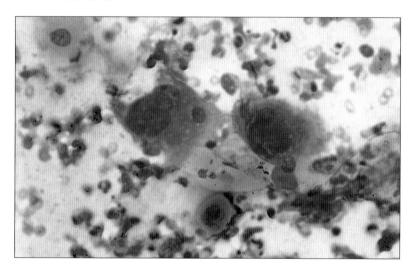

Fig. 17.39 Squamous cell carcinoma – MGG x40. This field shows single carcinoma cells, the smallest one being keratinized, thus providing a clue to the diagnosis.

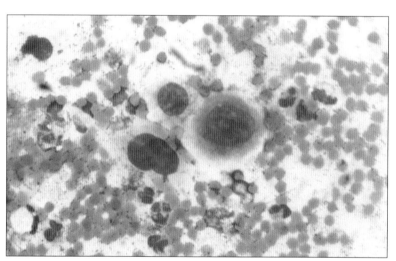

Fig. 17.40 Squamous cell carcinoma – MGG x40. The malignant cells in this field have little cytoplasm, with no evidence of keratinization, suggestive of a poorly differentiated neoplasm.

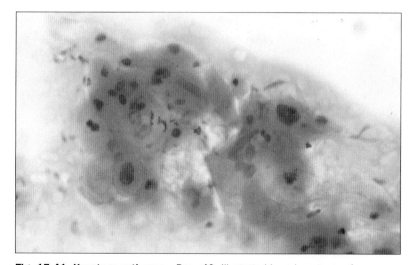

Fig. 17.41 Keratoacanthoma – Pap x40. Illustrated here is a group of abnormal, keratinized squamous cells from a lesion that was demonstrated to be a keratoacanthoma on histology. The cells are indistinguishable from squamous carcinoma cells.

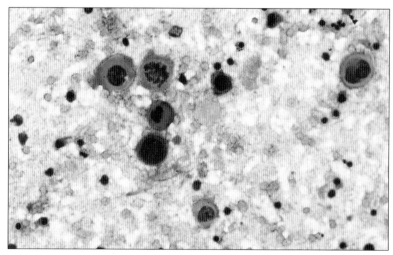

Fig. 17.42 Keratoacanthoma – MGG x40. The neoplastic cells seen here have keratinized cytoplasm and abnormal hyperchromatic nuclei, identical to those of squamous cell carcinomas. Note the mitotic figure.

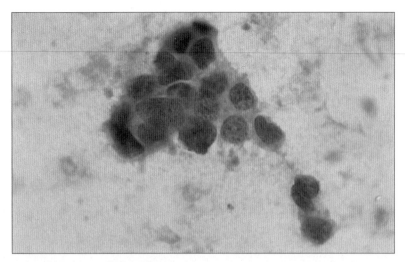

Fig. 17.43 Merkel cell tumour – Pap x100. These tumours are composed of small cells with rounded nuclei and stippled or speckled chromatin, with very little cytoplasm. They are slightly larger than lymphocytes.

and, occasionally, indistinguishable from small cell carcinoma. The cells do not have prominent nucleoli and have very little cytoplasm, but usually occur in clusters. Unfortunately, there is usually insufficient spare material to perform immunocytochemical stains for a definitive diagnosis.

Granular cell tumour has been described in Chapter 8 (see **Figures 8.121–8.124**).

Metastatic tumours are common in the skin and subcutaneous tissues. It is helpful to have clinical information about a previous neoplasm when examining an aspirate to determine the type of malignancy present. Commonly metastasing tumours include **melanoma (Figs 17.45, 17.46)** and **adenocarcinoma** from a variety of primary sites, such as the breast **(Figs 17.47, 17.48)**, bronchus **(Fig. 17.49)**, gastrointestinal tract **(Figs 17.50, 17.51)**, and kidney **(Figs 17.52, 17.53)**. **Transitional cell carcinoma** frequently metastasizes to the skin **(Figs 17.54, 17.55)** and may show squamous differentiation **(Figs 17.56, 17.57)**. **Small cell carcinoma** of the lung may spread to the skin **(Fig. 17.58)**. Aspirates of recurrent **meningioma** following surgery characteristically exhibit whorls and flat groups of cells with blunt-ended, spindle-shaped nuclei **(Figs 17.59–17.61)**. Psammoma bodies may occasionally be seen.

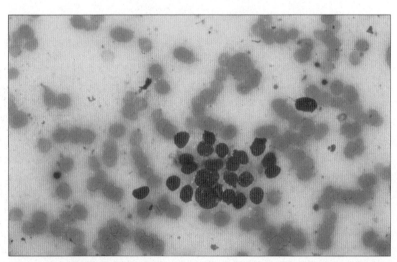

Fig. 17.44 Merkel cell tumour – MGG x100. This air-dried smear of an aspirate from a Merkel cell tumour contains a group of small cells with hyperchromatic nuclei, showing some variability in nuclear size. The cells are slightly larger than the surrounding erythrocytes, but show no specific features that would distinguish them from any other small, round cell tumour in this preparation.

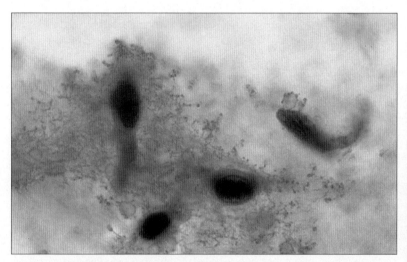

Fig. 17.45 Metastatic malignant melanoma – Pap x100. The spindle cells seen here are from a melanoma deposit in skin above the site of a previously excised melanoma. Intranuclear inclusions, prominent nucleoli, and pigment are not obvious in this aspirate, but a review of the original biopsy specimen showed a spindle-cell melanoma.

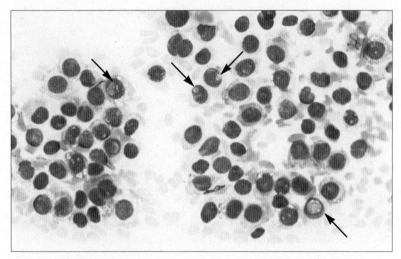

Fig. 17.46 Metastatic malignant melanoma – MGG x40. This field shows another appearance of metastatic melanoma, with cells containing rounded nuclei and striking intranuclear inclusions (arrows). No pigment is seen.

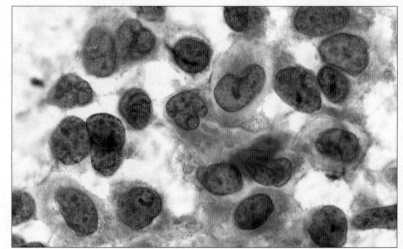

Fig. 17.47 Metastatic adenocarcinoma of the breast – Pap x100. Illustrated here is an aspirate of a skin metastasis from a grade 3 carcinoma of the breast. Note the marked budding and clefting of the nuclear margins, prominent nucleoli, and clumping and clearing of chromatin. The features in this case are identical to those of the primary ductal carcinoma.

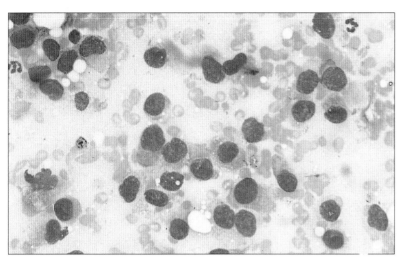

Fig. 17.48 Metastatic adenocarcinoma of the breast – MGG x63. This air-dried smear is from the same aspirate as that shown in **Figure 17.47**. Note the smoothing out of the nuclear outlines due to air drying, and also the absence of nucleoli and unremarkable chromatin pattern. This field incorrectly suggests a lower grade tumour, emphasizing the point that grading of breast carcinomas should be performed on wet-fixed, well-preserved material (see Chapter 9).

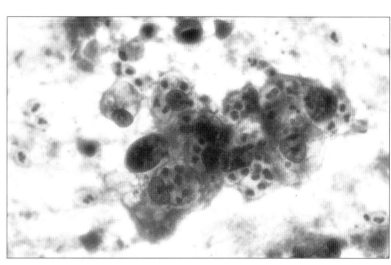

Fig. 17.49 Metastatic adenocarcinoma of the lung – Pap x40. The aspirate seen here is from a skin nodule in the forearm in a patient with adenocarcinoma of the lung. The cells shown in this cluster have large, red central nucleoli and vacuoles containing neutrophils – a feature commonly associated with endometrial carcinoma, but also seen occasionally in other adenocarcinomas.

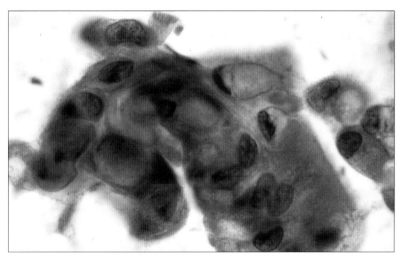

Fig. 17.50 Metastatic adenocarcinoma of the rectum – Pap x100. This group of adenocarcinoma cells contains intracellular mucin. Abnormal nuclei and nucleoli are also seen.

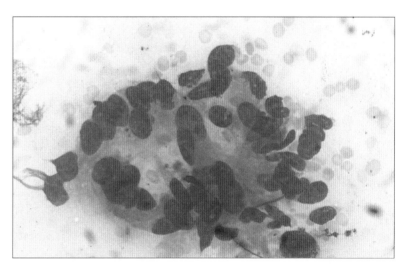

Fig. 17.51 Metastatic adenocarcinoma of the colon – MGG x40. Illustrated are adenocarcinoma cells arranged in acinar fashion. The nuclei are somewhat elongated and nucleoli are visible in some of the cells.

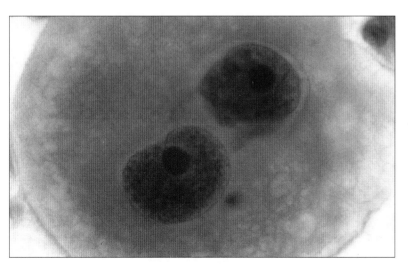

Fig. 17.52 Metastatic renal cell carcinoma – Pap x100. The large cell shown here is binucleate with huge red nucleoli and abnormally clumped chromatin. The cytoplasm is abundant and foamy.

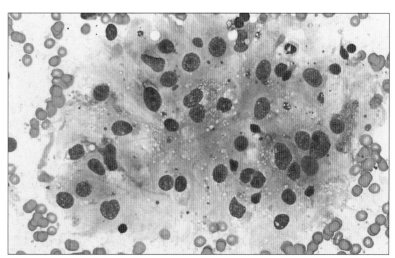

Fig. 17.53 Metastatic renal cell carcinoma – MGG x40. This field demonstrates the characteristic appearance of renal cell carcinoma cells, with abundant pale foamy cytoplasm, relatively rounded nuclei, and prominent nucleoli.

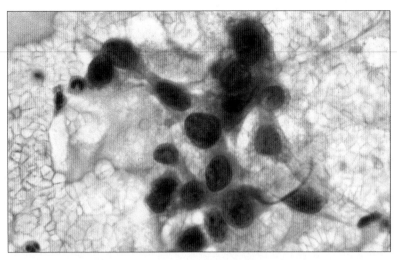

Fig. 17.54 Metastatic transitional cell carcinoma – Pap x40. The epithelial cells seen here show pleomorphism and ill-defined cytoplasm. Without a history of a primary urothelial carcinoma, it would be difficult to correctly classify these cells.

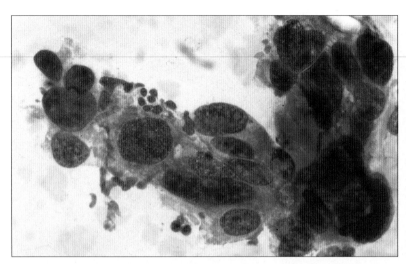

Fig. 17.55 Metastatic transitional cell carcinoma – MGG x40. These are large cells with pleomorphic nuclei and ill-defined cytoplasm, arranged in small sheets.

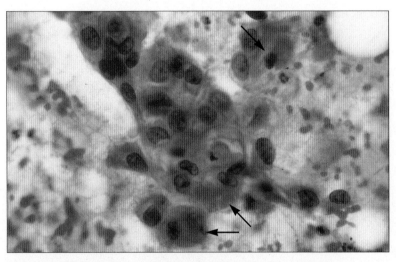

Fig. 17.56 Metastatic transitional cell carcinoma with squamous differentiation – Pap x40. This fine needle aspirate of a skin metastasis shows a cluster of malignant cells with round-to-ovoid nuclei and prominent nucleoli. Most of the cells have delicate cytoplasm, but a few show the dense orange keratinization characteristic of squamous differentiation (arrows).

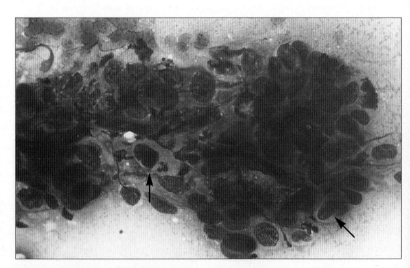

Fig. 17.57 Metastatic transitional cell carcinoma with squamous differentiation – MGG x40. The cluster of carcinoma cells seen here includes two cells with bright blue keratinized cytoplasm (arrows).

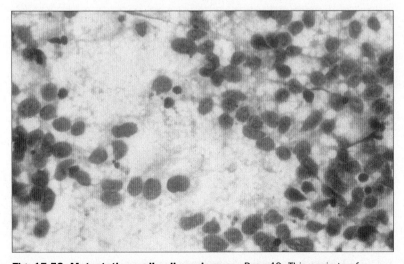

Fig. 17.58 Metastatic small cell carcinoma – Pap x40. This aspirate of a metastatic small cell carcinoma in the skin of the chest wall shows small malignant cells with faintly speckled chromatin and very little cytoplasm. The preservation is poor.

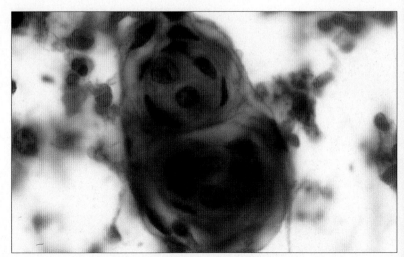

Fig. 17.59 Meningioma – Pap x63. Illustrated here is the characteristic appearance of meningioma cells, arranged in whorls.

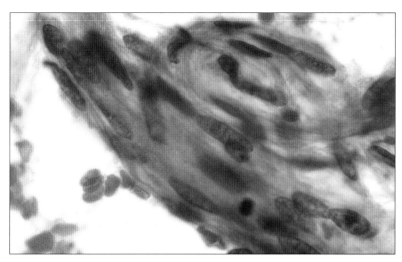

Fig. 17.60 Meningioma – Pap x63. Occasionally the meningioma cells are arranged in longitudinal groups; the nuclei here appear to be more elongated than the ovoid nuclei seen in the whorls.

FINE NEEDLE ASPIRATES OF SOFT TISSUE LESIONS

Most soft tissue lesions cannot be classified confidently on cytological material as sampling may be limited. Reactive conditions, such as **nodular fasciitis** and **fibromatosis,** are often poorly cellular; the former, on occasion, contains myxoid material and abnormal spindle cells. **Neurilemmoma (Schwannoma)** is not uncommon. Histologically, it is composed of spindle-celled and myxoid areas (**Fig. 17.62**). Aspirates of neurilemmomas are often insufficient for diagnosis, but can be cellular, showing the features seen on histology. These are spindle cells arranged in a palisading fashion (**Fig. 17.63**), with some myxoid material (**Fig. 17,64**). The cells are occasionally ovoid (**Fig. 17.65**). **Sarcomas** present as soft-tissue masses, usually composed of spindle cells and abnormal rounded, enlarged cells without the characteristics of epithelial cells (**Fig. 17.66**). They

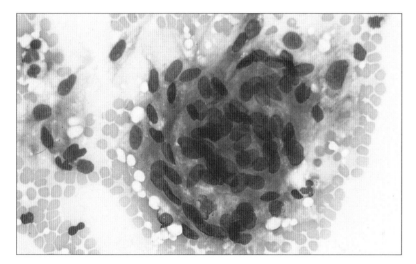

Fig. 17.61 Meningioma – MGG x40. The whorls typical of this tumour are not as well preserved in the air-dried smear as in wet-fixed material.

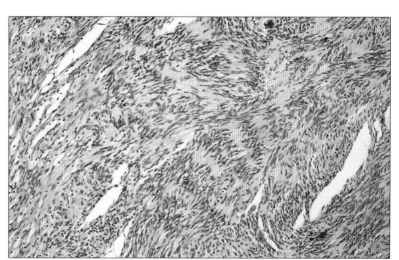

Fig. 17.62 Neurilemmoma – H&E x40. This histological section shows the characteristic palisaded spindle cells which comprise this tumour. (Courtesy of Dr A Salerno, Bolzano, Italy.)

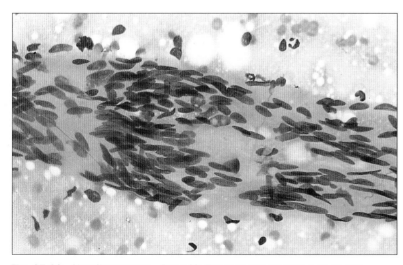

Fig. 17.63 Neurilemmoma – Pap x40. The thin spindle cells seen in this aspirate show palisading. (Courtesy of Dr A Salerno, Bolzano, Italy.)

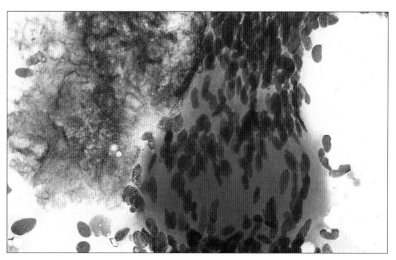

Fig. 17.64 Neurilemmoma – MGG x40. In this field there are spindle cells in a palisade arrangement and some magenta-coloured myxoid stroma. (Courtesy of Dr A Salerno, Bolzano, Italy.)

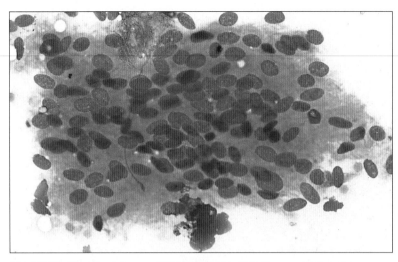

Fig. 17.65 Neurilemmoma – MGG x40. In this field the neoplastic cells are ovoid rather than spindle-shaped. (Courtesy of Dr A Salerno, Bolzano, Italy.)

often contain large red nucleoli, which are sometimes multiple, and may be multinucleated **(Figs 17.67, 17.68)**. Myxoid material may be found. **Liposarcomas** show characteristic features, such as crow's foot blood vessels and lipoblasts on histological sections **(Fig. 17.69)**, but these are difficult to identify in cytological material. The aspirates are usually cellular, composed of pleomorphic cells, both spindle-shaped and round, often with intranuclear inclusions **(Fig. 17.70)**,

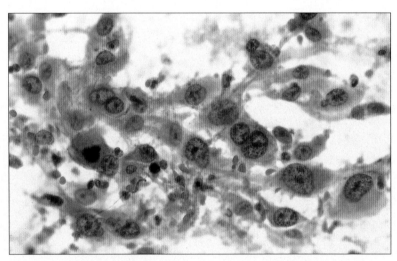

Fig. 17.66 Sarcoma NOS – Pap x40. The cells illustrated here are large, round to spindle-shaped, with pleomorphic nuclei, large irregular nucleoli, and abnormal clumping and clearing of the chromatin.

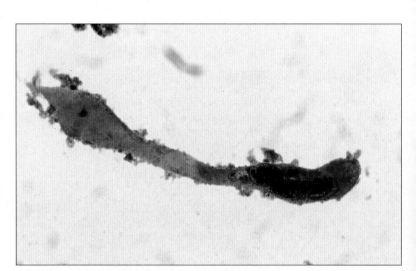

Fig. 17.67 Sarcoma NOS – Pap x40. This elongated neoplastic cell contains three nuclei at one end and abundant cytoplasm.

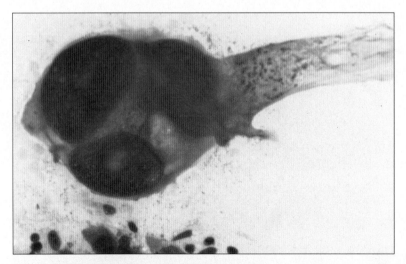

Fig. 17.68 Sarcoma NOS – MGG x40. Seen here is an enormous tadpole cell with three large nuclei at one end.

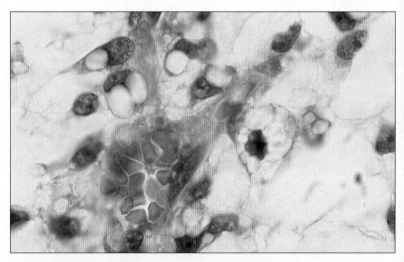

Fig. 17.69 Liposarcoma – H&E x40. This histological section of a myxoid liposarcoma demonstrates the diagnostic features of this neoplasm, namely crow's foot blood vessels and lipoblasts. The nuclei are indented and scalloped by the cytoplasmic vacuoles.

and they may show multinucleation (**Figs 17.71, 17.72**) as well as myxoid background material (**Fig. 17.73**). Cells of extremely bizarre shapes may seen in pleomorphic liposarcoma (**Fig. 17.74**). **Angiosarcoma** may sometimes develop following radiotherapy for carcinoma of the breast. The aspirate is often heavily blood-stained with no diagnostic cells. Rarely, a few malignant cells may be seen, usually with rounded nuclei, abnormal enlarged nucleoli, and very little

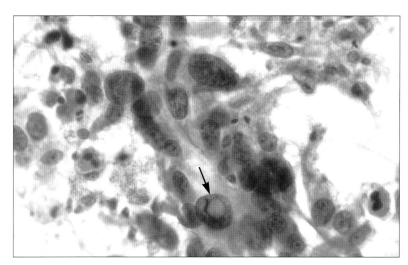

Fig. 17.70 Liposarcoma – Pap x40. This cellular aspirate from a sarcoma, which was classified on histology as a liposarcoma, contains a mixture of large and small malignant cells, some with rounded nuclei and others spindle-shaped. Note the intranuclear inclusion (arrow). It is not possible to type sarcomas from cytological material alone and they should be reported as being consistent with a sarcoma NOS.

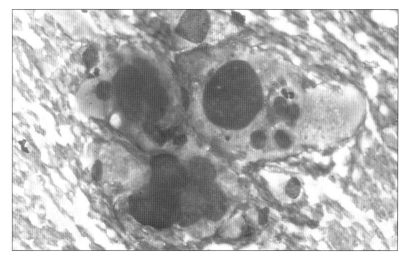

Fig. 17.71 Liposarcoma – MGG x63. The sarcoma cells illustrated here are large with translucent cytoplasm; two are multinucleated.

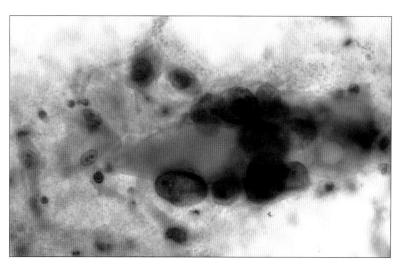

Fig. 17.72 Liposarcoma – Pap x63. This field shows a large multinucleated cell with vacuolated cytoplasm. Smaller tumour cells are seen in the background. There are no specific features to help type this neoplasm.

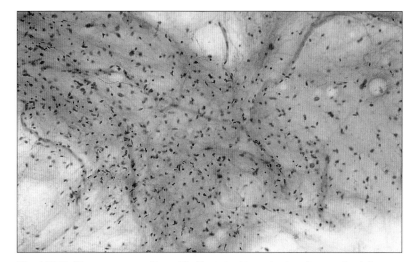

Fig. 17.73 Liposarcoma – Pap x10. Illustrated here is abundant, pale pink myxoid material traversed by blood vessels, with a scattering of spindle-shaped and rounded nuclei. Crow's foot blood vessels are not identifiable in cytological material.

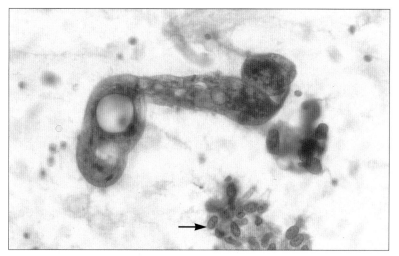

Fig. 17.74 Pleomorphic liposarcoma – Pap x40. The large bizarre-shaped nucleus in this illustration contains several intranuclear inclusions (intranuclear cytoplasmic invaginations). There are clusters of smaller neoplastic cells nearby – one group resembles histiocytes with bean-shaped nuclei (arrow).

cytoplasm (**Figs 17.75, 17.76**). They cannot be distinguished reliably from other sarcomas using smears. Aspirates from **embryonal rhabdomyosarcoma** contain small round cells which resemble lymphoid cells (**Fig. 17.77**). All soft-tissue neoplasms should be examined histologically for a definitive diagnosis.

Plasmacytomas (**Fig. 17.78**) may present as soft tissue masses. Aspirates from these lesions are usually cellular (**Figs 17.79, 17.80**) and contain pleomorphic

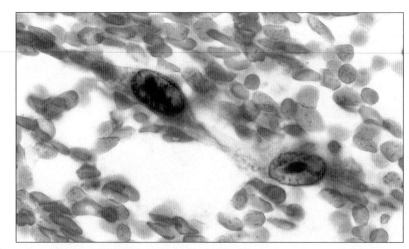

Fig. 17.75 Angiosarcoma – Pap x100. This field contains many erythrocytes and two spindle-shaped cells with very delicate cytoplasm, ovoid nuclei, and abnormal red nucleoli. These tumours are usually very scanty in cellularity; the cells are not specific, but are consistent with the clinical diagnosis of angiosarcoma. This specimen is an imprint smear of the excised tumour, which was confirmed to be an angiosarcoma on histology.

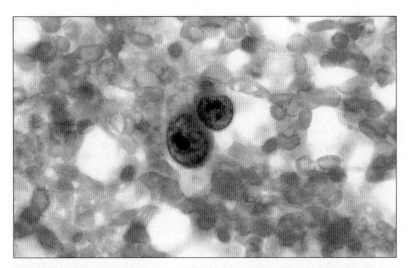

Fig. 17.76 Angiosarcoma – Pap x100. The two neoplastic cells seen in this aspirate (same case as shown in **Figure 17.71**) have rounded nuclei, large red nucleoli, and chromatin, which shows clumping with areas of clearing. Cytoplasm is not clearly visible.

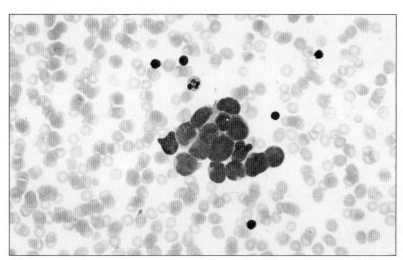

Fig. 17.77 Embryonal rhabdomyosarcoma – MGG x40. These round cells have nuclei which are about 3–4 times the size of an erythrocyte and very little cytoplasm. There appears to be some moulding between adjacent nuclei, simulating small-cell carcinoma. The clinical details are important, this case being an aspirated from a soft tissue mass in a 13-year-old girl. The report should give a differential diagnosis only, as the neoplasm cannot be typed from cytology alone.

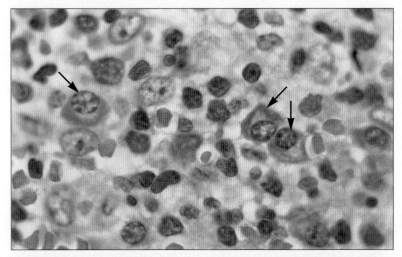

Fig. 17.78 Plasmacytoma – H&E x100. This high-power view of a histological section of a plasmacytoma shows at least three plasma cells with cart-wheel chromatin and a clear 'hof'(arrows). Lymphocytes and histiocytes are also visible here.

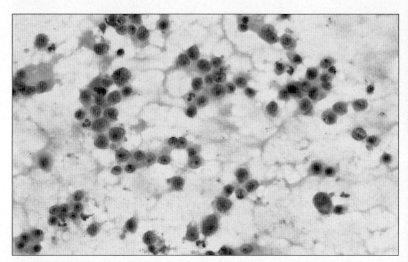

Fig. 17.79 Plasmacytoma – MGP x40. This cellular aspirate from a plasmacytoma of the chest wall shows numerous abnormal plasma cells with prominent nucleoli and occasional 'hofs'.

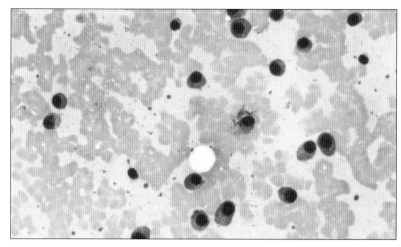

plasmacytoid cells, each with an eccentric nucleus and a 'hof' representing the Golgi body **(Fig. 17.81)**. Mitoses may be seen **(Fig. 17.82)**. A methyl green pyronin (MGP) stain is usually strongly positive **(Fig. 17.83)**. Binucleate plasma cells are often noted. **Lymphoma** deposits yield cellular aspirates with enlarged, abnormal lymphoid cells, often with multiple nucleoli, depending on the type of lymphoma **(Fig. 17.84)**.

Fig. 17.80 Plasmacytoma – MGG x40. The air-dried smear from the same case as in **Figure 17.75** shows plasma cells, each with an eccentric nucleus and a faint 'hof'. The clock-face chromatin is not apparent with this preparation.

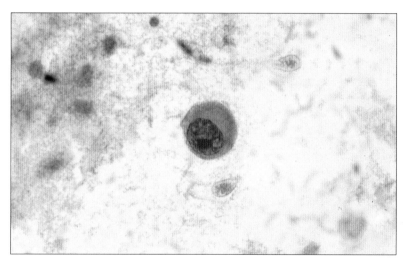

Fig. 17.81 Plasmacytoma – Pap x100. The plasma cell illustrated is abnormal, in spite of its eccentric nucleus and pale 'hof', as it also has a huge red nucleolus.

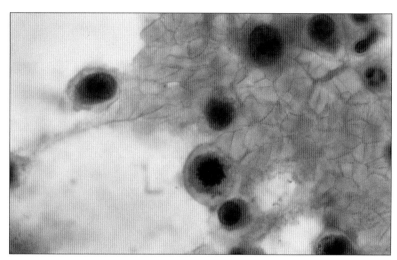

Fig. 17.82 Plasmacytoma – Pap x100. These neoplastic plasma cells seen here do not exhibit the characteristic clock-face chromatin and are variable in nuclear size. Note the mitotic figure.

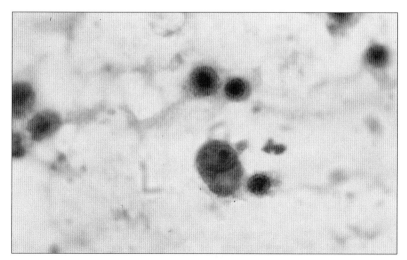

Fig. 17.83 Plasmacytoma – MGP x100. The methyl green pyronin stain shows strong granular positivity in this aspirate. Note the large red nucleolus in the cell in the centre of the field.

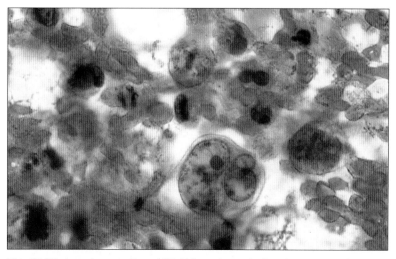

Fig. 17.84 Lymphoma – Pap x100. This aspirate of a lymphomatous soft tissue mass shows abnormal enlarged lymphoid cells with prominent nucleoli and large areas of chromatin clearing. This is a high-grade non-Hodgkin's lymphoma.

FINE NEEDLE ASPIRATES OF BONE

Most bony lesions are accessible to the radiologist's needle. The most common bone lesion to be sampled for cytological diagnosis is metastatic malignancy. Bone aspirates commonly contain **normal bone marrow constituents**, such as the precursors of blood cells, **megakaryocytes (Figs 17.85, 17.86)**, and **osteoclasts (Figs 17.87, 17.88)**.

Aspirates from inflammatory lesions, such as **osteomyelitis**, contain inflammatory cells and debris. **Tuberculosis** should be considered if the smears contain multinucleated (Langhans' type) giant cells **(Figs 17.89, 17.90)** and epithelioid histiocytes **(Fig. 17.91)**. A Papanicolaou-stained smear may be restained with Ziehl–Neelsen's stain to demonstrate acid-fast bacilli **(Fig. 17.92)**.

Aneurysmal bone cyst aspirates are usually heavily blood-stained and contain numerous giant cells **(Fig. 17.93)**, but these features are not specific.

Aspirates in **acute lymphoblastic leukaemias** contain blast cells **(Fig. 17.94)**, which may exhibit PAS-positive granules **(Fig. 17.95)**.

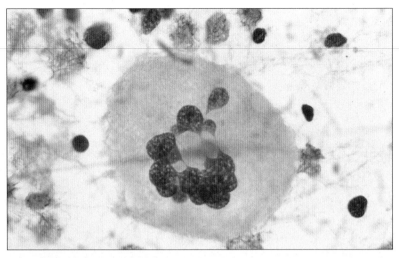

Fig. 17.85 Megakaryocyte – Pap x63. Illustrated here is a large megakaryocyte with multiple hyperchromatic nuclei.

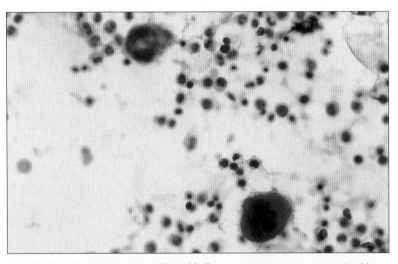

Fig. 17.86 Megakaryocytes – Pap x40. Two megakaryocytes are seen in this field, demonstrating the variation in nuclear appearances – one is binucleate and the other has a huge horseshoe-shaped nucleus.

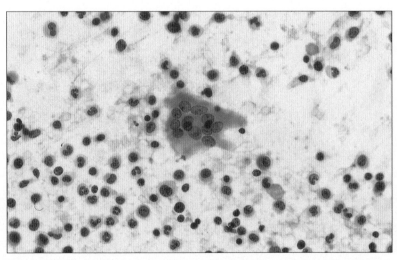

Fig. 17.87 Osteoclast – Pap x40. This cellular aspirate of a vertebral lesion shows normal constituents of bone marrow, such as the precursors of blood cells, and also a multinucleated osteoclast. This multinucleated cell has several small, vesicular, uniform nuclei, unlike the hyperchromatic nuclei seen in megakaryocytes.

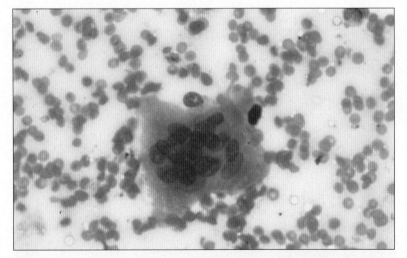

Fig. 17.88 Osteoclast – MGG x40. This megakaryocyte in the corresponding air-dried smear is multinucleated and has foamy cytoplasm, with ill-defined cytoplasmic borders.

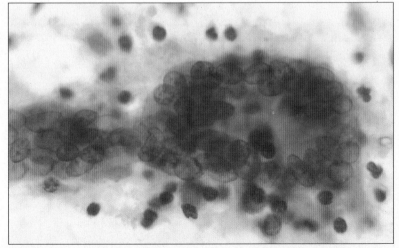

Fig. 17.89 Tuberculosis, Langhans' giant cell – Ziehl–Neelsen over Pap x40. This bone aspirate, which was stained with the Ziehl–Neelsen stain after a Papanicolaou stain, revealed this Langhans' giant cell with its peripheral nuclei.

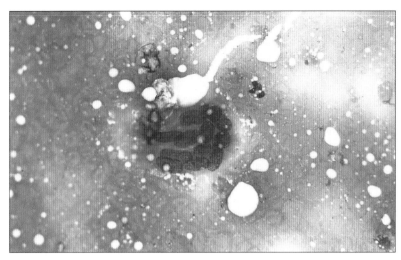

Fig. 17.90 Tuberculosis, Langhans' giant cell – MGG x40. The air-dried smear from the same case as that shown in **Figure 17.85** shows a Langhans' giant cell with multiple nuclei.

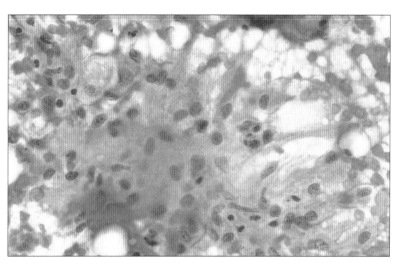

Fig. 17.91 Tuberculosis, epithelioid histiocytes – Pap x40. Illustrated here is a granuloma composed of epithelioid histiocytes, with ill-defined cytoplasmic margins and elongated nuclei. Caseation necrosis is not as easy to identify in these specimens as it is in lymph node aspirates.

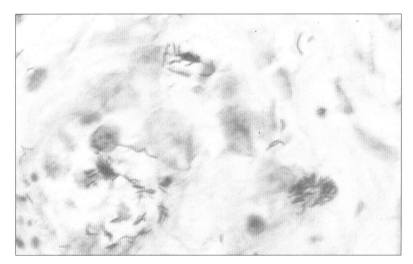

Fig. 17.92 Tuberculosis, mycobacteria – Ziehl–Neelsen over Pap x100. Acid-fast bacilli are occasionally seen in aspirates, as illustrated here.

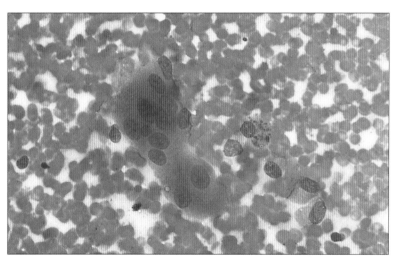

Fig. 17.93 Aneurysmal bone cyst – MGG x40. Illustrated here is a large multinucleated giant cell. This case was shown to be an aneurysmal bone cyst from the histological specimen.

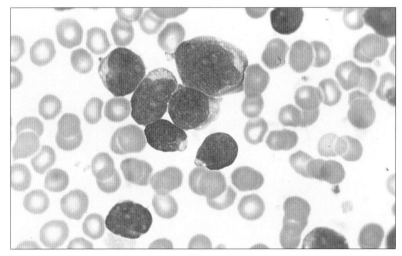

Fig. 17.94 Acute lymphoblastic leukaemia – MGG x100. This bone marrow aspirate contains abnormal, pleomorphic blast cells.

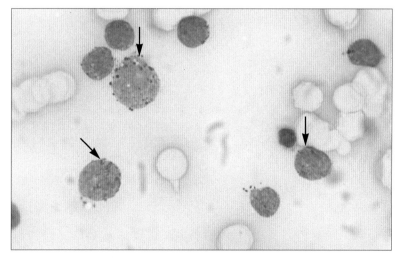

Fig. 17.95 Acute lymphoblastic leukaemia – PAS x100. This field shows the PAS-positive granules characteristic of the blast cells in this disease (arrows).

Histological sections of bone marrow in **myeloma** reveal large numbers of plasma cells, many of them abnormal. The fine needle aspirate is correspondingly cellular, with abnormal plasma cells ranging from those with a single nucleus and prominent nucleolus to binucleate forms **(Fig. 17.96)** and even multinucleated cells, all with clock-face chromatin **(Fig. 17.97)**. The cells may appear to have distended cytoplasm with a decreased nuclear–cytoplasmic ratio **(Fig. 17.98)**.

Osteosarcoma aspirates are often very cellular and composed of large pleomorphic cells with abundant, fairly dense cytoplasm **(Figs 17.99, 17.100)**. Large

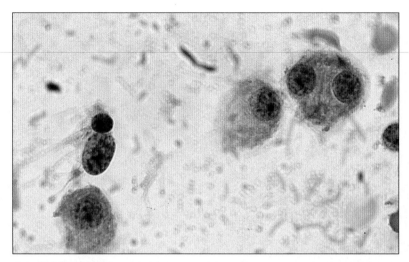

Fig. 17.96 Multiple myeloma – Pap x100. In this field there are abnormal plasma cells with prominent nucleoli and clock-face chromatin. Note the binucleate form.

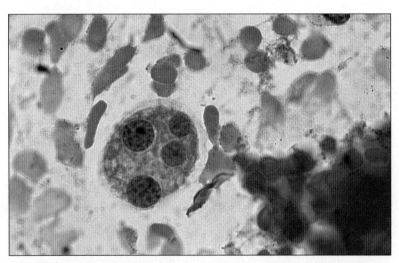

Fig. 17.97 Multiple myeloma – Pap x100. The large cell pictured here contains four nuclei, each with a cart-wheel chromatin pattern. Nucleoli are present.

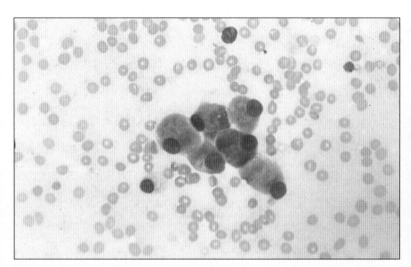

Fig. 17.98 Multiple myeloma – MGG x40. This air-dried smear from the same case as shown in **Figures 17.92, 17.93** shows abnormal plasma cells with distended cytoplasm and eccentric nuclei. The chromatin pattern is not identifiable in air-dried preparations.

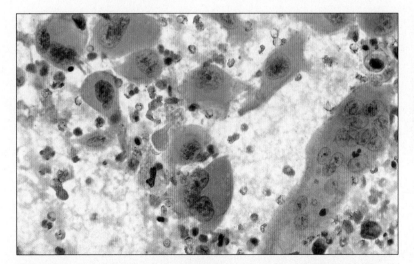

Fig. 17.99 Osteosarcoma – Pap x40. This is a very cellular aspirate consisting of pleomorphic malignant cells with fairly dense cytoplasm and irregular nuclei with clumped chromatin. The cells have sharp, well-defined cytoplasmic borders. A multinucleated giant cell is also seen containing small, uniform, vesicular nuclei; it may represent an osteoclast rather than a tumour giant cell.

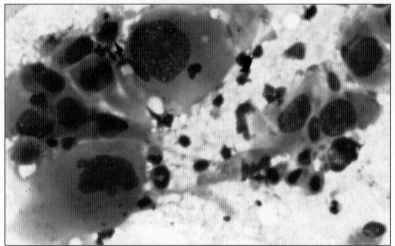

Fig. 17.100 Osteosarcoma – MGG x40. The extreme pleomorphism of this neoplasm is well-illustrated here. The cells have huge, irregular nuclei and prominent nucleoli.

nucleoli may be visible and mitoses are often seen (**Fig. 17.101**). Spindle-cell forms may occur (**Fig. 17.102**) and osteoid is a frequent constituent, which is pale in wet-fixed smears and magenta in air-dried preparations (**Figs 17.103, 17.104**). **Chondrosarcoma** aspirates contain fibrillary chondroid material with large abnormal cells, which are not always identifiable as chondrocytes (**Fig. 17.105**), unless the characteristic perinuclear haloes are seen.

Aspirates from **Ewing's sarcoma** are cellular, containing small dissociated cells with rounded nuclei slightly larger than the erythrocytes, vesicular chromatin, and

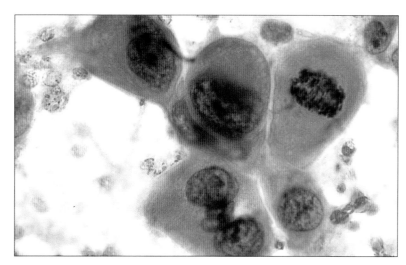

Fig. 17.101 Osteosarcoma – Pap x100. This field displays large pleomorphic tumour cells with irregular nuclei, clumped chromatin, abnormal nucleoli, and dense cytoplasm with well-defined cell margins. Note the mitotic figure.

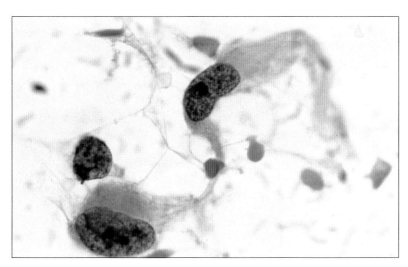

Fig. 17.102 Osteosarcoma – Pap x63. The cells in this case are spindle-shaped with delicate cytoplasm. The nuclei are irregular with coarsely clumped chromatin and large nucleoli.

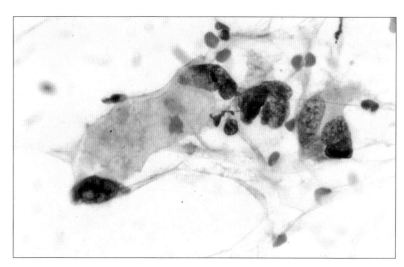

Fig. 17.103 Osteosarcoma – Pap x63. The pale pink material in this field is osteoid, not uncommonly seen in aspirates of this neoplasm. The tumour cells have spindle-shaped nuclei with irregular margins.

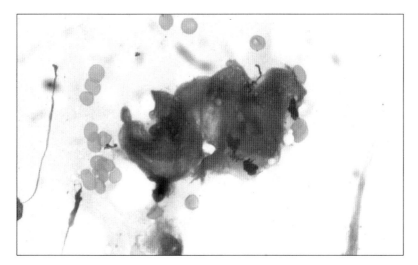

Fig. 17.104. Osteosarcoma – MGG x40. Osteoid stains a magenta shade with May Grunwald Giemsa. The neoplastic cell in the field has an irregular nucleus and wispy cytoplasm.

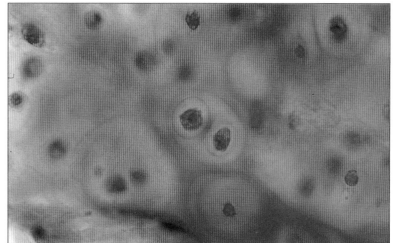

Fig. 17.105 Chondrosarcoma – Pap x40. The magenta-coloured background material seen here is chondroid, within which are neoplastic cells, including binucleate forms. The cells are typical of chondrocytes, as they exhibit perinuclear haloes. (Courtesy of Dr J Scurr, Princess Margaret Hospital, Swindon, UK.)

visible nucleoli. The cytoplasm is delicate and may appear to be drawn out, possibly by smearing, making the nuclei appear eccentric in some cells **(Fig. 17.106)**. These malignant cells are strongly PAS-positive **(Fig. 17.107)**.

Metastatic tumours are common in bones, so cells in the aspirates usually exhibit the features of the primary neoplasm. Tumours commonly seen are metastases from **adenocarcinoma of the breast (Fig. 17.108)**, **lung (Fig. 17.109)**, **prostate (Fig. 17.110)**, **kidney (Figs 17.111)**, and **gastrointestinal tract (Fig. 17.112)**. The features are sometimes those of a poorly differentiated neoplasm

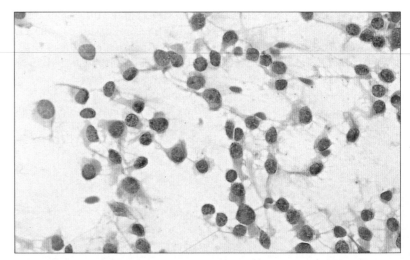

Fig. 17.106 Ewing's sarcoma – Pap x63. Illustrated here are the small cells of Ewing's sarcoma, showing dissociation, vesicular chromatin, and fragile cytoplasm, which appears to be drawn out by smearing. Occasional cells display nucleoli. The cells are not as clustered as those in embryonal rhabdomyosarcoma, although they are the same size.

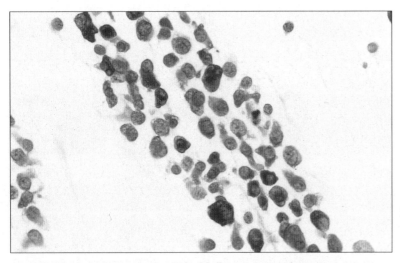

Fig. 17.107 Ewing's sarcoma – PAS x63. This aspirate is from the same case as shown in **Figure 17.102** and shows a strong cytoplasmic positivity with PAS, which is characteristic of this neoplasm. Note the vesicular chromatin and small nucleoli.

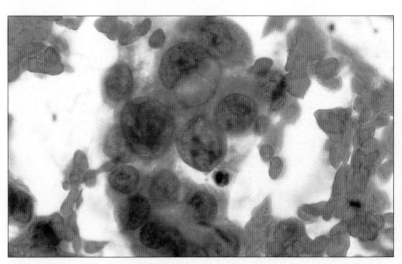

Fig. 17.108 Metastatic adenocarcinoma of the breast – Pap x100. This cluster of adenocarcinoma cells in a vertebral aspirate shows pleomorphism, red nucleoli, and abnormal chromatin. Note the vacuole in one of the cells. It is not possible to diagnose confidently the site of the primary tumour from cytology samples.

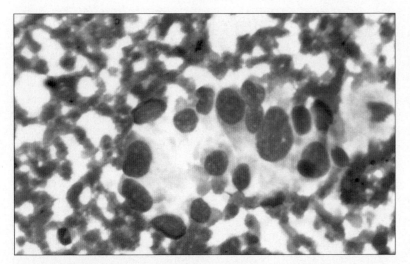

Fig. 17.109 Metastatic adenocarcinoma of the lung – MGG x40. The tumour cells seen here are forming an acinar pattern, but no mucin is evident.

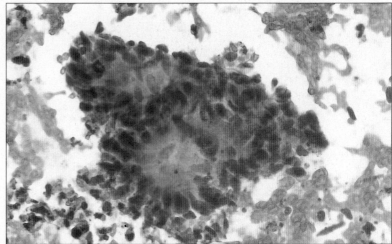

Fig. 17.110 Metastatic adenocarcinoma of the prostate – Pap x40. This group of small adenocarcinoma cells in a sacral fine needle aspirate is metastatic from carcinoma of the prostate. The nuclei are fairly small and nucleoli are not prominent. If enough material is available immunocytochemical stains may be performed to confirm the diagnosis.

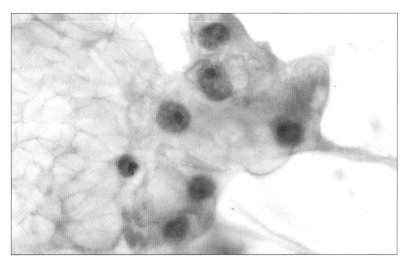

(Fig. 17.113), so cells in the aspirate should be compared with the histological sections of the primary tumour for an accurate diagnosis. Cells from **malignant melanoma** metastases may contain pigment and usually show prominent nuclei with abundant cytoplasm (**Fig. 17.114**).

Chordomas may present as soft tissue masses; for example, a tumour arising in the sacrum may appear as a mass in the buttock. The aspirate contains abundant myxoid material, which is pale pink and may be missed on the wet-fixed smear (**Fig. 17.115**), but is a bright magenta on air-dried material (**Fig. 17.116**).

Fig. 17.111 Metastatic renal cell carcinoma – Pap x100. The abundant delicate foamy cytoplasm, round nuclei, and prominent nucleoli seen in these cells characterize them as metastasis from a renal cell carcinoma.

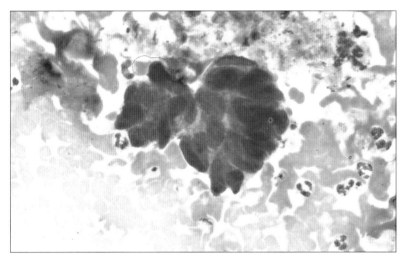

Fig. 17.112 Metastatic adenocarcinoma of ampulla of Vater – MGG x40. The tumour cells seen here have elongated nuclei, but show no evidence of mucin production. The features are consistent with the history of a primary tumour in the ampulla of Vater.

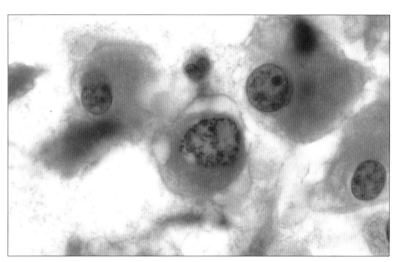

Fig. 17.113 Metastatic high-grade renal cell carcinoma – Pap x100. These malignant cells have round nuclei, markedly abnormal chromatin, and prominent nucleoli. The cytoplasm is dense rather than vacuolated; it was only by comparison with the histology of the original tumour that this was shown to be consistent with metastatic renal cell carcinoma.

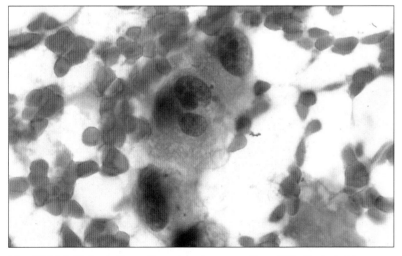

Fig. 17.114 Metastatic malignant melanoma – Pap x100. Illustrated here are neoplastic cells with large nuclei and prominent nucleoli. The cytoplasm is not as dense as is usually seen in these neoplasms, but the cells contain coarse intracytoplasmic pigment granules. Intranuclear inclusions are not seen.

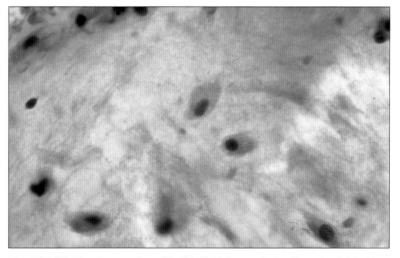

Fig. 17.115 Chordoma – Pap x40. This field demonstrates the pale pink to blue myxoid material characteristic of this neoplasm. Scattered within it are single cells with delicate cytoplasm and central nuclei. The differential diagnosis would be sarcoma NOS.

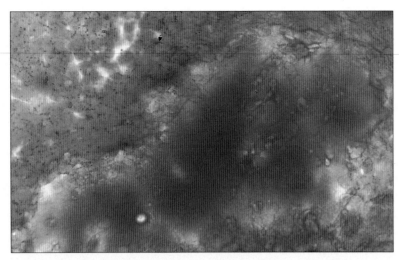

Fig. 17.116 Chordoma – MGG x40. The myxoid material in chordoma stains magenta with May Grunwald Giemsa, as seen here. There is no fibrillary appearance to the material.

The material may appear dense and chondroid in some aspirates (**Fig. 17.117**). The characteristic cell of which this tumour is composed is the physaliferous cell, large cell with a small central nucleus and abundant foamy cytoplasm (**Figs 17.118, 17.119**), sometimes with definite vacuoles (**Fig. 17.120**). Binucleation is not uncommon (**Fig. 17.121**) and cells with hyperchromatic nuclei and darker-staining cytoplasm may also be found (**Fig. 17.122**).

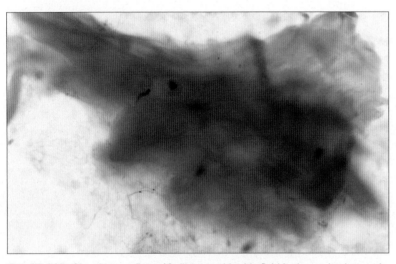

Fig. 17.117 Chordoma – Pap x40. Illustrated in this field is denser background material with more well-defined edges than the usual myxoid material seen in these tumours. This represents chondroid change.

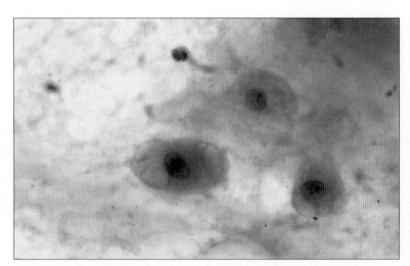

Fig. 17.118 Chordoma – Pap x63. The cells demonstrated here have abundant foamy cytoplasm and central nuclei, with vesicular chromatin and a small nucleolus. They are very similar to histiocytes, but do not have bean-shaped nuclei or intracytoplasmic debris.

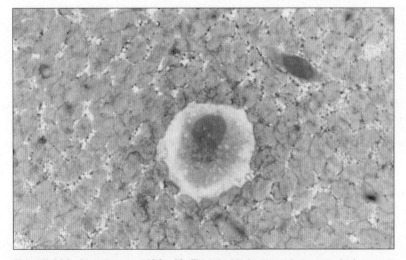

Fig. 17.119 Chordoma – MGG x40. This air-dried smear shows a typical physaliferous cell with foamy cytoplasm and a rounded nucleus in the centre of the field.

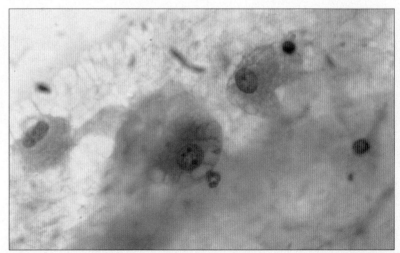

Fig. 17.120 Chordoma – Pap x63. The physaliferous cells seen here contain several intracytoplasmic vacuoles and have ill-defined cellular borders. The myxoid material varies in shade from pale blue to pale pink.

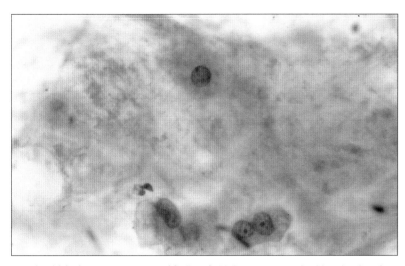

Fig. 17.121 Chordoma – Pap x63. This field demonstrates the binucleation that is occasionally seen in physaliferous cells.

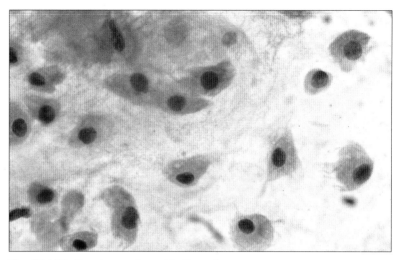

Fig. 17.122 Chordoma – Pap x63. Physaliferous cells are not always pale and delicate. Here the cells contain darker-staining cytoplasm and hyperchromatic nuclei.

SUGGESTED READING

Akhtar M, Ali M, Bakry M, *et al*. Fine needle aspiration biopsy diagnosis of rhabdomyosarcoma. Cytologic, histologic and ultrastructural correlations. *Diagn Cytopathol* 1992; **8**: 465–474.

Akhtar M, Ali A, Sabbah R, *et al*. Aspiration cytology of neuroblastoma. Light and electron microscopic correlations. *Cancer* 1986; **57**: 797–803.

Gupta R, Naran S, Dowle C. Needle aspiration cytology and immunocytochemical study in a case of angiosarcoma of the breast. *Diagn Cytopathol* 1991; **7**: 363–365.

Lundgren L, Kindblom L-G, Willems J, *et al*. Proliferative myositis and fasciitis. A light and electron microscopic, cytologic, DNA–cytometric and immunohistochemical study. *APMIS* 1992; **100**: 437–448.

Malberger E, Tillinger R, Lichtig C. Diagnosis of basal cell carcinoma with aspiration cytology. *Acta Cytol* 1984; **28**: 301–304.

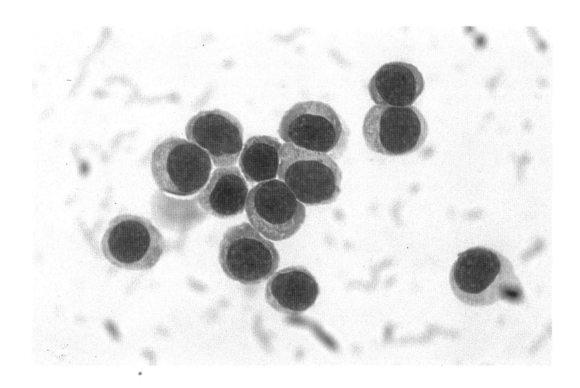

CEREBROSPINAL FLUID

18

Cerebrospinal fluid (CSF) cytology is useful when used in conjunction with micro-biological and biochemical examination. Its primary role is in the diagnosis of meningitis, but it is also of use in excluding meningeal involvement by metasta-tic neoplasms, and in monitoring the effect of treatment on patients with meningeal lymphoma. Its value in the diagnosis of primary brain tumours in the cytology laboratory of most hospitals is somewhat limited, as patients with this disease are usually referred to specialist centres.

It is essential that cerebrospinal fluid is sent fresh to the cytology laboratory as the cells start to degenerate quite quickly. If delay is unavoidable a small amount of alcohol may be added to the specimen to preserve the cells. There are several methods of preparation, including sedimentation, use of a Millipore filter, and cytocentrifugation. It is important not to spin the samples at too rapid a speed as this disrupts and distorts the cells. Fixation and staining preferences also vary, both Papanicolaou and May Grunwald Giemsa stains being used. The latter is favoured in some laboratories, as the cells are easier to spot in scanty samples.

Normal CSF obtained by lumbar puncture contains very few cells, the accept-able number being about 5–10 cells/mm³. These comprise mainly lymphocytes and monocytes, the latter being quite variable in nuclear shape (Figs 18.1–18.3). Rarely, normal cells, such as ependymal (Fig. 18.4) and choroid plexus cells, may be seen in the CSF. Glove powder (starch granules) is not infrequently pre-sent; the granules exhibit a Maltese cross appearance under polarized light. A traumatic tap is unsatisfactory for evaluation as the blood obscures all other cel-lular detail. Cartilage cells are occasionally seen in CSF samples; they may have one or two nuclei surrounded by a clear halo (Fig. 18.5).

Increased numbers of lymphocytes and monocytes are not infrequently found in CSF samples, with no specific features to enable identification of a pathological process (Figs 18.6, 18.7). Such findings have to be reported as non-specific reactive lymphocytosis.

A **subarachnoid haemorrhage** results in xanthochromic CSF, which on examination contains siderophages (macrophages containing intracytoplasmic

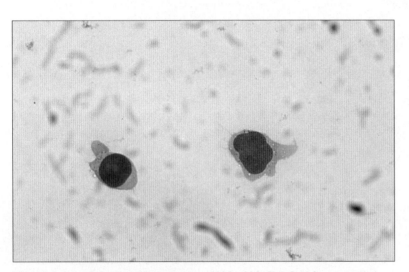

Fig. 18.1 Lymphocyte and monocyte – MGG x100. This field from a normal CSF sample illustrates a lymphocyte with a round nucleus and scanty cytoplasm, adjacent to a monocyte with an irregular nucleus. The amount of cytoplasm seen in monocytes is variable.

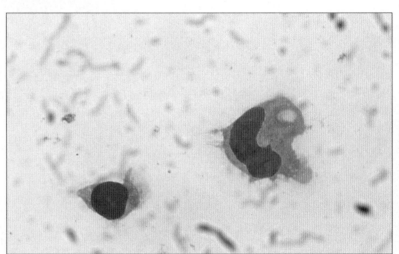

Fig. 18.2 Lymphocyte and monocyte – MGG x100. The monocyte in this illustration displays a bean-shaped nucleus and abundant cytoplasm. The lymphocyte next to it has very little cytoplasm in comparison.

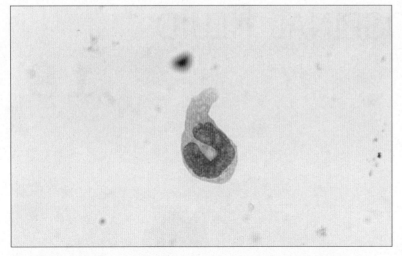

Fig. 18.3 Monocyte – MGG x100. This monocyte has a horseshoe-shaped nucleus and delicate cytoplasm.

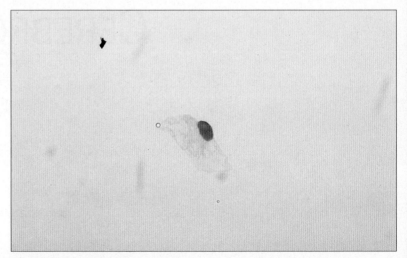

Fig. 18.4 Ependymal cell – MGG x100. Ependymal cells are seen very occasionally in CSF. The cytoplasm is pale and abundant.

haemosiderin) and, occasionally, macrophages with phagocytosed erythrocytes.

Bacterial meningitis is usually diagnosed clinically, with CSF being dispatched to the laboratory to confirm the diagnosis. The fluid contains many acute inflammatory cells, the majority being neutrophil polymorphs. A similar picture may be found in fluid from an infected shunt **(Fig. 18.8)**.

Viral meningitis in the early stages may display both polymorphs and lymphocytes in the CSF **(Fig. 18.9)**. In the later stages, lymphocytes predominate **(Fig. 18.10)**. Tuberculous meningitis may present similar findings, with monocytes, lymphocytes, and very occasional neutrophils **(Figs 18.11, 18.12)**.

Immunocompromised patients are susceptible to infections with fungi such as *Candida* and *Cryptococcus neoformans*. The budding yeast forms of the latter can be identified in CSF using India ink **(Fig. 18.13)** or mucicarmine stains **(Fig. 18.14)**.

In **multiple sclerosis** there is often an increased number of lymphocytes **(Fig. 18.15)** with occasional plasma cells **(Fig. 18.16)**, the latter being diagnostic.

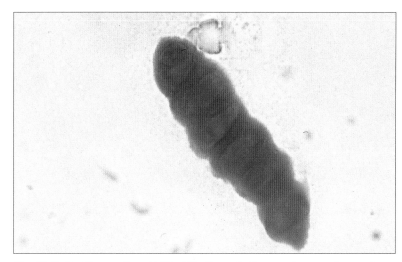

Fig. 18.5 Cartilage cells – MGG x100. The cells illustrated are cartilage cells with dark nuclei and a distinct perinuclear halo. They are not infrequently seen in CSF samples.

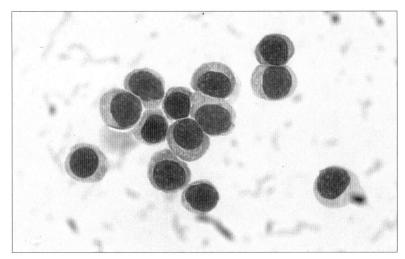

Fig. 18.6 Reactive lymphocytosis – MGG x100. These beautifully preserved lymphocytes have uniform hyperchromatic nuclei and a thin rim of cytoplasm. No specific features are visible.

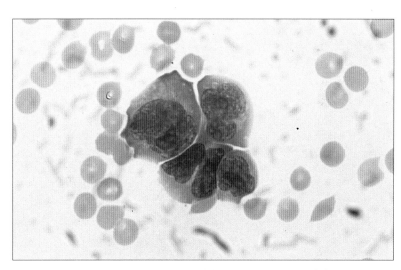

Fig. 18.7 Reactive lymphocytosis – MGG x100. The lymphocytes seen in this field show marked variability in nuclear size and shape. However, the next few samples examined showed a normal scanty population of lymphocytes and the patient became asymptomatic, suggesting that this was a reactive lymphocytosis.

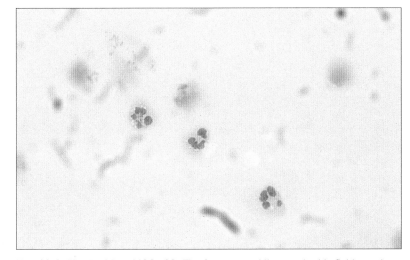

Fig. 18.8 Meningitis – MGG x63. The few neutrophils seen in this field may be due to early bacterial meningitis, early viral meningitis, or an infected shunt. In full-blown bacterial meningitis, large numbers of polymorphs are present.

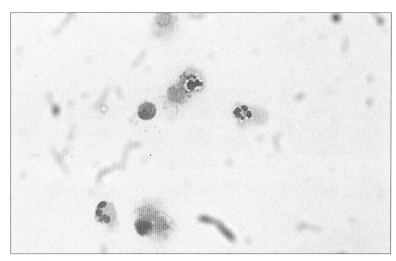

Fig. 18.9 Viral meningitis – MGG x63. This CSF contains polymorphs, occasional lymphocytes, and monocytes. In the later stages of viral meningitis lymphocytes predominate.

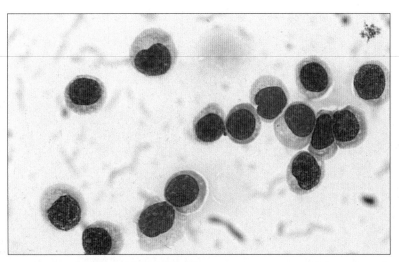

Fig. 18.10 Viral meningitis – MGG x100. This field illustrates the abundance of lymphocytes seen in viral meningitis.

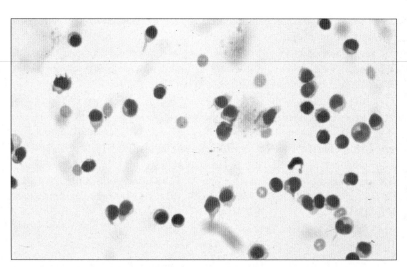

Fig. 18.11 Tuberculous meningitis – MGG x40. This CSF contains numerous lymphocytes and an occasional monocyte. A few neutrophils may also be seen in some cases. The appearances are not specific and should be interpreted in conjunction with the clinical details, and biochemical and bacteriological tests.

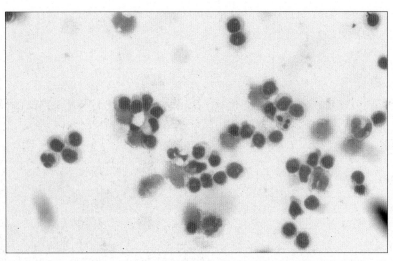

Fig. 18.12 Tuberculous meningitis – MGG x40. This CSF is another sample from the same patient as shown in **Figure 18.11** and illustrates a few neutrophils with abundant lymphocytes and a few monocytes.

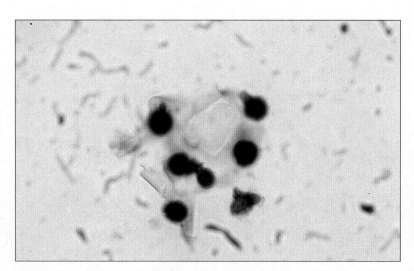

Fig. 18.13 Cryptococcal infection – India ink preparation x100. In this preparation the budding yeast forms are seen stained black. The clear capsule around the yeast cells cannot be identified properly. (Courtesy of The Department of Microbiology, St Luke's Hospital, Guildford, UK.)

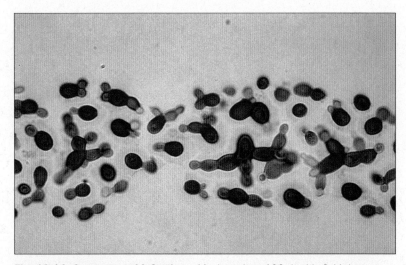

Fig. 18.14 Cryptococcal infection – Mucicarmine x100. In this field there are numerous yeast cells with clearly visible capsules, showing varying degrees of budding. (Courtesy of Professor S Lucas, St Thomas' Hospital, London, UK.)

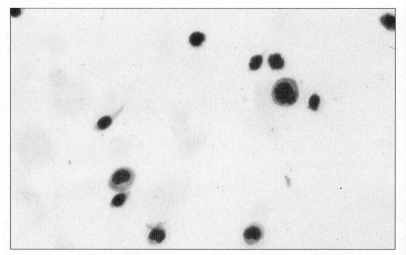

Fig. 18.15 Multiple sclerosis – MGG x40. In this condition there is an increased number of cells in the CSF, predominantly lymphocytes, but the diagnostic cell is the plasma cell. This field displays lymphoid cells which show variability in size, but no plasma cells are seen.

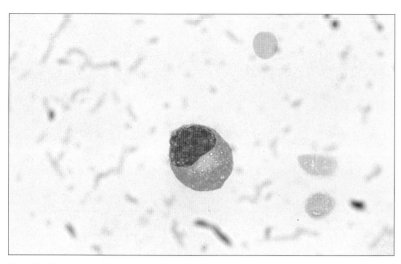

Fig. 18.16 Multiple sclerosis – MGG x100. The cell in the centre of the field is a plasma cell with an eccentric nucleus displaying a 'clock-face' or 'cart-wheel' chromatin pattern. Note the prominent 'hof' adjacent to the nucleus.

Leukaemias and **lymphocytes** can involve the meninges, so neoplastic cells are then seen in the CSF. The predominant cells in leukaemias are blast cells **(Fig. 18.17)**. Lymphomatous involvement produces a very cellular fluid which, under high magnification, is found to be composed of a monotonous population of abnormal lymphoid cells **(Figs 18.18, 18.19)**. Immunocytochemical markers may be necessary to identify the cell type, but occasionally the morphology of the cell establishes the type, as for plasmacytoid lymphomas.

Primary CNS tumours may exfoliate cells infrequently into the CSF, but these are not always easy to classify.

Metastatic carcinoma cells in CSF, such as breast carcinoma cells, are often difficult to identify as they do not retain their morphological characteristics **(Fig. 18.20)**, but occasionally they may display similarities to the primary neoplasm

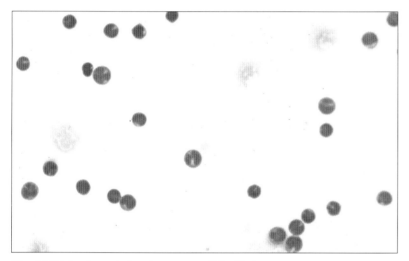

Fig. 18.17 Leukaemic involvement – MGG x40. Many abnormal lymphocytes are seen in this field.

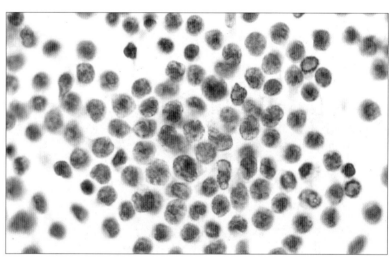

Fig. 18.18 CNS lymphoma – Pap x100. This CSF is hypercellular, being composed of a uniform population of abnormal lymphoid cells. The nuclear outlines are irregular, rather than smooth and round as in normal lymphocytes. This particular case was investigated further and found to be a T cell lymphoma.

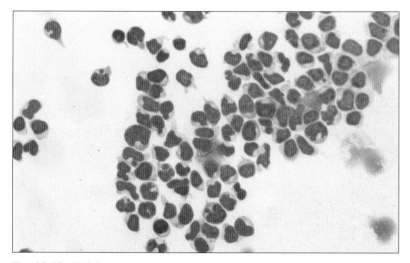

Fig. 18.19 CNS lymphoma – MGG x40. This air-dried preparation of the same sample as shown in **Figure 18.18** exhibits the markedly convoluted nuclei characteristic of T cells.

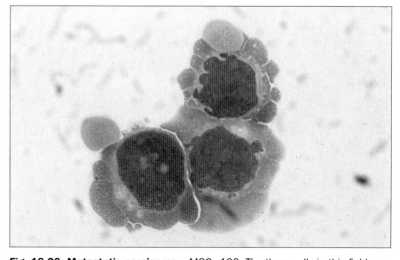

Fig. 18.20 Metastatic carcinoma – MGG x100. The three cells in this field are abnormal with large irregular nuclei, but are difficult to classify as carcinoma cells. The cytoplasmic borders appear to show blebs, simulating the frilly borders of mesothelial cells in serous effusions. The erythrocytes adjacent to the cells are a guide to the large size of the nuclei. These cells were metastatic from carcinoma of the breast.

(Fig. 18.21), including cytoplasmic vacuolation (Fig. 18.22). Other tumours which metastasize to the meninges include rhabdomyosarcoma (Fig. 18.23), testicular teratomas (Fig. 18.24), and medulloblastoma, with its characteristically lobulated nuclei (Fig. 18.25).

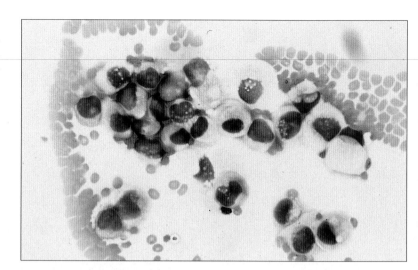

Fig. 18.21 **Metastatic carcinoma** – MGG x40. This cellular CSF contains large carcinoma cells in clusters, with clear cytoplasm. This is another example of metastatic carcinoma of the breast, in this case the cells being identifiable as epithelial.

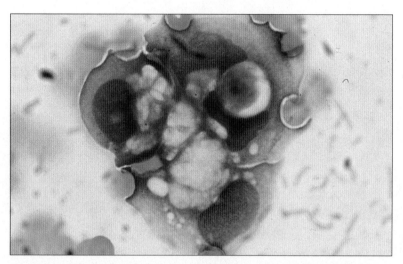

Fig. 18.22 **Metastatic carcinoma** – MGG x100. In this sample, also from a patient with breast carcinoma, the cells illustrated are vacuolated, with the vacuoles slightly indenting the nuclei.

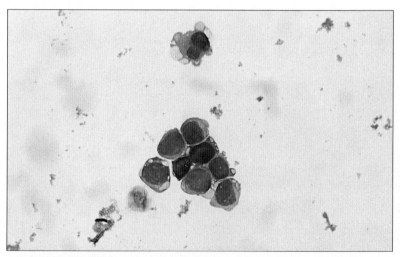

Fig. 18.23 **Metastatic rhabdomyosarcoma** – MGG x40. This field illustrates the difficulty that arises in categorizing metastatic tumour cells in the CSF. These are rhabdomyosarcoma cells with little cytoplasm and mildly pleomorphic nuclei, resembling lymphocytes.

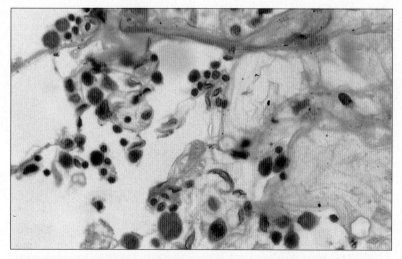

Fig. 18.24 **Metastatic teratoma** – Pap x40. This very cellular specimen, from a patient with metastases from a testicular teratoma, is composed of a mixture of large and small pleomorphic tumour cells, lymphocytes, and histiocytes.

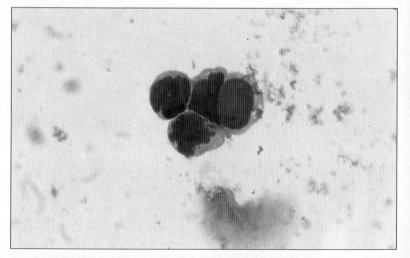

Fig. 18.25 **Medulloblastoma** – MGG x100. Illustrated here are medulloblastoma cells which have characteristically lobulated nuclei and a thin rim of cytoplasm.

SUGGESTED READING

Bigner SH, Johnston WW. *Cytopathology of the Central Nervous System.* London: Edward Arnold; 1994: 47–97.

Dee AL. Carcinoma of the breast present initially in cerebrospinal fluid. *Acta Cytol* 1985; **29**: 909–910.

Ringenberg SQ, Francis R, Doll DC. Meningeal carcinomatosis as the presenting manifestation of tumors of unknown origin, *Acta Cytol* 1990; **34**: 590–592.

Timperley WR. Cerebrospinal fluid examination and direct brain preparations. In: Gray W, ed. *Diagnostic Cytopathology.* Edinburgh: Churchill Livingstone; 1995: 901–913.

INDEX

Note: textual references are shown in normal type, chapters in *italics* and figure numbers in **bold**.